Brain Tumors in Children

Amar Gajjar • Gregory H. Reaman
Judy M. Racadio • Franklin O. Smith
Editors

Brain Tumors in Children

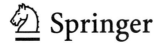 Springer

Editors
Amar Gajjar
Department of Oncology
St. Jude Children's Research Hospital
Memphis, TN
USA

Gregory H. Reaman
Children's National Medical Center
George Washington University
Silver Spring, WA
USA

Judy M. Racadio
Cincinnati, OH
USA

Franklin O. Smith
Medpace
Cincinnati, OH
USA

ISBN 978-3-030-13258-3   ISBN 978-3-319-43205-2   (eBook)
https://doi.org/10.1007/978-3-319-43205-2

Printed on acid-free paper

This Springer imprint is published by the registered company Springer Nature Switzerland AG
The registered company address is: Gewerbestrasse 11, 6330 Cham, Switzerland

Preface

Brain tumor programs are like orchestras—several components all working together seamlessly to provide optimal clinical care and conduct basic, translational, and clinical research, and thus advance the field. The last decade has witnessed unprecedented advances in the field of neuro-oncology that have impacted the entire practice of treating children with brain tumors. Using modern molecular technologies that have facilitated a unique insight into the genomic make up of pediatric brain tumors, we have gained in-depth knowledge into the genetic heterogeneity of these tumors. This knowledge has also generated a new classification that is gradually being implemented by the World Health Organization (WHO). The fields of neurosurgery, neuroimaging, and radiation oncology have witnessed technological advances that have revolutionized how these modalities have been deployed in the treatment of children. The introduction of targeted therapies based on tumor molecular profiling has injected a new era of hope for curing brain tumors that were incurable in the past. Neurocognitive deficits, which are a significant concern in children treated for brain tumors, are being addressed with interventions that promise to remediate some of the damage. Long-term follow-up of brain tumor survivors has documented the unique health risk profile that these children carry for their life based on their treatment history. The recognition that more than two-thirds of the burden of pediatric cancer occurs in developing countries raises unique challenges regarding delivery of adequate therapy to this disadvantaged population. The authors of the individual chapters, all experts in their own domains, have done an outstanding job of succinctly documenting the recent advances and providing a glimpse of where the field is headed over the next few years. This book is a must-read for trainees, junior and seasoned practitioners in the field as it provides a lucid update in a rapidly emerging field.

Memphis, TN, USA   Amar Gajjar
Silver Spring, WA, USA   Gregory H. Reaman
Cincinnati, OH, USA   Judy M. Racadio
Cincinnati, OH, USA   Franklin O. Smith

Contents

Epidemiology of Pediatric Central Nervous System Tumors

Nicholas A. Vitanza, Cynthia J. Campen, and Paul G. Fisher

1.1 Introduction

Tumors of the central nervous system (CNS) comprise a broad and diverse collection of neoplasms within pediatric oncology. Yet when taken together pediatric brain and spine tumors represent the most common childhood cancer with an incidence of 5.57 per 100,000 annually and are a leading cause of cancer-related death in patients under 19 years of age (Ostrom et al. 2014; Siegel et al. 2015). Factors such as genetic predisposition, age, and sex play an increasingly significant role in understanding presentation, management, and etiology of childhood brain tumors. Although long-standing observations regarding general patterns of CNS tumors continue to be clinically useful, the introduction of molecular subtypes, such as in medulloblastoma and ependymoma, and the discovery of epigenetic regulators, such as in diffuse intrinsic pontine gliomas (DIPG) and other diffuse midline gliomas with H3K27M mutations, have repurposed epidemiological findings and reconceptualized CNS tumor classification (Louis et al. 2016). The elucidation of the molecular profile of pediatric CNS tumors has made it clear that epidemiology, viewed through a prism of genetics and epigenetics, can offer even greater insights into this incredibly challenging group of tumors. Epidemiology today considers not only environmental, parental, and birth factors that may increase the risk of pediatric CNS tumors, but also germline and molecular features that are causal or pathognomonic of tumor types and subtypes.

1.2 Astrocytomas and Other Gliomas

The gliomas are a heterogeneous group of tumors, comprised mostly of astrocytomas. Pediatric astrocytomas are divided into four grades by the World Health Organization (WHO), with pilocytic astrocytomas (WHO grade I) being the most common subtype of pediatric CNS tumor, comprising approximately 15% (Ostrom et al. 2014; Louis et al. 2007). The incidence of pilocytic astrocytomas in children in England and the USA is 0.75–0.97 per 100,000, and these tumors have an exceedingly low incidence of metastasis or malignant transformation (Ostrom et al. 2014; Stokland et al. 2010; Fisher et al. 2008; Arora et al. 2009). Although they may occur in any CNS location including the spine, they most commonly arise from the posterior fossa, optic pathway and hypothalamus, or brain stem (Fernandez et al. 2003; Gajjar et al. 1997;

N. A. Vitanza
Division of Pediatric Hematology/Oncology, Seattle Children's Hospital, University of Washington School of Medicine, Seattle, WA, USA

C. J. Campen · P. G. Fisher (✉)
Division of Child Neurology, Department of Neurology, Lucile Packard Children's Hospital at Stanford, Stanford University, Palo Alto, CA, USA
e-mail: pfisher@stanford.edu

Hayostek et al. 1993; Khatib et al. 1994). Diffuse astrocytomas (WHO grade II), anaplastic astrocytomas (WHO grade III), and glioblastomas (WHO grade IV) have an incidence of 0.27, 0.08, and 0.15 per 100,000 children 0–14 years of age, respectively. Low-grade gliomas, which are comprised of WHO grade I and II astrocytomas as well as WHO grade I gangliogliomas, most commonly present with greater than 6 months of symptoms (Fisher et al. 2008). The incorporation of molecular characteristics in the 2016 WHO classification of tumors of the CNS will assist in a deeper epidemiological understanding by addressing distinct biologic entities, such as diffuse gliomas with IDH mutations and diffuse midline gliomas with H3K27M mutations (Louis et al. 2016).

Children with pilocytic astrocytomas have excellent outcomes of >96% overall survival (OS) at 10 years, and patients with subtotal resections do not do significantly worse than patients with gross total resections (Ostrom et al. 2014; Gajjar et al. 1997). Posterior fossa tumors are common in children, with pilocytic astrocytomas being the second most common tumor arising in that location, behind only medulloblastoma; mean age of occurrence is 7.1 years (Smoots et al. 1998). Up to 60% of pilocytic astrocytomas are associated with a KIAA1549:BRAF fusion, which is associated with a better outcome (Becker et al. 2015; Jones et al. 2008). Optic pathway and hypothalamic astrocytomas are most often pilocytic astrocytomas, but other subtypes of low-grade gliomas also account for a small number of cases (Hoffman et al. 1993; Laithier et al. 2003). Optic pathway gliomas (OPGs) occur in approximately 15% of patients with neurofibromatosis type 1 (NF1), though they most often occur sporadically (Listernick et al. 1989). OPGs are reported to have a broad median age between 4.3 and 8.8 years, and those occurring in patients with NF1 present at a significantly earlier age than sporadic cases (Listernick et al. 1989; Nicolin et al. 2009; Singhal et al. 2002; Ahn et al. 2006; Janss et al. 1995; Khafaga et al. 2003; Jahraus and Tarbell 2006; Avery et al. 2011). The variation in age of presentation may be secondary to the presence of a cancer predisposition syn-

drome in NF1 patients, as well as the practice of asymptomatic surveillance imaging in that group, while 90% of sporadic cases present with new neurologic symptoms. Subependymal giant cell astrocytomas (SEGAs) are another WHO grade I astrocytoma subtype that develop almost exclusively in patients with tuberous sclerosis (TS), which occurs in 1 in 5600 live births (O'Callaghan et al. 1998). Five to twenty percent of patients with TS develop SEGAs, often in adolescence, but congenital cases have also been reported (Adriaensen et al. 2009; O'Callaghan et al. 2008; Hahn et al. 1991).

Several WHO grade II subtypes can be distinguished by histology and presentation. Pilomyxoid astrocytomas (WHO grade II) have a more aggressive course than pilocytic astrocytomas (WHO grade I), a greater propensity for growing in the hypothalamochiasmatic region, and often present earlier with a mean age of 3.3 years (Bhargava et al. 2013). Pleomorphic xanthoastrocytomas (WHO grade II) are typically located in the superficial temporal lobe; they classically present with seizures and have a median age at diagnosis of 20.5 years and an approximately 75% overall survival (Gallo et al. 2013; Perkins et al. 2012). These can rarely transform into a high-grade glioma.

Low-grade gliomas of the brain stem can be pilocytic astrocytomas or gangliogliomas, which typically occur dorsally and have the possibility of long-term cure. WHO grade II, III, and IV gliomas of the brain stem have dismal outcomes and together comprise diffuse intrinsic pontine glioma (DIPG). The 2016 WHO classification has adjusted that nomenclature in favor of diffuse midline gliomas, as diffuse gliomas of the pons, thalamus, and spinal cord may form a more biologically distinct category when H3K27M mutations are present (Louis et al. 2016; Shankar et al. 2016).

DIPGs arise most commonly in the ventral pons and comprise 10–15% of all pediatric CNS tumors and 80% of brain stem gliomas, affecting roughly 300 children in the USA each year (Ostrom et al. 2014; Ramos et al. 2013; Smith et al. 1998). Males and females are affected equally and the median age of presentation is

7 years (Lassiter et al. 1971; Lober et al. 2014; Veldhuijzen van Zanten et al. 2014). Presentation usually consists of a classic triad of ataxia, cranial nerve palsies, and pyramidal tract signs developing over 1 month, although atypical cases can present more slowly over several months (Fisher et al. 2000). It is now recognized that approximately 17% of patients undergo both local and distant neuraxis dissemination by 15 months, which is not far beyond the median overall survival of patients with DIPG, as only 10% of patients survive beyond 2 years and only 2–3% are considered long-term survivors (Gururangan et al. 2006; Hargrave et al. 2006; Jackson et al. 2013). Recently, 80% of DIPGs have been found to harbor mutations in K27M of histone 3.1 or 3.3, which are associated with mutations in *ACVR1* and *p53*, respectively (Taylor et al. 2014; Wu et al. 2012).

High-grade gliomas (HGGs) occur much more frequently in adults, with an increasing incidence with age to a peak between the ages of 75 and 85 years (Ostrom et al. 2014). The outcomes of patients with high-grade gliomas appear to be inverse to patient age, as 5-year overall survivals for children less than three and those 3–14 years of age are 31–66% and 19%, respectively (Mathew et al. 2014). Glioblastoma has been reported in classic CNS tumor predisposition syndromes, such as neurofibromatosis, Li–Fraumeni, and Turcot syndromes, as well as in several genitourinary syndromes, such as Turner and Mayer–Rokitansky–Küster–Hauser syndrome, though the majority of cases are believed to be sporadic (Hanaei et al. 2015; Jeong and Yee 2014; Macy et al. 2012; Gonzalez and Prayson 2013).

1.3 Embryonal Tumors

Embryonal brain tumors are a diverse group of aggressive neoplasms, including medulloblastoma, primary neuroectodermal tumors (PNET), atypical rhabdoid/teratoid tumors (ATRT), and pineoblastoma, which share high mitotic activity and a predilection for dissemination throughout the neuraxis, and are all WHO grade IV (Louis

et al. 2007). They account for 15% of CNS tumors in patients 0–14 years of age and 12% in those 0–19 years of age, with incidences of 0.78 and 0.64 per 100,000, respectively; these incidences have remained unchanged since at least 1990 (Ostrom et al. 2014; Johnston et al. 2014). Embryonal CNS tumors rarely occur outside of childhood with the median age at presentation being 7.3 years, and 44% of them being diagnosed between the ages of 4 and 9 years (Ostrom et al. 2014; Kool et al. 2012). Medulloblastomas, the most common malignant brain tumor in pediatrics, histologically appear as PNETs specifically arising in the posterior fossa (Northcott et al. 2011). A minority of medulloblastoma cases have been reported in patients with genetic predisposition syndromes such as Gorlin, Turcot B, Li–Fraumeni, ataxia telangiectasia, Nijmegen breakage, Rubenstein–Taybi, and Coffin–Siris syndromes (Distel et al. 2003; Hart et al. 1987; Larsen et al. 2014; Skomorowski et al. 2012; Taylor et al. 2001; Rogers et al. 1988). Overall, there is a male predominance of 1.5:1, with females reported to have superior outcomes, although again this is likely subgroup dependent, as there are fewer females in the higher risk Group 3 and 4, while more young females have sonic hedgehog (SHH) driven tumors (Louis et al. 2007; Northcott et al. 2011). Historically, patients clinically classified as average-risk had a 5-year OS of roughly 85%, while high-risk patients suffered poorer outcomes with near 70% OS and patients with large-cell anaplastic histology had particularly dismal outcomes (Kool et al. 2012; Gajjar et al. 2006; Packer et al. 2006; Tarbell et al. 2013; Ramaswamy et al. 2013). Overall, long-term survival in patients with medulloblastoma is achieved in only 66% of patients, with 10% suffering from secondary malignancies, 32% of which are secondary brain tumors (Ning et al. 2015).

Although particular subsets of medulloblastoma have long been suspected to behave differently, it is now commonly accepted that there are four distinct molecular subgroups: WNT, SHH, Group 3, and Group 4, which account for 11%, 28%, 27%, and 34% of cases, respectively (Kool et al. 2012; Northcott et al. 2011; Badiali et al. 1991).

Prodromes may vary among the groups, ranging from only 2 weeks in patients with SHH tumors, to 4 weeks in patients with Group 3 tumors and 8 weeks in patients with WNT or Group 4 tumors (Ramaswamy et al. 2014). Furthermore, age of presentation varies as the incidence of SHH medulloblastomas is bimodal, peaking under 3 years and again over 15 years of age (Northcott et al. 2011). WNT and Group 4 both peak around age 11, but WNT tumors are essentially absent in infancy (Kool et al. 2012; Northcott et al. 2011). WNT tumors have no gender predominance, are the least frequent subgroup, and experience the best outcomes with greater than 90% overall survival (Ellison et al. 2011, 2011). Outcomes in patients with SHH tumors are inferior, though strongly age-dependent as the 10-year OS is 77% and 51% in infants and children, respectively (Kool et al. 2012; Ramaswamy et al. 2013). Despite presenting with metastatic disease in 17% of infants and 22% of children, SHH tumors most often recur locally (Kool et al. 2012; Ramaswamy et al. 2013). Group 3 and Group 4 occur nearly twice as often in males, accounting for the male predominance in medulloblastoma as a whole. Forty-seven percent of Group 3 medulloblastomas present with metastases and, while they do not have significantly worse prognoses than those without metastases, this subgroup overall suffers the poorest outcomes with long-term survival in less than 50% of patients (Kool et al. 2012; Northcott et al. 2011). Group 4 patients, on the other hand, have significantly different outcomes associated with the presence of metastases, ranging from nearly 40% OS (metastases present) to greater than 70% (metastases absent) (Kool et al. 2012). In patients that experience recurrence, the molecular subgroup remains consistent, and although outcomes are uniformly poor, Group 4 patients have the longest survival following recurrence (Ramaswamy et al. 2013).

Atypical teratoid/rhabdoid tumors (ATRTs) are embryonal CNS tumors with rhabdoid features that were initially described in the 1990s (Zuccoli et al. 1999). Since their initial description their incidence has increased, while the incidence of other PNETs has declined, more likely representative of a change in classification than a change in biological patterns of disease (Ostrom

et al. 2014). The incidence of ATRT in childhood is approximately 0.1 per 100,000 with a peak between 1 and 2 years of age and no gender predisposition observed in the USA (Ostrom et al. 2014, b; Hilden et al. 2004; von Hoff et al. 2011; Woehrer et al. 2010). They account for 10% of CNS tumors in patients less than 1 year of age, but only 1.6% of all childhood brain tumors (Ostrom et al. 2014). The wide range of reported OS, between 28 and 48%, may be affected by delays in appropriate diagnosis, as one report noted a 5-year OS of only 15% in patients who were initially misdiagnosed (Ostrom et al. 2014; Hilden et al. 2004; von Hoff et al. 2011; Woehrer et al. 2010; Athale et al. 2009; Lafay-Cousin et al. 2012). Most reports conclude that metastatic disease at presentation is not prognostic, while descriptions of the prognostic impact of age differ (Ostrom et al. 2014; Hilden et al. 2004; von Hoff et al. 2011; Woehrer et al. 2010; Athale et al. 2009; Lafay-Cousin et al. 2012). The location of ATRTs, however, does appear to change with age, as patients under 1 year of age most commonly have infratentorial disease and the incidence of supratentorial disease increases with age (Ostrom et al. 2014). The characteristic loss of *INI1* in these tumors is most commonly somatic, although germline mutations have been reported and can result in a rhabdoid tumor predisposition syndrome (RTPS) (Sredni and Tomita 2015; Taylor et al. 2000). The development of ATRTs has also been associated with low birth weight and twin pregnancies (Heck et al. 2013).

Pineoblastomas are malignant tumors of the pineal gland that, like other PNETs, are histologically similar to medulloblastomas, but display a distinct biology (Li et al. 2005). While some pineal tumors, such as germ cell tumors, occur more commonly in males, reports suggest pineoblastoma may be more common in females (Villa et al. 2012; Fauchon et al. 2000). Although patients with bilateral retinoblastomas may develop a pineoblastoma, "trilateral retinoblastoma" occurs in only 1% of patients with bilateral retinoblastoma and only in the setting of germline mutations (Ramasubramanian et al. 2013). While the majority of pineoblastoma cases appear sporadic, cases also have been reported as part of Turcot syndrome and with germline *DICER1* mutations (Ikeda et al. 1998; Gadish et al. 2005; Sabbaghian et al. 2012).

1.4   Ependymoma

Virchow initially described ependymomas in the nineteenth century as CNS tumors originating from the walls of the ventricular system (Virchow 1863–67). Though ependymomas likely consist of several discrete subgroups that can be distinguished by location and molecular profile, most reports evaluate ependymomas as a whole or by grade, leaving their epidemiologic understanding incomplete. Ependymoma incidence in the USA is 0.3 and 0.29 per 100,000 children aged 0–14 years and 0–19 years, respectively, and has not increased since 1973; nearly one-third of cases occur in children under the age of 4 years (Ostrom et al. 2014; McGuire et al. 2009). Although 46% of ependymomas in adults are spinal, location varies according to age in children (Vera-Bolanos et al. 2015). The mean age for spinal, supratentorial, and infratentorial ependymomas are 12.2, 7.8, and 5 years, respectively (McGuire et al. 2009). The gender incidence may be affected by age and location, as the overall male-to-female ratio is 1.3:1, though males are more commonly affected by supratentorial ependymomas (1.4:1) and less commonly affected by spinal ependymoma (0.7:1) than females (McGuire et al. 2009; Dohrmann and Farwell 1976). Presentation with metastatic disease is rare in pediatric ependymomas but is more common in infants, although reports vary on whether supratentorial or infratentorial tumors are more likely to metastasize (Zacharoulis et al. 2008; Allen et al. 1998).

Currently, the treatment of ependymoma primarily varies according to age, grade, and location. In 2015, a new molecular classification was proposed though it has yet to be validated. It divides ependymomas into anatomical compartments: supratentorial (ST), posterior fossa (PF), and spinal (SP); tumors in each compartment are then divided into one of three subgroups: a subependymoma group and two other genetic or epigenetic subgroups (Pajtler et al. 2015).

Supratentorial ependymomas are distinguished by either *RELA* fusions (ST-EPN-RELA), which occur at a median age of 8 years and result in frequent disease progressions, or *YAP1* fusions (ST-EPN-YAP1), which occur at a median age of 1.4 years (Pajtler et al. 2015). Posterior fossa ependymomas are subdivided into those with a CpG methylator phenotype (PF-EPN-A), which account for 48% of all pediatric ependymomas and experience poor outcomes, and those that are not hypermethylated (PF-EPN-B), which often occur in older patients (EPN-PFB) (Pajtler et al. 2015; Parker et al. 2014; Witt et al. 2011).

Although histologic classification of WHO grade II or III in pediatric ependymoma may not offer prognostic significance, several WHO grade I subsets are clearly less aggressive neoplasms (Perilongo et al. 1997; Ross and Rubinstein 1989; Robertson et al. 1998). Subependymomas represent less than 1% of CNS tumors in children, are designated WHO grade I, and have essentially no metastatic potential (Scheinker 1945; Ragel et al. 2006). Myxopapillary ependymomas, also WHO grade I, have a median age of presentation of 36 years, yet are not uncommon in children with reports of patients as young as 6 years old being affected (Barton et al. 2010; Woesler et al. 1998). Despite their WHO grade I designation, the pediatric variant may be more aggressive than that seen in adults with a suggestion of dissemination in as many as 58% of patients (Fassett et al. 2005). Neurofibromatosis type II (NF2) is the most common hereditary predisposition for ependymoma, most often causing intramedullary spinal tumors of the cervical spine (Bianchi et al. 1994; Plotkin et al. 2011). Pediatric ependymomas have also been reported in Turcot B, MEN1, and Li–Fraumeni syndromes (Chan et al. 1999; Metzger et al. 1991).

1.5   Germ Cell Tumors

Germ cell tumors (GCTs) are a heterogeneous group of cancers with variable classification and nomenclature depending on the particular organ involvement. In the CNS, they are divided into germinomas, non-germinomatous germ cell tumors (NGGCT), and teratomas. The most common locations for GCTs are the suprasellar and pineal regions. GCTs account for 4% of pediatric CNS tumors with an incidence of 0.2 and 0.22 per 100,000 in children aged 0–14 and 0–19 years, respectively (Ostrom et al. 2014). Males account for 76% of all CNS GCTs, 58% of pituitary GCTs, and a remarkable 93% of pineal GCTs (Goodwin et al. 2009). In both sexes there is a small spike at birth and a much greater spike in adolescence with incidences peaking at roughly age 15. Race also influences incidence patterns, as in the USA nearly 20% of patients were Asian or Pacific Islander with an incidence of 0.26 per 100,000, double the 0.13 per 100,000 in white children 0–15 years of age (Goodwin et al. 2009). CNS GCTs also account for a greater percentage of pediatric CNS tumors in Japan, Korea, Taiwan, and China at 7.8%, 11.2%, 14%, and 7.9%, respectively (Cho et al. 2002; Mori and Kurisaka 1986; Wong et al. 2005; Zhou et al. 2008). Klinefelter syndrome is associated with the development of pediatric germ cell tumors including intracranial germinomas (Arens et al. 1988). Down syndrome and NF1 have also been reported in patients with intracranial germinomas (Hashimoto et al. 1995; Wong et al. 1995).

1.6 Family History

Despite the increasing awareness of CNS tumor genetic predispositions, further discussed within another chapter, there is still little evidence of the development of CNS tumors in the parents or siblings of affected children. The studies reporting increased pediatric CNS tumor incidence among siblings have been plagued by small numbers and an inability to exclude genetic predisposition syndromes; however, a larger Nordic cohort of patients showed no association among siblings outside of genetic predisposition syndromes (Draper et al. 1977; Farwell and Flannery 1984; Miller 1971; Winther et al. 2001). There have been several reports regarding the association of parental age with pediatric CNS tumors: two studies identified increased parental age as a risk factor, while one found only advanced maternal age to be a significant risk (Hemminki et al. 1999; Johnson et al. 2009; Yip et al. 2006). A review of Sweden's Family-Cancer Database, consisting of over 13,000 CNS tumor diagnoses, found that oldest siblings were at increased risk for several childhood malignancies and this risk increased with the number of younger siblings (Altieri et al. 2006). The existence of three or more younger siblings resulted in a relative risk of 1.34, 2.3, 2.61, and 3.71 of astrocytoma, medulloblastoma, ependymoma, and meningioma, respectively (Altieri et al. 2006).

1.7 Birth History

As early as 1968, Kobayashi had published a report of the association between congenital anomalies and childhood cancer (Kobayashi et al. 1968). A review of 90,400 children found patients with congenital anomalies had a risk ratio of 5.8 (CI 3.7–9.1) of developing cancer in their first year of life (Agha et al. 2005). The risk was also increased for central nervous system and sympathetic nervous system tumors individually at a risk ratio of 2.5 (CI 1.8–3.4) and 2.2 (CI 1.4–3.4), respectively. A Bjørge et al. study of 5.2 million children and their families in Norway and Sweden also found patients with congenital anomalies had an increased cancer risk that extended into early adulthood (Bjorge et al. 2008). Furthermore, patients with CNS malformations were also at the highest risk of developing CNS malignancies, with a standardized incidence rate (SIR) of 58 (CI 41–80) and 8.3 (Louis et al. 2007; Stokland et al. 2010; Fisher et al. 2008; Arora et al. 2009; Fernandez et al. 2003; Gajjar et al. 1997; Hayostek et al. 1993; Khatib et al. 1994; Smoots et al. 1998; Becker et al. 2015; Jones et al. 2008; Hoffman et al. 1993) in Norway and Sweden, respectively. To assess potential cancer risk associated with congenital anomalies even outside of the setting of chromosomal defects, a review of the California Cancer Registry (CCR) found that between 1988 and 2004, children with congenital anomalies without chromosomal defects had a 1.8-fold increased risk of CNS cancer (Fisher et al. 2012).

A further examination found a particularly increased risk in medulloblastoma (OR 1.7, CI 1.1–2.6), PNET (OR 3.64, CI 1.5–8.6), and germ cell tumors (OR 6.4, CI 2.1–19.6), as well as an increased risk in mothers with greater than two fetal losses after 20 weeks of gestation (OR 3.13, CI 1.3–7.4) (Partap et al. 2011).

Many large studies have evaluated the impact of birth weight on the risk of developing CNS tumors, with several suggesting an increased birth weight carries a greater relative risk, although the most common specific tumors types varied among studies (Bjorge et al. 2013; Harder et al. 2008; MacLean et al. 2010; Milne et al. 2008; Schmidt et al. 2010). In an examination matching each case (17,698) to 10 controls, Bjørge found an increased childhood cancer risk for higher birth weight infants, and also infants with larger head circumferences (Bjorge et al. 2013). Additionally, in an evaluation of Nordic children, Schmidt found a gestational age-adjusted birth weight of greater than 4.5 kg increased the risk of all CNS tumors (OR 1.27, CI 1.03–1.6), with the greatest increase among embryonal tumors (Schmidt et al. 2010). When 3733 CNS tumors from the CCR were matched to controls, Maclean et al. found an increased birth weight of 4 kg associated with an increased risk of CNS tumors, especially HGGs (MacLean et al. 2010). A meta-analysis of eight studies found that increased birth weight was associated with increased incidence of astrocytomas and medulloblastomas, but not ependymomas (Harder et al. 2008). Conversely, a study of over 600,000 live births in Western Australia between 1980 and 2004 found no association between birth size and the development of CNS tumors prior to age 14 (Milne et al. 2008).

1.8   Immune System

Although allergic conditions have been consistently reported as inversely associated with adult gliomas, reports in children have varied (Chen et al. 2011). In pediatrics, an initial report from the United Kingdom found that maternal asthma resulted in a decreased relative risk of their children developing a CNS tumor, particularly PNETs (Harding et al. 2008). Another study evaluating 272 matched case–control pairs in Canada found asthma associated inversely with the development of CNS tumors, especially ependymomas, while the relationship with eczema was not significant (Roncarolo and Infante-Rivard 2012). Furthermore, the use of asthma controller medications was found to be associated with an increased risk. However, a study of 352 pediatric brain tumors in Denmark, Norway, Sweden, and Switzerland found no association with asthma or eczema (Shu et al. 2014).

Studies evaluating the influence of prior infectious history on the development of pediatric CNS tumors have been conflicting. Harding et al. found infants without social interaction with other infants in the first year of life had an increased risk (OR 1.37, CI 1.08–1.75) of CNS tumors, especially PNET, compared to those who had such interaction (Harding et al. 2009). Attendance in day care also appeared to show a protective benefit, though not statistically significant. A Canadian study also found a reduced risk in patients with day care attendance, and, unlike Harding's study, breastfeeding was found to be protective against the development of brain tumors (Shaw et al. 2006; Harding et al. 2007). Conversely, Anderson et al. found no association with day care attendance but that patients with more frequent sick days in the first 6 years of life had an increased incidence of gliomas and embryonal tumors (Andersen et al. 2013).

1.9   Environmental Exposure

Radiation therapy (RT), used decades ago to treat tinea capitis and more recently to treat childhood acute lymphoblastic leukemia (ALL), is known to cause secondary CNS tumors, especially meningiomas, *p53* mutated glioblastomas, and PNETs (Kleinerman 2006; Ohgaki and Kleihues 2005). Fifty-three percent of secondary neoplasms in survivors of childhood ALL occur in the CNS and 89% of those are associated with prior cranial irradiation (Mody et al. 2008; Schmiegelow et al. 2013). The timing and outcome are dependent on pathology, as non-meningioma CNS tumors occur between 6.5 and 9.8 years and meningiomas occurred between 12.3 and 18.3 years after treatment, with OS of 18% and 96%, respectively (Schmiegelow et al. 2013). Prenatal diagnostic imaging has been evaluated as a potential cancer risk, but studies from the United Kingdom, Sweden, and Denmark did not describe a significant increase in pediatric CNS tumors in patients exposed to prenatal X-rays compared to controls (Mellemkjaer et al. 2006; Rajaraman et al. 2011; Stalberg et al. 2007). Diagnostic head X-rays also have not been associated with the development of CNS tumors (Khan et al. 2010). However, CT scans contribute to a slightly elevated risk of CNS tumors, with risk decreasing with increasing age at first CT scan exposure (Pearce et al. 2012; Mathews et al. 2013).

Magnetic fields, radio waves, and mobile phone use have not been found to be associated with an increase in pediatric brain tumors (Aydin et al. 2011; Elliott et al. 2010; Ha et al. 2007; Kheifets et al. 2010).

Although many different maternal medications have been evaluated, none have been found to consistently increase the risk of pediatric CNS tumors in offspring. A German study found an association between maternal prenatal antibiotic use and an increased risk of medulloblastoma (OR 2.07, CI 1.03–4.17) and astrocytoma (OR 2.26, CI 1.09–4.69) (Kaatsch et al. 2010). Although the odds ratio was similarly elevated in a Canadian study, the results were not statistically significant (OR 1.7, CI 0.8–3.6) (Shaw et al. 2006). A 2010 Swedish study evaluating potential associations with prenatal medications and the development of pediatric CNS tumors in children 0–14 years of age found no association with antibiotics, antifungals, antacids, analgesics, antiasthmatics, antiemetics, antihistamines, diuretics, folic acid, iron, laxatives, or vitamins, but did find an association with antihypertensives (OR 2.7, CI 1.1–6.5), particularly β-blockers (OR 5.3, CI 1.2–24.8) (Stalberg et al. 2010). An association between prenatal antihypertensive use and the development of pediatric CNS tumors, however, was not found in a German study evaluating pediatric CNS tumors diagnosed between

1992 and 1997 (Schuz et al. 2007). Amide or amine-containing medications can potentially be carcinogenic after conversion to N-nitroso compounds (NOCs) in the stomach, though three studies have all found little or no support for an association between maternal exposure and central nervous system tumors in subsequent children (Cardy et al. 2006; Carozza et al. 1995).

Prenatal vitamins, especially iron and folic acid, consistently have been shown to decrease the risk of pediatric CNS tumors (Bunin et al. 2005, 2006; Ortega-Garcia et al. 2010; Milne et al. 2012).

Although prenatal alcohol exposure can have a variety of toxic effects on the developing child, there is no clear increased risk of pediatric CNS tumors (Infante-Rivard and El-Zein 2007; Milne et al. 2013). The role of maternal tobacco smoking during pregnancy is unclear, as several reports have found no association (Filippini et al. 2002; Huncharek et al. 2002; Norman et al. 1996), while a review of the Swedish Birth Register of births between 1983 and 1997 found a hazard ratio of 1.24 (CI 1.01–1.53) (Brooks et al. 2004).

Pesticide exposure may have an association with pediatric CNS tumors. A review of 4723 patients from the North of England found no significant relationship between occupational exposure to pesticides and risk of any childhood cancer (Pearce et al. 2006). In contrast, a study from the USA found that paternal pesticide exposure was associated with an increased risk of his child developing an astrocytoma (OR 1.8, CI 1.1–31), but not PNET (Shim et al. 2009). A separate study investigating paternal hobbies did identify exposure to pesticides as increasing the risk of medulloblastoma and PNET (Rosso et al. 2008). An Australian study also found preconception exposure to pesticides increased the risk of pediatric CNS tumors (Greenop et al. 2013). The effect of residential pesticides may be contingent on particular predispositions as polymorphisms in *PON1*, a gene responsible for organophosphorous metabolism, may increase the risk of pediatric CNS tumors in exposed patients (Searles Nielsen et al. 2010).

An investigation of the risk of pediatric CNS tumors among children of parents working in a wide variety of occupations found no clear associations (Mazumdar et al. 2008). However, a separate analysis found that brain tumors were more common in children of mothers working in electronic component manufacturing (OR 13.78, CI 1.45–129) and garment and textile workers (IR 7.25, CI 1.42–37) (Ali et al. 2004). There also appears to be an increased incidence of CNS tumors among children whose parents are exposed to diesel fuel, but not other exhausts (Peters et al. 2013). Paternal polycyclic aromatic hydrocarbon exposure has also been linked to a subsequent increase in pediatric CNS tumors (OR 1.4, CI 1.1–1.7) (Cordier et al. 2004).

In conclusion, pediatric neuro-oncology is a rapidly evolving field in which molecular investigations are fueling a restructuring of tumor subgroups. Although pediatric CNS tumors have historically been distinguished by histopathology and location, driving mutations and epigenetic profiles are proving to not only be attractive therapeutic targets but also epicenters for new classifications. The challenge will be to integrate former classification systems with the latter, and, perhaps just as importantly, to frame our historical data according to the new groupings so that the decades of lessons learned in epidemiology can continue to be applied in the pursuit of improving outcomes for children with CNS tumors.

References

Adriaensen ME, Schaefer-Prokop CM, Stijnen T, Duyndam DA, Zonnenberg BA, Prokop M (2009) Prevalence of subependymal giant cell tumors in patients with tuberous sclerosis and a review of the literature. Eur J Neurol 16(6):691–696

Agha MM, Williams JI, Marrett L, To T, Zipursky A, Dodds L (2005) Congenital abnormalities and childhood cancer. Cancer 103(9):1939–1948

Ahn Y, Cho BK, Kim SK, Chung YN, Lee CS, Kim IH et al (2006) Optic pathway glioma: outcome and prognostic factors in a surgical series. Childs Nerv Syst 22(9):1136–1142

Ali R, Yu CL, Wu MT, Ho CK, Pan BJ, Smith T et al (2004) A case-control study of parental occupation, leukemia, and brain tumors in an industrial city in Taiwan. J Occup Environ Med 46(9):985–992

Allen JC, Siffert J, Hukin J (1998) Clinical manifestations of childhood ependymoma: a multitude of syndromes. Pediatr Neurosurg 28(1):49–55

Altieri A, Castro F, Bermejo JL, Hemminki K (2006) Association between number of siblings and nervous system tumors suggests an infectious etiology. Neurology 67(11):1979–1983

Andersen TV, Schmidt LS, Poulsen AH, Feychting M, Roosli M, Tynes T et al (2013) Patterns of exposure to infectious diseases and social contacts in early life and risk of brain tumours in children and adolescents: an International Case-Control Study (CEFALO). Br J Cancer 108(11):2346–2353

Arens R, Marcus D, Engelberg S, Findler G, Goodman RM, Passwell JH (1988) Cerebral germinomas and Klinefelter syndrome. A review. Cancer 61(6):1228–1231

Arora RS, Alston RD, Eden TO, Estlin EJ, Moran A, Birch JM (2009) Age-incidence patterns of primary CNS tumors in children, adolescents, and adults in England. Neuro-Oncology 11(4):403–413

Athale UH, Duckworth J, Odame I, Barr R (2009) Childhood atypical teratoid rhabdoid tumor of the central nervous system: a meta-analysis of observational studies. J Pediatr Hematol Oncol 31(9):651–663

Avery RA, Fisher MJ, Liu GT (2011) Optic pathway gliomas. J Neuroophthalmol 31(3):269–278

Aydin D, Feychting M, Schuz J, Tynes T, Andersen TV, Schmidt LS et al (2011) Mobile phone use and brain tumors in children and adolescents: a multicenter case-control study. J Natl Cancer Inst 103(16):1264–1276

Badiali M, Pession A, Basso G, Andreini L, Rigobello L, Galassi E et al (1991) N-myc and c-myc oncogenes amplification in medulloblastomas. Evidence of particularly aggressive behavior of a tumor with c-myc amplification. Tumori 77(2):118–121

Barton VN, Donson AM, Kleinschmidt-DeMasters BK, Birks DK, Handler MH, Foreman NK (2010) Unique molecular characteristics of pediatric myxopapillary ependymoma. Brain Pathol 20(3):560–570

Becker AP, Scapulatempo-Neto C, Carloni AC, Paulino A, Sheren J, Aisner DL et al (2015) KIAA1549: BRAF gene fusion and FGFR1 hotspot mutations are prognostic factors in pilocytic astrocytomas. J Neuropathol Exp Neurol 74(7):743–754

Bhargava D, Sinha P, Chumas P, Al-Tamimi Y, Shivane A, Chakrabarty A et al (2013) Occurrence and distribution of pilomyxoid astrocytoma. Br J Neurosurg 27(4):413–418

Bianchi AB, Hara T, Ramesh V, Gao J, Klein-Szanto AJ, Morin F et al (1994) Mutations in transcript isoforms of the neurofibromatosis 2 gene in multiple human tumour types. Nat Genet 6(2):185–192

Bjorge T, Cnattingius S, Lie RT, Tretli S, Engeland A (2008) Cancer risk in children with birth defects and in their families: a population based cohort study of 5.2 million children from Norway and Sweden. Cancer Epidemiol Biomark Prev 17(3):500–506

Bjorge T, Sorensen HT, Grotmol T, Engeland A, Stephansson O, Gissler M et al (2013) Fetal growth and childhood cancer: a population-based study. Pediatrics 132(5):e1265–e1275

Brooks DR, Mucci LA, Hatch EE, Cnattingius S (2004) Maternal smoking during pregnancy and risk of brain tumors in the offspring. A prospective study of 1.4 million Swedish births. Cancer Causes Control 15(10):997–1005

Bunin GR, Gallagher PR, Rorke-Adams LB, Robison LL, Cnaan A (2006) Maternal supplement, micronutrient, and cured meat intake during pregnancy and risk of medulloblastoma during childhood: a children's oncology group study. Cancer Epidemiol Biomark Prev 15(9):1660–1667

Bunin GR, Kushi LH, Gallagher PR, Rorke-Adams LB, McBride ML, Cnaan A (2005) Maternal diet during pregnancy and its association with medulloblastoma in children: a children's oncology group study (United States). Cancer Causes Control 16(7):877–891

Cardy AH, Little J, McKean-Cowdin R, Lijinsky W, Choi NW, Cordier S et al (2006) Maternal medication use and the risk of brain tumors in the offspring: the SEARCH international case-control study. Int J Cancer 118(5):1302–1308

Carozza SE, Olshan AF, Faustman EM, Gula MJ, Kolonel LN, Austin DF et al (1995) Maternal exposure to N-nitrosatable drugs as a risk factor for childhood brain tumours. Int J Epidemiol 24(2):308–312

Chan TL, Yuen ST, Chung LP, Ho JW, Kwan K, Fan YW et al (1999) Germline hMSH2 and differential somatic mutations in patients with Turcot's syndrome. Genes Chromosomes Cancer 25(2):75–81

Chen C, Xu T, Chen J, Zhou J, Yan Y, Lu Y et al (2011) Allergy and risk of glioma: a meta-analysis. Eur J Neurol 18(3):387–395

Cho KT, Wang KC, Kim SK, Shin SH, Chi JG, Cho BK (2002) Pediatric brain tumors: statistics of SNUH, Korea (1959–2000). Childs Nerv Syst 18(1–2):30–37

Cordier S, Monfort C, Filippini G, Preston-Martin S, Lubin F, Mueller BA et al (2004) Parental exposure to polycyclic aromatic hydrocarbons and the risk of childhood brain tumors: the SEARCH International Childhood Brain Tumor Study. Am J Epidemiol 159(12):1109–1116

Distel L, Neubauer S, Varon R, Holter W, Grabenbauer G (2003) Fatal toxicity following radio- and chemotherapy of medulloblastoma in a child with unrecognized Nijmegen breakage syndrome. Med Pediatr Oncol 41(1):44–48

Dohrmann GJ, Farwell JR (1976) Ependymal neoplasms in children. Trans Am Neurol Assoc 101:125–129

Draper GJ, Heaf MM, Kinnier Wilson LM (1977) Occurrence of childhood cancers among sibs and estimation of familial risks. J Med Genet 14(2):81–90

Elliott P, Toledano MB, Bennett J, Beale L, de Hoogh K, Best N et al (2010) Mobile phone base stations and early childhood cancers: case-control study. BMJ 340:c3077

Ellison DW, Dalton J, Kocak M, Nicholson SL, Fraga C, Neale G et al (2011) Medulloblastoma: clinicopathological correlates of SHH, WNT, and non-SHH/WNT molecular subgroups. Acta Neuropathol 121(3):381–396

Ellison DW, Kocak M, Dalton J, Megahed H, Lusher ME, Ryan SL et al (2011) Definition of disease-risk stratification groups in childhood medulloblastoma using combined clinical, pathologic, and molecular variables. J Clin Oncol 29(11):1400–1407

Farwell J, Flannery JT (1984) Cancer in relatives of children with central-nervous-system neoplasms. N Engl J Med 311(12):749–753

Fassett DR, Pingree J, Kestle JR (2005) The high incidence of tumor dissemination in myxopapillary ependymoma in pediatric patients. Report of five cases and review of the literature. J Neurosurg 102(1 Suppl):59–64

Fauchon F, Jouvet A, Paquis P, Saint-Pierre G, Mottolese C, Ben Hassel M et al (2000) Parenchymal pineal tumors: a clinicopathological study of 76 cases. Int J Radiat Oncol Biol Phys 46(4):959–968

Fernandez C, Figarella-Branger D, Girard N, Bouvier-Labit C, Gouvernet J, Paz Paredes A et al (2003) Pilocytic astrocytomas in children: prognostic factors--a retrospective study of 80 cases. Neurosurgery 53(3):544–553. discussion 54–5

Filippini G, Maisonneuve P, McCredie M, Peris-Bonet R, Modan B, Preston-Martin S et al (2002) Relation of childhood brain tumors to exposure of parents and children to tobacco smoke: the SEARCH international case-control study. Surveillance of Environmental Aspects Related to Cancer in Humans. Int J Cancer 100(2):206–213

Fisher PG, Breiter SN, Carson BS, Wharam MD, Williams JA, Weingart JD et al (2000) A clinicopathologic reappraisal of brain stem tumor classification. Identification of pilocystic astrocytoma and fibrillary astrocytoma as distinct entities. Cancer 89(7):1569–1576

Fisher PG, Reynolds P, Von Behren J, Carmichael SL, Rasmussen SA, Shaw GM (2012) Cancer in children with nonchromosomal birth defects. J Pediatr 160(6):978–984

Fisher PG, Tihan T, Goldthwaite PT, Wharam MD, Carson BS, Weingart JD et al (2008) Outcome analysis of childhood low-grade astrocytomas. Pediatr Blood Cancer 51(2):245–250

Gadish T, Tulchinsky H, Deutsch AA, Rabau M (2005) Pinealoblastoma in a patient with familial adenomatous polyposis: variant of Turcot syndrome type 2? Report of a case and review of the literature. Dis Colon Rectum 48(12):2343–2346

Gajjar A, Chintagumpala M, Ashley D, Kellie S, Kun LE, Merchant TE et al (2006) Risk-adapted craniospinal radiotherapy followed by high-dose chemotherapy and stem-cell rescue in children with newly diagnosed medulloblastoma (St Jude Medulloblastoma-96): long-term results from a prospective, multicentre trial. Lancet Oncol 7(10):813–820

Gajjar A, Sanford RA, Heideman R, Jenkins JJ, Walter A, Li Y et al (1997) Low-grade astrocytoma: a decade of experience at St. Jude Children's Research Hospital. J Clin Oncol 15(8):2792–2799

Gallo P, Cecchi PC, Locatelli F, Rizzo P, Ghimenton C, Gerosa M et al (2013) Pleomorphic xanthoastrocytoma: long-term results of surgical treatment and analysis of prognostic factors. Br J Neurosurg 27(6):759–764

Gonzalez EM, Prayson RA (2013) Glioblastoma arising in a patient with Mayer-Rokitansky-Kuster-Hauser syndrome. J Clin Neurosci 20(10):1464–1465

Goodwin TL, Sainani K, Fisher PG (2009) Incidence patterns of central nervous system germ cell tumors: a SEER Study. J Pediatr Hematol Oncol 31(8):541–544

Greenop KR, Peters S, Bailey HD, Fritschi L, Attia J, Scott RJ et al (2013) Exposure to pesticides and the risk of childhood brain tumors. Cancer Causes Control 24(7):1269–1278

Gururangan S, McLaughlin CA, Brashears J, Watral MA, Provenzale J, Coleman RE et al (2006) Incidence and patterns of neuraxis metastases in children with diffuse pontine glioma. J Neuro-Oncol 77(2):207–212

Ha M, Im H, Lee M, Kim HJ, Kim BC, Gimm YM et al (2007) Radio-frequency radiation exposure from AM radio transmitters and childhood leukemia and brain cancer. Am J Epidemiol 166(3):270–279

Hahn JS, Bejar R, Gladson CL (1991) Neonatal subependymal giant cell astrocytoma associated with tuberous sclerosis: MRI, CT, and ultrasound correlation. Neurology 41(1):124–128

Hanaei S, Habibi Z, Nejat F, Sayarifard F, Vasei M (2015) Pediatric glioblastoma multiforme in association with Turner's syndrome: a case report. Pediatr Neurosurg 50(1):38–41

Harder T, Plagemann A, Harder A (2008) Birth weight and subsequent risk of childhood primary brain tumors: a meta-analysis. Am J Epidemiol 168(4):366–373

Harding NJ, Birch JM, Hepworth SJ, McKinney PA (2008) Atopic dysfunction and risk of central nervous system tumours in children. Eur J Cancer 44(1):92–99

Harding NJ, Birch JM, Hepworth SJ, McKinney PA (2009) Infectious exposure in the first year of life and risk of central nervous system tumors in children: analysis of day care, social contact, and overcrowding. Cancer Causes Control 20(2):129–136

Harding NJ, Birch JM, Hepworth SJ, McKinney PA, Investigators U (2007) Breastfeeding and risk of childhood CNS tumours. Br J Cancer 96(5):815–817

Hargrave D, Bartels U, Bouffet E (2006) Diffuse brainstem glioma in children: critical review of clinical trials. Lancet Oncol 7(3):241–248

Hart RM, Kimler BF, Evans RG, Park CH (1987) Radiotherapeutic management of medulloblastoma in a pediatric patient with ataxia telangiectasia. Int J Radiat Oncol Biol Phys 13(8):1237–1240

Hashimoto T, Sasagawa I, Ishigooka M, Kubota Y, Nakada T, Fujita T et al (1995) Down's syndrome associated with intracranial germinoma and testicular embryonal carcinoma. Urol Int 55(2):120–122

Hayostek CJ, Shaw EG, Scheithauer B, O'Fallon JR, Weiland TL, Schomberg PJ et al (1993) Astrocytomas of the cerebellum. A comparative clinicopathologic study of pilocytic and diffuse astrocytomas. Cancer 72(3):856–869

Heck JE, Lombardi CA, Cockburn M, Meyers TJ, Wilhelm M, Ritz B (2013) Epidemiology of rhabdoid tumors of early childhood. Pediatr Blood Cancer 60(1):77–81

Hemminki K, Kyyronen P, Vaittinen P (1999) Parental age as a risk factor for childhood leukemia and brain cancer in offspring. Epidemiology 10(3):271–275

Hilden JM, Meerbaum S, Burger P, Finlay J, Janss A, Scheithauer BW et al (2004) Central nervous system atypical teratoid/rhabdoid tumor: results of therapy in children enrolled in a registry. J Clin Oncol 22(14):2877–2884

Hoffman HJ, Soloniuk DS, Humphreys RP, Drake JM, Becker LE, De Lima BO et al (1993) Management and outcome of low-grade astrocytomas of the midline in children: a retrospective review. Neurosurgery 33(6):964–971

Huncharek M, Kupelnick B, Klassen H (2002) Maternal smoking during pregnancy and the risk of childhood brain tumors: a meta-analysis of 6566 subjects from twelve epidemiological studies. J Neuro-Oncol 57(1):51–57

Ikeda J, Sawamura Y, van Meir EG (1998) Pineoblastoma presenting in familial adenomatous polyposis (FAP): random association, FAP variant or Turcot syndrome? Br J Neurosurg 12(6):576–578

Infante-Rivard C, El-Zein M (2007) Parental alcohol consumption and childhood cancers: a review. J Toxicol Environ Health B Crit Rev 10(1–2):101–129

Jackson S, Patay Z, Howarth R, Pai Panandiker AS, Onar-Thomas A, Gajjar A et al (2013) Clinico-radiologic characteristics of long-term survivors of diffuse intrinsic pontine glioma. J Neuro-Oncol 114(3):339–344

Jahraus CD, Tarbell NJ (2006) Optic pathway gliomas. Pediatr Blood Cancer 46(5):586–596

Janss AJ, Grundy R, Cnaan A, Savino PJ, Packer RJ, Zackai EH et al (1995) Optic pathway and hypothalamic/chiasmatic gliomas in children younger than age 5 years with a 6-year follow-up. Cancer 75(4):1051–1059

Jeong TS, Yee GT (2014) Glioblastoma in a patient with neurofibromatosis type 1: a case report and review of the literature. Brain Tumor Res Treat 2(1):36–38

Johnson KJ, Carozza SE, Chow EJ, Fox EE, Horel S, McLaughlin CC et al (2009) Parental age and risk of childhood cancer: a pooled analysis. Epidemiology 20(4):475–483

Johnston DL, Keene D, Kostova M, Strother D, Lafay-Cousin L, Fryer C et al (2014) Incidence of medulloblastoma in Canadian children. J Neuro-Oncol 120(3):575–579

Jones DT, Kocialkowski S, Liu L, Pearson DM, Backlund LM, Ichimura K et al (2008) Tandem duplication producing a novel oncogenic BRAF fusion gene defines the majority of pilocytic astrocytomas. Cancer Res 68(21):8673–8677

Kaatsch P, Scheidemann-Wesp U, Schuz J (2010) Maternal use of antibiotics and cancer in the offspring:

results of a case-control study in Germany. Cancer Causes Control 21(8):1335–1345

Khafaga Y, Hassounah M, Kandil A, Kanaan I, Allam A, El Husseiny G et al (2003) Optic gliomas: a retrospective analysis of 50 cases. Int J Radiat Oncol Biol Phys 56(3):807–812

Khan S, Evans AA, Rorke-Adams L, Orjuela MA, Shiminski-Maher T, Bunin GR (2010) Head injury, diagnostic X-rays, and risk of medulloblastoma and primitive neuroectodermal tumor: a Children's Oncology Group study. Cancer Causes Control 21(7):1017–1023

Khatib ZA, Heideman RL, Kovnar EH, Langston JA, Sanford RA, Douglas EC et al (1994) Predominance of pilocytic histology in dorsally exophytic brain stem tumors. Pediatr Neurosurg 20(1):2–10

Kheifets L, Ahlbom A, Crespi CM, Feychting M, Johansen C, Monroe J et al (2010) A pooled analysis of extremely low-frequency magnetic fields and childhood brain tumors. Am J Epidemiol 172(7):752–761

Kleinerman RA (2006) Cancer risks following diagnostic and therapeutic radiation exposure in children. Pediatr Radiol 36(Suppl 2):121–125

Kobayashi N, Furukawa T, Takatsu T (1968) Congenital anomalies in children with malignancy. Paediatr Univ Tokyo 16:31–37

Kool M, Korshunov A, Remke M, Jones DT, Schlanstein M, Northcott PA et al (2012) Molecular subgroups of medulloblastoma: an international meta-analysis of transcriptome, genetic aberrations, and clinical data of WNT, SHH, group 3, and group 4 medulloblastomas. Acta Neuropathol 123(4):473–484

Lafay-Cousin L, Hawkins C, Carret AS, Johnston D, Zelcer S, Wilson B et al (2012) Central nervous system atypical teratoid rhabdoid tumours: the Canadian paediatric brain tumour consortium experience. Eur J Cancer 48(3):353–359

Laithier V, Grill J, Le Deley MC, Ruchoux MM, Couanet D, Doz F et al (2003) Progression-free survival in children with optic pathway tumors: dependence on age and the quality of the response to chemotherapy-results of the first French prospective study for the French Society of Pediatric Oncology. J Clin Oncol 21(24):4572–4578

Larsen AK, Mikkelsen DB, Hertz JM, Bygum A (2014) Manifestations of Gorlin-Goltz syndrome. Dan Med J 61(5):A4829

Lassiter KR, Alexander E Jr, Davis CH Jr, Kelly DL Jr (1971) Surgical treatment of brain stem gliomas. J Neurosurg 34(6):719–725

Li MH, Bouffet E, Hawkins CE, Squire JA, Huang A (2005) Molecular genetics of supratentorial primitive neuroectodermal tumors and pineoblastoma. Neurosurg Focus 19(5):E3

Listernick R, Charrow J, Greenwald MJ, Esterly NB (1989) Optic gliomas in children with neurofibromatosis type 1. J Pediatr 114(5):788–792

Lober RM, Cho YJ, Tang Y, Barnes PD, Edwards MS, Vogel H et al (2014) Diffusion-weighted MRI derived apparent diffusion coefficient identifies prognostically

distinct subgroups of pediatric diffuse intrinsic pontine glioma. J Neuro-Oncol 117(1):175–182

Louis DN, Ohgaki H, Wiestler OD, Cavenee WK, Burger PC, Jouvet A et al (2007) The 2007 WHO classification of tumours of the central nervous system. Acta Neuropathol 114(2):97–109

Louis DN, Perry A, Reifenberger G, von Deimling A, Figarella-Branger D, Cavenee WK et al (2016) The 2016 World Health Organization classification of tumors of the central nervous system: a summary. Acta Neuropathol 131(6):803–820

MacLean J, Partap S, Reynolds P, Von Behren J, Fisher PG (2010) Birth weight and order as risk factors for childhood central nervous system tumors. J Pediatr 157(3):450–455

Macy ME, Birks DK, Barton VN, Chan MH, Donson AM, Kleinschmidt-Demasters BK et al (2012) Clinical and molecular characteristics of congenital glioblastoma. Neuro-Oncology 14(7):931–941

Mathew RK, O'Kane R, Parslow R, Stiller C, Kenny T, Picton S et al (2014) Comparison of survival between the UK and US after surgery for most common pediatric CNS tumors. Neuro-Oncology 16(8):1137–1145

Mathews JD, Forsythe AV, Brady Z, Butler MW, Goergen SK, Byrnes GB et al (2013) Cancer risk in 680,000 people exposed to computed tomography scans in childhood or adolescence: data linkage study of 11 million Australians. BMJ 346:f2360

Mazumdar M, Liu CY, Wang SF, Pan PC, Wu MT, Christiani DC et al (2008) No association between parental or subject occupation and brain tumor risk. Cancer Epidemiol Biomark Prev 17(7):1835–1837

McGuire CS, Sainani KL, Fisher PG (2009) Incidence patterns for ependymoma: a surveillance, epidemiology, and end results study. J Neurosurg 110(4):725–729

Mellemkjaer L, Hasle H, Gridley G, Johansen C, Kjaer SK, Frederiksen K et al (2006) Risk of cancer in children with the diagnosis immaturity at birth. Paediatr Perinat Epidemiol 20(3):231–237

Metzger AK, Sheffield VC, Duyk G, Daneshvar L, Edwards MS, Cogen PH (1991) Identification of a germ-line mutation in the p53 gene in a patient with an intracranial ependymoma. Proc Natl Acad Sci U S A 88(17):7825–7829

Miller RW (1971) Deaths from childhood leukemia and solid tumors among twins and other sibs in the United States, 1960–67. J Natl Cancer Inst 46(1):203–209

Milne E, Greenop KR, Bower C, Miller M, van Bockxmeer FM, Scott RJ et al (2012) Maternal use of folic acid and other supplements and risk of childhood brain tumors. Cancer Epidemiol Biomark Prev 21(11):1933–1941

Milne E, Greenop KR, Scott RJ, de Klerk NH, Bower C, Ashton LJ et al (2013) Parental alcohol consumption and risk of childhood acute lymphoblastic leukemia and brain tumors. Cancer Causes Control 24(2):391–402

Milne E, Laurvick CL, Blair E, de Klerk N, Charles AK, Bower C (2008) Fetal growth and the risk of childhood CNS tumors and lymphomas in Western Australia. Int J Cancer 123(2):436–443

Mody R, Li S, Dover DC, Sallan S, Leisenring W, Oeffinger KC et al (2008) Twenty-five-year follow-up among survivors of childhood acute lymphoblastic leukemia: a report from the Childhood Cancer Survivor Study. Blood 111(12):5515–5523

Mori K, Kurisaka M (1986) Brain tumors in childhood: statistical analysis of cases from the brain tumor registry of Japan. Childs Nerv Syst 2(5):233–237

Nicolin G, Parkin P, Mabbott D, Hargrave D, Bartels U, Tabori U et al (2009) Natural history and outcome of optic pathway gliomas in children. Pediatr Blood Cancer 53(7):1231–1237

Ning MS, Perkins SM, Dewees T, Shinohara ET (2015) Evidence of high mortality in long term survivors of childhood medulloblastoma. J Neuro-Oncol 122(2):321–327

Norman MA, Holly EA, Ahn DK, Preston-Martin S, Mueller BA, Bracci PM (1996) Prenatal exposure to tobacco smoke and childhood brain tumors: results from the United States West Coast childhood brain tumor study. Cancer Epidemiol Biomark Prev 5(2):127–133

Northcott PA, Korshunov A, Witt H, Hielscher T, Eberhart CG, Mack S et al (2011) Medulloblastoma comprises four distinct molecular variants. J Clin Oncol 29(11):1408–1414

O'Callaghan FJ, Martyn CN, Renowden S, Noakes M, Presdee D, Osborne JP (2008) Subependymal nodules, giant cell astrocytomas and the tuberous sclerosis complex: a population-based study. Arch Dis Child 93(9):751–754

O'Callaghan FJ, Shiell AW, Osborne JP, Martyn CN (1998) Prevalence of tuberous sclerosis estimated by capture-recapture analysis. Lancet 351(9114):1490

Ohgaki H, Kleihues P (2005) Epidemiology and etiology of gliomas. Acta Neuropathol 109(1):93–108

Ortega-Garcia JA, Ferris-Tortajada J, Claudio L, Soldin OP, Sanchez-Sauco MF, Fuster-Soler JL et al (2010) Case control study of periconceptional folic acid intake and nervous system tumors in children. Childs Nerv Syst 26(12):1727–1733

Ostrom QT, Chen Y, MdB P, Ondracek A, Farah P, Gittleman H et al (2014) The descriptive epidemiology of atypical teratoid/rhabdoid tumors in the United States, 2001–2010. Neuro-Oncology 16(10):1392–1399

Ostrom QT, Gittleman H, Liao P, Rouse C, Chen Y, Dowling J et al (2014) CBTRUS statistical report: primary brain and central nervous system tumors diagnosed in the United States in 2007–2011. Neuro-Oncology 16(Suppl 4):iv1–i63

Packer RJ, Gajjar A, Vezina G, Rorke-Adams L, Burger PC, Robertson PL et al (2006) Phase III study of craniospinal radiation therapy followed by adjuvant chemotherapy for newly diagnosed average-risk medulloblastoma. J Clin Oncol 24(25):4202–4208

Pajtler KW, Witt H, Sill M, Jones DT, Hovestadt V, Kratochwil F et al (2015) Molecular classification of ependymal tumors across all CNS compartments, histopathological grades, and age groups. Cancer Cell 27(5):728–743

Parker M, Mohankumar KM, Punchihewa C, Weinlich R, Dalton JD, Li Y et al (2014) C11orf95-RELA fusions drive oncogenic NF-kappaB signalling in ependymoma. Nature 506(7489):451–455

Partap S, MacLean J, Von Behren J, Reynolds P, Fisher PG (2011) Birth anomalies and obstetric history as risks for childhood tumors of the central nervous system. Pediatrics 128(3):e652–e657

Pearce MS, Hammal DM, Dorak MT, McNally RJ, Parker L (2006) Paternal occupational exposure to pesticides or herbicides as risk factors for cancer in children and young adults: a case-control study from the North of England. Arch Environ Occup Health 61(3):138–144

Pearce MS, Salotti JA, Little MP, McHugh K, Lee C, Kim KP et al (2012) Radiation exposure from CT scans in childhood and subsequent risk of leukaemia and brain tumours: a retrospective cohort study. Lancet 380(9840):499–505

Perilongo G, Massimino M, Sotti G, Belfontali T, Masiero L, Rigobello L et al (1997) Analyses of prognostic factors in a retrospective review of 92 children with ependymoma: Italian Pediatric Neuro-Oncology Group. Med Pediatr Oncol 29(2):79–85

Perkins SM, Mitra N, Fei W, Shinohara ET (2012) Patterns of care and outcomes of patients with pleomorphic xanthoastrocytoma: a SEER analysis. J Neuro-Oncol 110(1):99–104

Peters S, Glass DC, Reid A, de Klerk N, Armstrong BK, Kellie S et al (2013) Parental occupational exposure to engine exhausts and childhood brain tumors. Int J Cancer 132(12):2975–2979

Plotkin SR, O'Donnell CC, Curry WT, Bove CM, MacCollin M, Nunes FP (2011) Spinal ependymomas in neurofibromatosis type 2: a retrospective analysis of 55 patients. J Neurosurg Spine 14(4):543–547

Ragel BT, Osborn AG, Whang K, Townsend JJ, Jensen RL, Couldwell WT (2006) Subependymomas: an analysis of clinical and imaging features. Neurosurgery 58(5):881–890. discussion 90

Rajaraman P, Simpson J, Neta G, Berrington de Gonzalez A, Ansell P, Linet MS et al (2011) Early life exposure to diagnostic radiation and ultrasound scans and risk of childhood cancer: case-control study. BMJ 342:d472

Ramasubramanian A, Kytasty C, Meadows AT, Shields JA, Leahey A, Shields CL (2013) Incidence of pineal gland cyst and pineoblastoma in children with retinoblastoma during the chemoreduction era. Am J Ophthalmol 156(4):825–829

Ramaswamy V, Remke M, Bouffet E, Faria CC, Perreault S, Cho YJ et al (2013) Recurrence patterns across medulloblastoma subgroups: an integrated clinical and molecular analysis. Lancet Oncol 14(12):1200–1207

Ramaswamy V, Remke M, Shih D, Wang X, Northcott PA, Faria CC et al (2014) Duration of the pre-diagnostic interval in medulloblastoma is subgroup dependent. Pediatr Blood Cancer 61(7):1190–1194

Ramos A, Hilario A, Lagares A, Salvador E, Perez-Nunez A, Sepulveda J (2013) Brainstem gliomas. Semin Ultrasound CT MR 34(2):104–112

Robertson PL, Zeltzer PM, Boyett JM, Rorke LB, Allen JC, Geyer JR et al (1998) Survival and prognostic factors following radiation therapy and chemotherapy for ependymomas in children: a report of the Children's Cancer Group. J Neurosurg 88(4):695–703

Rogers L, Pattisapu J, Smith RR, Parker P (1988) Medulloblastoma in association with the Coffin-Siris syndrome. Childs Nerv Syst 4(1):41–44

Roncarolo F, Infante-Rivard C (2012) Asthma and risk of brain cancer in children. Cancer Causes Control 23(4):617–623

Ross GW, Rubinstein LJ (1989) Lack of histopathological correlation of malignant ependymomas with postoperative survival. J Neurosurg 70(1):31–36

Rosso AL, Hovinga ME, Rorke-Adams LB, Spector LG, Bunin GR, Children's Oncology G (2008) A case-control study of childhood brain tumors and fathers' hobbies: a Children's Oncology Group study. Cancer Causes Control 19(10):1201–1207

Sabbaghian N, Hamel N, Srivastava A, Albrecht S, Priest JR, Foulkes WD (2012) Germline DICER1 mutation and associated loss of heterozygosity in a pineoblastoma. J Med Genet 49(7):417–419

Scheinker I (1945) Subependymoma: a newly recognized tumor of subependymal derivation. J Neurosurg 2:232–240

Schmidt LS, Schuz J, Lahteenmaki P, Trager C, Stokland T, Gustafson G et al (2010) Fetal growth, preterm birth, neonatal stress and risk for CNS tumors in children: a Nordic population- and register-based case-control study. Cancer Epidemiol Biomark Prev 19(4):1042–1052

Schmiegelow K, Levinsen MF, Attarbaschi A, Baruchel A, Devidas M, Escherich G et al (2013) Second malignant neoplasms after treatment of childhood acute lymphoblastic leukemia. J Clin Oncol 31(19):2469–2476

Schuz J, Weihkopf T, Kaatsch P (2007) Medication use during pregnancy and the risk of childhood cancer in the offspring. Eur J Pediatr 166(5):433–441

Searles Nielsen S, McKean-Cowdin R, Farin FM, Holly EA, Preston-Martin S, Mueller BA (2010) Childhood brain tumors, residential insecticide exposure, and pesticide metabolism genes. Environ Health Perspect 118(1):144–149

Shankar GM, Lelic N, Gill CM, Thorner AR, Van Hummelen P, Wisoff JH et al (2016) BRAF alteration status and the histone H3F3A gene K27M mutation segregate spinal cord astrocytoma histology. Acta Neuropathol 131(1):147–150

Shaw AK, Li P, Infante-Rivard C (2006) Early infection and risk of childhood brain tumors (Canada). Cancer Causes Control 17(10):1267–1274

Shim YK, Mlynarek SP, van Wijngaarden E (2009) Parental exposure to pesticides and childhood brain cancer: U.S. Atlantic coast childhood brain cancer study. Environ Health Perspect 117(6):1002–1006

Shu X, Prochazka M, Lannering B, Schuz J, Roosli M, Tynes T et al (2014) Atopic conditions and brain tumor risk in children and adolescents--an international case-control study (CEFALO). Ann Oncol 25(4):902–908

Siegel RL, Miller KD, Jemal A (2015) Cancer statistics, 2015. CA Cancer J Clin 65(1):5–29

Singhal S, Birch JM, Kerr B, Lashford L, Evans DG (2002) Neurofibromatosis type 1 and sporadic optic gliomas. Arch Dis Child 87(1):65–70

Skomorowski M, Taxier M, Wise W Jr (2012) Turcot syndrome type 2: medulloblastoma with multiple colorectal adenomas. Clin Gastroenterol Hepatol 10(10):A24

Smith MA, Freidlin B, Ries LA, Simon R (1998) Trends in reported incidence of primary malignant brain tumors in children in the United States. J Natl Cancer Inst 90(17):1269–1277

Smoots DW, Geyer JR, Lieberman DM, Berger MS (1998) Predicting disease progression in childhood cerebellar astrocytoma. Childs Nerv Syst 14(11):636–648

Sredni ST, Tomita T (2015) Rhabdoid tumor predisposition syndrome. Pediatr Dev Pathol 18(1):49–58

Stalberg K, Haglund B, Axelsson O, Cnattingius S, Pfeifer S, Kieler H (2007) Prenatal X-ray exposure and childhood brain tumours: a population-based case-control study on tumour subtypes. Br J Cancer 97(11):1583–1587

Stalberg K, Haglund B, Stromberg B, Kieler H (2010) Prenatal exposure to medicines and the risk of childhood brain tumor. Cancer Epidemiol 34(4):400–404

Stokland T, Liu JF, Ironside JW, Ellison DW, Taylor R, Robinson KJ et al (2010) A multivariate analysis of factors determining tumor progression in childhood low-grade glioma: a population-based cohort study (CCLG CNS9702). Neuro-Oncology 12(12):1257–1268

Tarbell NJ, Friedman H, Polkinghorn WR, Yock T, Zhou T, Chen Z et al (2013) High-risk medulloblastoma: a pediatric oncology group randomized trial of chemotherapy before or after radiation therapy (POG 9031). J Clin Oncol 31(23):2936–2941

Taylor MD, Gokgoz N, Andrulis IL, Mainprize TG, Drake JM, Rutka JT (2000) Familial posterior fossa brain tumors of infancy secondary to germline mutation of the hSNF5 gene. Am J Hum Genet 66(4):1403–1406

Taylor KR, Mackay A, Truffaux N, Butterfield YS, Morozova O, Philippe C et al (2014) Recurrent activating ACVR1 mutations in diffuse intrinsic pontine glioma. Nat Genet 46(5):457–461

Taylor MD, Mainprize TG, Rutka JT, Becker L, Bayani J, Drake JM (2001) Medulloblastoma in a child with Rubenstein-Taybi syndrome: case report and review of the literature. Pediatr Neurosurg 35(5):235–238

Veldhuijzen van Zanten SE, Jansen MH, Sanchez Aliaga E, van Vuurden DG, Vandertop WP, Kaspers GJ (2014) A twenty-year review of diagnosing and treating children with diffuse intrinsic pontine glioma in The Netherlands. Expert Rev Anticancer Ther:1–8

Vera-Bolanos E, Aldape K, Yuan Y, Wu J, Wani K, Necesito-Reyes MJ et al (2015) Clinical course and progression-free survival of adult intracranial and spinal ependymoma patients. Neuro-Oncology 17(3):440–447

Villa S, Miller RC, Krengli M, Abusaris H, Baumert BG, Servagi-Vernat S et al (2012) Primary pineal tumors: outcome and prognostic factors--a study from the Rare Cancer Network (RCN). Clin Transl Oncol 14(11):827–834

Virchow R (1863–67) Die krankhaften Geschwülste, vol 3. August Hirschwald, Berlin

von Hoff K, Hinkes B, Dannenmann-Stern E, von Bueren AO, Warmuth-Metz M, Soerensen N et al (2011) Frequency, risk-factors and survival of children with atypical teratoid rhabdoid tumors (AT/RT) of the CNS diagnosed between 1988 and 2004, and registered to the German HIT database. Pediatr Blood Cancer 57(6):978–985

Winther JF, Sankila R, Boice JD, Tulinius H, Bautz A, Barlow L et al (2001) Cancer in siblings of children with cancer in the Nordic countries: a population-based cohort study. Lancet 358(9283):711–717

Witt H, Mack SC, Ryzhova M, Bender S, Sill M, Isserlin R et al (2011) Delineation of two clinically and molecularly distinct subgroups of posterior fossa ependymoma. Cancer Cell 20(2):143–157

Woehrer A, Slavc I, Waldhoer T, Heinzl H, Zielonke N, Czech T et al (2010) Incidence of atypical teratoid/rhabdoid tumors in children: a population-based study by the Austrian brain tumor registry, 1996–2006. Cancer 116(24):5725–5732

Woesler B, Moskopp D, Kuchelmeister K, Schul C, Wassmann H (1998) Intracranial metastasis of a spinal myxopapillary ependymoma. A case report. Neurosurg Rev 21(1):62–65

Wong TT, Ho DM, Chang TK, Yang DD, Lee LS (1995) Familial neurofibromatosis 1 with germinoma involving the basal ganglion and thalamus. Childs Nerv Syst 11(8):456–458

Wong TT, Ho DM, Chang KP, Yen SH, Guo WY, Chang FC et al (2005) Primary pediatric brain tumors: statistics of Taipei VGH, Taiwan (1975–2004). Cancer 104(10):2156–2167

Wu G, Broniscer A, McEachron TA, Lu C, Paugh BS, Becksfort J et al (2012) Somatic histone H3 alterations in pediatric diffuse intrinsic pontine gliomas and non-brainstem glioblastomas. Nat Genet 44(3):251–253

Yip BH, Pawitan Y, Czene K (2006) Parental age and risk of childhood cancers: a population-based cohort study from Sweden. Int J Epidemiol 35(6):1495–1503

Zacharoulis S, Ji L, Pollack IF, Duffner P, Geyer R, Grill J et al (2008) Metastatic ependymoma: a multi-institutional retrospective analysis of prognostic factors. Pediatr Blood Cancer 50(2):231–235

Zhou D, Zhang Y, Liu H, Luo S, Luo L, Dai K (2008) Epidemiology of nervous system tumors in children: a survey of 1,485 cases in Beijing Tiantan Hospital from 2001 to 2005. Pediatr Neurosurg 44(2):97–103

Zuccoli G, Izzi G, Bacchini E, Tondelli MT, Ferrozzi F, Bellomi M (1999) Central nervous system atypical teratoid/rhabdoid tumour of infancy. CT and mr findings. Clin Imaging 23(6):356–360

Principles of Pediatric Neurosurgery

2

P. Ryan Lingo, Asim F. Choudhri, and Paul Klimo Jr

2.1 Introduction

The incidence of primary malignant and nonmalignant central nervous system (CNS) tumors in children and adolescents aged 0–19 years in the US is 5.42 per 100,000, and approximately 4620 new cases are expected to be diagnosed in the US in 2015 (Ostrom et al. 2014). There is a rich variety of brain tumors found in children which is primarily a function of the patient's age and location of origin, with the overall most common being pilocytic astrocytoma (Ostrom et al. 2014). It has been traditionally taught that approximately 60% of pediatric brain tumors are infratentorial, but the actual ratio of supratentorial to infratentorial pediatric tumors is dependent on the specific age group (Ostrom et al. 2015). Tumors can be broadly categorized as glial (e.g., astrocytomas, ependymomas), embryo-

nal (e.g., medulloblastomas, pineoblastoma), germ cell (e.g., germinoma, teratoma), and other (e.g., choroid plexus tumors, craniopharyngiomas).

Neurosurgery represents one of the main pillars of pediatric neurooncologic care, along with medical and radiation oncology, pathology, and neuroradiology. Neurosurgical interventions include management of hydrocephalus, obtaining tissue for histopathological and molecular diagnosis, and tumor resection for oncologic (i.e., survival) and/or neurologic (e.g. seizure control) benefit. In this chapter, we will take the reader through the surgical management of pediatric neurooncologic patients from the preoperative, intraoperative, and postoperative phases of care.

2.2 Initial Evaluation

2.2.1 History and Examination

Clinical presentation is variable and dependent on the location of the tumor and the age of the patient. Most children will present with hydrocephalus, symptoms of raised intracranial pressure, focal neurologic deficit, or a seizure. Some tumors will be incidentally found as part of a workup for nonspecific symptoms, such as headaches or after a minor traumatic event. A detailed neurological exam should be performed on all patients; a thorough knowledge of neuroanatomy can help qualitatively detail preoperative deficits, both minor and major. This is easier in older children, but

P. Ryan Lingo · A. F. Choudhri
Department of Neurosurgery,
University of Tennessee, Memphis, TN, USA

Neuroscience Institute, Le Bonheur Children's
Hospital, Memphis, TN, USA

P. Klimo Jr (✉)
Department of Neurosurgery, University of
Tennessee, Memphis, TN, USA

Neuroscience Institute, Le Bonheur Children's
Hospital, Memphis, TN, USA

St. Jude Children's Research Hospital,
Memphis, TN, USA

Semmes Murphey, Memphis, TN, USA
e-mail: pklimo@semmes-murphey.com

© Springer International Publishing AG, part of Springer Nature 2018
A. Gajjar et al. (eds.), *Brain Tumors in Children*, https://doi.org/10.1007/978-3-319-43205-2_2

there are specific signs and symptoms that can be revealing in younger children.

Headache is a common symptom among patients with brain tumors and occurs with, or without, elevated intracranial pressure (ICP). These headaches are classically described as being worse in the morning and exacerbated by straining, coughing, or placing the head in a dependent location. Brain tumor headaches are frequently associated with nausea and may be temporarily relieved by the hyperventilation that occurs with vomiting. In a large study examining the epidemiology of headaches associated with pediatric brain tumors, approximately two-thirds of patients had chronic or frequent headaches prior to their first admission (The epidemiology of headache among children with brain tumor. Headache in children with brain tumors. The Childhood Brain Tumor Consortium 1991). In this study, headaches tended to be triggered by straining, coughing, or sneezing, to gradually worsen over time, to cause vomiting followed by relief, and to be severe enough to wake the child from sleep. Personality changes, school problems, and focal neurologic deficits were also associated with headaches. In a similar study, the most common symptom at presentation in children with brain tumors was headache; all of the patients with headaches also had other symptoms, including mental status changes, papilledema, eye movement derangements, hemimotor or sensory abnormalities, tandem gait difficulty, or abnormal deep tendon reflexes, present at the time of diagnosis (Wilne et al. 2006).

The two cranial nerves that can be affected by hydrocephalus or elevated ICP are the trochlear (4th) and abducens (6th). The trochlear nerve innervates the superior oblique muscle, which intorts, depresses, and adducts the eye. Patients with acquired weakness of the 4th nerve report vertical and oblique diplopia that is worse in down-gaze and gaze away from the affected eye, resulting in difficulty reading. Patients will adopt a characteristic head tilt away from their affected eye to reduce their diplopia, which is called the Bielschowsky's sign. The abducens nerve innervates the lateral rectus, which abducts the eye. Weakness of the 6th cranial nerve results in a lateral gaze palsy and horizontal diplopia that is worse with gaze toward the affected eye.

Posterior fossa tumors often present with symptoms of obstructive hydrocephalus, which in turn leads to elevated intracranial pressure. Headache and vomiting are hallmark features, particularly if present in the morning. In infants, hydrocephalus presents with a full or bulging fontanelle, separation of sutures, rapid head growth, macrocephaly, irritability, lethargy, or poor feeding/failure to thrive. Sundowning—or setting sun sign—describes downward deviation of both eyes, revealing an area of sclera above the irises. This usually occurs with advanced hydrocephalus with stretching of the third ventricle and upper brainstem. The pupils are sluggish and respond to light unequally.

Pineal region tumors can result in hydrocephalus and Parinaud's syndrome. Parinaud's syndrome, or dorsal midbrain syndrome, is a constellation of eye findings that includes upgaze palsy, convergence-retraction nystagmus, light-near pupillary dissociation (Argyll Robertson pupil), and lid retraction called Collier's sign (Baloh et al. 1985). When upgaze palsy is combined with lid retraction, it produces the setting sun sign. This syndrome is often seen with pineal region tumors that place pressure on the rostral interstitial nucleus of the medial longitudinal fasciculus and the posterior commissure, which mediate upgaze and the consensual pupillary light reflex, respectively.

Diencephalic syndrome, also known as Russell's syndrome, is characterized by progressive and severe failure to thrive (Zafeiriou et al. 2001). It is seen exclusively with suprasellar pilocytic astrocytoma tumors affecting the anterior hypothalamus. The child often appears emaciated despite being alert and active and has a "pseudohydrocephalic" face from severe loss of adipose tissue and a normal head circumference. Neurocutaneous syndromes—such as the neurofibromatoses, tuberous sclerosis, and Von Hippel-Lindau disease—are characterized by specific nervous system tumors associated with clinical exam findings. The details of these syndromes are beyond the scope of this chapter.

2.2.2 Seizures

Supratentorial tumor location, age < 2 years, and hyponatremia are independent risk factors for a first-time seizure in pediatric patients with a brain tumor (Hardesty et al. 2011). Seizures cause cerebral hyperemia and can thus precipitate a herniation event in the setting of preexisting increased intracranial pressure. They can also be the clinical manifestation of an intratumoral hemorrhage. If the patient is in status epilepticus, secondary brain damage may also occur through tissue hypoxia or acidosis. Guidelines are available that detail when imaging should be conducted in a child with a first-time nonfebrile seizure (Hirtz et al. 2000).

Antiepileptic drugs (AED)—such as phenytoin, phenobarbital, and carbamazeipine—induce the cytochrome P450 system and can reduce the efficacy of many common chemotherapeutics (Guerrini et al. 2013). Conversely, valproic acid inhibits the cytochrome P450 system and can increase levels of chemotherapeutics. Levetiracetam is a newer AED that has proven efficacious in preventing tumoral seizures with a low side-effect profile and no significant induction of the cytochrome P450 system (Zachenhofer et al. 2011). It is the first-line AED at our institution for children who suffer from seizures caused by a brain tumor.

2.2.3 Cerebral Edema

Brain tumors can cause vasogenic (i.e., interstitial) edema, which results from breakdown of the tight junctions between brain capillary endothelial cells and leakage of plasma filtrate into the interstitial space. Vasogenic edema is more marked in the white matter than the gray matter. Children are often started on steroids (e.g., dexamethasone) shortly after being diagnosed with a brain tumor. Steroids help with vasogenic edema, hydrocephalus (headaches, nausea/vomiting), and poor appetite, all of which cause the child to feel and look significantly better.

2.2.4 Preparation for Tumor Resection: Management of Hydrocephalus

For the vast majority of children, treatment of hydrocephalus is done by resecting the tumor. Prophylactic endoscopic third ventriculostomy (ETV) at the time of surgery has been shown to reduce the risk of post-resection hydrocephalus from approximately 27 to 6% in patients with posterior fossa tumors and hydrocephalus (Sainte-Rose et al. 2001). However, since resection alone effectively treats the majority of patients with posterior fossa tumor-induced hydrocephalus, pre-resection ETV is an unnecessary surgery, if tumor resection is to be carried out in a timely manner. However, if the patient's hydrocephalus will not resolve with resection (e.g., CSF dissemination), or there is no immediate role for resection (e.g., pineal mass), or no resection at all (e.g., diffuse pontine glioma), then long-term hydrocephalus management can be achieved either by placing a ventricular shunt or by performing an ETV. The ETV Success Score was developed to help surgeons determine the likelihood of ETV succeeding in a particular child, taking into consideration age, hydrocephalus etiology, and whether the child currently has a shunt or not.

Patients who present in extremis from severe hydrocephalus may require emergent placement of an external ventricular drain (EVD) (Lin and Riva-Cambrin 2015; El-Gaidi et al. 2015). Care must be taken not to drain too much cerebrospinal fluid in patients with posterior fossa tumors as this can precipitate upward transtentorial herniation (Osborn et al. 1978). Ascending transtentorial herniation results in a clinical syndrome of nausea and vomiting, followed by progression to stupor and coma with small nonreactive pupils and loss of vertical gaze. Radiographically, there is displacement of the midbrain and cerebellum through the tentorial notch, causing flattening of the quadrigeminal cistern and a "spinning top" appearance to the midbrain from compression of the posterior aspect of the midbrain.

2.2.5 Preparation for Tumor Resection: Neuroimaging

Computed tomography (CT) scans are very useful in the initial evaluation because they are quick and sensitive for detecting hydrocephalus, hemorrhage, edema, and ectopic calcifications. Once the child is deemed stable, he or she should have a magnetic resonance image (MRI) of the brain both with and without contrast. Unless the index of suspicion is low, an MRI of the full spine (with and without contrast) should also be obtained to look for leptomeningeal—or "drop"—metastases. Standard MRI brain sequences include T1 (with and without contrast), T2, FLAIR, diffusion weighted imaging (DWI) with the apparent diffusion coefficient map (ADC), and susceptibility weighted imaging (SWI). ADC maps have been shown to correlate with tumor cellularity in pediatric brain tumors (Choudhri et al. 2015a). Sometimes brain tumors can resemble other pathologies, such as infection or demyelinating disease. Magnetic resonance (MR) perfusion and spectroscopy can help distinguish tumors from other such conditions by highlighting increased blood flow and products of cell turnover, like elevated choline and depressed N-acetylaspartate, respectively.

Vascular imaging studies, such as MR or CT angiogram/venogram, are useful if tumors involve major intracranial arteries, veins, or sinovenous structures. Traditional angiography is also a valuable preoperative tool when tumors are felt to be hypervascular and may benefit from preoperative embolization (Fig. 2.1). If such

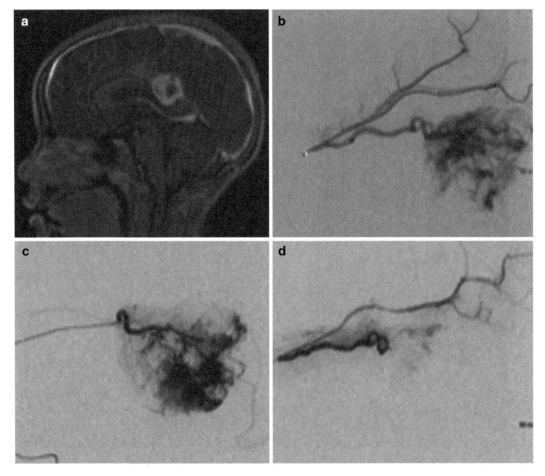

Fig. 2.1 T1 weighted (T1W) MRI with contrast of an interhemispheric hemangioma (**a**). Angiogram demonstrates vascular supply through the pericallosal artery (**b**). Microcatheterization of the tumor for embolization (**c**). Post embolization angiogram (**d**)

embolization is performed, resection should follow within 24–48 h as the embolization may cause new or worsening cerebral edema.

Eloquent location of a tumor is particularly challenging for the surgeon. Functional MRI (fMRI), magnetoencephalography (MEG), transcranial magnetic stimulation (TMS), and diffusion tensor imaging (DTI) are modalities that provide further knowledge of the patient's functional neuroanatomy (Ottenhausen et al. 2015). These imaging studies may localize elo-

quent regions, such as the primary motor cortex, Broca's and Wernicke's area, or subcortical tracts like the corticospinal, geniculocalcarine, or arcuate fasciculus. Functional MRI relies on the theory of neurovascular coupling and assumes that when functional networks within the brain are activated, perfusion-induced changes occur regionally in the blood oxygen-level that can be detected by MRI. In young children, motor mapping can be performed with passive movement (Fig. 2.2) (Choudhri et al. 2015c). MEG detects

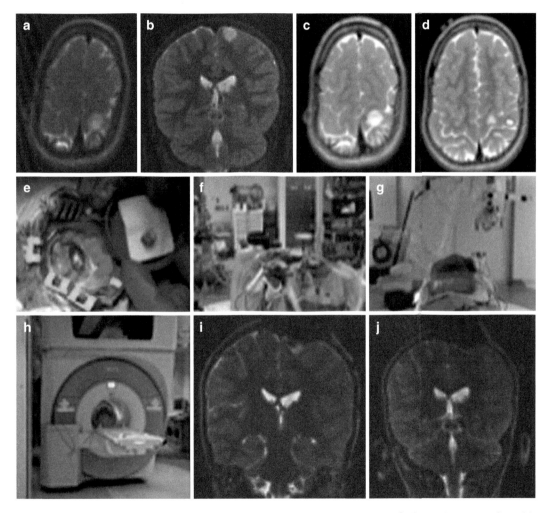

Fig. 2.2 Axial and coronal T2 weighted (T2W) MRI shows a low-grade glioma within the left precentral gyrus (**a**, **b**). Axial T2W image with functional MRI (fMRI) overlay from passive movement of the right lower extremity shows cortical activation along the medial margin of the tumor within the precentral gyrus near the vertex (**c**). Axial T2W image with fMRI overlay from passive movement of the right upper extremity shows cortical activation in the precentral gyrus inferolateral to the tumor (**d**). Resected tumor specimen (**e**). Operative setup utilizing frameless neuronavigation and a surgical microscope with the patient's head positioned 180° away from anesthesia to facilitate intraoperative MRI (iMRI) scanning (**f**, **g**). iMRI suite and scanner (**h**). Coronal T2W image from initial iMRI demonstrates residual tumor (**i**). Coronal T2W image from second iMRI after further resection demonstrates a gross total resection (**j**)

the magnetic fields created by bioelectrical currents as a result of neuronal activation and is, therefore, a direct marker of neuronal activity. Navigated TMS uses a magnetic field to induce a cortical electrical field and thus elicits or inhibits neuronal activity. A single pulse is used to elicit a motor response, or repetitive pulses are used to inhibit language function thereby mapping functional motor and language areas that are sufficient—and possibly necessary—to evoke a physiological response. DTI is the only preoperative method for visualizing subcortical white mater tracts (Fig. 2.3) (Choudhri et al. 2014b). All of these functional imaging techniques are more accurate for mapping motor areas than language areas.

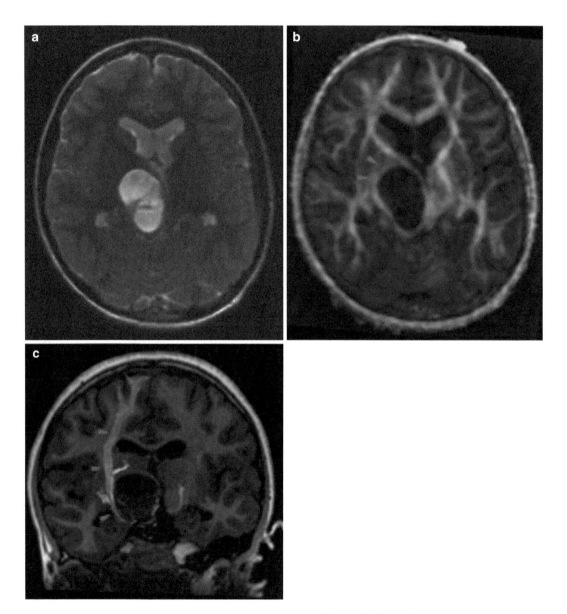

Fig. 2.3 Axial T2W image in a 5-year-old male shows a multicystic lesion centered in the right cerebral peduncle, consistent with a thalamopeduncular glioma (**a**). Axial T1W image with overlay of DTI data shows anterolateral displacement of the posterior limb of the internal capsule (red arrowheads) (**b**). Coronal T1W image with "tractography" overlay shows the course of the fibers of the corticospinal tract along the lateral aspect of the lesion (*red arrowheads*) (**c**)

2.2.6 Preparation for Tumor Resection: Neoadjuvant Chemotherapy

In some tumors found in newborns, infants, and young children, the risk of excessive blood loss with resection is great; the best example of this is choroid plexus carcinoma. Infants have small blood volumes; transfusing multiple blood volumes can lead to coagulopathy and electrolyte imbalance. Therefore, these patients may be best served by first treating the tumor with chemotherapy (i.e., neoadjuvant chemotherapy) before pursuing resection. Tumors will often shrink and become cystic and the reduction in vascularity is notable, resulting in safer and more complete tumor removal (Iwama et al. 2015; Van Poppel et al. 2011).

2.2.7 Preparation for Tumor Resection: Family Counseling

One of the most important steps in preparing a pediatric patient for a brain tumor resection is talking with the parents and family about the patient's prognosis, the risks, and the goals of surgery without overwhelming and confusing them with statistics and medical terminology. While there are general risks associated with any craniotomy, such as bleeding and wound infection, it is more important to stress the potential—or even anticipated—neurologic deficits specific to the location and size of the tumor. Neurologic injury may occur as a result of the surgical approach or during extirpation of the mass. Examples include Parinaud's syndrome with a pineoblastoma, posterior fossa syndrome in a young boy with a medulloblastoma, or cranial neuropathies with a cerebellopontine angle ependymoma. It is usually easier for the family to psychologically deal with new postoperative neurologic deficits if they've learned about them before surgery. It is equally important to define the expectations of surgery, such as total resection, subtotal resection, or biopsy, as well as the potential need for further surgical procedures (e.g., ventriculoperitoneal shunt, feeding tube),

therapies (e.g., physical, speech), and expected length of hospital stay.

2.2.8 Preparation for Tumor Resection: Teamwork

Orchestrating a successful surgery requires the integration of multiple individuals and services, including anesthesiology, operating room nurses and technologists, and neuroradiology for intraoperative MRI cases. It is important to have a preoperative "huddle" with all team members to discuss positioning, need for vascular access, estimated length of surgery, anticipated blood loss, specific blood pressure management, need for any intraoperative neuromonitoring, and airway management (i.e., whether the patient will be extubated or remain intubated after surgery). One way to set a preoperative threshold for blood transfusion is to define the maximal allowable blood loss. Maximal allowable blood loss is the estimated blood volume of the patient multiplied by the difference between the patient's starting and minimal allowable hematocrits, divided by the starting hematocrit. For example, a 5 kg infant with an estimated blood volume of 75 cc/kg, a starting hematocrit of 30, and a minimal acceptable hematocrit of 22 would have a maximal allowable blood loss of approximately 100 cc. If further bleeding is anticipated, transfusion of blood should be initiated.

2.3 Tumor Resection

In this section we will discuss surgical management and approaches to the more common locations and types of pediatric brain tumors, such as the pineal region/posterior third ventricle, posterior fossa, and suprasellar area. Each child's brain tumor is unique; in many respects, its surgical management should be as well. Much of what can be done by the neurosurgeon depends on the age of the child, the type of tumor, its location and therefore the risks associated with resection, and whether or not there are local or distant metastases. For many nonmetastatic childhood intracranial neoplasms, the goal of initial surgery is complete resection (i.e., gross total resection (GTR)), defined as no conclusive evidence of residual tumor on the intra- or immediate postoperative MRI, when deemed feasible. Such philosophy applies to tumors like medulloblastoma, ependymoma (infra- and supratentorial), primitive neuroectodermal tumor (PNET), and virtually all low-grade tumors.

Intraoperative magnetic resonance imaging (iMRI) has revolutionized surgical management of pediatric brain tumors by allowing the surgeon to confirm a gross total resection, while the patient is still under general anesthesia and their wound is open (Choudhri et al. 2014a, 2015b). This high-dollar technology greatly reduces the risk of having to take the child back to the operating room for continued resection, but with the drawbacks of added operating room (OR) time, challenges in interpreting the intraoperative images, and significant new safety issues (Shah et al. 2012). It also requires close cooperation and communication with the anesthesiology team, MR technologist, OR safety officer, and neuroradiologist.

2.3.1 Posterior Fossa (Excluding Brainstem Tumors)

The posterior fossa, as mentioned previously, is a common site for pediatric tumors. The "big 3" tumors are medulloblastoma, ependymoma, and pilocytic astrocytoma. Each has their own unique imaging features. Medulloblastomas and ependymomas are typically found within the 4th ventricle, whereas pilocytic astrocytomas are most often located within the cerebellum (i.e., the vermis or hemispheres). Medulloblastomas are hypercellular and therefore appear hyperdense on the initial CT. Pilocytic astrocytomas often have a cystic component with enhancing nodule(s). Ependymomas classically project through the foramen Luschka into the cerebellopontine angle, or through the foramen magnum into the cervical spinal canal (i.e., "plastic ependymoma"). Midline or fourth ventricular tumors are approached via a standard midline

suboccipital craniotomy, whereas hemispheric tumors require a lateral suboccipital approach. Although we have seen the dawn of a new era in which tumors are being classified at the molecular level, resulting in subclassification and novel "targeted" chemotherapeutic options, the surgical goal of these tumors remains maximal safe resection (Gajjar et al. 2014).

2.3.2 Brainstem Tumors

Brainstem tumors can be broadly categorized as being radiographically focal or diffuse/infiltrative (Green and Kieran 2015). The classic example of an infiltrative pediatric brainstem tumor is a diffuse intrinsic pontine glioma (DIPG). Children with these tumors are typically young and present with a combination of long-tract and cranial nerve findings. DIPG is a radiographic diagnosis, surgery is relegated to the management of hydrocephalus, and the only known treatment that has some effect, albeit temporary, is radiation (Bredlau and Korones 2014). For pontine tumors that are "atypical" in appearance, a biopsy is warranted. Focal tumors are more often low-grade, and most commonly are pilocytic astrocytomas. All focal tumors (with the exception of tectal gliomas), whether benign or malignant, should be considered for resection (Klimo et al. 2013, 2015a). Tectal gliomas have a well-known indolent biologic behavior, and like DIPG, surgery is limited to the treatment of hydrocephalus. Resection of focal brainstem tumors requires careful planning, high-quality preoperative imaging (including tractography), and detailed discussions with the parents on what neurologic deficits to expect.

2.3.3 Pineal Region/Posterior Third Ventricle

There is a wide variety of tumors that may arise in this region of the brain; examples include pineoblastoma and germ cell tumors (Fig. 2.4). Because these patients often present with obstructive hydrocephalus secondary to occlusion of the

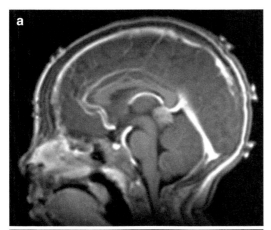

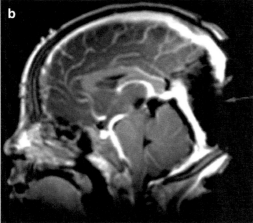

Fig. 2.4 Sagittal T1W + C image in a 2.5-year-old girl with a history of bilateral retinoblastoma shows an enhancing pineal mass (red arrowhead), consistent with a "tri-lateral" retinoblastoma (**a**). Sagittal T1W + C image from an iMRI scan shows successful resection of the tumor (*red arrowhead*). Note the open craniotomy (*red arrow*), which would have facilitated further resection, if needed (**b**)

aqueduct of Sylvius, surgical management is most often directed at treating the hydrocephalus by way of an endoscopic third ventriculostomy, obtaining cerebrospinal fluid (CSF) for germ cell markers (i.e., beta human chorionic gonadotropin, alfa fetoprotein), and angling the endoscope posteriorly to obtain tissue for biopsy. If the germ cell markers are elevated, then by definition the child has a non-germinomatous germ cell tumor (e.g., choriocarcinoma, endodermal sinus tumor) and initial treatment is chemotherapy. If the germ cell markers are negative and the biopsy is consistent with a germinoma, then the child is

treated with radiation with or without chemotherapy with a very high chance of cure, even with metastatic disease. A nondiagnostic biopsy with negative CSF markers usually requires an open biopsy. The three surgical approaches that we use to resect or biopsy tumors in the pineal region/posterior third ventricle are the supracerebellar-infratentorial, the occipital-transtentorial, and the posterior transcallosal (Kennedy and Bruce 2011).

2.3.4 Sellar/Suprasellar

The two most common suprasellar tumors in children are craniopharyngiomas and optic pathway-hypothalamic astrocytomas. Children who present with diabetes insipidus (DI) and an enhancing mass along the pituitary stalk or hypothalamic region typically have one of two pathologies: germinoma or eosinophilic granuloma (histiocytosis X). It is exceedingly rare for optic pathway-hypothalamic astrocytomas or craniopharyngiomas to present with DI. Pure sellar lesions are rare, but may include craniopharyngioma, micro- or macroadenomas (functioning or non-functioning) in older children, and the non-neoplastic Rathke's cleft cyst.

Controversy continues among neurosurgeons as to the role of surgery with craniopharyngiomas. There are those who feel that craniopharyngiomas should be maximally resected without adjuvant therapy (Elliott et al. 2010); others believe in a less aggressive surgical approach in order to avoid significant morbidity (i.e., neurologic, endocrine, or cognitive dysfunction) followed by radiotherapy (Klimo et al. 2015b). We generally ascribe to the latter philosophy. Purely cystic craniopharyngiomas can be treated with placement of an Ommaya catheter to aspirate the tumor cyst, followed by radiotherapy or the injection of intracystic chemotherapy (e.g., bleomycin), immunotherapy (e.g., interferon), or radioactive agents (e.g., P-32) (Cavalheiro et al. 2010; Mottolese et al. 2001; Zhao et al. 2010). Surgical approaches for craniopharyngiomas are dictated by the location of the tumor (Fig. 2.5) and include subfrontal, transsylvian, and anterior

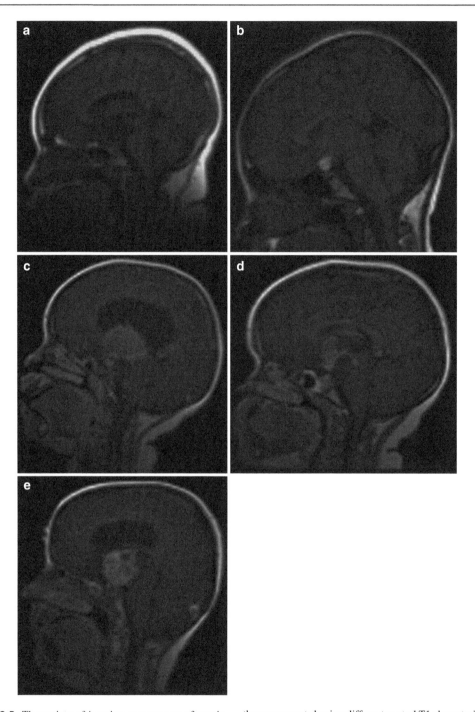

Fig. 2.5 The variety of imaging appearances of cranio-pharyngioma. This variety underscores the need for patient-specific surgical and treatment plans. Sagittal T1W image shows a cystic suprasellar lesion (**a**). Sagittal T1W image shows a suprasellar cystic lesion with intrinsic T1 hyperintense signal, representing proteinaceous secretions (**b**). Sagittal T1W image post contrast shows a multicystic suprasellar lesion with enhancing rims, with the components having different central T1 characteristics related to different proteinaceous contents (**c**). There is also caudal retroclival extension. Sagittal T1W image post contrast shows a central solid enhancing component with multiple smaller cystic components (**d**). Sagittal T1W image post contrast shows a large central solid enhancing component, with several internal cystic areas and a single posteriorly directed cyst within the third ventricle (**e**)

transcallosal approaches. Intrasellar craniopharyngiomas can be resected through a transnasal-transsphenoidal route, using a microscope or endoscope (Jane et al. 2010).

Optic pathway-hypothalamic tumors are generally not thought to be curable by surgery alone, except in the rare case of a prechiasmatic optic nerve glioma with no functional vision. These tumors originate from non-resectable areas of the brain and can often be diagnosed by imaging alone. They are associated with neurofibromatosis type I (i.e., von Recklinghausen disease). Surgery is reserved for biopsy or subtotal resection in those cases where there is significant symptomatic mass effect or where the tumor has caused obstructive hydrocephalus by growing cephalad into the third ventricle (Goodden et al. 2014). The primary treatment modalities for these tumors are chemotherapy and/or radiotherapy. The same approaches used for craniopharyngioma can be used for this tumor, with the exception of the transnasal approach.

2.3.5 Supratentorial

The goal of surgery for most supratentorial tumors should be maximal resection. Extraaxial tumors, such as meningiomas, are rare in children. As previously discussed, functional imaging modalities should be used in cases where the tumor is in close proximity to eloquent areas (Fig. 2.2). Awake craniotomy is difficult to perform in a child, so we rely heavily on these preoperative mapping tests. For a child whose tumor cannot be completely resected but who has debilitating seizures as a result of it, surgery to resect the epileptogenic part of the tumor (e.g., temporal lobectomy) can have a substantial positive impact on the quality of that child's life.

2.4 Postoperative Care

After tumor resection, patients are brought to the intensive care unit (ICU) for close neurologic and cardiorespiratory monitoring. Almost all patients are extubated while still deeply sedated in the OR so as to avoid any coughing or bucking as they awaken with the endotracheal tube in place and during transport to the ICU. Such reflexes can rapidly increase the patient's systemic blood pressure and intracranial venous pressure, which could lead to hemorrhage within the fresh resection cavity, especially if there is a raw, residual tumor surface. For excessively long cases or those with high volume fluid resuscitation, extubation may be delayed until neurologic and cardiopulmonary systems are assessed and stabilized.

The most common immediate postoperative issues that require close monitoring are intracranial hemorrhage, seizure, hydrocephalus, and endocrinologic derangements. Strict blood pressure control is paramount since postoperative hypertension can result in hemorrhage within the resection cavity (Basali et al. 2000). Prompt and adequate treatment for pain and agitation often improves the patient's blood pressure. A maximum allowable systolic blood pressure is typically set for the first 24–48 h after surgery, followed by gradual relaxation of the parameter. The blood pressure limit is age dependent, but an oft-recommended limit is less than 140 mmHg. We consider a nicardipine drip an easy and effective method of titrating the patient's blood pressure. Hypotension is to be avoided, particularly in cases in which there was significant brainstem or spinal cord compression by the tumor, or if there was manipulation/dissection of major arteries so as to maintain adequate tissue perfusion. Patients should be kept euvolemic to mildly hypervolemic.

As discussed previously, obstructive hydrocephalus is a common presenting condition in children with brain tumors. Our general approach to such children is to resect the tumor in order to relieve the hydrocephalus, which we are successful in achieving in many cases. Mechanisms of post-resection hydrocephalus include obstruction from residual tumor and subarachnoid block caused by leptomeningeal metastasis, operative blood products, or proteinaceous CSF. All patients with preoperative hydrocephalus, or who are at risk of developing hydrocephalus postoperatively (e.g., intraventricular tumor), need to be carefully monitored for persistent or new hydrocephalus, respectively. Such evidence would include increase in ventricular size, inability to wean an external ventricular drain (EVD), development of a new or growing subdural hygroma or pseudomeningocele, and clinical changes, such as irritability, headaches, emesis, full fontanelle, or depressed level of arousal. Postoperative hydrocephalus is treated with either an EVD, a shunt, or ETV.

The Canadian Preoperative Prediction Rule for Hydrocephalus (CPPRH) was devised in an attempt to identify patients before resection who are at risk for post-resection hydrocephalus (Riva-Cambrin et al. 2009). Variables predictive of post-resection hydrocephalus include age less than 2 (score of 3), papilledema (score of 1), moderate to severe hydrocephalus (score of 2), cerebral metastasis (score of 3), and specific estimated tumor pathologies (score of 1). A total score of ≥5 places the patient at high risk. Estimated preoperative tumor pathologies based on imaging and clinical information that qualify for a score of 1 include medulloblastoma, ependymoma, and dorsally exophytic brainstem glioma. The modified CPPRH also adds the presence of transependymal edema as a risk factor (Foreman et al. 2013). For children with favorable age (>2 years), pathology (e.g., tectal glioma, pineal tumors), anatomy, and site of CSF blockage (obstruction between the third ventricle and the interpeduncular cistern), ETV is preferred over shunting as shunts are generally viewed as life-long implants that come with high risk of one or more shunt malfunction(s) (Gupta et al. 2007; Vogel et al. 2013). In cases where ETV is not appropriate or if the ETV fails, then ventricular shunting is the sole option.

If the patient has a postoperative seizure and is not already on an AED, then electrolytes and blood glucose should be checked expeditiously and any abnormalities should be promptly corrected, especially low sodium and magnesium; a non-contrast CT scan of the head should be obtained to rule out any new hemorrhage, edema, or hydrocephalus and the patient should be given a bolus of an AED, such as phosphenytoin or levetiracetam (both ~ 20 mg/kg), followed by maintenance therapy. If the patient's seizure lasts more than 5 min or if multiple seizures occur without full neurologic recovery in the interictal period, then the patient is considered to be in status epilepticus, which is a medical emergency (Claassen et al. 2015).

Removal of sellar and suprasellar tumors, such as optic pathway gliomas or craniopharyngiomas, may lead to transient or permanent disruption of the hypothalamic-pituitary axis, and subsequent anterior and posterior pituitary lobe dysfunction. The endocrinopathies that are most problematic for neurosurgeons are the ones that can cause dramatic changes in the serum sodium level: central diabetes insipidus (DI), cerebral salt wasting (CSW), or the syndrome of inappropriate antidiuretic hormone release (SIADH). Central DI is caused by inadequate antidiuretic hormone release and results in excessive production of dilute urine and resultant hypernatremia. Urine output continuously exceeding 3 cc/kg/h with a specific gravity of 1.005 or less with a concurrent elevation in serum sodium above 145 is diagnostic. Without close monitoring of urine output and sodium levels in patients with or at risk for DI, sodium levels can easily exceed 160 mEq/L, resulting in severe dehydration, mental status changes, and seizures. The treatment is desmopressin and free water replacement titrated to the patient's urine output.

SIADH and CSW both cause hyponatremia. With severe hyponatremia (<125 mEq/L) or rapid drops in sodium, headache, confusion, seizures, and cerebral edema can occur. SIADH results from an abnormal release of antidiuretic hormone (ADH) in the absence of a physiologic osmotic stimulus, resulting in excess water retention. Patients are either hypervolemic from the retained water or sometimes euvolemic. Serum osmolality is low (<275 mOsm/kg of water) while the urine is concentrated (>100 mOsm/kg of water). Cerebral salt wasting also produces hyponatremia and low serum osmolality in the presence of concentrated urine; but unlike SIADH, patients are hypovolemic. Intracranial disease results in failure of the kidneys to conserve sodium by an unknown mechanism. The key difference is the treatment. Fluid restriction effectively corrects the hyponatremia caused by SIADH while volume replacement with gentle sodium support treats CSW. In the setting of a malignancy, SIADH is more common. Cerebral salt wasting will also respond to a fluid challenge. Regardless of the etiology, if the hyponatremia is severe (Na < 125 mEq/L) or symptomatic (i.e., confusion, seizures or coma), then correction with hypertonic (e.g., 3%) saline is indicated. However, care must be taken not to correct the sodium too quickly. In general, if the sodium level changed rapidly then the patient can tolerate rapid correction. The serum sodium must be checked every 2–6 h. The goal is to correct the serum sodium 1–2 mEq/L/h and limit the correction to 8–10 mEq/L in 24 h. If the sodium is corrected too quickly, central pontine myelinolysis can rarely occur. Conversely, rapid correction of hypernatremia can cause or exacerbate cerebral edema.

Given the high frequency of posterior fossa tumors, posterior fossa syndrome (PFS) deserves special mention. It is a syndrome consisting of mutism, oromotor and oculomotor apraxia, emotional lability, axial hypotonia, and cerebellar/brainstem dysfunction following resection of infratentorial tumors (Robertson et al. 2006). Risk factors include young age, male sex, large midline tumors, brainstem invasion, and medulloblastoma. It is thought to result from bilateral surgical damage to the proximal efferent cerebellar pathways (Patay 2015). Most patients wake-up from surgery with intact speech but develop mutism within 1–4 days after surgery. Most recover fluent speech within 4 months with average duration of 6 weeks. Recovery begins with clumsy and broken speech slowly progressing to full sentences. However, up to one-third of children will have lasting dysarthria after surgery. Irritability, inconsolable crying, impulsiveness, and disinhibition are the most frequent changes in affect. IQ and school performance are also affected, more commonly when the deep cerebellar nuclei are damaged. Treatment generally requires prolonged rehabilitation, including physical, occupational, and speech therapy. Overall, improvement is universal but the degree of recovery is variable. Mutism and emotional lability are generally transient but long-term cognitive and motor deficits are frequently recognized in these children.

References

Anon (1991) The epidemiology of headache among children with brain tumor. Headache in children with brain tumors. The Childhood Brain Tumor Consortium. J Neuro-Oncol 10(1):31–46

Baloh RW, Furman JM, Yee RD (1985) Dorsal midbrain syndrome: clinical and oculographic findings. Neurology 35(1):54–60

Basali A, Mascha EJ, Kalfas I, Schubert A (2000) Relation between perioperative hypertension and intracranial hemorrhage after craniotomy. Anesthesiology 93(1):48–54

Bredlau AL, Korones DN (2014) Diffuse intrinsic pontine gliomas: treatments and controversies. Adv Cancer Res 121:235–259. https://doi.org/10.1016/B978-0-12-800249-0.00006-8

Cavalheiro S, Di Rocco C, Valenzuela S, Dastoli PA, Tamburrini G, Massimi L, Nicacio JM, Faquini IV, Ierardi DF, Silva NS, Pettorini BL, Toledo SR (2010) Craniopharyngiomas: intratumoral chemotherapy with interferon-alpha: a multicenter preliminary study with 60 cases. Neurosurg Focus 28(4):E12. https://doi.org/10.3171/2010.1.FOCUS09310

Choudhri AF, Klimo P Jr, Auschwitz TS, Whitehead MT, Boop FA (2014a) 3T intraoperative MRI for management of pediatric CNS neoplasms. AJNR Am J Neuroradiol 35(12):2382–2387. https://doi.org/10.3174/ajnr.A4040

Choudhri AF, Chin EM, Blitz AM, Gandhi D (2014b) Diffusion tensor imaging of cerebral white matter: technique, anatomy, and pathologic patterns. Radiol Clin North Am 52(2):413–425. https://doi.org/10.1016/j.rcl.2013.11.005

Choudhri AF, Whitehead MT, Siddiqui A, Klimo P Jr, Boop FA (2015a) Diffusion characteristics of pediatric pineal tumors. Neuroradiol J 28(2):209–216. https://doi.org/10.1177/1971400915581741

Choudhri AF, Siddiqui A, Klimo P Jr, Boop FA (2015b) Intraoperative MRI in pediatric brain tumors. Pediatr Radiol 45(Suppl 3):397–405. https://doi.org/10.1007/s00247-015-3322-z

Choudhri AF, Patel RM, Siddiqui A, Whitehead MT, Wheless JW (2015c) Cortical activation through passive-motion functional MRI. AJNR Am J Neuroradiol 36(9):1675–1681. https://doi.org/10.3174/ajnr.A4345

Claassen J, Riviello JJ Jr, Silbergleit R (2015) Emergency neurological life support: status epilepticus. Neurocrit Care 23(Suppl 2):136–142. https://doi.org/10.1007/s12028-015-0172-3

El-Gaidi MA, El-Nasr AH, Eissa EM (2015) Infratentorial complications following preresection CSF diversion in children with posterior fossa tumors. J Neurosurg Pediatr 15(1):4–11. https://doi.org/10.3171/2014.8.PEDS14146

Elliott RE, Hsieh K, Hochm T, Belitskaya-Levy I, Wisoff J, Wisoff JH (2010) Efficacy and safety of radical resection of primary and recurrent craniopharyngiomas in 86 children. J Neurosurg Pediatr 5(1):30–48. https://doi.org/10.3171/2009.7.PEDS09215

Foreman P, McClugage S 3rd, Naftel R, Griessenauer CJ, Ditty BJ, Agee BS, Riva-Cambrin J, Wellons J 3rd (2013) Validation and modification of a predictive model of postresection hydrocephalus in pediatric patients with posterior fossa tumors. J Neurosurg Pediatr 12(3):220–226. https://doi.org/10.3171/2013.5.PEDS1371

Gajjar A, Pfister SM, Taylor MD, Gilbertson RJ (2014) Molecular insights into pediatric brain tumors have the potential to transform therapy. Clin Cancer Res 20(22):5630–5640. https://doi.org/10.1158/1078-0432.CCR-14-0833

Goodden J, Pizer B, Pettorini B, Williams D, Blair J, Didi M, Thorp N, Mallucci C (2014) The role of surgery in optic pathway/hypothalamic gliomas in children. J Neurosurg Pediatr 13(1):1–12. https://doi.org/10.3171/2013.8.PEDS12546

Green AL, Kieran MW (2015) Pediatric brainstem gliomas: new understanding leads to potential new treatments for two very different tumors. Curr Oncol Rep 17(3):436. https://doi.org/10.1007/s11912-014-0436-7

Guerrini R, Rosati A, Giordano F, Genitori L, Barba C (2013) The medical and surgical treatment of tumoral seizures: current and future perspectives. Epilepsia 54(Suppl 9):84–90. https://doi.org/10.1111/epi.12450

Gupta N, Park J, Solomon C, Kranz DA, Wrensch M, Wu YW (2007) Long-term outcomes in patients with treated childhood hydrocephalus. J Neurosurg 106(5 Suppl):334–339. https://doi.org/10.3171/ped.2007.106.5.334

Hardesty DA, Sanborn MR, Parker WE, Storm PB (2011) Perioperative seizure incidence and risk factors in 223 pediatric brain tumor patients without prior seizures. J Neurosurg Pediatr 7(6):609–615. https://doi.org/10.3171/2011.3.PEDS1120

Hirtz D, Ashwal S, Berg A, Bettis D, Camfield C, Camfield P, Crumrine P, Elterman R, Schneider S, Shinnar S (2000) Practice parameter: evaluating a first nonfebrile seizure in children: report of the quality standards subcommittee of the American Academy of Neurology, The Child Neurology Society, and The American Epilepsy Society. Neurology 55(5):616–623

Iwama J, Ogiwara H, Kiyotani C, Terashima K, Matsuoka K, Iwafuchi H, Morota N (2015) Neoadjuvant chemotherapy for brain tumors in infants and young children. J Neurosurg Pediatr 15(5):488–492. https://doi.org/10.3171/2014.11.PEDS14334

Jane JA Jr, Prevedello DM, Alden TD, Laws ER Jr (2010) The transsphenoidal resection of pediatric craniopharyngiomas: a case series. J Neurosurg Pediatr 5(1):49–60. https://doi.org/10.3171/2009.7.PEDS09252

Kennedy BC, Bruce JN (2011) Surgical approaches to the pineal region. Neurosurg Clin N Am 22(3):367–380., viii. https://doi.org/10.1016/j.nec.2011.05.007

Klimo P Jr, Pai Panandiker AS, Thompson CJ, Boop FA, Qaddoumi I, Gajjar A, Armstrong GT, Ellison DW, Kun LE, Ogg RJ, Sanford RA (2013) Management and outcome of focal low-grade brainstem tumors in pediatric patients: the St. Jude experience. J Neurosurg Pediatr 11(3):274–281. https://doi.org/10.3171/2012.11.PEDS12317

Klimo P Jr, Nesvick CL, Broniscer A, Orr BA, Choudhri AF (2015a) Malignant brainstem tumors in children, excluding diffuse intrinsic pontine gliomas. J Neurosurg Pediatr 17:1–9. https://doi.org/10.3171/2015.6.PEDS15166

Klimo P Jr, Venable GT, Boop FA, Merchant TE (2015b) Recurrent craniopharyngioma after conformal radiation in children and the burden of treatment. J Neurosurg Pediatr 15(5):499–505. https://doi.org/10.3171/2014.10.PEDS14384

Lin CT, Riva-Cambrin JK (2015) Management of posterior fossa tumors and hydrocephalus in children: a review. Childs Nerv Syst 31(10):1781–1789. https://doi.org/10.1007/s00381-015-2781-8

Mottolese C, Stan H, Hermier M, Berlier P, Convert J, Frappaz D, Lapras C (2001) Intracystic chemotherapy with bleomycin in the treatment of craniopharyngiomas. Childs Nerv Syst 17(12):724–730. https://doi.org/10.1007/s00381-001-0524-5

Osborn AG, Heaston DK, Wing SD (1978) Diagnosis of ascending transtentorial herniation by cranial computed tomography. AJR Am J Roentgenol 130(4):755–760. https://doi.org/10.2214/ajr.130.4.755

Ostrom QT, Gittleman H, Liao P, Rouse C, Chen Y, Dowling J, Wolinsky Y, Kruchko C, Barnholtz-Sloan J (2014) CBTRUS statistical report: primary brain and central nervous system tumors diagnosed in the United States in 2007–2011. Neuro-Oncology 16(Suppl 4):iv1–i63. https://doi.org/10.1093/neuonc/nou223

Ostrom QT, de Blank PM, Kruchko C, Petersen CM, Liao P, Finlay JL, Stearns DS, Wolff JE, Wolinsky Y, Letterio JJ, Barnholtz-Sloan JS (2015) Alex's lemonade stand foundation infant and childhood primary brain and central nervous system tumors diagnosed in the United States in 2007–2011. Neuro-Oncology 16(Suppl 10):x1–x36. https://doi.org/10.1093/neuonc/nou327

Ottenhausen M, Krieg SM, Meyer B, Ringel F (2015) Functional preoperative and intraoperative mapping and monitoring: increasing safety and efficacy in glioma surgery. Neurosurg Focus 38(1):E3. https://doi.org/10.3171/2014.10.FOCUS14611

Patay Z (2015) Postoperative posterior fossa syndrome: unraveling the etiology and underlying pathophysiology by using magnetic resonance imaging. Childs Nerv Syst 31(10):1853–1858. https://doi.org/10.1007/s00381-015-2796-1

Pittman T, Williams D, Weber TR, Steinhardt G, Tracy T Jr (1992) The risk of abdominal operations in children with ventriculoperitoneal shunts. J Pediatr Surg 27(8):1051–1053

Riva-Cambrin J, Detsky AS, Lamberti-Pasculli M, Sargent MA, Armstrong D, Moineddin R, Cochrane DD, Drake JM (2009) Predicting postresection hydrocephalus in pediatric patients with posterior fossa tumors. J Neurosurg Pediatr 3(5):378–385. https://doi.org/10.3171/2009.1.PEDS08298

Robertson PL, Muraszko KM, Holmes EJ, Sposto R, Packer RJ, Gajjar A, Dias MS, Allen JC, Children's Oncology G (2006) Incidence and severity of postoperative cerebellar mutism syndrome in children with medulloblastoma: a prospective study by the Children's Oncology Group. J Neurosurg 105(6 Suppl):444–451. https://doi.org/10.3171/ped.2006.105.6.444

Sainte-Rose C, Cinalli G, Roux FE, Maixner R, Chumas PD, Mansour M, Carpentier A, Bourgeois M, Zerah M, Pierre-Kahn A, Renier D (2001) Management of hydrocephalus in pediatric patients with posterior fossa tumors: the role of endoscopic third ventriculostomy. J Neurosurg 95(5):791–797. https://doi.org/10.3171/jns.2001.95.5.0791

Shah MN, Leonard JR, Inder G, Gao F, Geske M, Haydon DH, Omodon ME, Evans J, Morales D, Dacey RG, Smyth MD, Chicoine MR, Limbrick DD (2012) Intraoperative magnetic resonance imaging to reduce the rate of early reoperation for lesion resection in pediatric neurosurgery. J Neurosurg Pediatr 9(3):259–264. https://doi.org/10.3171/2011.12.PEDS11227

Van Poppel M, Klimo P Jr, Dewire M, Sanford RA, Boop F, Broniscer A, Wright K, Gajjar AJ (2011) Resection of infantile brain tumors after neoadjuvant chemotherapy: the St. Jude experience. J Neurosurg Pediatr 8(3):251–256. https://doi.org/10.3171/2011.6.PEDS11158

Vogel TW, Bahuleyan B, Robinson S, Cohen AR (2013) The role of endoscopic third ventriculostomy in the treatment of hydrocephalus. J Neurosurg Pediatr 12(1):54–61. https://doi.org/10.3171/2013.4.PEDS12481

Wilne SH, Ferris RC, Nathwani A, Kennedy CR (2006) The presenting features of brain tumours: a review of 200 cases. Arch Dis Child 91(6):502–506. https://doi.org/10.1136/adc.2005.090266

Zachenhofer I, Donat M, Oberndorfer S, Roessler K (2011) Perioperative levetiracetam for prevention of seizures in supratentorial brain tumor surgery. J Neuro-Oncol 101(1):101–106. https://doi.org/10.1007/s11060-010-0235-4

Zafeiriou DI, Koliouskas D, Vargiami E, Gombakis N (2001) Russell's diencephalic syndrome. Neurology 57(5):932

Zhao R, Deng J, Liang X, Zeng J, Chen X, Wang J (2010) Treatment of cystic craniopharyngioma with phosphorus-32 intracavitary irradiation. Childs Nerv Syst 26(5):669–674. https://doi.org/10.1007/s00381-009-1025-1

Principles of Radiation Oncology

3

Shannon M. MacDonald, Ranjit S. Bindra,
Roshan Sethi, and Matthew Ladra

3.1 Introduction

Radiation therapy plays an important role in the management of pediatric brain tumors. Despite advances in the fields of pediatric and medical oncology and neurosurgery, radiation is still a necessary treatment for local control and cure for most central nervous system (CNS) malignancies. Brain tumors, a heterogeneous group of diseases, together represent the most common disease site encountered by radiation oncologists. The eloquent areas from which these tumors arise makes the balance between the risks of life-altering side effects of radiation and the likelihood of local control and/or cure a difficult one to strike. While often we consider the main goal of our treatment to be cure, we must keep in mind the additional goal of allowing these children to grow and continue to live meaningful lives without a significant burden of major medical complications resulting from treatment. Technical and biological advances have enabled radiation oncologists to decrease the amount of healthy, uninvolved brain tissue and nearby organs that receive radiation. Trials that combine radiation with chemotherapy have allowed for a decrease in the dose and/or volume of radiation for some pediatric brain tumors. Neurosurgical advances have allowed for avoidance of radiation for selected tumors. In addition, advances in neuroradiology have led to better visualization of tumors and CNS structures. Advances in treatment planning software and the development of new radiation modalities have allowed for improvements in dose delivery.

S. M. MacDonald (✉)
Pediatric Radiation Oncology, Massachusetts General Hospital, Boston, MA, USA

Harvard Medical School, Boston, MA, USA
e-mail: SMACDONALD@mgh.harvard.edu

R. S. Bindra
Therapeutic Radiology and Experimental Pathology,
Yale School of Medicine, New Haven, CT, USA

R. Sethi
Harvard Radiation Oncology Program, Department of Radiation Oncology, Massachusetts General Hospital, Boston, MA, USA

M. Ladra
Radiation Oncology and Molecular Radiation Sciences, Johns Hopkins School of Medicine, Baltimore, MD, USA

3.2 Pediatric Radiation Therapy Delivery

Radiation therapy has evolved greatly in the past three decades. Advances in diagnostic imaging and radiation delivery have led to improved tumor targeting and reduced doses of radiation to critical structures outside of the treatment fields. Historically, radiation planning was performed using X-rays, termed "two-dimensional planning," and large geometric fields delivered treatment with excess doses to areas uninvolved by tumor. The widespread availability of computed tomography

© Springer International Publishing AG, part of Springer Nature 2018
A. Gajjar et al. (eds.), *Brain Tumors in Children*, https://doi.org/10.1007/978-3-319-43205-2_3

(CT) and magnetic resonance imaging (MRI) has allowed for more precise delineation of the "at-risk" tumor or tumor bed and adjacent normal anatomy. Modern "three-dimensional" (3D) planning now includes a planning CT acquired during the radiation simulation, and in most CNS cases, an MRI is fused to the CT for target delineation and treatment planning. Using these imaging modalities, the target area is better visualized and margins for setup error and target uncertainty around the volume can be made smaller, allowing for complete coverage of the target and minimization of doses to uninvolved tissues.

3.2.1 Intensity-Modulated Radiation Therapy

Until the late 1990s, 3D planning utilized single or multiple static beams with set blocks or collimation to shape the treatment fields. The development of more powerful treatment planning software led to the ability to generate more conformal plans with complex photon beam arrangements. Further gains in target volume conformality have come with the advent of intensity-modulated radiation therapy (IMRT), which uses dynamic collimation during treatment to deliver multiple small beamlets of photon radiation of various intensities from multiple angles to shape high dose to the target volume. This sophisticated treatment planning software also allows for the weighting of critical normal structures that create plans with the reduction of moderate to high-dose radiation to adjacent normal structures. The IMRT planning is also more labor intensive for the physician, as it requires the delineation of all desired structures and targets, the specification of desired target dose and of dose and volume limitations for normal structures, and the ultimate prioritization of dose to each. Multiple iterations of the radiation plan are run by the treatment planning software program until the best possible fit to the physician-defined parameters is found. IMRT allows for highly conformal photon plans with the high-dose isodose lines closely surrounding the target volume. This conformality does usually come with a cost, and the increased number of beams utilized to create highly conformal shapes also increases the amount of low-dose radiation delivered compared to 3D plans. Therefore, although the risk of toxicity to nearby structures is lower due to the more rapid fall off of dose, the increase in low-dose radiation may also increase the risk of a radiation-induced malignancy from the greater amount of normal tissue exposed to radiation. Figure 3.1 shows an IMRT plan for a suprasellar region tumor treated with involved-field radiation.

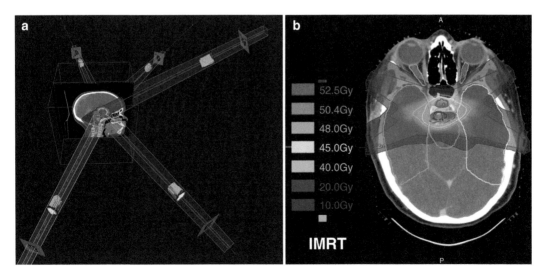

Fig. 3.1 Intensity-modulated radiation therapy (IMRT) plan for a suprasellar tumor. (**a**) shows beams directions and intensity modulation of the beams. (**b**) shows the dosimetry for this plan in the axial plane

3.2.2 Stereotactic Radiosurgery/ Stereotactic Radiation Therapy

Stereotactic radiation uses image guidance and a 3D coordinate system to deliver high doses of radiation to very precise target volumes. Stereotactic Radiosurgery (SRS) refers to the delivery of a single treatment while Stereotactic Radiation Therapy (SRT) refers to multiple fractionated doses of radiation. With SRS, multiple small beams of radiation are focused on the tumor, delivering a very high dose to the target while depositing a low dose to the surrounding tissues. Because these treatments are given in a single or very few doses, a high dose is delivered with each fraction and accurate targeting is critical. Rigid immobilizations and fiducial markers are typically used to account for patient motion and image guidance is used prior to the delivery of each fraction. There are several available systems for photon SRS/SRT delivery. Newer systems have been developed for the delivery of stereotactic proton therapy as well. Within the pediatric population, the extensive immobilization requirements and long treatment often require sedation, even in older children, and may be impractical in certain cases.

3.2.3 Proton Radiation

The use of proton radiation in pediatric CNS malignancies has gained widespread acceptance over the last decade due to the ability to dramatically reduce excess dose deposited outside of the target volume. Currently, there are more than 65 proton centers worldwide, including 27 active centers in the US with several more US centers under construction and many more in development. Compared to photon radiation, which has a higher entrance dose and a longer dose fall off, protons deposit a lower and nearly constant quantity of radiation until the end of the beam range, where the majority of energy is quickly released over a short area called the Bragg Peak, approximately 5–10 mm in length (MacDonald et al. 2006). Thus, the lower entrance dose and abrupt dose fall off allows for CNS tumors to be treated with a reduction of radiation dose delivered to the uninvolved CNS tissue.

To date more than 80,000 patients have received proton therapy. Proton radiation can be delivered using three-dimensional conformal proton radiation (3DCPT), sometimes called double-scattered protons. With 3DCPT, individual proton beams are attenuated to create a modulated beam or Spread Out Bragg Peak (SOBP). The individual beams are shaped by brass apertures to conform to the tumor volume and a Lucite compensator modulates the distal end of the beam. New proton delivery systems have developed a scanning technique, often called pencil beam scanning (PBS) (Trofimov and Bortfeld 2003). PBS uses a small diameter proton beam deflected by magnets in the X and Y-axis to "paint" dose layer by layer over the tumor volume. This technique creates more conformal treatment volumes and reduces the entrance dose and may have greater beam penumbra due to the absence of brass apertures.

Previously, dosimetric studies predominated the proton literature and clinical data was sparse. In recent years, a number of studies have emerged showing comparable disease control and favorable toxicity profiles in a variety of tumor types, including ependymoma, medulloblastoma, and low-grade glioma (Ladra et al. 2014; Greenberger et al. 2014; Fitzek et al. 2006; Childs et al. 2012; Cotter et al. 2011; DeLaney et al. 2005; Gray et al. 2009; Rombi et al. 2012).

3.3 Ependymoma

Ependymoma accounts for 5% of pediatric brain tumors. Approximately two-thirds develop in the fourth ventricle and cerebellopontine angle. The remaining third are found in the supratentorium and spine, the latter often in older patients (Merchant and Fouladi 2005; Phi et al. 2012; CBTRUS 2012). Localized disease is treated with surgical resection followed by postoperative radiotherapy (RT). While some centers have attempted to give chemotherapy to children ≤3 years of age (to delay RT), the relapse rate is unacceptably high and surgery and localized modern RT is the preferred standard in the US. Chemotherapy is used for patients with residual disease after primary resection; this is typically a short course, used prior to performing a second surgery in an attempt to achieve a gross total resection (Merchant and Fouladi 2005; Needle et al. 1997; Shu et al. 2007; Timmermann et al. 2000, 2005; Zacharoulis et al. 2007). The advantage of this treatment modality remains unclear, as discussed further below. In photon series, 5-year progression-free survival (PFS) ranges from 41 to 58%, while 5-year overall survival (OS) ranges from 54 to 71% (Perilongo et al. 1997; Oya et al. 2002; Shu et al. 2007; Jaing et al. 2004; Mansur et al. 2005). Similar results have been reported for patients treated with proton therapy (MacDonald et al. 2008, 2013). In the largest single-institution prospective cohort study, Merchant et al. followed 153 ependymoma patients treated at St. Jude's Children's Hospital. They found a 5-year PFS of 74% and a 5-year OS of 85% in a cohort with a high rate of total resection (Merchant et al. 2009c).

The efficacy of postoperative RT was established by retrospective data cohorts, and confirmed by improved survival in prospective cohorts treated with RT as standard of care (Phi et al. 2012; Perilongo et al. 1997; Merchant 2009; Mansur et al. 2005; Koshy et al. 2011; Schild et al. 1998; Shu et al. 2007; Timmermann et al. 2000; Merchant et al. 2009c). Craniospinal irradiation (CSI) was initially delivered to all patients because of concern for tumor dissemination along the neuroaxis (Merchant 2009). However, because the majority of relapses in ependymoma were found to be local, metastatic disease at diagnosis was rare, and prophylactic spinal doses between 20 and 40 Gy did not improve distant control, the standard of care shifted to treatment of the tumor bed with a margin (Oya et al. 2002; Mansur et al. 2005; Merchant et al. 1997).

For patients with localized disease, the tumor bed and residual tumor are considered the gross tumor volume (GTV). The clinical target volume (CTV) is a 0.5–1 cm extension of the GTV, with expansion limited by bony constraints. The prescribed dose delivered to the CTV varies between 54 and 59.4 Gy, depending on the physician's comfort level, modality, the presence of residual disease after resection, and the age of the patient (lower doses favored for children under 3 years of age). In the large prospective cohort study discussed above, Merchant et al. delivered 59.4 Gy to all patients except those under 18 months who underwent gross total resection; patients in the latter category were treated with 54 Gy (Merchant et al. 2009c). Disseminated ependymoma, defined as the presence of more than one discrete disease site and/or positive cytology in the cerebrospinal fluid (CSF), is typically treated with CSI but outcomes are poor and it is unclear what CSI dose is required for control.

Prognosis depends significantly on the extent of resection (Phi et al. 2012; Perilongo et al. 1997; Koshy et al. 2011; Oya et al. 2002; Merchant et al. 2009c; Timmermann et al. 2005; Shu et al. 2007). Gross total resection, defined as no evidence of disease on postoperative MRI, may provide a significant survival advantage over near-total resection (<5 mm enhancing tumor) and subtotal resection (≥5 mm enhancing tumor). Second-look surgery is often used to optimize local control. Merchant et al., in their 2009 series, referred 43.1% of patients with less than a gross total resection for a second surgery. The major limiting factor for second surgery is concern regarding the level of morbidity, though Morris et al. found that most patients can tolerate the repeat operation (Morris et al. 2009). The majority of ependymomas have Classic (World Health Organization [WHO] Grade II) histology. Anaplastic (WHO Grade III) histology may worsen overall survival, though many series (most with small numbers of patients) have not found a statistically significant difference (Phi et al. 2012; Koshy et al. 2011; Oya et al. 2002; Merchant et al. 2009c; Shu et al. 2007; Schild et al. 1998; Mansur et al. 2005; Goldwein et al. 1990). Currently, ependymomas are not treated differently according to histology, though this approach may be refined with molecular techniques that identify genetic predispositions to relapse.

The most frequently used chemotherapy regimen is vincristine, carboplatin, cyclophosphamide, and etoposide. The value of this modality in the treatment of ependymoma is unclear (Merchant and Fouladi 2005; Zacharoulis et al. 2007; Timmermann et al. 2000, 2005; Needle et al. 1997). It has been frequently used as a tool to delay RT in patients under the age of 3 years. The cognitive effect of RT to the brain appears most potent in this age group. However, this approach has no proven benefit, and remains controversial (Merchant et al. 2009c; Timmermann et al. 2005; Zacharoulis et al. 2007; Koshy et al. 2011). It is also used to shrink disease after subtotal resections, an approach tested by the Children's Oncology Group (COG) protocol ACNS 0121. Although clinical response is often observed, this treatment strategy does not, at this point, appear to prolong survival. In addition, the use of chemotherapy often delays time to RT, the critical modality in the treatment of ependymoma (Shu et al. 2007). ACNS0831, a COG Phase III trial, studies the use of chemotherapy after surgery and radiation in patients who undergo a total or near total resection. It continues to accrue patients, and results are not currently available.

Focal radiotherapy to the developing brain is associated with several toxicities, including growth hormone deficiency (directly proportional to dose to the hypothalamus), central hypothyroidism, and hearing loss (rare, but more common when tumor extension into the foramina of Luschka brings high dose close to the cochlea) (Hancock et al. 1995; Merchant et al. 2002a, 2004a; Rappaport and Brauner 1989). Many of these toxicities are potentiated by the administration of chemotherapy. Cognitive function appears relatively stable with conformal photon therapy (Di Pinto et al. 2010; Conklin et al. 2008; Merchant et al. 2004b). Proton RT, by sparing more healthy brain tissue, may decrease the risk of these toxicities, though that has not been demonstrated in a prospective setting (MacDonald et al. 2008, 2013). Figure 3.2 shows a proton plan for a posterior fossa ependymoma.

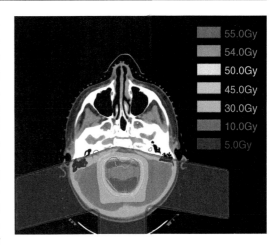

Fig. 3.2 3D conformal proton plan for a posterior fossa ependymoma demonstrating near complete sparing of the cochlea

3.4 Germ Cell Tumors

Germ cell tumors (GCTs) grow from embryonic remnants, and occur at their highest incidence at the time of puberty (Villano et al. 2008). While these tumors are rare, they are more likely to occur in males and, for still unclear reasons, among patients born in Japan. In the brain, primary GCTs develop primarily in the pineal and suprasellar regions; they obey the midline predilection of all GCTs, which also occur in the mediastinum, the spine, and the gonads. There are multiple subtypes, but the major histological distinction is between pure germinoma and non-germinomatous germ cell tumors. The latter category encompasses multiple histologies, including embryonal carcinoma, endodermal sinus tumor (also known as yolk sac), choriocarcinoma, and teratoma. Teratomas may be further divided into mature, immature, and teratoma with malignant transformation. Finally, there are "mixed" GCTs, which contain germinomatous and non-germinomatous components (Dearnaley et al. 1990; Jennings et al. 1985; Matsutani et al. 1987, 1997, 1998; Modak et al. 2004; Robertson et al. 1997; Smith et al. 2004). Non-germinomatous elements generally secrete alpha-fetoprotein (AFP) and human chorionic gonadotropin (HCG) into both the CSF and the serum; the concentration of these markers may correlate with tumor aggression, though this has not been definitively demonstrated (Baranzelli et al. 1999; Chang et al. 1995). Pure germinomas, by definition, are associated with normal-range AFP, though they may secrete HCG up to approximately 100 IU/dL (this definition varies).

Although primary surgical resection is not a component of treatment, neuro-endoscopic biopsy is critical if markers are not elevated, given that histology drives treatment and correlates specifically to prognosis. In 1997, Matsutani et al. classified CNS GCTs according to prognosis as "Good" (germinoma, mature teratoma, HCG-secreting germinoma), "Intermediate" (mixed teratoma or immature teratoma), or "Poor" (choriocarcinoma, yolk sac tumor, embryonal carcinoma and teratoma with malignant elements) (Matsutani et al. 1997). Overall survival at 3 years varied between 9.3 and 94.1% according to these prognostic groups, though a variety of treatment methods (including the omission of radiation therapy) were used. Resection was performed in this series. In the US, it is rare to perform more than a biopsy at diagnosis as the preference is to avoid surgical morbidity associated with resection of the pineal or suprasellar region.

3.4.1 Pure Germinoma

Pure CNS germinomas are considered highly curable. RT alone is associated with 10-year OS greater than 90% in most series (Rogers et al. 2005; MacDonald et al. 2011; Matsutani et al. 1997). The standard of care for germinomas, like for ependymomas, was formerly relatively high-dose CSI followed by a boost to the tumor site. Rogers et al., in a review of 20 studies, found that the rate of isolated spinal relapse was similar among patients treated with CSI versus a smaller field, generally whole brain RT (WBRT) or whole ventricle RT (WVRT). While there remains no clear consensus, most centers now treat localized disease with WVRT followed by a boost to the involved-field. For select cases with basal ganglia primary or involvement, whole brain RT may be favored (Shirato et al. 1997). Most centers deliver chemotherapy prior to RT, as discussed below.

WVRT encompasses the third and fourth ventricles, the lateral ventricles +/− the prepontine cistern, and is considered a CTV. Figure 3.3 shows the whole ventricle volume. The GTV for primary disease is defined as the pre-chemotherapy volume. The CTV is a 1–1.5 cm margin around the GTV and this CTV should be planned

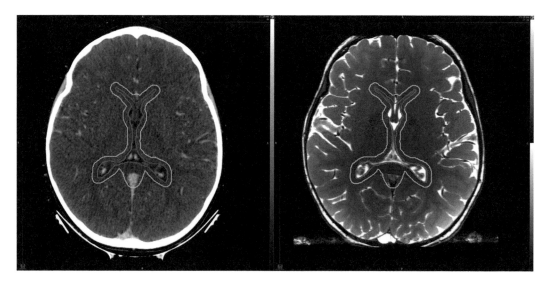

Fig. 3.3 Whole ventricular volume at the level of the lateral ventricles in the axial plane. Clinical target volume (CTV) shown in magenta. Planning target volume (PTV) shown in cyan

up-front to ensure that it is included in the whole ventricular CTV. Doses vary widely, but the COG protocol ACNS 0232 defined standard of care as 24 Gy WVRT followed by a 21 Gy boost to the involved-field. If the patient received chemotherapy (which is increasingly common, as mentioned below), the WVRT dose is 24 Gy (or 18 Gy on COG protocol ACNS1123), and the total dose to the involved-field is 30–36 Gy. Metastatic disease, defined as the presence of satellite lesions in the brain and/or spine, positive CSF cytology, visible seeding during neuro-endoscopy, or brain invasion >1 cm adjacent to a suprasellar or pineal mass, is typically treated with 24 Gy CSI followed by a 21 Gy boost to the involved-field(s) or chemotherapy followed by 21 Gy CSI followed by a boost to 30–36 Gy.

A subset of GCTs occur in *both* the pineal and suprasellar regions without interlinking tumor extension. Sometimes both lesions are observed on MRI, or sometimes the presence of the infundibular or pituitary axis lesion is inferred by clinical evidence of diabetes insipidus, or shrinkage of the pineal gland during chemotherapy infers pineal occult disease. These "bifocal" lesions are considered locoregional disease rather than metastatic, and are treated according to the same guidelines above (Aizer et al. 2013; Lafay-Cousin et al. 2006). The majority are pure germinoma. However, despite the predominance of this histology, it is not clear if the requirement for biopsy can be waived, even in the setting of normal serological markers. "Occult" non-germinomatous elements do occur, and drastically change treatment and prognosis (Aizer et al. 2013).

Currently, chemotherapy (typically carboplatin and etoposide) is often used prior to RT to reduce RT doses. The value of this approach has been suggested by retrospective studies and Phase II investigations, but not confirmed by a prospective, randomized trial (Kretschmar et al. 2007; Eom et al. 2008; Khatua et al. 2010; Finlay et al. 2008). Based on these results, the current ACNS 1123 trial treats patients with reduced-dose "response-based" WVRT and involved-field boost after chemotherapy. Patients with complete response to 4 cycles of carboplatin/etoposide are eligible for 18 Gy WVRT followed by a 12 Gy boost to the involved-field. Partial response or progressive disease is treated with 24 Gy WVRT and 12 Gy boost to the involved-field. A select subset of patients with incomplete response to chemotherapy may be referred to second-look surgery for attempted resection of residual disease.

Attempts to shrink RT fields or omit RT altogether following chemotherapy have not been clearly successful. Chemotherapy alone was found to be associated with an unacceptably high rate of relapse (Balmaceda et al. 1996). The results of pre-radiotherapy chemotherapy followed by involved-field-only RT were also equivocal with higher than anticipated rates of failure in the ventricular system (Baranzelli et al. 1997; Fouladi et al. 1998). An arm of the COG ACNS 0232 protocol investigated this particular approach, but had to close due to poor accrual.

3.4.2 Non-germinomatous GCTs

Unlike pure germinomas, non-germinomatous germ cell tumors (NGGCT) require both chemotherapy and radiotherapy to achieve acceptable cure rates. RT alone is associated with poor 5-year survival rates (Dearnaley et al. 1990; Hoffman et al. 1991; Matsutani et al. 1997). Chemotherapy alone is similarly associated with poor outcomes (Balmaceda et al. 1996; Baranzelli et al. 1999; Chang et al. 1995). COG ACNS 0122, a Phase II protocol, administered 6 cycles of carboplatin/etoposide followed by 36 Gy CSI and involved-field radiation to 54 Gy to 103 patients. This regimen also included referral to second-look surgery for patients with incomplete response to induction chemotherapy (15 patients were referred, only 2 had evidence of residual disease), and peripheral blood stem cell rescue (only 2 patients, both of whom achieved complete response). The majority (69%) of patients achieved complete response or partial response. At a median follow-up of 5.1 years, the 5-year OS was 93% and the event-free survival (EFS) was 84% with no treatment-related deaths. This approach is now considered the current standard-of-care off study in North America (Goldman et al. 2015). The SIOP-CNS-GCT-96 trial for NGGCT was recently published good results using a Cisplatin based chemotherapy regimen followed by involved field radiation therapy and this regimen is frequently used in Europe (Calaminus et al. 2017).

As in pure germinomas, the GTV is considered the pre-chemotherapy tumor volume and residual tumor. The CTV is a 1.0 cm expansion of the GTV. CSI follows conventional borders, both the whole brain (including frontal lobe and cribriform plate regions) and spine (including the vertebral bodies). The dose (36 Gy CSI, 54 Gy to primary disease) is delivered in fractions of 1.8 Gy. Spine metastases are boosted to 9 Gy (obeying cord tolerance at 45 Gy).

The COG ACNS1123, a Phase II protocol, treating patients with NGGCT with response-based post-chemotherapy RT. Those patients who achieve a complete remission with 6 cycles of carboplatin/etoposide alternating with ifosfamide/etoposide receive 30.6 Gy WVRT followed by a 23.4 Gy boost to the involved-field. Unfortunately, in September 2016, ACNS1123 NGGCT arm closed to accrual due to exceeding the number of relapses allowable based on statistical design. Ten patients had developed recurrence at the time of evaluation. After thorough evaluation of all patients enrolled, 2 of the 10 patients with relapse were found to be ineligible as they did not meet the definition of response required to move on to WVI. Of the 8 remaining patients, all had distant recurrence with a component in the spine and 6 patients had isolated spinal failures. Given these results, in the US most physicians recommend CSI as per the Goldman study (Goldman et al. 2015).

3.5 Low-Grade Glioma

As the most common pediatric CNS malignancy, low-grade gliomas comprise a variety of histologic subtypes. They can arise anywhere in the CNS, and specific histologies have a propensity for various locations. Regardless of histology, surgical resection, when possible, represents the preferred initial intervention and leads to excellent long-term outcomes. After complete resection, the 10-year OS is approximately 90% and PFS ranges from 75 to 90%, depending on histology and location (Pollack et al. 1995; Fisher et al. 2001, 2008; Gajjar et al. 1997; Pencalet et al. 1999). For patients with a subtotal resection or those with deep brain, brainstem, spinal, or optic pathway and hypothalamic tumors in whom resection is not possible, treatment decisions become more complex and management is best determined in a multidisciplinary setting.

Many children with incomplete resections will not need further therapy, and several large series have shown the rate of progression to be 45–65% after surgery alone (Gajjar et al. 1997; Fisher et al. 2001; Shaw and Wisoff 2003). Therefore, a "wait-and-see" approach is often adopted in these patients, using routine neuroimaging and clinical assessment to monitor status and delay chemotherapy or radiation until progression or clinical symptoms appear. At the time of progression, chemotherapy is most often the treatment of choice in children without significant symptoms, due to concerns of neurocognitive decline with the use of radiation, especially in children 5 years or younger. Carboplatin and vincristine are currently used in the majority of children as front-line adjuvant therapy after Packer et al. reported a 68% three-year PFS rate with this regimen (Packer et al. 1997). In this series, age was a significant prognostic factor of response, with children 5 years of age or younger having a 3-year PFS of 74% and children over the age of 5 having a 3-year PFS of 39%. Alternatively, multi-agent therapy using thioguanine, procarbazine, lomustine, and vincristine (TPCV) has shown efficacy, and a randomized COG A9952 trial showed the 5-year PFS for TPCV to be 52 versus 39% for carboplatin and vincristine, although the difference lacked statistical significance (Ater et al. 2012).

Chemotherapy is effective in delaying progression, and remains the preferred nonsurgical therapy in children vulnerable to the effects of radiation, allowing for continued brain development and endocrine maturation. However, in many children, radiation is ultimately required for definitive treatment. The largest radiation series to date was published by Merchant and colleagues, who reported on the St. Jude experience with 78 supratentorial and infratentorial low-grade gliomas. After irradiation, the 10-year PFS rate was 74% and local control rate was 84% (Merchant et al. 2009b). The incidence of vasculopathy was also reported and was seen in 5% of children at 6 years. None of the patients with neurofibromatosis type 1 ($n = 13$) developed recurrence or secondary malignancy. Other institutions have reported on similar cohorts with 10-year EFS ranging from 65 to 77% and local control rates of 85 to 88% following radiation therapy (Marcus et al. 2005; Grabenbauer et al. 2000; Erkal et al. 1997). More recently, Greenberger et al. published the long-term results for 32 children with low-grade gliomas of the brain or spine treated at Massachusetts General Hospital with proton therapy (Greenberger et al. 2014). At a median follow-up of 8 years, OS was 100% and EFS was 83%. Prospective neurocognitive evaluations were available for 12 of the 32 patients and overall did not show any statistically significant losses, though the subset of patients treated before the age of 7 years showed statistically significant losses in verbal comprehension and the subset who received high doses to the left temporal lobe and/or hippocampus had significant Full Scale IQ and verbal comprehension losses as well. For those patients with tumors arising from or in close proximity to the optic pathway, stabilization or improvement of visual acuity was achieved in 83%. Previously, Tao et al. published the outcomes for 42 children with optic chiasm gliomas treated with photon radiation at what was then the Joint Center for Radiation Therapy in Boston, and showed that at 10 years, 81% of patients had stabilization or improvement of vision (Tao et al. 1997). In this series the 10-year OS and PFS were 100% and 89%, respectively.

Radiation volumes for low-grade gliomas have steadily decreased over time with the realization that these tumors are not typically highly infiltrative. The GTV consists of visible tumor (both enhancing and non-enhancing) as well as any cystic components of the tumor. The CTV includes the GTV plus a small margin of 5 mm. Standard radiation doses range from 50.4 to 54 Gy for intracranial disease and 45 to 50.4 for spinal tumors. In cases of leptomeningeal or metastatic disease, the entire craniospinal axis is radiated to a dose of 36 Gy followed by involved-field treatment to 45–54 Gy, depending on tumor location.

Adverse late effects from radiation can include cognitive decline, endocrine deficiencies, and less commonly hearing loss, vasculopathy, and second malignancy. In a separate publication, Merchant et al. reported the incidence of late effects for the 78 low-grade glioma patients treated on study with radiation (Merchant et al. 2009a). Cognitive function was assessed at 60 months after radiation, and for the entire cohort, only the decline in spelling scores was clinically significant, with average patient scores decreasing from 98 to 90 points (with an average control score being 85 to 115). Most striking, though, was the effect of age on cognitive dysfunction. Each year of increasing age reduced the IQ loss by 0.026 points; whereas a child who was age 5 when irradiated could expect a 10-point IQ decline at 5 years, at 12 years of age no significant IQ loss was observed. As expected, hearing loss and endocrinopathies were directly related to the cochlear and hypothalamic doses, respectively; increasing rates for hearing loss were noted with prior chemotherapy use, and pretreatment hydrocephalus contributed to baseline endocrine deficits.

Therefore, the decision to pursue chemotherapy in lieu of radiation should be made when the adverse effects are minimal and a meaningful delay to irradiation can be achieved without loss of function. As discussed above, prospective trial results show that 35–48% of treated patients will achieve 5 years of PFS with chemotherapy as initial adjuvant treatment (Ater et al. 2012). The choice of chemotherapy as an alternative to radiotherapy as the primary intervention may risk neurologic deterioration in patients who are not closely monitored, and may lead to irreparable functional loss, as in those with optic pathway tumors.

3.6   Medulloblastoma

Radiation therapy plays an integral role in the curative treatment of most children with medulloblastoma. Currently, children <36 months of age receive intensive multi-agent chemotherapy with or without high-dose chemotherapy and stem cell rescue (HDCSCR). In these young children, radiation is omitted due to the concern of severe cognitive impairment from the craniospinal portion of RT. Survival in young children treated with chemotherapy alone is typically lower than in their older counterparts who receive combined modality therapy with chemotherapy and RT. EFS at 5 years in children with nonmetastatic disease (M0) after chemotherapy alone is approximately 32–54%, although with favorable histologic subtypes such as desmoplastic tumors, EFS rates can reach up to 77% (Leary et al. 2011; Geyer et al. 2005; Rutkowski et al. 2010; Dhall et al. 2008; Rutkowski et al. 2005). Failure in these children is still predominately local and therefore the current COG study ACNS0334 for children <36 months does allow for primary site irradiation (50.4–54 Gy). The St. Jude SJYC07 protocol is currently exploring the use of limited radiation to the resection bed only in young children with medulloblastoma following surgical resection and multi-agent chemotherapy. For favorable histologies, such as desmoplastic nodular tumors or those with extensive nodularity, the more recent COG ACNS1121 study utilizes intensive chemotherapy without any radiation (Rutkowski et al. 2010).

For children old enough to receive radiation, treatment strategies are based on risk classification. Currently the COG stratifies children into two risk groups: "high-risk" or "standard-risk." Standard-risk patients are defined as those over the age of 3 years with ≤1.5 cm^2 of residual disease following surgery and no metastatic disease (grossly or in CSF). All others are considered high-risk. Recently, the COG has updated the risk stratification for protocols to specify for frankly anaplastic/large cell histologies, which tend to have poorer outcomes compared to classic and desmoplastic histologies (Packer et al. 2006; Brown et al. 2000). Children with anaplastic/large cell tumors are considered "other than average risk" and are treated per the high-risk protocols. Multiple studies utilizing gene expression profiles to characterize medulloblastoma have been published over the past decade, demonstrating that histologically similar tumors can frequently be divided into four distinct molecular subgroups with significantly different prognoses (Northcott et al. 2011; Jones et al. 2012; Remke et al. 2011; Cho et al. 2011). The four groups include WNT (wingless), SHH (sonic hedgehog), Group 3, and Group 4. Improved understanding of the molecular nature of medulloblastoma is rapidly improving our ability to classify failure risk and it is likely that in the near future a revised classification system for medulloblastoma will incorporate molecular stratification. Institutional trials, such as the St. Jude SJMB12 protocol, have already begun to use these groups to tailor radiation dose, and discussions regarding the next COG trial for medulloblastoma have proposed modification based on molecular classification.

At present, standard-risk medulloblastoma patients receive 23.4 Gy to the craniospinal axis followed by a boost to the posterior fossa or tumor bed to a total dose of 54 Gy. This is usually started within 31 days of surgery, given concurrently with weekly vincristine, and followed by maintenance chemotherapy (cisplatin, lomustine, vincristine) after radiation. For standard-risk disease, the disease-free survival (DFS) of children treated with chemotherapy and radiation is in excess of 80% (Packer et al. 2006). The need to treat the entire posterior fossa versus just the involved-field tumor resection bed during the boost portion of RT is currently being explored in the recently closed COG ACNS0331 study. This study randomized children to receive boosts to the posterior fossa or involved-field in a 1:1 ratio, and the results should be forthcoming. Off study, it is the practice of many centers to treat just the involved-field with a boost, based on three single institution studies that showed no increase in PF failures using this technique (Wolden et al. 2003; Douglas et al. 2004; Merchant et al. 1999). In addition to randomizing patients to involved-field versus posterior fossa boost volumes, ACNS0331 also randomized children <8 years of age with standard-risk medulloblastoma to reduced-dose CSI of 18 Gy versus the standard 23.4 Gy. The use of 18 Gy stems from favorable results of a limited series at Children's Hospital of Philadelphia that demonstrated comparable long-term outcomes and improved neurocognitive results for young children (Goldwein et al. 1996; Packer et al. 1999). Currently, 23.4 Gy still represents the standard for care for children with average risk medulloblastoma, but results from the ACNS0331 may show that a reduction in craniospinal dose is possible in younger patients. Though this study has only been presented in abstract form, initial results show equivalence for treatment of the involved field versus treatment of whole posterior fossa. Unofrtunately, 18 CSI was inferior compared with 23.4 CSI (J Michalski, ASTRO 2016).

For high-risk patients or "other than average risk" medulloblastoma, the craniospinal dose is increased to 36 Gy and, in the recently closed COG study ACNS0332, patients were randomized to weekly vincristine +/− daily carboplatin as a potential radiosensitizing agent. The entire PF was treated with a boost to 55.8 Gy, though 54 Gy is routinely used off study. Children with metastases receive 55.8 Gy to intracranial sites and 45–50.4 Gy to spinal sites, depending on whether these sites are above or below the terminus of the spinal cord. For diffusely involved spinal cord lesions (radiographically visible lesions in ≥3 of 4 spinal cord sections) the entire cord may be treated to 39.6 Gy. ACNS0332 also included maintenance chemotherapy with cisplatin, cyclophosphamide, and vincristine and children were randomized to receive posttreatment isotretinoin. Survival rates for high-risk disease are approximately 50–70% (Tarbell et al. 2013; Zeltzer et al. 1999). Children with standard-risk disease and anaplastic histology have a slightly improved DFS of approximately 73% (Packer et al. 2006).

Radiation treatment volumes include the entire brain and spine for the CSI treatments. Special attention should be paid in the brain to coverage of the cribriform plate, posterior orbits, and internal auditory canals, all of which can harbor microscopic disease outside of the cranium. In the spine, a margin of approximately one vertebral body below the end of thecal sac, typically located at S2/S3, should be given. An MRI may be useful for confirming thecal sac termination. 3D conformal photon techniques are standard for the CSI portion, but do deliver excess radiation to the esophagus, thyroid, heart, bone marrow, ovaries, and bowel. The use of IMRT or Volumetric Modulated Arc Therapy (VMAT) can decrease the heart and bone marrow dose but leads to increased lung and kidney doses, as well as an increase in total volume irradiated, which can increase the risk for secondary malignancies (Brodin et al. 2011; St Clair et al. 2004; Lomax et al. 1999). Proton therapy is being used with increasing frequency in CSI treatments, as the absence of exit dose spares the thyroid, heart, lungs, abdominal organs, and gonads from radiation.

For the boost component, the posterior fossa volume extends from the tentorium superiorly to C1 inferiorly. Laterally the posterior fossa volume includes the entire cerebellum and extends to the bony occiput and anteriorly this volume includes the brainstem and lower midbrain. For involved-field treatment, the volume should include the tumor bed (paying close attention to any presurgery extension into the foramen of Luschka) and any residual gross disease. The volume should also account for anatomical shifts following surgery, as re-expansion of compressed cerebellum occurs following surgery. A margin of 0.5–1.5 cm is typically added to the tumor bed, depending on the method of daily image localization and the invasive characteristics of the tumor. Again, conformal techniques such as IMRT and VMAT used during the boost can reduce dose to critical structures such as the cochlea, hypothalamus, and temporal lobes. Further dose reductions to these structures can be achieved with proton therapy and there is now clinical data to suggest that use of proton therapy may translate to improved cognitive and endocrine outcomes (Eaton et al).

3.7 Supratentorial Primitive Neuroectodermal Tumors

Supratentorial primitive neuroectodermal tumors (PNETs) are, by definition, small round blue cell tumors that occur within the supratentorial brain. The incidence is less than that of medulloblastoma, comprising 2–3% of primary brain tumors versus 20% for medulloblastoma (Gaffney et al. 1985). The metastatic rate for SPNET is similar to medulloblastoma, but these tumors portend a worse prognosis with increased local failure compared to their medulloblastoma counterparts (Timmermann et al. 2002; Reddy et al. 2000). The 5-year PFS ranges from 37 to 48%, although patients with pineoblastomas and patients without metastatic disease have slightly better outcomes (Jakacki 1999; Jakacki et al. 1995; Cohen et al. 1995; Reddy et al. 2000; Timmermann et al. 2002). Treatment algorithms are similar to medulloblastoma, with maximal resection as the initial intervention, followed by craniospinal radiation and chemotherapy. Because of the increased rate of disease recurrence, all children who present with SPNET are considered "high-risk" and are treated as such on the high-risk COG medulloblastoma/PNET protocols (currently ACNS0332 and ACNS0334). As in medulloblastoma, children <3 years of age with SPNET have been treated without radiation therapy but have had dismal outcomes and focal radiation should be strongly considered for children under the age of three (Timmermann et al. 2006; Jakacki et al. 1995; Duffner et al. 1995). Due to the rarity of these tumors, SPNET specific radiation recommendations do not exist and treatments are the same as for high-risk medulloblastoma, with

36 Gy CSI and a 54 Gy boost to the resection bed.

3.8 Craniopharyngioma

Craniopharyngiomas are benign tumors of epithelial origin arising from the suprasellar region, believed to be remnants of Rathke's pouch. The role of RT in craniopharyngioma is controversial and management decisions depend heavily on endocrine status and tumor size and extent. Survival in children with craniopharyngioma is excellent and therefore treatment options focus heavily on the preservation of quality of life. Surgical excision is often curative if gross total resection can be achieved, but craniopharyngiomas are highly adherent tumors and arise in close proximity to the brainstem, hypothalamus, optic chiasm and nerves, and critical vascular structures. Local control at 10 years following radiographically confirmed gross total resection can be as high as 80%; however, radiographic gross total resection is only achieved in 50–80% of attempts (Hoffman et al. 1992; Fahlbusch et al. 1999; De Vile et al. 1996; Stripp et al. 2004). The risk of endocrine deficits, cognitive dysfunction, visual deficits, and hypothalamic obesity following surgery rises significantly as the extent of resection increases and, therefore, a limited surgical approach with postoperative RT has been adopted at most pediatric centers.

Cyst decompression (which improves the tumor geometry allowing for smaller radiation fields) with endoscopic biopsy or partial resection followed by radiation therapy has led to excellent results in children. With limited resection and RT, PFS ranges between 80 and 90% (Fitzek et al. 2006; Regine and Kramer 1992; Merchant et al. 2013; Rajan et al. 1993; Hetelekidis et al. 1993). Toxicity following combined modality treatment is favorable. In the Boston Children's Hospital and Joint Center review of 20-year outcomes for 15 children treated with surgery alone and 37 children treated with limited surgery and RT, the incidence of visual loss and diabetes insipidus was significantly lower for the combined modality arm (Hetelekidis et al. 1993). Similarly, the St. Jude experience for craniopharyngioma found that the surgery alone cohort experienced more frequent neurologic, visual, and endocrine effects than the surgery and RT patients and that the full scale IQ loss was larger (a mean of 9.8 points lost for surgery alone vs. 1.3 points for surgery plus RT, $P < 0.06$) (Merchant et al. 2002b). Finally, compared to surgery plus RT, memory, problem solving, and performance IQ scores have been found to be lower with surgery alone in pediatric and adult cohorts (Carpentieri et al. 2001; Cavazzuti et al. 1983; Clopper et al. 1977).

The radiation target volume for craniopharyngiomas should include both solid and cystic components as well as any area of the brain in contact with the tumor or tumor cyst prior to surgical resection. Doses of 50.4–54 Gy at daily fractions of 1.8 Gy are recommended. Some series have used higher doses of radiation, but due to concerns for optic structure tolerance and lack of convincing evidence that an increased dose provides greater tumor control, higher doses are not generally recommended. During

radiation, the re-accumulation of fluid in existing cysts may occur and therefore re-imaging with cone beam CT or a T2-weighted non-contrast MRI every 7–14 days for monitoring should be considered.

Various radiation techniques, including IMRT, Fractionated Stereotactic Radiation Therapy (FSRT), VMAT, SRS, and Gamma Knife (GK), have all been used with good success. The choice between fractionated techniques such as IMRT and VMAT versus single fraction treatment with SRS or GK depends on the initial extent of tumor and proximity of residual tumor to critical structures such as the brainstem, optic chiasm and optic nerves. Proton therapy, either with passively scattered 3D techniques or Intensity-Modulated Proton Therapy (IMPT), has been used with increasing frequency in pediatric craniopharyngiomas requiring fractionated treatment, due to the ability to reduce dose to the temporal lobes, hippocampi, and surrounding vasculature compared to photon techniques (Boehling et al. 2012). Figure 3.4 shows a proton beam scanning plan for craniopharyngioma.

3.9 Atypical Teratoid Rhabdoid Tumor

Atypical teratoid/rhabdoid (AT/RT) tumors are rare malignant embryonal tumors of the CNS, which primarily affect children less than 5 years of age. Although they account for less than 5% of all pediatric CNS tumors, it has been estimated that up to 20% of malignant CNS tumors diagnosed in patients 3 years and younger are AT/RTs (Packer et al. 2002). These tumors are aggressive and are associated with a poor prognosis, with median survivals historically ranging between 6 and 12 months (Burger et al. 1998).

Because of the rarity of this tumor and its predominant presentation in younger children, there is ongoing controversy regarding the optimal treatment for this disease. Substantial evidence supports the importance of a maximal

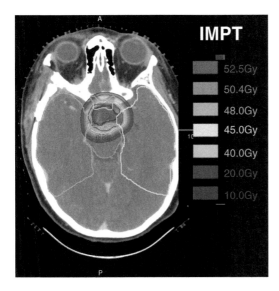

Fig. 3.4 Proton scanning beam plan for a craniopharyngioma

safe resection, which is prognostic for OS (Hilden et al. 2004; Zimmerman et al. 2005). The role of chemotherapy has been studied extensively and appears to provide a benefit (Gardner et al. 2008). In the past, RT was avoided or delayed for the treatment of AT/RT, because it was believed that any possible benefits were far outweighed by the late toxicities of this modality in young children (Duffner et al. 1993). However, more recent data has suggested that early RT can significantly increase local control and prolong OS, even in very young patients (McGovern et al. 2014; Chi et al. 2009; Squire et al. 2007; De Amorim Bernstein et al. 2013). In parallel, the emergence of newer RT modalities, such as proton therapy, has facilitated the treatment of younger children with significantly less exposure of normal tissues to RT. As such, the role of RT in the treatment of AT/RT is evolving, and it likely will play a more prominent role in the adjuvant treatment regimen for these tumors, regardless of patient age.

AT/RTs primarily are composed of rhabdoid cells, and often they contain areas that closely resemble classical primitive neuroectodermal tumors (Kleihues et al. 2002). As a result, it is thought that many cases of AT/RT were misdiagnosed as medulloblastomas, especially in younger patients (Rorke et al. 1996). The discovery that nearly all AT/RTs have a deletion or mutation in the hSNF5/INI1 gene, which is not typically seen in medulloblastoma/PNET, has significantly aided in the distinction between these two tumor types (Haberler et al. 2006). Immunohistochemical staining for INI1 is now commonly performed to confirm the diagnosis of AT/RT, which has led to an increase in the identification of cases at first diagnosis. Approximately two-thirds of AT/RTs present in the posterior fossa, with other locations including the cerebral hemispheres and the spine (Hilden et al. 1998). Up to one-third of patients present with neuraxis dissemination at diagnosis (Hilden et al. 2004).

Similar to the case for medulloblastoma, there are two rationales for including RT in the adjuvant treatment regimen for AT/RT: (1) to prevent local recurrence at the primary site and (2) to prevent leptomeningeal spread of occult, microscopic disease that may be present at initial diagnosis. In both cases, the decision to offer RT is balanced against the toxicities of CNS RT exposure in very young children. This issue, coupled with the rarity of these tumors and the consequent lack of randomized trials to guide treatment, has resulted in substantial controversy regarding the use of RT for this disease. Further complicating the matter is the finding that AT/RTs are resistant to many conventional chemotherapy regimens used to treat other CNS tumors. Analysis of misclassified AT/RT cases treated on PNET/medulloblastoma and other Pediatric Oncology Group (POG) protocols revealed an extremely poor response rate to traditional chemotherapy regimens, including even "eight-in-one" intensive strategies (Burger et al. 1998). These findings led to the testing of even more intensive regimens, which typically incorporated intrathecal chemotherapy, and some of which reserved RT only for recurrent disease (Gardner et al. 2008; Zaky et al. 2014; Zimmerman et al. 2005; Olson et al. 1995).

In parallel, emerging evidence at the time suggested a compelling association between the use of up-front RT and long-term AT/RT survivors, even in very young children. In the AT/RT registry created by Hilden et al., 8 of the 13 patients with a durable response to therapy were treated with RT as part of the treatment regimen (Hilden et al. 2004). A review of AT/RT patients treated at the St. Jude's Children's Research Hospital by Tekautz et al. revealed only two long-term survivors, both of whom received up-front RT (Tekautz et al. 2005). In this particular study, 1-year EFS and 2-year OS in AT/RT patients treated with chemotherapy alone were 0% and 12%, respectively. This compared with 90% 2-year PFS and OS rates for those treated with chemotherapy and RT. A retrospective study of AT/RT patients treated at the Taipai Veterans General Hospital in Taiwan found a statistically significant correlation between delays in RT and adverse patient outcomes. Two Surveillance Epidemiology and End Results (SEER)-based studies also revealed statistically significant links between OS and RT in AT/RT patients younger than 3 years old (Buscariollo et al. 2012;

Bishop et al. 2012). More recently, initial results from AT/RT patients treated with proton-based RT modalities have been reported. Bernstein et al. reported on the Massachusetts General Hospital (MGH) experience with ten consecutive patients (De Amorim Bernstein et al. 2013), and McGovern et al. reported on the results of 31 patients treated at the MD Anderson Cancer Center (MDACC) (McGovern et al. 2014). Both studies utilized proton-based RT; selected patients received involved-field RT (IFRT) versus CSI, and the majority of patients were under 3 years of age. These studies were notable for acceptable rates of toxicity and favorable responses. In particular, the MDACC study reported a median PFS of 20.8 months and a median OS of 34.3 months, which are promising in comparison to historic results (McGovern et al. 2014).

Based on the promising results above, which suggest that RT can improve EFS and OS, RT was made a backbone of the ongoing non-randomized Phase III COG trial for AT/RT (ACNS0333; NCT00653068). In this trial, patients initially undergo resection followed by induction chemotherapy with a stem cell harvest, and they are then stratified into two groups of patients: (1) younger patients with localized disease (M0) in which chemotherapy to delay RT is desired, or patients in which disease is disseminated (M+) and up-front intensive chemotherapy is indicated, and (2) older M0 patients in whom focal RT can be given with acceptable late toxicities. Both groups are allowed a second-look surgery. The age cutoffs to define younger patients are <6 months and <12 months for infratentorial and supratentorial tumors, respectively. Group 1 patients move on directly to consolidation chemotherapy and stem cell rescue, followed by RT. Group 2 patients move on to focal RT followed by chemotherapy and stem cell rescue. CSI is not mandated in this study.

Despite a growing momentum towardsw the incorporation of RT into the up-front setting for AT/RT, the optimal RT treatment volumes and doses remain undefined. Burger et al. reviewed AT/RT patterns of relapse in 52 cases, and noted 24 cases of primary site only relapses, and 9 cases of combined local and craniospinal (distant) relapses (Burger et al. 1998). Similar results were observed in the St. Jude's Children's Research Hospital experience (Tekautz et al. 2005). Although these results highlight a clear role for focal RT to the primary site, another study reviewed 52 AT/RT cases and found that approximately 34% of them presented with leptomeningeal dissemination based on imaging or CSF analysis (Rorke et al. 1996). The latter study suggests that these tumors have a predilection for early seeding of the neuraxis, in a manner similar to that observed in medulloblastoma. The decision to utilize CSI as part of the RT approach is highly dependent on the age of the patient, the stage of the disease, and institutional preferences. Further studies are needed to determine whether focal RT will be equal to CSI in terms of disease control for AT/RT. RT doses largely have been extrapolated from medulloblastoma. In ACNS0333, M0 patients are treated with between 50.4 and 54 Gy to the primary site without CSI depending on age. Patients with M+ disease who are 3 years of age or younger receive a CSI dose of 23.4 Gy, followed by a primary boost to 50.4 Gy. Patients older than 3 years of age are treated with 36 Gy CSI followed by a primary site boost to 54 Gy. However, as noted earlier, the decision to treat M+ patients with CSI is left to the discretion of the treating radiation oncologist. Also discussed earlier, proton therapy is of great interest for the treatment of AT/RT because of the relatively young age at disease presentation (De Amorim Bernstein et al. 2013; McGovern et al. 2014). The benefits of this modality apply to both CSI and focal RT to the primary site, as in both cases substantial sparing of normal tissue can be achieved.

3.10 Choroid Plexus Tumors

Choroid plexus tumors are rare neoplasms in the CNS; they account for less than 1% of all brain tumors. As such, there is a paucity of large-scale clinical trials specifically addressing the most optimal treatment regimen for this disease. Clinical decisions thus have been primarily based on data from institutional series and literature reviews. While surgical resection is considered standard as the first and most important intervention, there is continued controversy regarding the roles of adjuvant chemotherapy and radiotherapy for the treatment of this disease.

Choroid plexus tumors are classified by the WHO into three categories: choroid plexus papilloma (CPP; grade I), atypical CPP (grade II), and choroid plexus carcinoma (CPC; grade III) (Louis et al. 2007). As expected, CPCs are the most aggressive tumors among the choroid neoplasms, with 5-year OS rates ranging between 20 and 40% (Berger et al. 1998). The majority of choroid plexus tumors develop in childhood (over 70%). In the pediatric population, these tumors most commonly arise in the lateral ventricles, followed by the fourth ventricle, and the third ventricle (approximately 80%, 15% and 5%, respectively) (Thompson et al. 1973).

There has been only one randomized trial completed for choroid plexus tumors, the International Society of Paediatric Oncology (SIOP) trial CPT-SIOP-2000. This study evaluated specific treatment regimens for CPPs, atypical CPPs, and CPCs, and it included localized and metastatic disease in both children and adults. Initial results from the atypical CPP group were reported, which suggested a favorable response to chemotherapy (Wrede et al. 2009). Local RT or CSI for CPP tumors typically was reserved only for progressive disease that could not be addressed with a re-resection or chemotherapy, and these decisions were also guided by patient age. However, radiotherapy was an integral part of the treatment regimen for CPCs in this protocol. Patients with either localized or metastatic CPC first underwent a maximal possible resection, followed by 2 cycles of chemotherapy. All patients over the age of 3 years with either a complete response or partial response/stable disease then received CSI with a primary site RT boost, followed by additional chemotherapy. Younger patients received additional chemotherapy in an effort to either delay or to exclude RT. More recently, CPT-SIOP-2009 has been initiated, which also includes RT in subsets of patients with choroid plexus tumors, based on age, histology, staging, and response to chemotherapy (NCT01014767). While there are no published data regarding the efficacy of RT from these SIOP trials to date, they highlight the important role of this modality in the treatment of choroid plexus tumors.

Wolff et al. published results from a meta-analysis of 566 patients; these results provided compelling evidence for the role of RT in the treatment of CPCs (Wolff et al. 1999, 2002). Although this study included adult patients, the majority of the subjects were children, with a mean age at diagnosis of 3.5 years. This study demonstrated a statistically significant OS benefit in CPC patients who received postoperative RT versus those who did not. This benefit was observed in patients who received a gross total resection, and also in the setting of residual disease (Wolff et al. 1999, 2002). Of note, this study did not distinguish patients who received RT alone versus RT and chemotherapy. More recently, however, another group reported a systematic review to assess the effects of chemotherapy and RT on OS for patients with CPC, focusing specifically on pediatric tumors (Sun et al. 2014). This study demonstrated improved OS with chemotherapy alone, and also with combined chemotherapy and RT, but not with RT alone. Interestingly, a multivariate Cox regression analysis indicated that combined chemotherapy and RT provided the greatest OS, but the Kaplan-Meier OS curves overlapped. Both studies suffer from the limitations associated with literature reviews, but they are nonetheless notable for an OS benefit associated with the addition of RT to the adjuvant treatment regimen.

The optimal RT fields for CPC remain controversial, with some practitioners advocating IFRT, WBRT, or CSI. Mazloom et al. recently performed a comprehensive literature review to determine the most effective RT fields for the treatment of CPC (Mazloom et al. 2010). A total of 56 patients were identified from 33 articles with sufficient information regarding the type of radiation fields and the treatment outcome. Approximately 70% of the patients were treated with CSI, 15% received WBRT, and 15% received a focal treatment to the tumor bed. The authors found that the use of CSI versus more localized RT had a statistically significant PFS benefit (5-year PFS was 44% vs. 15%, respectively). This also correlated with a significant increase in OS (5-year OS was 68% vs. 28%, respectively).

Consistent with the study discussed above and others (Fitzpatrick et al. 2002), most major centers in the US recommend CSI as part of the adjuvant CPC treatment regimen for patients 3 years and older. Chemotherapy-based strategies to delay RT are recommended for younger patients, although some institutions also treat younger patients with CSI, recognizing the aggressive nature of the disease. It should be noted once again that due to the rarity of this disease, there is no clear consensus on the optimal RT fields and doses for CPC. The CSI dose typically is 36 Gy with a boost to the primary site of 18 Gy (54 Gy total), and CSI doses have been reduced to 23.4 Gy for younger patients. A standard CSI technique and primary site boost is utilized for CPC, as described for other posterior fossa tumors presented earlier. Exceptions to the use of RT for CPC in patients 3 years and older may include Li-Fraumeni Syndrome (LFS) patients. LFS often is caused by a TP53 mutation, and it has been associated with CPCs. TP53 mutations can induce radioresistance, and one recent study suggested a detrimental effect on OS in a small series of LFS patients with CPC who received RT as part of their treatment regimen (Bahar et al. 2015). However, further studies are needed to confirm this association.

3.11 Supratentorial High-Grade Glioma

Approximately 6% of pediatric brain tumors are comprised of supratentorial high-grade gliomas. As in the adult setting, high-grade gliomas are devastating, aggressive tumors in children. The 5-year OS for children with these tumors ranges between 15 and 30% and has not improved over the last 3 decades (Cohen et al. 2011b). It is well established that a maximally safe resection is the most important first step in the management of these tumors, and studies have demonstrated a direct correlation between the extent of resection and outcomes, specifically in the pediatric population (Finlay et al. 1995). RT is the backbone of adjuvant treatment for pediatric high-grade glioma, at least in patients 3 years and older. The rationale is that microscopic disease is found well beyond the resection cavities of gross totally resected tumors, such that locoregional control with RT is needed to prevent tumor recurrence. The role of chemotherapy in pediatric high-grade glioma is less well-defined, but nonetheless remains important in the adjuvant setting. While concurrent and adjuvant temozolomide chemotherapy is part of the standard of care in adult GBM, it appears to have less of a benefit in pediatric high-grade gliomas (Cohen et al. 2011b). Numerous experimental agents have been tested either concurrently with RT or adjuvantly, but they have not yielded any benefits in OS. Thus, better therapies are needed to treat pediatric high-grade gliomas.

The term high-grade glioma often is used synonymously with malignant gliomas, and it includes WHO grade III (most commonly anaplastic astrocytoma) and grade IV (glioblastoma multiforme) tumors (Louis et al. 2007). These tumors appear as centrally necrotic, contrast-enhancing lesions on T1 imaging sequences and are accompanied by surrounding abnormal T2 signal changes representing a mix of edema and microscopic disease. The majority of supratentorial gliomas present in the cerebral hemispheres, although 20–30% can present in other structures, such as the thalamus and basal ganglia (Kramm et al. 2011). In contrast to medulloblastomas and other "seeding" tumors, leptomeningeal spread of disease is not common in pediatric high-grade gliomas. As such, current therapies are directed at aggressive local control, which is discussed further below.

The addition of chemotherapy to RT showed great promise for pediatric high-grade gliomas in early clinical trials, such as CCG-943, which tested the addition of vincristine concurrently with RT followed by adjuvant prednisone, lomustine, and vincristine (pCV) (Finlay et al. 1995).

This trial reported impressive, statistically significant 5-year EFS of 46% with the addition of chemotherapy to RT, versus 5-year EFS of 18% with RT alone. However, it is likely that many patients in this study actually had low-grade gliomas, which may have skewed the results (Finlay and Zacharoulis 2005). CCG-945 then tested whether intensification of chemotherapy could increase treatment efficacy in addition to RT, and it tested the CCG-9545 chemotherapy regimen versus an "8-in-1" chemotherapy regimen (Finlay et al. 1995). The latter regimen was not better with regard to EFS or OS, and most importantly the former regimen was nearly half as efficacious as shown previously in CCG-943; the use of pCV-based chemotherapy had a 5-year PFS of 26% in CCG-945, versus the aforementioned 5-year EFS of 46% in CCG-943. This further highlighted the possibility that the results of CCG-943 were confounded by the inclusion of lower grade tumors. Indeed, a central pathology review of CCG-945 patients revealed that approximately 30% of cases classified as high-grade tumors were actually lower grade histologies (Batra et al. 2014; Pollack et al. 2003). Attempts were then made to intensify chemotherapy prior to RT as in CCG 9933 (MacDonald et al. 2005). In this trial, approximately 42% of patients progressed before the initiation of RT, and over 20% of patients were unable to proceed to RT.

The current standard of care for adult GBM is resection followed by RT with concurrent and adjuvant temozolomide, based on the results of a randomized, Phase III trial published by Stupp et al. in 2005. Temozolomide is orally administered and well tolerated, and thus there was great hope that it would show efficacy in children with malignant gliomas. ACNS0126 tested this hypothesis, although unlike the "Stupp trial," it was a Phase II trial testing the efficacy of RT and temozolomide in children (Cohen et al. 2011b). This trial unfortunately was negative, as the addition of temozolomide to RT showed no benefit to historical controls. However, it should be noted that the data from ACNS0126 was compared to data from CCG-945, which also tested chemotherapy with RT. Thus, ACNS0126 did not necessarily disprove the benefit of adding chemotherapy to the treatment regimen in children with malignant gliomas. Indeed, many practitioners continue to treat pediatric patients with RT and temozolomide off-protocol when there are no clinical trials available for enrollment (Fangusaro and Warren 2013).

Many other novel systemic agents have been tested with RT, either concurrently or in the adjuvant setting, but unfortunately with limited success (reviewed in (Fangusaro 2012)). Many of these agents were tested based on evidence of efficacy from adult GBM studies. However, we now understand that pediatric malignant gliomas are genetically unique tumors when compared to their adult counterparts (Huse and Rosenblum 2015). This critical finding suggests an opportunity may exist to develop novel therapies for pediatric gliomas in the future. Nonetheless, a common theme in the trials presented above is the importance of RT as the backbone of the adjuvant treatment regimen for this tumor, which will be discussed further below.

There are three key aspects of RT delivery for supratentorial malignant gliomas that have evolved over time, and that have largely been extrapolated from the adult setting: (1) delineation of the volumes for treatment, (2) selection of the most appropriate RT dose, and (3) determination of the most optimal fractionation regimens. Each topic is discussed in greater detail below.

The primary GTV (GTV1) typically is defined as the resection bed, gross residual tumor as seen on gadolinium-enhanced T1 and/or T2 MRI sequences, and also any other suspicious abnormalities seen on the T2 MRI sequences. A primary CTV (CTV1) is then defined based on an anatomically confined 2-cm expansion off this GTV. The corresponding primary planning target volume (PTV1) typically is defined as CTV1 plus 0.3–0.5 cm, depending on the image-guided RT protocols at the treating institution. This volume is taken to 54 Gy in 1.80 Gy fractions. A second GTV (GTV2) is defined that can be limited to the postoperative bed alone, any residual tumor, or which is identical to GTV1 if this initial volume is considered small. CTV2 typically is delineated by a smaller expansion off GTV2,

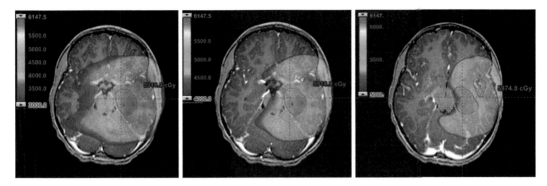

Fig. 3.5 Example of a highly conformal, intensity-modulated radiation therapy (IMRT)-based treatment plan for a pediatric supratentorial glioblastoma multiforme. The minimum doses shown are 3000, 4000 and 5000 cGy (left, middle, and right panels, respectively)

typically in the range of 0.5–1 cm, followed by a 0.3–0.5 cm expansion for PTV2. This volume is referred to as "the boost" or "cone-down," and it is taken to 5940 cGy. This approach is most commonly used in COG protocols, and bears resemblance to the Radiation Therapy Oncology Group (RTOG)-based protocols for target delineation in adult GBM. One key difference is that the RTOG-based approach for adult GBM involves an initial volume that is taken to 46 Gy, followed by a boost to 60 Gy, in 2 Gy fractions (Gilbert et al. 2014). In contrast, the RT guidelines in the Stupp trial specified a dose of 60 Gy to the postoperative bed and any enhancing disease seen on CT or MRI (Stupp et al. 2009; Stupp et al. 2005). The rather large, 2 cm CTV expansion presented above is based on previous imaging and histologic studies in adult glioma, which suggest that microscopic glioma cells are found within this region beyond the resection cavity, typically within the surrounding edema seen on T2 sequences (Halperin et al. 1989). Nonetheless, studies have shown that recurrences are almost universally in the central region of the original tumor site, or close to the resection cavity, despite high doses of RT to these areas (Wallner et al. 1989). Hyperfractionation has been tested in pediatric gliomas with limited success (Fallai and Olmi 1997), and thus conventional fractionation is considered standard for this disease. Total doses above 60 Gy were tested in the adult setting for malignant glioma, either during the initial treatment or as an additional boost, but unfortunately they also did not yield any clear benefits (Biswas et al. 2009; Shrieve et al. 1999). Either 3D-conformal or IMRT-based RT planning is recommended in almost all cases, in order to reduce normal tissue exposure to radiation. An example of a case treated at our institution is shown in Fig. 3.5. This case is notable for considerable sparing of normal structures, including the brainstem, at higher RT doses.

3.12 Diffuse Intrinsic Pontine Glioma

Approximately 15–20% of pediatric CNS tumors arise in the brainstem, and 80% of them are diffuse intrinsic pontine gliomas (DIPGs) (Stiller and Nectoux 1994). Survival rates for this disease have been stagnant for over 30 years, with a median survival of less than 1 year from diagnosis (Cohen et al. 2011b). DIPGs are considered surgically unresectable, and the diagnosis generally is made based on characteristic findings on MRI combined with clinical presentation. In the past, it was considered that the risks of tumor biopsies outweighed the benefits, since histologic confirmation rarely changed management for this disease. However, the discovery of unique mutations in DIPG subsets, coupled with more advanced stereotactic biopsy techniques, has reignited the question of whether these interventions should be performed in newly diagnosed patients (MacDonald 2012). RT is the only modality that appears to improve OS for this disease, with early studies indicating a doubling of OS with the addition of this modality in newly diagnosed patients (Langmoen et al. 1991). In contrast, multiple conventional chemotherapies and novel biologic agents have been tested in DIPG patients with no clear OS gains. A recent review reported 55 clinical trials since 1984 that tested novel therapies over RT alone, with no improvement in OS for DIPG (Jansen et al. 2012). Thus, additional approaches are desperately needed for this devastating disease.

Since biopsies have been relatively uncommon to confirm the initial diagnosis of DIPG, most information about the histologies associated with this tumor type have been gleaned from autopsy specimens. The majority of DIPGs are fibrillary astrocytomas with varying degrees of higher-grade features, such as anaplasia and tumor necrosis (Schumacher et al. 2007). As such, WHO grading ranges from II to IV, although the significance of these classifications has been questioned, because they do not necessarily change prognosis (Grigsby et al. 1989; Laigle-Donadey et al. 2008). More recently, there has been an explosion in our understanding of the molecular changes that underlie DIPGs. A wide range of novel gene mutations that are not observed in adult gliomas have been identified in subsets of DIPG tumors; these mutations are even distinct from those in pediatric supratentorial tumors (reviewed in (Morales La Madrid et al. 2015)). These mutations are important because they suggest distinct molecular subtypes of DIPG, with clear differences in prognosis and possibly treatment response (Buczkowicz et al. 2014). Examples include the K27 M and G34R point mutations in the H3F3A gene, truncating mutations in the PPM1D gene, and activating mutations in the ACVR1 gene (Morales La Madrid et al. 2015). As can be gleaned from the name, DIPG tumors arise in the pons, but they tend to extend directly into the midbrain, medulla, and the cerebellar peduncles (Grigsby

et al. 1989). Of note, up to a third of patients may have leptomeningeal disease at the time of initial diagnosis (Buczkowicz et al. 2014; Donahue et al. 1998). These findings highlight an important role for both locoregional disease control and prevention of distant disease relapse, therefore highlighting the important roles for both RT and systemic therapies, respectively, but additional targeted therapies likely will also be needed. The evidence supporting these modalities is discussed further below.

Brainstem tumors were treated with RT from the early 1940s onwards (Peirce and Bouchard 1950). Jenkin et al. reported one of the first trials that tested the addition of chemotherapy to RT in 1987. The addition of chemotherapy was associated with a dismal 5-year OS rate of 20%, which was not significant over RT alone (Jenkin et al. 1987). CCG-9941 tested two different pre-irradiation chemotherapy regimens, which also were negative when compared to historical series using RT alone (Jennings et al. 2002). More intensive, high-dose chemotherapy regimens were subsequently tested, but unfortunately they also failed to increase OS for this disease (Bouffet et al. 2000; Dunkel et al. 1998).

More recently, the ACNS0126 trial tested the role of temozolomide for DIPG, based on the promising results in the treatment of adult GBM as presented above (Cohen et al. 2011a). This was a Phase II trial in which patients received 59.4 Gy to the tumor with concurrent and adjuvant temozolomide, which was essentially identical to the Stupp regimen for adult GBM (Stupp et al. 2009). There was great hope that this trial would yield positive results, as many practitioners were already prescribing this regimen by extrapolation from the adult GBM experience for the reasons described earlier. However, the 1-year EFS rate in ACNS0126 was 14% for DIPG patients, which unfortunately was not superior to historical controls (Cohen et al. 2011a). Several other studies yielded similar results around this time, providing evidence that temozolomide does not have a role in the treatment of DIPG (Rizzo et al. 2015; Chassot et al. 2012; Jalali et al. 2010; Chiang et al. 2010).

Many other novel systemic therapies have been tested in combination with RT, but unfortunately they also have not shown great success in the treatment of DIPG (reviewed in (Jansen et al. 2012)). A major concern regarding the use of systemic agents is whether they penetrate the blood–brain barrier (BBB), although to some degree RT may enhance permeability (Warren 2012). The common theme among these studies is that no additional intervention beyond RT has further improved survival for DIPG. However, survival for this disease remains dismal, with 2-year OS rates in the range of 10% and lower. Thus, additional therapies are needed, but RT likely will continue to play an integral role in the management of this disease.

Similar to the case for supratentorial gliomas, there are several key aspects related to the use of RT to treat DIPG that have evolved over decades: (1) selection of the appropriate RT dose, (2) the role of altered fractionation schemes, and (3) definition of the most optimal treatment volumes. While DIPG is a relatively rare disease, and there are limited randomized data guiding treatments, it is important to note that these three aspects have been addressed in clinical trials and studies of limited patient series. Each topic is discussed in greater detail below.

The relatively high dose of RT for DIPG and other brainstem tumors was supported by Lee et al. in a study published in 1975, which looked at outcomes for infratentorial and supratentorial brain tumors treated with a range of RT doses (Lee 1975). Although the series was small (24 patients), and it included both pediatric and adult patients, it was nonetheless informative because the authors found a striking dose threshold; zero of 11 patients treated with an RT dose of less than 50 Gy were alive at 3 years, while 6 of 13 treated with >50 Gy were alive during this same time. A subsequent study by Kim et al. examined a larger group of brainstem tumors, and also found a trend for improved survival in patients treated with greater than 50 Gy of RT to the primary site (Kim et al. 1980).

Another related question was whether altered fractionation schemes would be more advantageous as a means to dose escalate while minimizing normal tissue toxicity for DIPG. Initial studies testing 1 Gy twice daily fractions to 72 Gy were promising (Packer et al. 1993; Edwards et al. 1989). However, further escalation up to 78 Gy in a similar manner suggested there was no clear benefit to this approach over conventionally fractionated RT regimens (Packer et al. 1994; Freeman et al. 1993; Mandell et al. 1999). These data have led to a general consensus that outside of a clinical trial, a standard RT dose for DIPG is 54 Gy in 1.8 or 2 Gy fractions. Most clinicians seek to start RT as soon as possible, after there is sufficient evidence to make a DIPG diagnosis. Interestingly, a recent study reported no effect of the time from diagnosis to the start of RT on EFS or OS in children with DIPG (Pai Panandiker et al. 2014). In recent years, hypofractionated RT regimens have also been proposed for DIPG. In contrast to hyperfractionation as a means to dose escalate RT, these studies were designed to minimize the amount of time that patients spend receiving their actual treatment, given the extremely poor OS for this disease. Results from these studies have suggested that this approach is similar in outcomes to conventionally fractionated RT (Janssens et al. 2009; Janssens et al. 2013; Zaghloul et al. 2014). However, this approach warrants considerable pause and thought within our academic community, as it would essentially represent a palliative approach with no intent for a long-term cure.

As mentioned earlier, most DIPGs are localized to the pons, but they extend radially in all directions. As such, a standard approach for volume delineation in the 3D treatment planning era is to contour the primary tumor as the GTV, followed by a 1 cm CTV expansion to account for microscopic disease. Gross tumor typically is identified as a T2- or FLAIR-based abnormality on the corresponding MRI sequence. A standard PTV margin is then

Opposed Lateral RT Fields   IMRT

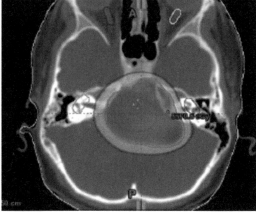

Fig. 3.6 Comparison of RT treatment plans utilizing opposed lateral fields versus IMRT for a DIPG. The minimum dose shown is 4600 cGy (blue shading) for to contrast the differences between the two approaches in these two panels

applied, which ranges between 0.3 and 0.5 cm based on institutional image-guided RT standards. Historically, these tumors were treated with parallel-opposed laterals using large treatment portals (Freeman et al. 1993). However, with the advent and relative ease of 3D conformal- and IMRT-based approaches, many clinicians utilize these more sophisticated techniques for this disease. Indeed, these more conformal approaches can significantly reduce dose to the bilateral cochlea and temporal lobes. A side-by-side comparison of two such RT plans for a patient treated at our institution is shown in Fig. 3.6. The potential for late RT toxicities in this patient population may be less relevant given their poor overall survival, which may raise questions of whether more complicated and expensive treatment modalities should be employed. However, there remains a small subset of patients who survive beyond 1–2 years, either because they are true DIPG outliers, or they actually had a less aggressive tumor (that was never biopsied) (MacDonald 2012). Thus, strong arguments can be made to treat DIPG patients with 3D conformal RT or IMRT, regardless of resource utilization concerns.

Conclusions

The potentially curative applications of radiation therapy in pediatric tumors are often avoided due to the fear of severe late complications, and attempts have been made to omit radiation for young brain tumor patients, even in the face of substantially poorer outcomes. Although the late effects of radiation can lead to profound cognitive and physical changes, advances in neuroimaging and radiation delivery have led to the ability to minimize the risk of late effects in many children. Smaller target volumes, radiation dose reduction with combined chemotherapy use, and more conformal radiation techniques now allow for children to receive localized treatment with the expectation of a good quality of life for many patients. Therefore, delaying or omitting radiation is very reasonable to consider in selected patients, but physicians must weigh the consequence of tumor progression, additional chemotherapeutic agents and surgeries, and the possibility that radiation volumes and dose may increase at the time of eventual treatment if initial radiation is deferred. Additional research is still needed to further decrease late side effects of therapy and improve disease outcomes for children afflicted with brain tumors.

References

Aizer AA, Sethi RV, Hedley-Whyte ET, Ebb D, Tarbell NJ, Yock TI, Macdonald SM (2013) Bifocal intracranial tumors of nongerminomatous germ cell etiology: diagnostic and therapeutic implications. Neuro-Oncology 15(7):955–960. https://doi.org/10.1093/neuonc/not050

Ater JL, Zhou T, Holmes E, Mazewski CM, Booth TN, Freyer DR, Lazarus KH, Packer RJ, Prados M, Sposto R, Vezina G, Wisoff JH, Pollack IF (2012) Randomized study of two chemotherapy regimens for treatment of low-grade glioma in young children: a report from the Children's Oncology Group. J Clin Oncol 30(21):2641–2647. https://doi.org/10.1200/JCO.2011.36.6054

Bahar M, Kordes U, Tekautz T, Wolff J (2015) Radiation therapy for choroid plexus carcinoma patients with Li-Fraumeni syndrome: advantageous or detrimental? Anticancer Res 35(5):3013–3017

Balmaceda C, Heller G, Rosenblum M, Diez B, Villablanca JG, Kellie S, Maher P, Vlamis V, Walker RW, Leibel S, Finlay JL (1996) Chemotherapy without irradiation--a novel approach for newly diagnosed CNS germ cell tumors: results of an international cooperative trial. The first international central nervous system germ cell tumor study. J Clin Oncol 14(11):2908–2915

Baranzelli MC, Patte C, Bouffet E, Couanet D, Habrand JL, Portas M, Lejars O, Lutz P, Le Gall E, Kalifa C (1997) Nonmetastatic intracranial germinoma: the experience of the French Society of Pediatric Oncology. Cancer 80(9):1792–1797

Baranzelli MC, Kramar A, Bouffet E, Quintana E, Rubie H, Edan C, Patte C (1999) Prognostic factors in children with localized malignant nonseminomatous germ cell tumors. J Clin Oncol 17(4):1212

Batra V, Sands SA, Holmes E, Geyer JR, Yates A, Becker L, Burger P, Gilles F, Wisoff J, Allen JC, Pollack IF, Finlay JL (2014) Long-term survival of children less than six years of age enrolled on the CCG-945 phase III trial for newly-diagnosed high-grade glioma: a report from the Children's Oncology Group. Pediatr Blood Cancer 61(1):151–157. https://doi.org/10.1002/pbc.24718

Berger C, Thiesse P, Lellouch-Tubiana A, Kalifa C, Pierre-Kahn A, Bouffet E (1998) Choroid plexus carcinomas in childhood: clinical features and prognostic factors. Neurosurgery 42(3):470–475

Bishop AJ, McDonald MW, Chang AL, Esiashvili N (2012) Infant brain tumors: incidence, survival, and the role of radiation based on Surveillance, Epidemiology, and End Results (SEER) Data. Int J Radiat Oncol Biol Phys 82(1):341–347. https://doi.org/10.1016/j.ijrobp.2010.08.020

Biswas T, Okunieff P, Schell MC, Smudzin T, Pilcher WH, Bakos RS, Vates GE, Walter KA, Wensel A, Korones DN, Milano MT (2009) Stereotactic radiosurgery for glioblastoma: retrospective analysis. Radiat Oncol 4:11. https://doi.org/10.1186/1748-717X-4-11

Boehling NS, Grosshans DR, Bluett JB, Palmer MT, Song X, Amos RA, Sahoo N, Meyer JJ, Mahajan A, Woo SY (2012) Dosimetric comparison of three-dimensional conformal proton radiotherapy, intensity-modulated proton therapy, and intensity-modulated radiotherapy for treatment of pediatric craniopharyngiomas. Int J Radiat Oncol Biol Phys 82(2):643–652. https://doi.org/10.1016/j.ijrobp.2010.11.027

Bouffet E, Raquin M, Doz F, Gentet JC, Rodary C, Demeocq F, Chastagner P, Lutz P, Hartmann O, Kalifa C (2000) Radiotherapy followed by high dose busulfan and thiotepa: a prospective assessment of high dose chemotherapy in children with diffuse pontine gliomas. Cancer 88(3):685–692

Brodin NP, Munck Af Rosenschold P, Aznar MC, Kiil-Berthelsen A, Vogelius IR, Nilsson P, Lannering B, Bjork-Eriksson T (2011) Radiobiological risk estimates of adverse events and secondary cancer for proton and photon radiation therapy of pediatric medulloblastoma. Acta Oncol 50(6):806–816. https://doi.org/10.3109/0284186X.2011.582514

Brown HG, Kepner JL, Perlman EJ, Friedman HS, Strother DR, Duffner PK, Kun LE, Goldthwaite PT, Burger PC (2000) "Large cell/anaplastic" medulloblastomas: a Pediatric Oncology Group Study. J Neuropathol Exp Neurol 59(10):857–865

Buczkowicz P, Bartels U, Bouffet E, Becher O, Hawkins C (2014) Histopathological spectrum of paediatric diffuse intrinsic pontine glioma: diagnostic and therapeutic implications. Acta Neuropathol 128(4):573–581. https://doi.org/10.1007/s00401-014-1319-6

Burger PC, Yu IT, Tihan T, Friedman HS, Strother DR, Kepner JL, Duffner PK, Kun LE, Perlman EJ (1998) Atypical teratoid/rhabdoid tumor of the central nervous system: a highly malignant tumor of infancy and childhood frequently mistaken for medulloblastoma: a Pediatric Oncology Group study. Am J Surg Pathol 22(9):1083–1092

Buscariollo DL, Park HS, Roberts KB, Yu JB (2012) Survival outcomes in atypical teratoid rhabdoid tumor for patients undergoing radiotherapy in a surveillance, epidemiology, and end results analysis. Cancer 118(17):4212–4219. https://doi.org/10.1002/cncr.27373

Calaminus G, Frappaz D, Kortmann RD et al (2017) Outcome of patients with intracranial non-germinomatous germ cell tumors-lessons from the SIOP-CNS-GCT-96 trial. Neuro Oncol 19(12):1661–1672

Carpentieri SC, Waber DP, Scott RM, Goumnerova LC, Kieran MW, Cohen LE, Kim F, Billett AL, Tarbell NJ, Pomeroy SL (2001) Memory deficits among children with craniopharyngiomas. Neurosurgery 49(5):1053–1057. discussion 1057–1058

Cavazzuti V, Fischer EG, Welch K, Belli JA, Winston KR (1983) Neurological and psychophysiological sequelae following different treatments of craniopharyngioma in children. J Neurosurg 59(3):409–417. https://doi.org/10.3171/jns.1983.59.3.0409

CBTRUS Statistical Report: Primary Brain and Central Nervous System Tumors Diagnosed in the United

States in 2004–2008 (2012) Central brain tumor registry of the United States. www.cbtrus.com

Chang TK, Wong TT, Hwang B (1995) Combination chemotherapy with vinblastine, bleomycin, cisplatin, and etoposide (VBPE) in children with primary intracranial germ cell tumors. Med Pediatr Oncol 24(6):368–372

Chassot A, Canale S, Varlet P, Puget S, Roujeau T, Negretti L, Dhermain F, Rialland X, Raquin MA, Grill J, Dufour C (2012) Radiotherapy with concurrent and adjuvant temozolomide in children with newly diagnosed diffuse intrinsic pontine glioma. J Neuro-Oncol 106(2):399–407. https://doi.org/10.1007/s11060-011-0681-7

Chi SN, Zimmerman MA, Yao X, Cohen KJ, Burger P, Biegel JA, Rorke-Adams LB, Fisher MJ, Janss A, Mazewski C, Goldman S, Manley PE, Bowers DC, Bendel A, Rubin J, Turner CD, Marcus KJ, Goumnerova L, Ullrich NJ, Kieran MW (2009) Intensive multimodality treatment for children with newly diagnosed CNS atypical teratoid rhabdoid tumor. J Clin Oncol 27(3):385–389. https://doi.org/10.1200/JCO.2008.18.7724

Chiang KL, Chang KP, Lee YY, Huang PI, Hsu TR, Chen YW, Chang FC, Wong TT (2010) Role of temozolomide in the treatment of newly diagnosed diffuse brainstem glioma in children: experience at a single institution. Childs Nerv Syst 26(8):1035–1041. https://doi.org/10.1007/s00381-010-1106-1

Childs SK, Kozak KR, Friedmann AM, Yeap BY, Adams J, MacDonald SM, Liebsch NJ, Tarbell NJ, Yock TI (2012) Proton radiotherapy for parameningeal rhabdomyosarcoma: clinical outcomes and late effects. Int J Radiat Oncol Biol Phys 82(2):635–642. https://doi.org/10.1016/j.ijrobp.2010.11.048

Cho YJ, Tsherniak A, Tamayo P, Santagata S, Ligon A, Greulich H, Berhoukim R, Amani V, Goumnerova L, Eberhart CG, Lau CC, Olson JM, Gilbertson RJ, Gajjar A, Delattre O, Kool M, Ligon K, Meyerson M, Mesirov JP, Pomeroy SL (2011) Integrative genomic analysis of medulloblastoma identifies a molecular subgroup that drives poor clinical outcome. J Clin Oncol 29(11):1424–1430. https://doi.org/10.1200/JCO.2010.28.5148

Clopper RR, Meyer WJ 3rd, Udvarhelyi GB, Money J, Aarabi B, Mulvihill JJ, Piasio M (1977) Postsurgical IQ and behavioral data on twenty patients with a history of childhood craniopharyngioma. Psychoneuroendocrinology 2(4):365–372

Cohen BH, Zeltzer PM, Boyett JM, Geyer JR, Allen JC, Finlay JL, McGuire-Cullen P, Milstein JM, Rorke LB, Stanley P et al (1995) Prognostic factors and treatment results for supratentorial primitive neuroectodermal tumors in children using radiation and chemotherapy: a Children's Cancer Group randomized trial. J Clin Oncol 13(7):1687–1696

Cohen KJ, Heideman RL, Zhou T, Holmes EJ, Lavey RS, Bouffet E, Pollack IF (2011a) Temozolomide in the treatment of children with newly diagnosed diffuse intrinsic pontine gliomas: a report from the Children's Oncology Group. Neuro-Oncology 13(4):410–416. https://doi.org/10.1093/neuonc/noq205

Cohen KJ, Pollack IF, Zhou T, Buxton A, Holmes EJ, Burger PC, Brat DJ, Rosenblum MK, Hamilton RL, Lavey RS, Heideman RL (2011b) Temozolomide in the treatment of high-grade gliomas in children: a report from the Children's Oncology Group. Neuro-Oncology 13(3):317–323. https://doi.org/10.1093/neuonc/noq191

Conklin HM, Li C, Xiong X, Ogg RJ, Merchant TE (2008) Predicting change in academic abilities after conformal radiation therapy for localized ependymoma. J Clin Oncol 26(24):3965–3970. https://doi.org/10.1200/JCO.2007.15.9970

Cotter SE, Herrup DA, Friedmann A, Macdonald SM, Pieretti RV, Robinson G, Adams J, Tarbell NJ, Yock TI (2011) Proton radiotherapy for pediatric bladder/prostate rhabdomyosarcoma: clinical outcomes and dosimetry compared to intensity-modulated radiation therapy. Int J Radiat Oncol Biol Phys 81(5):1367–1373. https://doi.org/10.1016/j.ijrobp.2010.07.1989

De Amorim Bernstein K, Sethi R, Trofimov A, Zeng C, Fullerton B, Yeap BY, Ebb D, Tarbell NJ, Yock TI, MacDonald SM (2013) Early clinical outcomes using proton radiation for children with central nervous system atypical teratoid rhabdoid tumors. Int J Radiat Oncol Biol Phys 86(1):114–120. https://doi.org/10.1016/j.ijrobp.2012.12.004

De Vile CJ, Grant DB, Kendall BE, Neville BG, Stanhope R, Watkins KE, Hayward RD (1996) Management of childhood craniopharyngioma: can the morbidity of radical surgery be predicted? J Neurosurg 85(1):73–81. https://doi.org/10.3171/jns.1996.85.1.0073

Dearnaley DP, A'Hern RP, Whittaker S, Bloom HJ (1990) Pineal and CNS germ cell tumors: Royal Marsden Hospital experience 1962–1987. Int J Radiat Oncol Biol Phys 18(4):773–781

DeLaney TF, Park L, Goldberg SI, Hug EB, Liebsch NJ, Munzenrider JE, Suit HD (2005) Radiotherapy for local control of osteosarcoma. Int J Radiat Oncol Biol Phys 61(2):492–498. https://doi.org/10.1016/j.ijrobp.2004.05.051

Dhall G, Grodman H, Ji L, Sands S, Gardner S, Dunkel IJ, McCowage GB, Diez B, Allen JC, Gopalan A, Cornelius AS, Termuhlen A, Abromowitch M, Sposto R, Finlay JL (2008) Outcome of children less than three years old at diagnosis with non-metastatic medulloblastoma treated with chemotherapy on the "head start" I and II protocols. Pediatr Blood Cancer 50(6):1169–1175. https://doi.org/10.1002/pbc.21525

Di Pinto M, Conklin HM, Li C, Xiong X, Merchant TE (2010) Investigating verbal and visual auditory learning after conformal radiation therapy for childhood ependymoma. Int J Radiat Oncol Biol Phys 77(4):1002–1008. https://doi.org/10.1016/j.ijrobp.2009.06.003

Donahue B, Allen J, Siffert J, Rosovsky M, Pinto R (1998) Patterns of recurrence in brain stem gliomas: evidence for craniospinal dissemination. Int J Radiat Oncol Biol Phys 40(3):677–680

Douglas JG, Barker JL, Ellenbogen RG, Geyer JR (2004) Concurrent chemotherapy and reduced-dose cranial spinal irradiation followed by conformal posterior fossa tumor bed boost for average-risk medulloblastoma: efficacy and patterns of failure. Int J Radiat Oncol Biol Phys 58(4):1161–1164. https://doi.org/10.1016/j.ijrobp.2003.09.010

Duffner PK, Horowitz ME, Krischer JP, Friedman HS, Burger PC, Cohen ME, Sanford RA, Mulhern RK, James HE, Freeman CR et al (1993) Postoperative chemotherapy and delayed radiation in children less than three years of age with malignant brain tumors. N Engl J Med 328(24):1725–1731. https://doi.org/10.1056/NEJM199306173282401

Duffner PK, Cohen ME, Sanford RA, Horowitz ME, Krischer JP, Burger PC, Friedman HS, Kun LE (1995) Lack of efficacy of postoperative chemotherapy and delayed radiation in very young children with pineoblastoma. Pediatric Oncology Group. Med Pediatr Oncol 25(1):38–44

Dunkel IJ, Garvin JH Jr, Goldman S, Ettinger LJ, Kaplan AM, Cairo M, Li H, Boyett JM, Finlay JL (1998) High dose chemotherapy with autologous bone marrow rescue for children with diffuse pontine brain stem tumors. Children's cancer group. J Neuro-Oncol 37(1):67–73

Edwards MS, Wara WM, Urtasun RC, Prados M, Levin VA, Fulton D, Wilson CB, Hannigan J, Silver P (1989) Hyperfractionated radiation therapy for brain-stem glioma: a phase I–II trial. J Neurosurg 70(5):691–700. https://doi.org/10.3171/jns.1989.70.5.0691

Eom KY, Kim IH, Park CI, Kim HJ, Kim JH, Kim K, Kim SK, Wang KC, Cho BG, Jung HW, Heo DS, Kang HJ, Shin HY, Ahn HS (2008) Upfront chemotherapy and involved-field radiotherapy results in more relapses than extended radiotherapy for intracranial germinomas: modification in radiotherapy volume might be needed. Int J Radiat Oncol Biol Phys 71(3):667–671. https://doi.org/10.1016/j.ijrobp.2008.01.061

Erkal HS, Serin M, Cakmak A (1997) Management of optic pathway and chiasmatic-hypothalamic gliomas in children with radiation therapy. Radiother Oncol 45(1):11–15

Fahlbusch R, Honegger J, Paulus W, Huk W, Buchfelder M (1999) Surgical treatment of craniopharyngiomas: experience with 168 patients. J Neurosurg 90(2):237–250. https://doi.org/10.3171/jns.1999.90.2.0237

Fallai C, Olmi P (1997) Hyperfractionated and accelerated radiation therapy in central nervous system tumors (malignant gliomas, pediatric tumors, and brain metastases). Radiother Oncol 43(3):235–246

Fangusaro J (2012) Pediatric high grade glioma: a review and update on tumor clinical characteristics and biology. Front Oncol 2:105. https://doi.org/10.3389/fonc.2012.00105

Fangusaro J, Warren KE (2013) Unclear standard of care for pediatric high grade glioma patients. J Neuro-Oncol 113(2):341–342. https://doi.org/10.1007/s11060-013-1104-8

Finlay JL, Zacharoulis S (2005) The treatment of high grade gliomas and diffuse intrinsic pontine tumors of childhood and adolescence: a historical - and futuristic - perspective. J Neuro-Oncol 75(3):253–266. https://doi.org/10.1007/s11060-005-6747-7

Finlay JL, Boyett JM, Yates AJ, Wisoff JH, Milstein JM, Geyer JR, Bertolone SJ, McGuire P, Cherlow JM, Tefft M et al (1995) Randomized phase III trial in childhood high-grade astrocytoma comparing vincristine, lomustine, and prednisone with the eight-drugs-in-1-day regimen. Children's Cancer Group. J Clin Oncol 13(1):112–123

Finlay J, da Silva NS, Lavey R, Bouffet E, Kellie SJ, Shaw E, Saran F, Matsutani M (2008) The management of patients with primary central nervous system (CNS) germinoma: current controversies requiring resolution. Pediatr Blood Cancer 51(2):313–316. https://doi.org/10.1002/pbc.21555

Fisher BJ, Leighton CC, Vujovic O, Macdonald DR, Stitt L (2001) Results of a policy of surveillance alone after surgical management of pediatric low grade gliomas. Int J Radiat Oncol Biol Phys 51(3):704–710

Fisher PG, Tihan T, Goldthwaite PT, Wharam MD, Carson BS, Weingart JD, Repka MX, Cohen KJ, Burger PC (2008) Outcome analysis of childhood low-grade astrocytomas. Pediatr Blood Cancer 51(2):245–250. https://doi.org/10.1002/pbc.21563

Fitzek MM, Linggood RM, Adams J, Munzenrider JE (2006) Combined proton and photon irradiation for craniopharyngioma: long-term results of the early cohort of patients treated at Harvard cyclotron laboratory and Massachusetts General Hospital. Int J Radiat Oncol Biol Phys 64(5):1348–1354. https://doi.org/10.1016/j.ijrobp.2005.09.034

Fitzpatrick LK, Aronson LJ, Cohen KJ (2002) Is there a requirement for adjuvant therapy for choroid plexus carcinoma that has been completely resected? J Neuro-Oncol 57(2):123–126

Fouladi M, Grant R, Baruchel S, Chan H, Malkin D, Weitzman S, Greenberg ML (1998) Comparison of survival outcomes in patients with intracranial germinomas treated with radiation alone versus reduced-dose radiation and chemotherapy. Childs Nerv Syst 14(10):596–601. https://doi.org/10.1007/s003810050279

Freeman CR, Krischer JP, Sanford RA, Cohen ME, Burger PC, del Carpio R, Halperin EC, Munoz L, Friedman HS, Kun LE (1993) Final results of a study of escalating doses of hyperfractionated radiotherapy in brain stem tumors in children: a Pediatric oncology group study. Int J Radiat Oncol Biol Phys 27(2):197–206

Gaffney CC, Sloane JP, Bradley NJ, Bloom HJ (1985) Primitive neuroectodermal tumours of the cerebrum. Pathology and treatment. J Neuro-Oncol 3(1):23–33

Gajjar A, Sanford RA, Heideman R, Jenkins JJ, Walter A, Li Y, Langston JW, Muhlbauer M, Boyett JM, Kun LE (1997) Low-grade astrocytoma: a decade of experience at St. Jude Children's Research Hospital. J Clin Oncol 15(8):2792–2799

Gardner SL, Asgharzadeh S, Green A, Horn B, McCowage G, Finlay J (2008) Intensive induction chemotherapy followed by high dose chemotherapy with autologous hematopoietic progenitor cell rescue in young children newly diagnosed with central nervous system atypical teratoid rhabdoid tumors. Pediatr Blood Cancer 51(2):235–240. https://doi.org/10.1002/pbc.21578

Geyer JR, Sposto R, Jennings M, Boyett JM, Axtell RA, Breiger D, Broxson E, Donahue B, Finlay JL, Goldwein JW, Heier LA, Johnson D, Mazewski C, Miller DC, Packer R, Puccetti D, Radcliffe J, Tao ML, Shiminski-Maher T (2005) Multiagent chemotherapy and deferred radiotherapy in infants with malignant brain tumors: a report from the Children's Cancer Group. J Clin Oncol 23(30):7621–7631. https://doi.org/10.1200/JCO.2005.09.095

Gilbert MR, Dignam JJ, Armstrong TS, Wefel JS, Blumenthal DT, Vogelbaum MA, Colman H, Chakravarti A, Pugh S, Won M, Jeraj R, Brown PD, Jaeckle KA, Schiff D, Stieber VW, Brachman DG, Werner-Wasik M, Tremont-Lukats IW, Sulman EP, Aldape KD, Curran WJ Jr, Mehta MP (2014) A randomized trial of bevacizumab for newly diagnosed glioblastoma. N Engl J Med 370(8):699–708. https://doi.org/10.1056/NEJMoa1308573

Goldman S, Bouffet E, Fisher PG, Allen JC, Robertson PL, Chuba PJ, Donahue B, Kretschmar CS, Zhou T, Buxton AB, Pollack IF (2015) Phase II trial assessing the ability of neoadjuvant chemotherapy with or without second-look surgery to eliminate measurable disease for nongerminomatous germ cell tumors: a Children's Oncology Group Study. J Clin Oncol 33(22):2464–2471. https://doi.org/10.1200/JCO.2014.59.5132

Goldwein JW, Leahy JM, Packer RJ, Sutton LN, Curran WJ, Rorke LB, Schut L, Littman PS, D'Angio GJ (1990) Intracranial ependymomas in children. Int J Radiat Oncol Biol Phys 19(6):1497–1502

Goldwein JW, Radcliffe J, Johnson J, Moshang T, Packer RJ, Sutton LN, Rorke LB, D'Angio GJ (1996) Updated results of a pilot study of low dose craniospinal irradiation plus chemotherapy for children under five with cerebellar primitive neuroectodermal tumors (medulloblastoma). Int J Radiat Oncol Biol Phys 34(4):899–904

Grabenbauer GG, Schuchardt U, Buchfelder M, Rodel CM, Gusek G, Marx M, Doerr HG, Fahlbusch R, Huk WJ, Wenzel D, Sauer R (2000) Radiation therapy of optico-hypothalamic gliomas (OHG)--radiographic response, vision and late toxicity. Radiother Oncol 54(3):239–245

Gray ST, Chen YL, Lin DT (2009) Efficacy of proton beam therapy in the treatment of Ewing's sarcoma of the paranasal sinuses and anterior skull base. Skull Base 19(6):409–416. https://doi.org/10.1055/s-0029-1220207

Greenberger BA, Pulsifer MB, Ebb DH, MacDonald SM, Jones RM, Butler WE, Huang MS, Marcus KJ, Oberg JA, Tarbell NJ, Yock TI (2014) Clinical outcomes and late endocrine, neurocognitive, and visual profiles of proton radiation for pediatric low-grade gliomas. Int J Radiat Oncol Biol Phys 89(5):1060–1068. https://doi.org/10.1016/j.ijrobp.2014.04.053

Grigsby PW, Garcia DM, Ghiselli R (1989) Analysis of autopsy findings in patients treated with irradiation for thalamic and brain stem tumors. Am J Clin Oncol 12(3):255–258

Haberler C, Laggner U, Slavc I, Czech T, Ambros IM, Ambros PF, Budka H, Hainfellner JA (2006) Immunohistochemical analysis of INI1 protein in malignant pediatric CNS tumors: lack of INI1 in atypical teratoid/rhabdoid tumors and in a fraction of primitive neuroectodermal tumors without rhabdoid phenotype. Am J Surg Pathol 30(11):1462–1468. https://doi.org/10.1097/01.pas.0000213329.71745.ef

Halperin EC, Bentel G, Heinz ER, Burger PC (1989) Radiation therapy treatment planning in supratentorial glioblastoma multiforme: an analysis based on post mortem topographic anatomy with CT correlations. Int J Radiat Oncol Biol Phys 17(6):1347–1350

Hancock SL, McDougall IR, Constine LS (1995) Thyroid abnormalities after therapeutic external radiation. Int J Radiat Oncol Biol Phys 31(5):1165–1170

Hetelekidis S, Barnes PD, Tao ML, Fischer EG, Schneider L, Scott RM, Tarbell NJ (1993) 20-year experience in childhood craniopharyngioma. Int J Radiat Oncol Biol Phys 27(2):189–195

Hilden JM, Watterson J, Longee DC, Moertel CL, Dunn ME, Kurtzberg J, Scheithauer BW (1998) Central nervous system atypical teratoid tumor/rhabdoid tumor: response to intensive therapy and review of the literature. J Neuro-Oncol 40(3):265–275

Hilden JM, Meerbaum S, Burger P, Finlay J, Janss A, Scheithauer BW, Walter AW, Rorke LB, Biegel JA (2004) Central nervous system atypical teratoid/rhabdoid tumor: results of therapy in children enrolled in a registry. J Clin Oncol 22(14):2877–2884. https://doi.org/10.1200/JCO.2004.07.073

Hoffman HJ, Otsubo H, Hendrick EB, Humphreys RP, Drake JM, Becker LE, Greenberg M, Jenkin D (1991) Intracranial germ-cell tumors in children. J Neurosurg 74(4):545–551. https://doi.org/10.3171/jns.1991.74.4.0545

Hoffman HJ, De Silva M, Humphreys RP, Drake JM, Smith ML, Blaser SI (1992) Aggressive surgical management of craniopharyngiomas in children. J Neurosurg 76(1):47–52. https://doi.org/10.3171/jns.1992.76.1.0047

Huse JT, Rosenblum MK (2015) The emerging molecular foundations of pediatric brain tumors. J Child Neurol. https://doi.org/10.1177/0883073815579709

Jaing TH, Wang HS, Tsay PK, Tseng CK, Jung SM, Lin KL, Lui TN (2004) Multivariate analysis of clinical prognostic factors in children with intracranial ependymomas. J Neuro-Oncol 68(3):255–261

Jakacki RI (1999) Pineal and nonpineal supratentorial primitive neuroectodermal tumors. Childs Nerv Syst 15(10):586–591. https://doi.org/10.1007/s003810050547

Jakacki RI, Zeltzer PM, Boyett JM, Albright AL, Allen JC, Geyer JR, Rorke LB, Stanley P, Stevens KR, Wisoff J et al (1995) Survival and prognostic factors following radiation and/or chemotherapy for primitive neuroectodermal tumors of the pineal region in infants and children: a report of the Children's Cancer Group. J Clin Oncol 13(6):1377–1383

Jalali R, Raut N, Arora B, Gupta T, Dutta D, Munshi A, Sarin R, Kurkure P (2010) Prospective evaluation of radiotherapy with concurrent and adjuvant temozolomide in children with newly diagnosed diffuse intrinsic pontine glioma. Int J Radiat Oncol Biol Phys 77(1):113–118. https://doi.org/10.1016/j.ijrobp.2009.04.031

Jansen MH, van Vuurden DG, Vandertop WP, Kaspers GJ (2012) Diffuse intrinsic pontine gliomas: a systematic update on clinical trials and biology. Cancer Treat Rev 38(1):27–35. https://doi.org/10.1016/j.ctrv.2011.06.007

Janssens GO, Gidding CE, Van Lindert EJ, Oldenburger FR, Erasmus CE, Schouten-Meeteren AY, Kaanders JH (2009) The role of hypofractionation radiotherapy for diffuse intrinsic brainstem glioma in children: a pilot study. Int J Radiat Oncol Biol Phys 73(3):722–726. https://doi.org/10.1016/j.ijrobp.2008.05.030

Janssens GO, Jansen MH, Lauwers SJ, Nowak PJ, Oldenburger FR, Bouffet E, Saran F, Kamphuis-van Ulzen K, van Lindert EJ, Schieving JH, Boterberg T, Kaspers GJ, Span PN, Kaanders JH, Gidding CE, Hargrave D (2013) Hypofractionation vs conventional radiation therapy for newly diagnosed diffuse intrinsic pontine glioma: a matched-cohort analysis. Int J Radiat Oncol Biol Phys 85(2):315–320. https://doi.org/10.1016/j.ijrobp.2012.04.006

Jenkin RD, Boesel C, Ertel I, Evans A, Hittle R, Ortega J, Sposto R, Wara W, Wilson C, Anderson J et al (1987) Brain-stem tumors in childhood: a prospective randomized trial of irradiation with and without adjuvant CCNU, VCR, and prednisone. A report of the Children's Cancer Study Group. J Neurosurg 66(2):227–233. https://doi.org/10.3171/jns.1987.66.2.0227

Jennings MT, Gelman R, Hochberg F (1985) Intracranial germ-cell tumors: natural history and pathogenesis. J Neurosurg 63(2):155–167. https://doi.org/10.3171/jns.1985.63.2.0155

Jennings MT, Sposto R, Boyett JM, Vezina LG, Holmes E, Berger MS, Bruggers CS, Bruner JM, Chan KW, Dusenbery KE, Ettinger LJ, Fitz CR, Lafond D, Mandelbaum DE, Massey V, McGuire W, McNeely L, Moulton T, Pollack IF, Shen V (2002) Preradiation chemotherapy in primary high-risk brainstem tumors: phase II study CCG-9941 of the Children's Cancer Group. J Clin Oncol 20(16):3431–3437

Jones DT, Jager N, Kool M, Zichner T, Hutter B, Sultan M, Cho YJ, Pugh TJ, Hovestadt V, Stutz AM, Rausch T, Warnatz HJ, Ryzhova M, Bender S, Sturm D, Pleier S, Cin H, Pfaff E, Sieber L, Wittmann A, Remke M, Witt H, Hutter S, Tzaridis T, Weischenfeldt J, Raeder B, Avci M, Amstislavskiy V, Zapatka M, Weber UD, Wang Q, Lasitschka B, Bartholomae CC, Schmidt M, von Kalle C, Ast V, Lawerenz C, Eils J, Kabbe R, Benes V, van Sluis P, Koster J, Volckmann R, Shih D, Betts MJ, Russell RB, Coco S, Tonini GP, Schuller U, Hans V, Graf N, Kim YJ, Monoranu C, Roggendorf W, Unterberg A, Herold-Mende C, Milde T, Kulozik AE, von Deimling A, Witt O, Maass E, Rossler J, Ebinger M, Schuhmann MU, Fruhwald MC, Hasselblatt M, Jabado N, Rutkowski S, von Bueren AO, Williamson D, Clifford SC, McCabe MG, Collins VP, Wolf S, Wiemann S, Lehrach H, Brors B, Scheurlen W, Felsberg J, Reifenberger G, Northcott PA, Taylor MD, Meyerson M, Pomeroy SL, Yaspo ML, Korbel JO, Korshunov A, Eils R, Pfister SM, Lichter P (2012) Dissecting the genomic complexity underlying medulloblastoma. Nature 488 (7409):100–105 https://doi.org/10.1038/nature11284

Khatua S, Dhall G, O'Neil S, Jubran R, Villablanca JG, Marachelian A, Nastia A, Lavey R, Olch AJ, Gonzalez I, Gilles F, Nelson M, Panigrahy A, McComb G, Krieger M, Fan J, Sposto R, Finlay JL (2010) Treatment of primary CNS germinomatous germ cell tumors with chemotherapy prior to reduced dose whole ventricular and local boost irradiation. Pediatr Blood Cancer 55(1):42–46. https://doi.org/10.1002/pbc.22468

Kim TH, Chin HW, Pollan S, Hazel JH, Webster JH (1980) Radiotherapy of primary brain stem tumors. Int J Radiat Oncol Biol Phys 6(1):51–57

Kleihues P, Louis DN, Scheithauer BW, Rorke LB, Reifenberger G, Burger PC, Cavenee WK (2002) The WHO classification of tumors of the nervous system. J Neuropathol Exp Neurol 61(3):215–225. discussion 226–219

Koshy M, Rich S, Merchant TE, Mahmood U, Regine WF, Kwok Y (2011) Post-operative radiation improves survival in children younger than 3 years with intracranial ependymoma. J Neuro-Oncol 105(3):583–590. https://doi.org/10.1007/s11060-011-0624-3

Kramm CM, Butenhoff S, Rausche U, Warmuth-Metz M, Kortmann RD, Pietsch T, Gnekow A, Jorch N, Janssen G, Berthold F, Wolff JE (2011) Thalamic high-grade gliomas in children: a distinct clinical subset? Neuro-Oncology 13(6):680–689. https://doi.org/10.1093/neuonc/nor045

Kretschmar C, Kleinberg L, Greenberg M, Burger P, Holmes E, Wharam M (2007) Pre-radiation chemotherapy with response-based radiation therapy in children with central nervous system germ cell tumors: a report from the Children's Oncology Group. Pediatr Blood Cancer 48(3):285–291. https://doi.org/10.1002/pbc.20815

Ladra MM, Szymonifka JD, Mahajan A, Friedmann AM, Yong Yeap B, Goebel CP, MacDonald SM, Grosshans DR, Rodriguez-Galindo C, Marcus KJ, Tarbell NJ, Yock TI (2014) Preliminary results of a phase II trial of proton radiotherapy for pediatric rhabdomyosarcoma. J Clin Oncol 32(33):3762–3770. https://doi.org/10.1200/JCO.2014.56.1548

Lafay-Cousin L, Millar BA, Mabbott D, Spiegler B, Drake J, Bartels U, Huang A, Bouffet E (2006) Limited-field radiation for bifocal germinoma. Int J Radiat Oncol Biol Phys 65(2):486–492. https://doi.org/10.1016/j.ijrobp.2005.12.011

Laigle-Donadey F, Doz F, Delattre JY (2008) Brainstem gliomas in children and adults. Curr Opin Oncol 20(6):662–667. https://doi.org/10.1097/CCO.0b013e32831186e0

Langmoen IA, Lundar T, Storm-Mathisen I, Lie SO, Hovind KH (1991) Management of pediatric pontine gliomas. Childs Nerv Syst 7(1):13–15

Leary SE, Zhou T, Holmes E, Geyer JR, Miller DC (2011) Histology predicts a favorable outcome in young children with desmoplastic medulloblastoma: a report from the Children's Oncology Group. Cancer 117(14):3262–3267. https://doi.org/10.1002/cncr.25856

Lee F (1975) Radiation of infratentorial and supratentorial brain-stem tumors. J Neurosurg 43(1):65–68. https://doi.org/10.3171/jns.1975.43.1.0065

Lomax AJ, Bortfeld T, Goitein G, Debus J, Dykstra C, Tercier PA, Coucke PA, Mirimanoff RO (1999) A treatment planning inter-comparison of proton and intensity modulated photon radiotherapy. Radiother Oncol 51(3):257–271

Louis DN, Ohgaki H, Wiestler OD, Cavenee WK, Burger PC, Jouvet A, Scheithauer BW, Kleihues P (2007) The 2007 WHO classification of tumours of the central nervous system. Acta Neuropathol 114(2):97–109. https://doi.org/10.1007/s00401-007-0243-4

MacDonald TJ (2012) Diffuse intrinsic pontine glioma (DIPG): time to biopsy again? Pediatr Blood Cancer 58(4):487–488. https://doi.org/10.1002/pbc.24090

MacDonald TJ, Arenson EB, Ater J, Sposto R, Bevan HE, Bruner J, Deutsch M, Kurczynski E, Luerssen T, McGuire-Cullen P, O'Brien R, Shah N, Steinbok P, Strain J, Thomson J, Holmes E, Vezina G, Yates A, Phillips P, Packer R (2005) Phase II study of high-dose chemotherapy before radiation in children with newly diagnosed high-grade astrocytoma: final analysis of Children's Cancer Group Study 9933. Cancer 104(12):2862–2871. https://doi.org/10.1002/cncr.21593

MacDonald SM, DeLaney TF, Loeffler JS (2006) Proton beam radiation therapy. Cancer Investig 24(2):199–208. https://doi.org/10.1080/07357900500524751

MacDonald SM, Safai S, Trofimov A, Wolfgang J, Fullerton B, Yeap BY, Bortfeld T, Tarbell NJ, Yock T (2008) Proton radiotherapy for childhood ependymoma: initial clinical outcomes and dose comparisons. Int J Radiat Oncol Biol Phys 71(4):979–986. https://doi.org/10.1016/j.ijrobp.2007.11.065

MacDonald SM, Trofimov A, Safai S, Adams J, Fullerton B, Ebb D, Tarbell NJ, Yock TI (2011) Proton radiotherapy for pediatric central nervous system germ cell tumors: early clinical outcomes. Int J Radiat Oncol Biol Phys 79(1):121–129. https://doi.org/10.1016/j.ijrobp.2009.10.069

MacDonald SM, Sethi R, Lavally B, Yeap BY, Marcus KJ, Caruso P, Pulsifer M, Huang M, Ebb D, Tarbell NJ, Yock TI (2013) Proton radiotherapy for pediatric central nervous system ependymoma: clinical outcomes for 70 patients. Neuro-Oncology 15(11):1552–1559. https://doi.org/10.1093/neuonc/not121

Mandell LR, Kadota R, Freeman C, Douglass EC, Fontanesi J, Cohen ME, Kovnar E, Burger P, Sanford RA, Kepner J, Friedman H, Kun LE (1999) There is no role for hyperfractionated radiotherapy in the management of children with newly diagnosed diffuse intrinsic brainstem tumors: results of a Pediatric oncology group phase III trial comparing conventional vs. hyperfractionated radiotherapy. Int J Radiat Oncol Biol Phys 43(5):959–964

Mansur DB, Perry A, Rajaram V, Michalski JM, Park TS, Leonard JR, Luchtman-Jones L, Rich KM, Grigsby PW, Lockett MA, Wahab SH, Simpson JR (2005) Postoperative radiation therapy for grade II and III intracranial ependymoma. Int J Radiat Oncol Biol Phys 61(2):387–391. https://doi.org/10.1016/j.ijrobp.2004.06.002

Marcus KJ, Goumnerova L, Billett AL, Lavally B, Scott RM, Bishop K, Xu R, Young Poussaint T, Kieran M, Kooy H, Pomeroy SL, Tarbell NJ (2005) Stereotactic radiotherapy for localized low-grade gliomas in children: final results of a prospective trial. Int J Radiat Oncol Biol Phys 61(2):374–379. https://doi.org/10.1016/j.ijrobp.2004.06.012

Matsutani M, Takakura K, Sano K (1987) Primary intracranial germ cell tumors: pathology and treatment. Prog Exp Tumor Res 30:307–312

Matsutani M, Sano K, Takakura K, Fujimaki T, Nakamura O, Funata N, Seto T (1997) Primary intracranial germ cell tumors: a clinical analysis of 153 histologically verified cases. J Neurosurg 86(3):446–455. https://doi.org/10.3171/jns.1997.86.3.0446

Matsutani M, Ushio Y, Abe H, Yamashita J, Shibui S, Fujimaki T, Takakura K, Nomura K, Tanaka R, Fukui M, Yoshimoto T, Hayakawa T, Nagashima T, Kurisu K, Kayama T (1998) Combined chemotherapy and radiation therapy for central nervous system germ cell tumors: preliminary results of a phase II study of the Japanese Pediatric brain tumor study group. Neurosurg Focus 5(1):e7

Mazloom A, Wolff JE, Paulino AC (2010) The impact of radiotherapy fields in the treatment of patients with choroid plexus carcinoma. Int J Radiat Oncol Biol Phys 78(1):79–84. https://doi.org/10.1016/j.ijrobp.2009.07.1701

McGovern SL, Okcu MF, Munsell MF, Kumbalasseriyil N, Grosshans DR, McAleer MF, Chintagumpala M, Khatua S, Mahajan A (2014) Outcomes and acute toxicities of proton therapy for pediatric atypical teratoid/rhabdoid tumor of the central nervous system. Int J Radiat Oncol Biol Phys 90(5):1143–1152. https://doi.org/10.1016/j.ijrobp.2014.08.354

Merchant TE (2009) Three-dimensional conformal radiation therapy for ependymoma. Childs Nerv Syst 25(10):1261–1268. https://doi.org/10.1007/s00381-009-0892-9

Merchant TE, Fouladi M (2005) Ependymoma: new therapeutic approaches including radiation and chemotherapy. J Neuro-Oncol 75(3):287–299

Merchant TE, Haida T, Wang MH, Finlay JL, Leibel SA (1997) Anaplastic ependymoma: treatment of pediatric patients with or without craniospinal radiation therapy. J Neurosurg 86(6):943–949. https://doi.org/10.3171/jns.1997.86.6.0943

Merchant TE, Happersett L, Finlay JL, Leibel SA (1999) Preliminary results of conformal radiation therapy for medulloblastoma. Neuro-Oncology 1(3):177–187

Merchant TE, Goloubeva O, Pritchard DL, Gaber MW, Xiong X, Danish RK, Lustig RH (2002a) Radiation dose-volume effects on growth hormone secretion. Int J Radiat Oncol Biol Phys 52(5):1264–1270

Merchant TE, Kiehna EN, Sanford RA, Mulhern RK, Thompson SJ, Wilson MW, Lustig RH, Kun LE (2002b) Craniopharyngioma: the St. Jude Children's Research Hospital experience 1984–2001. Int J Radiat Oncol Biol Phys 53(3):533–542

Merchant TE, Gould CJ, Xiong X, Robbins N, Zhu J, Pritchard DL, Khan R, Heideman RL, Krasin MJ, Kun LE (2004a) Early neuro-otologic effects of three-dimensional irradiation in children with primary brain tumors. Int J Radiat Oncol Biol Phys 58(4):1194–1207. https://doi.org/10.1016/j.ijrobp.2003.07.008

Merchant TE, Mulhern RK, Krasin MJ, Kun LE, Williams T, Li C, Xiong X, Khan RB, Lustig RH, Boop FA, Sanford RA (2004b) Preliminary results from a phase II trial of conformal radiation therapy and evaluation of radiation-related CNS effects for pediatric patients with localized ependymoma. J Clin Oncol 22(15):3156–3162. https://doi.org/10.1200/JCO.2004.11.142

Merchant TE, Conklin HM, Wu S, Lustig RH, Xiong X (2009a) Late effects of conformal radiation therapy for pediatric patients with low-grade glioma: prospective evaluation of cognitive, endocrine, and hearing deficits. J Clin Oncol 27(22):3691–3697. https://doi.org/10.1200/JCO.2008.21.2738

Merchant TE, Kun LE, Wu S, Xiong X, Sanford RA, Boop FA (2009b) Phase II trial of conformal radiation therapy for pediatric low-grade glioma. J Clin Oncol 27(22):3598–3604. https://doi.org/10.1200/JCO.2008.20.9494

Merchant TE, Li C, Xiong X, Kun LE, Boop FA, Sanford RA (2009c) Conformal radiotherapy after surgery for paediatric ependymoma: a prospective study. Lancet Oncol 10(3):258–266

Merchant TE, Kun LE, Hua CH, Wu S, Xiong X, Sanford RA, Boop FA (2013) Disease control after reduced volume conformal and intensity modulated radiation therapy for childhood craniopharyngioma. Int J Radiat Oncol Biol Phys 85(4):e187–e192. https://doi.org/10.1016/j.ijrobp.2012.10.030

Modak S, Gardner S, Dunkel IJ, Balmaceda C, Rosenblum MK, Miller DC, Halpern S, Finlay JL (2004) Thiotepa-based high-dose chemotherapy with autologous stem-cell rescue in patients with recurrent or progressive CNS germ cell tumors. J Clin Oncol 22(10):1934–1943. https://doi.org/10.1200/JCO.2004.11.053

Morales La Madrid A, Hashizume R, Kieran MW (2015) Future clinical trials in DIPG: bringing epigenetics to the clinic. Front Oncol 5:148. https://doi.org/10.3389/fonc.2015.00148

Morris EB, Li C, Khan RB, Sanford RA, Boop F, Pinlac R, Xiong X, Merchant TE (2009) Evolution of neurological impairment in pediatric infratentorial ependymoma patients. J Neuro-Oncol 94(3):391–398. https://doi.org/10.1007/s11060-009-9866-8

Needle MN, Molloy PT, Geyer JR, Herman-Liu A, Belasco JB, Goldwein JW, Sutton L, Phillips PC (1997) Phase II study of daily oral etoposide in children with recurrent brain tumors and other solid tumors. Med Pediatr Oncol 29(1):28–32

Northcott PA, Korshunov A, Witt H, Hielscher T, Eberhart CG, Mack S, Bouffet E, Clifford SC, Hawkins CE, French P, Rutka JT, Pfister S, Taylor MD (2011) Medulloblastoma comprises four distinct molecular variants. J Clin Oncol 29(11):1408–1414. https://doi.org/10.1200/JCO.2009.27.4324

Olson TA, Bayar E, Kosnik E, Hamoudi AB, Klopfenstein KJ, Pieters RS, Ruymann FB (1995) Successful treatment of disseminated central nervous system malignant rhabdoid tumor. J Pediatr Hematol Oncol 17(1):71–75

Oya N, Shibamoto Y, Nagata Y, Negoro Y, Hiraoka M (2002) Postoperative radiotherapy for intracranial ependymoma: analysis of prognostic factors and patterns of failure. J Neuro-Oncol 56(1):87–94

Packer RJ, Boyett JM, Zimmerman RA, Rorke LB, Kaplan AM, Albright AL, Selch MT, Finlay JL, Hammond GD, Wara WM (1993) Hyperfractionated radiation therapy (72 Gy) for children with brain stem gliomas. A Children's Cancer Group phase I/II trial. Cancer 72(4):1414–1421

Packer RJ, Boyett JM, Zimmerman RA, Albright AL, Kaplan AM, Rorke LB, Selch MT, Cherlow JM, Finlay JL, Wara WM (1994) Outcome of children with brain stem gliomas after treatment with 7800 cGy of hyperfractionated radiotherapy. A Children's Cancer Group phase I/II trial. Cancer 74(6):1827–1834

Packer RJ, Ater J, Allen J, Phillips P, Geyer R, Nicholson HS, Jakacki R, Kurczynski E, Needle M, Finlay J, Reaman G, Boyett JM (1997) Carboplatin and vincristine chemotherapy for children with newly diagnosed progressive low-grade gliomas. J Neurosurg 86(5):747–754. https://doi.org/10.3171/jns.1997.86.5.0747

Packer RJ, Goldwein J, Nicholson HS, Vezina LG, Allen JC, Ris MD, Muraszko K, Rorke LB, Wara WM, Cohen BH, Boyett JM (1999) Treatment of children with medulloblastomas with reduced-dose craniospinal radiation therapy and adjuvant chemotherapy: a Children's Cancer Group Study. J Clin Oncol 17(7):2127–2136

Packer RJ, Biegel JA, Blaney S, Finlay J, Geyer JR, Heideman R, Hilden J, Janss AJ, Kun L, Vezina G, Rorke LB, Smith M (2002) Atypical teratoid/rhabdoid tumor of the central nervous system: report on workshop. J Pediatr Hematol Oncol 24(5):337–342

Packer RJ, Gajjar A, Vezina G, Rorke-Adams L, Burger PC, Robertson PL, Bayer L, LaFond D, Donahue BR, Marymont MH, Muraszko K, Langston J, Sposto R (2006) Phase III study of craniospinal radiation therapy followed by adjuvant chemotherapy for newly diagnosed average-risk medulloblastoma. J Clin Oncol 24(25):4202–4208. https://doi.org/10.1200/JCO.2006.06.4980

Pai Panandiker AS, Wong JK, Nedelka MA, Wu S, Gajjar A, Broniscer A (2014) Effect of time from diagnosis to start of radiotherapy on children with diffuse intrinsic pontine glioma. Pediatr Blood Cancer 61(7):1180–1183. https://doi.org/10.1002/pbc.24971

Peirce CB, Bouchard J (1950) Role of radiation therapy in the control of malignant neoplasms of the brain and brain stem. Radiology 55(3):337–343. https://doi.org/10.1148/55.3.337

Pencalet P, Maixner W, Sainte-Rose C, Lellouch-Tubiana A, Cinalli G, Zerah M, Pierre-Kahn A, Hoppe-Hirsch E, Bourgeois M, Renier D (1999) Benign cerebellar astrocytomas in children. J Neurosurg 90(2):265–273. https://doi.org/10.3171/jns.1999.90.2.0265

Perilongo G, Massimino M, Sotti G, Belfontali T, Masiero L, Rigobello L, Garre L, Carli M, Lombardi F, Solero C, Sainati L, Canale V, del Prever AB, Giangaspero F, Andreussi L, Mazza C, Madon E (1997) Analyses of prognostic factors in a retrospective review of 92 children with ependymoma: Italian Pediatric Neurooncology Group. Med Pediatr Oncol 29(2):79–85

Phi JH, Wang KC, Park SH, Kim IH, Kim IO, Park KD, Ahn HS, Lee JY, Son YJ, Kim SK (2012) Pediatric infratentorial ependymoma: prognostic significance of anaplastic histology. J Neuro-Oncol 106(3):619–626. https://doi.org/10.1007/s11060-011-0699-x

Pollack IF, Claassen D, al-Shboul Q, Janosky JE, Deutsch M (1995) Low-grade gliomas of the cerebral hemispheres in children: an analysis of 71 cases. J Neurosurg 82(4):536–547. https://doi.org/10.3171/jns.1995.82.4.0536

Pollack IF, Boyett JM, Yates AJ, Burger PC, Gilles FH, Davis RL, Finlay JL, Children's Cancer G (2003) The influence of central review on outcome associations in childhood malignant gliomas: results from the CCG-945 experience. Neuro-Oncology 5(3):197–207. https://doi.org/10.1215/S1152-8517-03-00009-7

Rajan B, Ashley S, Gorman C, Jose CC, Horwich A, Bloom HJ, Marsh H, Brada M (1993) Craniopharyngioma--a long-term results following limited surgery and radiotherapy. Radiother Oncol 26(1):1–10

Rappaport R, Brauner R (1989) Growth and endocrine disorders secondary to cranial irradiation. Pediatr Res 25(6):561–567

Reddy AT, Janss AJ, Phillips PC, Weiss HL, Packer RJ (2000) Outcome for children with supratentorial prim-itive neuroectodermal tumors treated with surgery, radiation, and chemotherapy. Cancer 88(9):2189–2193

Regine WF, Kramer S (1992) Pediatric craniopharyngiomas: long term results of combined treatment with surgery and radiation. Int J Radiat Oncol Biol Phys 24(4):611–617

Remke M, Hielscher T, Korshunov A, Northcott PA, Bender S, Kool M, Westermann F, Benner A, Cin H, Ryzhova M, Sturm D, Witt H, Haag D, Toedt G, Wittmann A, Schottler A, von Bueren AO, von Deimling A, Rutkowski S, Scheurlen W, Kulozik AE, Taylor MD, Lichter P, Pfister SM (2011) FSTL5 is a marker of poor prognosis in non-WNT/non-SHH medulloblastoma. J Clin Oncol 29(29):3852–3861. https://doi.org/10.1200/JCO.2011.36.2798

Rizzo D, Scalzone M, Ruggiero A, Maurizi P, Attina G, Mastrangelo S, Lazzareschi I, Ridola V, Colosimo C, Caldarelli M, Balducci M, Riccardi R (2015) Temozolomide in the treatment of newly diagnosed diffuse brainstem glioma in children: a broken promise? J Chemother 27(2):106–110. https://doi.org/10.1179/1973947814Y.0000000228

Robertson PL, DaRosso RC, Allen JC (1997) Improved prognosis of intracranial non-germinoma germ cell tumors with multimodality therapy. J Neuro-Oncol 32(1):71–80

Rogers SJ, Mosleh-Shirazi MA, Saran FH (2005) Radiotherapy of localised intracranial germinoma: time to sever historical ties? Lancet Oncol 6(7):509–519. https://doi.org/10.1016/S1470-2045(05)70245-X

Rombi B, DeLaney TF, MacDonald SM, Huang MS, Ebb DH, Liebsch NJ, Raskin KA, Yeap BY, Marcus KJ, Tarbell NJ, Yock TI (2012) Proton radiotherapy for pediatric Ewing's sarcoma: initial clinical outcomes. Int J Radiat Oncol Biol Phys 82(3):1142–1148. https://doi.org/10.1016/j.ijrobp.2011.03.038

Rorke LB, Packer RJ, Biegel JA (1996) Central nervous system atypical teratoid/rhabdoid tumors of infancy and childhood: definition of an entity. J Neurosurg 85(1):56–65. https://doi.org/10.3171/jns.1996.85.1.0056

Rutkowski S, Bode U, Deinlein F, Ottensmeier H, Warmuth-Metz M, Soerensen N, Graf N, Emser A, Pietsch T, Wolff JE, Kortmann RD, Kuehl J (2005) Treatment of early childhood medulloblastoma by postoperative chemotherapy alone. N Engl J Med 352(10):978–986. https://doi.org/10.1056/NEJMoa042176

Rutkowski S, von Hoff K, Emser A, Zwiener I, Pietsch T, Figarella-Branger D, Giangaspero F, Ellison DW, Garre ML, Biassoni V, Grundy RG, Finlay JL, Dhall G, Raquin MA, Grill J (2010) Survival and prognostic factors of early childhood medulloblastoma: an international meta-analysis. J Clin Oncol 28(33):4961–4968. https://doi.org/10.1200/JCO.2010.30.2299

Schild SE, Nisi K, Scheithauer BW, Wong WW, Lyons MK, Schomberg PJ, Shaw EG (1998) The results of radiotherapy for ependymomas: the Mayo Clinic experience. Int J Radiat Oncol Biol Phys 42(5):953–958

Schumacher M, Schulte-Monting J, Stoeter P, Warmuth-Metz M, Solymosi L (2007) Magnetic resonance imaging compared with biopsy in the diagnosis of brainstem diseases of childhood: a multicenter review. J Neurosurg 106(2 Suppl):111–119. https://doi.org/10.3171/ped.2007.106.2.111

Shaw EG, Wisoff JH (2003) Prospective clinical trials of intracranial low-grade glioma in adults and children. Neuro-Oncology 5(3):153–160. https://doi.org/10.1215/S1152-8517-02-00060-1

Shirato H, Nishio M, Sawamura Y, Myohjin M, Kitahara T, Nishioka T, Mizutani Y, Abe H, Miyasaka K (1997) Analysis of long-term treatment of intracranial germinoma. Int J Radiat Oncol Biol Phys 37(3):511–515

Shrieve DC, Alexander E 3rd, Black PM, Wen PY, Fine HA, Kooy HM, Loeffler JS (1999) Treatment of patients with primary glioblastoma multiforme with standard postoperative radiotherapy and radiosurgical boost: prognostic factors and long-term outcome. J Neurosurg 90(1):72–77. https://doi.org/10.3171/jns.1999.90.1.0072

Shu HK, Sall WF, Maity A, Tochner ZA, Janss AJ, Belasco JB, Rorke-Adams LB, Phillips PC, Sutton LN, Fisher MJ (2007) Childhood intracranial ependymoma: twenty-year experience from a single institution. Cancer 110(2):432–441. https://doi.org/10.1002/cncr.22782

Smith AA, Weng E, Handler M, Foreman NK (2004) Intracranial germ cell tumors: a single institution experience and review of the literature. J Neuro-Oncol 68(2):153–159

Squire SE, Chan MD, Marcus KJ (2007) Atypical teratoid/rhabdoid tumor: the controversy behind radiation therapy. J Neuro-Oncol 81(1):97–111. https://doi.org/10.1007/s11060-006-9196-z

St Clair WH, Adams JA, Bues M, Fullerton BC, La Shell S, Kooy HM, Loeffler JS, Tarbell NJ (2004) Advantage of protons compared to conventional X-ray or IMRT in the treatment of a pediatric patient with medulloblastoma. Int J Radiat Oncol Biol Phys 58(3):727–734

Stiller CA, Nectoux J (1994) International incidence of childhood brain and spinal tumours. Int J Epidemiol 23(3):458–464

Stripp DC, Maity A, Janss AJ, Belasco JB, Tochner ZA, Goldwein JW, Moshang T, Rorke LB, Phillips PC, Sutton LN, Shu HK (2004) Surgery with or without radiation therapy in the management of craniopharyngiomas in children and young adults. Int J Radiat Oncol Biol Phys 58(3):714–720. https://doi.org/10.1016/S0360-3016(03)01570-0

Stupp R, Mason WP, van den Bent MJ, Weller M, Fisher B, Taphoorn MJ, Belanger K, Brandes AA, Marosi C, Bogdahn U, Curschmann J, Janzer RC, Ludwin SK, Gorlia T, Allgeier A, Lacombe D, Cairncross JG, Eisenhauer E, Mirimanoff RO, European Organisation for R, Treatment of Cancer Brain T, Radiotherapy G, National Cancer Institute of Canada Clinical Trials G (2005) Radiotherapy plus concomitant and adjuvant temozolomide for glioblastoma. N Engl J Med 352(10):987–996. https://doi.org/10.1056/NEJMoa043330

Stupp R, Hegi ME, Mason WP, van den Bent MJ, Taphoorn MJ, Janzer RC, Ludwin SK, Allgeier A, Fisher B, Belanger K, Hau P, Brandes AA, Gijtenbeek J, Marosi C, Vecht CJ, Mokhtari K, Wesseling P, Villa S, Eisenhauer E, Gorlia T, Weller M, Lacombe D, Cairncross JG, Mirimanoff RO, European Organisation for R, Treatment of Cancer Brain T, Radiation Oncology G, National Cancer Institute of Canada Clinical Trials G (2009) Effects of radiotherapy with concomitant and adjuvant temozolomide versus radiotherapy alone on survival in glioblastoma in a randomised phase III study: 5-year analysis of the EORTC-NCIC trial. Lancet Oncol 10(5):459–466. https://doi.org/10.1016/S1470-2045(09)70025-7

Sun MZ, Ivan ME, Oh MC, Delance AR, Clark AJ, Safaee M, Oh T, Kaur G, Molinaro A, Gupta N, Parsa AT (2014) Effects of adjuvant chemotherapy and radiation on overall survival in children with choroid plexus carcinoma. J Neuro-Oncol 120(2):353–360. https://doi.org/10.1007/s11060-014-1559-2

Tao ML, Barnes PD, Billett AL, Leong T, Shrieve DC, Scott RM, Tarbell NJ (1997) Childhood optic chiasm gliomas: radiographic response following radiotherapy and long-term clinical outcome. Int J Radiat Oncol Biol Phys 39(3):579–587

Tarbell NJ, Friedman H, Polkinghorn WR, Yock T, Zhou T, Chen Z, Burger P, Barnes P, Kun L (2013) High-risk medulloblastoma: a pediatric oncology group randomized trial of chemotherapy before or after radiation therapy (POG 9031). J Clin Oncol 31(23):2936–2941. https://doi.org/10.1200/JCO.2012.43.9984

Tekautz TM, Fuller CE, Blaney S, Fouladi M, Broniscer A, Merchant TE, Krasin M, Dalton J, Hale G, Kun LE, Wallace D, Gilbertson RJ, Gajjar A (2005) Atypical teratoid/rhabdoid tumors (ATRT): improved survival in children 3 years of age and older with radiation therapy and high-dose alkylator-based chemotherapy. J Clin Oncol 23(7):1491–1499. https://doi.org/10.1200/JCO.2005.05.187

Thompson JR, Harwood-Nash DC, Fitz CR (1973) The neuroradiology of childhood choroid plexus neoplasms. Am J Roentgenol Radium Therapy, Nucl Med 118(1):116–133

Timmermann B, Kortmann RD, Kuhl J, Meisner C, Slavc I, Pietsch T, Bamberg M (2000) Combined postoperative irradiation and chemotherapy for anaplastic ependymomas in childhood: results of the German prospective trials HIT 88/89 and HIT 91. Int J Radiat Oncol Biol Phys 46(2):287–295

Timmermann B, Kortmann RD, Kuhl J, Meisner C, Dieckmann K, Pietsch T, Bamberg M (2002) Role of radiotherapy in the treatment of supratentorial primitive neuroectodermal tumors in childhood: results of the prospective German brain tumor trials HIT 88/89 and 91. J Clin Oncol 20(3):842–849

Timmermann B, Kortmann RD, Kuhl J, Rutkowski S, Dieckmann K, Meisner C, Bamberg M (2005) Role of radiotherapy in anaplastic ependymoma in children under age of 3 years: results of the prospective German brain tumor trials HIT-SKK 87 and 92. Radiother Oncol 77(3):278–285

Timmermann B, Kortmann RD, Kuhl J, Rutkowski S, Meisner C, Pietsch T, Deinlein F, Urban C, Warmuth-Metz M, Bamberg M (2006) Role of radiotherapy in supratentorial primitive neuroectodermal tumor in young children: results of the German HIT-SKK87 and HIT-SKK92 trials. J Clin Oncol 24(10):1554–1560. https://doi.org/10.1200/JCO.2005.04.8074

Trofimov A, Bortfeld T (2003) Optimization of beam parameters and treatment planning for intensity modulated proton therapy. Technol Cancer Res Treat 2(5):437–444

Villano JL, Propp JM, Porter KR, Stewart AK, Valyi-Nagy T, Li X, Engelhard HH, McCarthy BJ (2008) Malignant pineal germ-cell tumors: an analysis of cases from three tumor registries. Neuro-Oncology 10(2):121–130. https://doi.org/10.1215/15228517-2007-054

Wallner KE, Galicich JH, Krol G, Arbit E, Malkin MG (1989) Patterns of failure following treatment for glioblastoma multiforme and anaplastic astrocytoma. Int J Radiat Oncol Biol Phys 16(6):1405–1409

Warren KE (2012) Diffuse intrinsic pontine glioma: poised for progress. Front Oncol 2:205. https://doi.org/10.3389/fonc.2012.00205

Wolden SL, Dunkel IJ, Souweidane MM, Happersett L, Khakoo Y, Schupak K, Lyden D, Leibel SA (2003) Patterns of failure using a conformal radiation therapy tumor bed boost for medulloblastoma. J Clin Oncol 21(16):3079–3083. https://doi.org/10.1200/JCO.2003.11.140

Wolff JE, Sajedi M, Coppes MJ, Anderson RA, Egeler RM (1999) Radiation therapy and survival in choroid plexus carcinoma. Lancet 353(9170):2126

Wolff JE, Sajedi M, Brant R, Coppes MJ, Egeler RM (2002) Choroid plexus tumours. Br J Cancer 87(10):1086–1091. https://doi.org/10.1038/sj.bjc.6600609

Wrede B, Hasselblatt M, Peters O, Thall PF, Kutluk T, Moghrabi A, Mahajan A, Rutkowski S, Diez B, Wang X, Pietsch T, Kortmann RD, Paulus W, Jeibmann A, Wolff JE (2009) Atypical choroid plexus papilloma: clinical experience in the CPT-SIOP-2000 study. J Neuro-Oncol 95(3):383–392. https://doi.org/10.1007/s11060-009-9936-y

Zacharoulis S, Levy A, Chi SN, Gardner S, Rosenblum M, Miller DC, Dunkel I, Diez B, Sposto R, Ji L, Asgharzadeh S, Hukin J, Belasco J, Dubowy R, Kellie S, Termuhlen A, Finlay J (2007) Outcome for young children newly diagnosed with ependymoma, treated with intensive induction chemotherapy followed by myeloablative chemotherapy and autologous stem cell rescue. Pediatr Blood Cancer 49(1):34–40. https://doi.org/10.1002/pbc.20935

Zaghloul MS, Eldebawy E, Ahmed S, Mousa AG, Amin A, Refaat A, Zaky I, Elkhateeb N, Sabry M (2014) Hypofractionated conformal radiotherapy for pediatric diffuse intrinsic pontine glioma (DIPG): a randomized controlled trial. Radiother Oncol 111(1):35–40. https://doi.org/10.1016/j.radonc.2014.01.013

Zaky W, Dhall G, Ji L, Haley K, Allen J, Atlas M, Bertolone S, Cornelius A, Gardner S, Patel R, Pradhan K, Shen V, Thompson S, Torkildson J, Sposto R, Finlay JL (2014) Intensive induction chemotherapy followed by myeloablative chemotherapy with autologous hematopoietic progenitor cell rescue for young children newly-diagnosed with central nervous system atypical teratoid/rhabdoid tumors: the head start III experience. Pediatr Blood Cancer 61(1):95–101. https://doi.org/10.1002/pbc.24648

Zeltzer PM, Boyett JM, Finlay JL, Albright AL, Rorke LB, Milstein JM, Allen JC, Stevens KR, Stanley P, Li H, Wisoff JH, Geyer JR, McGuire-Cullen P, Stehbens JA, Shurin SB, Packer RJ (1999) Metastasis stage, adjuvant treatment, and residual tumor are prognostic factors for medulloblastoma in children: conclusions from the Children's Cancer Group 921 randomized phase III study. J Clin Oncol 17(3):832–845

Zimmerman MA, Goumnerova LC, Proctor M, Scott RM, Marcus K, Pomeroy SL, Turner CD, Chi SN, Chordas C, Kieran MW (2005) Continuous remission of newly diagnosed and relapsed central nervous system atypical teratoid/rhabdoid tumor. J Neuro-Oncol 72(1):77–84. https://doi.org/10.1007/s11060-004-3115-y

Imaging Children with CNS Tumors

4

Julie H. Harreld

4.1 Introduction

Though many pediatric brain tumors are diagnosed by head computed tomography (CT) performed for emergent indications such as vomiting, ataxia, or altered mental status, CT, even with intravenous contrast, is insufficient for tumor characterization or metastasis detection. CT also carries a low risk of radiation-induced secondary cancers; this risk increases with cumulative dose without a threshold effect (Miglioretti et al. 2013). Furthermore, the eye lens, which may be exposed to radiation with head CT, is sensitive to radiation-induced cataract formation at doses as low as 0.5 Sv (Fish et al. 2011). Magnetic resonance imaging (MRI) offers far superior tissue contrast without radiation, and is therefore the gold-standard for diagnosis of central nervous system (CNS) tumors and metastases. As technology advances, MRI becomes increasingly important in diagnosing metastasis, since it detects leptomeningeal metastatic disease in up to 50% of those with false-negative cerebrospinal fluid (CSF) examination and better correlates with survival than CSF results (Maroldi et al. 2005; Terterov et al. 2010; Pang et al. 2008). MRI is particularly important in children with ependymomas, in whom CSF may

be negative despite the presence of extensive leptomeningeal involvement (Poltinnikov and Merchant 2006). It is therefore critical to optimize imaging for initial diagnosis and for detection of postsurgical resection residual tumor and leptomeningeal metastasis.

MRI, however, has its own challenges. MRI is more expensive and time-consuming than CT, and there may be significant technical variability in scans performed at different centers or on different equipment. Very young patients, and some older or apprehensive patients, require anesthesia in order to complete the scan and reduce motion degradation of the images. However, anesthesia can cause physiologic changes resulting in increased signal within the sulci on fluid-attenuated inversion recovery (FLAIR) imaging (Harreld et al. 2014), potentially mimicking or obscuring metastasis; recent awareness of potential long-term cognitive effects associated with early-childhood anesthesia (Sun 2010) drives the search for alternatives to anesthesia for motion control. Limitations on safe anesthesia time may also require minimizing the length of the MRI examination.

4.2 Brain Imaging Basics

Attention to certain basic principles can greatly enhance the utility of MR imaging in children with CNS tumors. Children are smaller than adults and have a much greater propensity than

J. H. Harreld, M.D.
Department of Diagnostic Imaging, St. Jude
Children's Research Hospital, Memphis, TN, USA
e-mail: julie.harreld@stjude.org

© Springer International Publishing AG, part of Springer Nature 2018
A. Gajjar et al. (eds.), *Brain Tumors in Children*, https://doi.org/10.1007/978-3-319-43205-2_4

adults to develop tumors prone to leptomeningeal (CSF) dissemination, requiring thinner slices (≤3–4 mm), no interslice "gap," and smaller fields of view for improved resolution and detection for accurate risk stratification (Engelhard and Corsten 2005). Sequences and parameters should be chosen to increase conspicuity of enhancement and exploit innate tumor characteristics, such as hypercellularity. Acquisition planes should be targeted to visualize tricky locations, and noncontributory sequences should be eliminated to minimize scan time (Fig. 4.1).

Isotropic volumetric T1-weighted images (WI) with contrast (MPRAGE, SPACE, CUBE) provide excellent resolution of the brain, and in the sagittal plane provide optimal visualization of the anterior recesses of the third ventricle, a common site of metastasis. However, because volumetric sequences are highly susceptible to patient motion (Ida et al. 2014), it may be necessary to

acquire sagittal 2D Spin Echo (SE) or gradient echo T1 post-contrast, with slice thickness ≤ 3 mm and 0 gap to maximize detection of leptomeningeal metastasis.

T1 subtraction images are created at the MRI console by subtracting pre-contrast T1WI from post-contrast T1WI and therefore require no additional scan time, and are helpful for detecting subtle enhancement, and differentiating between T1 shortening from blood or mineralization and true enhancement (Ellingson et al. 2014).

Hypercellular tumors and metastases are seen very well on diffusion-weighted imaging (DWI), which has been found to be useful in imaging pediatric brain tumors such as medulloblastoma, atypical teratoid/rhabdoid tumors (ATRT), and other embryonal tumors (Koral et al. 2014; Pierce et al. 2014; Pierce and Provenzale 2014; Yamashita et al. 2009). Acquisition of at least two levels of diffusion weighting, known as b-values

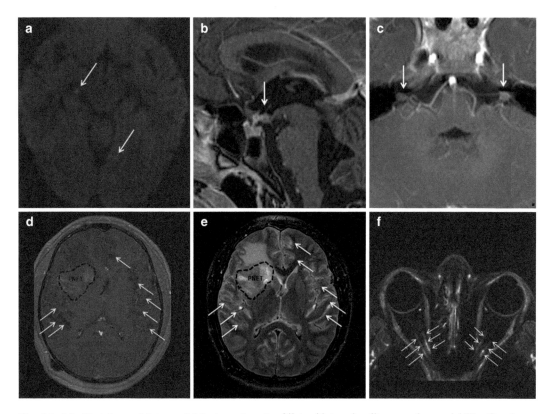

Fig. 4.1 Manifestations of intracranial leptomeningeal metastasis (arrows). (**a**) Hypercellular medulloblastoma metastases on DWI; (**b**) spinal cord astrocytoma metastases in the anterior 3rd ventricle on sagittal 3D T1 + C; (**c**) nodular choroid plexus carcinoma metastases within the bilateral internal auditory canals on axial T1 + C; enhancing embryonal tumor (PNET) and non-enhancing leptomeningeal metastases on (**d**) axial T1 + C and (**e**) FLAIR+C; (**f**) metastatic embryonal tumor within the CSF surrounding the optic nerves on subtracted T1 images

(0 and 1000 are recommended), permits calculation of apparent diffusion coefficient (ADC) maps, increasing diagnostic confidence (Mukherjee et al. 2008) (Fig. 4.1b).

Post-contrast fluid-attenuated inversion recovery (FLAIR) is useful for tumor detection and is now a common sequence performable on any platform. FLAIR imaging has been shown to be particularly sensitive for the detection of intracranial leptomeningeal metastasis (Kremer et al. 2006; Fukuoka et al. 2010; Griffiths et al. 2003). This is because gadolinium contrast is particularly bright on FLAIR, on which CSF in sulci is dark, accentuating conspicuity of enhancing leptomeningeal metastasis (Mathews et al. 1999). Typical T2 hyperintensity of metastases may also contribute to lesion conspicuity on FLAIR imaging. Fat saturation may further enhance metastasis conspicuity. Because delayed post-contrast FLAIR has been found to be more sensitive for metastasis detection (Kremer et al. 2006), it is recommended that FLAIR be performed last (Fig. 4.1e).

4.3 Spine Imaging Basics

Isolated spinal leptomeningeal metastasis of primary brain tumors, though infrequent, does occur (Perreault et al. 2014) and most children are asymptomatic (Bartels et al. 2006); thus, adequate spine imaging surveillance is crucial. High-quality, thin-slice ($\leq$3 mm, 0 gap) post-contrast sagittal and axial T1WI without fat saturation are a basic minimum for evaluation for potentially very small leptomeningeal metastases. Typical spin echo (SE) and fast/turbo spin-echo (FSE, TSE) techniques are subject to significant CSF pulsation artifact, which can obscure or mimic metastasis, and should be avoided (Larsen et al. 1996; Lisanti et al. 2007). This limitation is overcome by the use of fast T1 FLAIR, which shows significantly improved lesion-to-CSF contrast due to suppression of CSF, with similar acquisition times (Shah et al. 2011). Both CSF artifact and scan time of axial imaging may be significantly decreased through the use of three-dimensional (3D) techniques (Siemens: VIBE; GE: LAVA; Philips: THRIVE) (Cho et al. 2016). Detection of non-enhancing

metastasis may be enhanced by the addition of sagittal myelographic T2-weighted images (CISS/FIESTA/FISP), and diffusion-weighted imaging may be a useful adjunct for detection of hypercellular metastases, as may be seen with embryonal tumors (Fig. 4.2). Optimally, initial MRI screening for spinal leptomeningeal metastasis should be performed preoperatively due to the possibility of obscuration of metastases by postoperative sequelae, such as enhancing subdural collections (Harreld et al. 2015; Warmuth-Metz et al. 2004).

Diagnosis and follow-up for primary spinal cord tumors requires, at a minimum, pre- and post-contrast axial and sagittal thin slices ($\leq$3 mm, 0 gap) through the level of the tumor, as well as specific imaging for leptomeningeal metastasis as above. Diffusion-weighted imaging may be helpful for analysis of cellularity, and diffusion tensor imaging to assess for infiltration versus displacement of spinal tracts. Gradient echo images assist in detection of hemorrhage.

4.4 Advanced/Specialized/ Metabolic Imaging

4.4.1 Diffusion Tensor Imaging

In diffusion tensor imaging (DTI), directional diffusion gradients are applied to a T2-weighted (spin echo) echo-planar images (EPI) sequence before and after a 180° refocusing pulse. Water protons moving freely through these gradients acquire random spins and are thus dephased (unsynchronized), causing signal loss in voxels where water motion (diffusion) is significant. Conversely, stationary or slowly moving protons generate increased signal on diffusion-weighted images. The apparent diffusion coefficient (ADC) may be calculated from images acquired without and with a diffusion gradient and allows quantitation of the displacement of water molecules over time (mm^2/s) in a particular voxel (Mukherjee et al. 2008; McRobbie 2007).

In tissues, water mobility may be restricted by cell membranes, macromolecules, or decreased extracellular spaces. In such cases, signal on

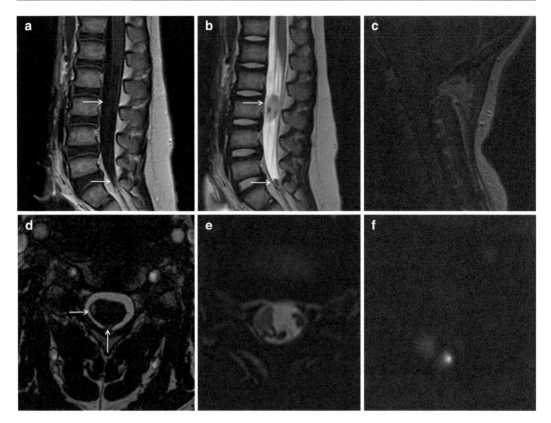

Fig. 4.2 Imaging spinal leptomeningeal metastasis. Non-enhancing ependymoma metastasis is not well seen on (**a**) sagittal T1 + C, but is well seen on (**b**) sagittal T2WI. CSF was negative. Metastatic pineoblastoma studs the spinal cord surface on (**c**) sagittal T1 + C images of the upper spine, an appearance sometimes called "sugar coating". Metastatic PNET/embryonal tumor is well seen on axial (**d**) CISS. Nodular medulloblastoma metastases on axial T2WI (**e**) are bright on DWI (**f**), which confirms hypercellularity

diffusion-weighted imaging (DWI) is increased, and the ADC is decreased. Tumors with high cell density, such as embryonal tumors like medulloblastoma and ATRT, have decreased or "restricted" water diffusion and therefore appear bright on DWI and dark on the ADC map. This is in contrast to vasogenic/peritumoral edema, in which there is an accumulation of extracellular water due to blood–brain barrier breakdown or osmotic shifts, causing increased ADC and facilitating differentiation from tumor (Liang et al. 2007).

Whereas water movement (diffusion) is apparently equal in all directions (isotropic) in gray matter, in white matter it is greatest parallel to the fiber bundles ("tracts") and restricted perpendicular to the tracts, a property known as anisotropy. This is exploited in diffusion tensor imaging (DTI) for fiber tracking, a technique that can be helpful in differentiating diffuse from focal tumor, and that may have surgical and prognostic implications. DTI measures such as fractional anisotropy and radial diffusivity may be useful for quantitative assessment of myelin damage, as may be seen following radiation therapy in children with brain tumors.

4.4.2 Perfusion Imaging

In dynamic susceptibility contrast (DSC) perfusion MRI, signal changes measured on images acquired repeatedly during circulation of contrast are used to calculate estimated cerebral blood flow (CBF), mean transit time (MTT), and cerebral blood volume (CBV), the amount of blood present in a given volume of tissue at a given time (mL/100 g). Because of the variability of absolute measurements of perfusion between scanners and changes in cerebral perfusion due to caffeine, opioids, and/or anesthesia, perfusion is quantified by ratios of tumor to normal brain. Elevations of CBV relative to normal brain >2 have been associated with poor prognosis (Law et al. 2008), diagnostic of high-grade tumor (Hakyemez et al. 2005), and indicative of tumor recurrence rather than radiation necrosis (Mitsuya et al. 2010). Though relative cerebral blood volume (rCBV) is a useful adjunct to anatomic features and diffusion characteristics, perfusion imaging is frequently nonspecific in pediatric tumors, since low-grade tumors such as pilocytic astrocytoma, oligodendroglioma, and choroid plexus papilloma may have significantly elevated rCBV (Borja et al. 2013; Brandao et al. 2013). However, identification of areas of increased rCBV within tumors, which reflect vascularity and frequently grade, may be useful in directing biopsy of large, infiltrating or heterogeneous tumors, and may be useful in following tumors through treatment.

Arterial Spin Labeling (ASL), a non-contrast technique, relies on magnetic "labeling" of protons entering the slice of interest, with the subsequent signal change as compared to a non-labeled control image reflecting capillary perfusion only (McRobbie et al. 2007). Quantitative maps of cerebral blood flow (CBF) and mean transit time (MTT) can be obtained if a quantitative scan that also includes apparent T1 map is acquired, but because CBV cannot be calculated its utility in assessing brain tumors has not been established. Both techniques are subject to variations in hemodynamic factors.

4.4.3 ^{1}H MR Spectroscopy

The application of a radiofrequency pulse attuned to protons in a volume of brain tissue causes the protons in that volume to absorb the energy and to change from a low to a high energy state, known as resonance. The energy given off as the protons return to their low-energy state can be measured. Because the magnetic resonance of each proton depends on its local milieu, the resonant signals given off by different molecules are "shifted" from one another by very small amounts on the frequency spectrum, allowing us to distinguish between them on MR spectroscopy. This shift is greater at higher magnetic field strengths, resulting in better separation of resonance peaks. In the brain, the molecules (metabolites) of interest are: choline (Cho), an indicator of membrane turnover (phosphocholines released during myelin breakdown); creatine (Cr), used as a reference, but low in high-grade tumors; N-acetyl aspartate (NAA), a marker of membrane integrity; lactate, a marker of cell death/necrosis; and myoinositol, a sugar alcohol product of myelin breakdown (McRobbie et al. 2007). Absolute quantification of these metabolites may not be reliable, but their ratios are deranged in disease processes in the brain. Though an elevated Cho:NAA ratio may be seen in many disorders due to increased membrane turnover and decreased neuronal integrity, this ratio has also been found useful in grading of gliomas; Cho:NAA >2.2 and Cho:Cr >2 are considered a threshold for higher-grade tumor (Zeng et al. 2011). MR spectroscopy is frequently nonspecific in pediatric brain tumors; for example, juvenile pilocytic astrocytomas (JPAs) have elevated Cho:NAA ratios of approximately 3.4 (Hwang et al. 1998), and inflammatory lesions may also have significantly elevated Cho:NAA ratios. However, MR spectroscopy may be useful for guiding biopsy to the most metabolically active region of a tumor or lesion, or for following changes in metabolism over time.

4.4.4 Functional MRI

Functional MR imaging (fMRI) of the brain depends on the coupling of local increases in cerebral metabolic rate of oxygen (CMRO$_2$) and cerebral blood flow (CBF) to neuronal activation. Because the inflow of oxygenated blood "overshoots" the increased oxygen requirement, there is a local excess of intravascular oxygenated blood, which generates increased signal on echoplanar images (EPI), known as the blood oxygen

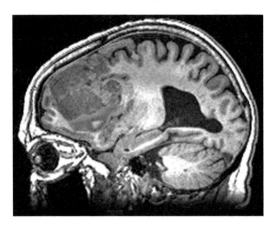

Fig. 4.3 fMRI shows inferior displacement of the activated dominant expressive speech area (red/yellow) by a large left frontal mass

level dependent (BOLD) response (Buxton 2010). fMRI may be task-based to identify centers key to motor function or memory, or may be performed at rest to determine baseline function. Because these signal changes may be dominated by changes in oxygenation of downstream venous blood, localization should be considered approximate. However, fMRI can be useful for preoperative assessment of feasibility of gross total resection of lesions in eloquent brain, by assessing proximity to language, memory, or motor centers (Fig. 4.3).

4.4.5 Positron Emission Tomography

F-18-labeled fluorodeoxyglucose positron emission tomography (^{18}FDG-PET), which relies upon the disproportionate uptake of fluorodeoxyglucose by glycolytically active tumors and the subsequent detection of positrons emitted by the radioactive ^{18}fluorine label, is not routinely performed for pediatric brain tumor diagnosis or surveillance. Although glucose uptake is theoretically proportional to tumor grade, grading of pediatric tumors is problematic as uptake values overlap in tumors of different grades; benign tumors such as pilocytic astrocytomas and choroid plexus papillomas may have high uptake, while higher-grade tumors such as epen-

dymoma may have low uptake (Stanescu et al. 2013; Zukotynski et al. 2014). It may also be difficult to distinguish tumors from normal brain, which has high background glucose uptake that may be focally increased by neuronal activation or regionally altered by anesthesia. However, like MR perfusion and spectroscopic imaging, ^{18}FDG-PET may be useful for guiding biopsy by identifying hypermetabolic tumor foci, differentiating tumor (increased uptake) from radiation necrosis (decreased uptake), and identifying subtle residual or recurrent tumor. Sensitivity and specificity of PET may be improved by registration to MRI rather than CT, improving anatomic visualization and reducing exposure to ionizing radiation (Zukotynski et al. 2014). Sensitivity and specificity may also be improved through the use of non-FDG radiotracers targeted toward detecting markers of tumor cell function, such as increased protein synthesis (radiolabeled amino acids and analogues such as ^{11}C-methionine and ^{18}F-DOPA), DNA synthesis (radiolabeled nucleosides such as ^{18}F-fluorodeoxythymidine), cell membrane synthesis (^{11}C-choline), and elevated oxidative metabolism (^{11}C-acetate) (Gulyas and Halldin 2012).

4.5 Imaging Features of Pediatric Brain and Spine Tumors

4.5.1 Infratentorial Brain Tumors

Although brain tumors are most frequently supratentorial in infants and older children, the posterior fossa is the most common location for brain tumors in children 2–11 years of age (Rickert and Paulus 2001; Ostrom et al. 2015). The most common tumors in the posterior fossa are gliomas (astrocytomas), medulloblastomas, atypical teratoid/rhabdoid tumors, and ependymomas.

4.5.1.1 Medulloblastoma
Medulloblastoma, the most common malignant tumor in children, is a World Health Organization (WHO) grade IV embryonal tumor with at least four molecular subtypes for which location may

be a marker. WNT-upregulated (wingless) tumors are the least common subtype (comprising about 10%), have the best prognosis (>90% 5-year survival) with rare metastasis, and tend to occur in older children and teenagers (Gajjar and Robinson 2014). WNT tumors are extra-axial and tend to involve the fourth ventricle and foramen of Luschka (unilaterally), and less commonly the cerebellopontine angle (Patay et al. 2015). Approximately 30% of medulloblastomas are of the sonic hedgehog (SHH) subtype, which have approximately 75% 5-year overall survival and tend to occur within the cerebellar hemisphere in children <5 years or > 16 years of age; 15–20% are metastatic at diagnosis, and recurrence may be local or metastatic (Gajjar and Robinson 2014; Ramaswamy et al. 2013; Gibson et al. 2010). Group 3 tumors (about 25%) occur in infants and children and have the poorest prognosis with approximately 50% 5-year survival. 40–45% have leptomeningeal metastases at diagnosis, which remains the most important negative prognostic factor (Gajjar and Robinson 2014; Ramaswamy et al. 2013). Group 4 tumors are most common (about 35%) and occur in all ages with male predominance and are metastatic at diagnosis in approximately 40%. Group 3 and 4 tumors tend to occur in the fourth ventricle (Perreault et al. 2014). Regardless of subtype, medulloblastomas tend to be T1 hypointense, T2 iso- or hyperintense to cerebellum, and diffusion-restricted; hemorrhage and/or cysts/necrosis may occur in any subtype, and though enhancement is variable overall, Group 4 tumors more commonly show little to no enhancement (Patay et al. 2015; Perreault et al. 2014) (Fig. 4.4). Metastasis is leptomeningeal; hematogenous metastasis is rare, and usually to bone.

Patients less than 5 years of age with medulloblastoma, particularly those less than 2 years with desmoplastic histology (most frequently the sonic hedgehog subtype), should be screened for Gorlin (basal cell nevus) syndrome, as they are at high risk for developing basal cell carcinomas in the radiation field (Bree and Shah 2011). Though dermoid cysts may be present in infancy, other manifestations such as odontogenic keratocysts and falcine calcifications may take years to develop and are not reliable early indicators (Kimonis et al. 1997).

4.5.1.2 Atypical Teratoid Rhabdoid Tumor

Atypical teratoid rhabdoid tumor (ATRT) is a grade IV embryonal tumor which was first considered a distinct entity by the WHO in 2000 (Ostrom et al. 2015). ATRT is a tumor of young children, presenting at a median age of 1 year; most present before 4 years of age, helping distinguish it from medulloblastoma, with which it is easily confused. About half occur in the posterior fossa, where they may occur in the cerebellar hemisphere or the fourth ventricle, with extension to the pineal recess occasionally raising the question of site of origin (Fig. 4.4). Leptomeningeal metastasis is common, and survival is poor; 5-year survival is only 27.5% (Poretti et al. 2012; Ostrom et al. 2015). On imaging, ATRTs have a variable appearance but are typically heterogeneous, with frequent cysts or necrosis and possible calcification and hemorrhage. Compared to gray matter, solid components are typically iso- to hyperdense on CT, hypo- to isointense on T1WI and iso- to hyperintense on T2WI. Restricted water diffusion is the rule, and may be more pronounced than with medulloblastoma, though definitive differentiation based on ADC is not possible (Koral et al. 2014) (Fig. 4.4). Like the original tumor, metastases are frequently diffusion-restricted and best seen on DWI. Attention should be paid to the kidneys when reviewing spine imaging, as patients may develop synchronous malignant rhabdoid renal tumors (Meyers et al. 2006).

4.5.1.3 Glioma

Gliomas arise from the support cells of the CNS (primarily astrocytes and oligodendrocytes), and account for almost 50% of brain and CNS tumors in children (Ostrom et al. 2014). Pilocytic astrocytoma, a WHO grade I neoplasm, is the most common pediatric glioma and the most common cerebellar neoplasm, accounting for approximately 85% of cerebellar astrocytomas (Koeller and Rushing 2004). Generally well-circumscribed, about two-thirds of pilocytic astrocytomas display

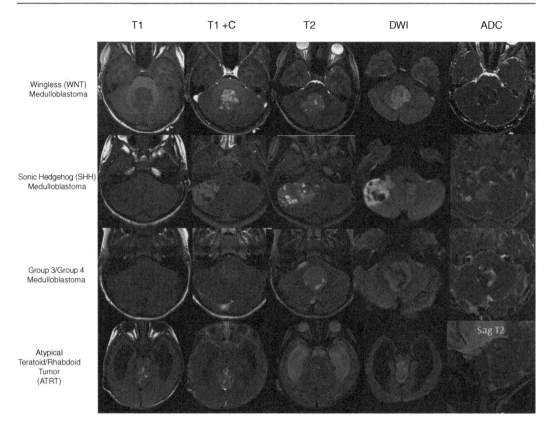

Fig. 4.4 Medulloblastomas and ATRT. While wingless (WNT), group 3 and group 4 medulloblastomas tend to occur within the fourth ventricle, the sonic hedgehog (SHH) subtype is usually hemispheric. Otherwise, imaging features are essentially the same for all subtypes, with T1 hypointensity, T2 hyperintensity, variable cysts and enhancement, and restricted diffusion (high signal on DWI, low signal on ADC) of solid components. ATRT shares the same signal characteristics; involvement of the pineal recess may raise the question of site of origin (Sag T2)

classic "cyst and enhancing nodule" morphology; the remainder appear necrotic or solid (Koeller and Rushing 2004). Despite their low-grade nature, pilocytic astrocytomas may metastasize via the CSF, without an associated increase in mortality (Koeller and Rushing 2004). Gross total resection is curative, but infiltrative tumor or involvement of the brainstem or vermis may limit resectability and predispose to progression. Though low-grade, pilocytic astrocytomas frequently demonstrate imaging features typically associated with high-grade gliomas including avid enhancement, elevated cerebral blood volume (CBV) and Cho:NAA ratios >2.2 on MR spectroscopy (Hwang et al. 1998; Zeng et al. 2011; Brandao et al. 2013). Solid components are typically T1 hypointense, T2 hyerintense, and rarely hemorrhagic or calcified. Diffusion restriction suggestive of hypercellularity is absent; in solid components, tumor-to-normal-brain ADC ratios tend to be ≥1.8 (Koral et al. 2014).

Ganglioglioma, a rare mixed glioneuronal tumor which is rarer still in the posterior fossa (comprising about 0.25% of all pediatric brain tumors) (Dudley et al. 2015; Rickert and Paulus 2001), may also appear solid, cystic/necrotic, or as cystic with a mural nodule like pilocytic astrocytoma, but may demonstrate hemorrhage and/or relatively low ADC values, assisting in differentiation (Gupta et al. 2014).

Ependymomas are WHO grade II neuroepithelial tumors comprising approximately 10% of intracranial neoplasms in children; two-thirds occur in the posterior fossa. Although they may occur at any age, including adulthood, they most frequently occur in young children (<5 years of age), in whom prognosis is poorest (Rickert and Paulus 2001; Poltinnikov and Merchant 2006; Pajtler et al. 2015). Posterior fossa ependymomas occur in the fourth ventricle and typically appear isodense to gray matter on CT and isointense to gray matter on T1WI and T2WI by MRI. They may appear either homogeneous or heterogeneous, with cystic/necrotic components and small calcifications frequently present; hemorrhage occurs more rarely. Though water diffusion (ADC) is gener-

ally increased compared to normal brain (Koral et al. 2014), restricted diffusion may be heterogeneously present, particularly in anaplastic (WHO grade III) ependymomas. Though the conventional MRI signal characteristics are nonspecific, characteristic protrusion through the foramina of Luschka and foramen magnum are highly suggestive; however, this appearance is not pathognomonic and can occur in medulloblastoma (Poretti et al. 2012). Leptomeningeal metastasis occurs in about 15% of patients and is typically CSF-negative, even in the presence of obvious metastasis on MRI (Poltinnikov and Merchant 2006).

Imaging features of posterior fossa pilocytic astrocytomas, ependymomas, and gangliogliomas are shown in Fig. 4.5.

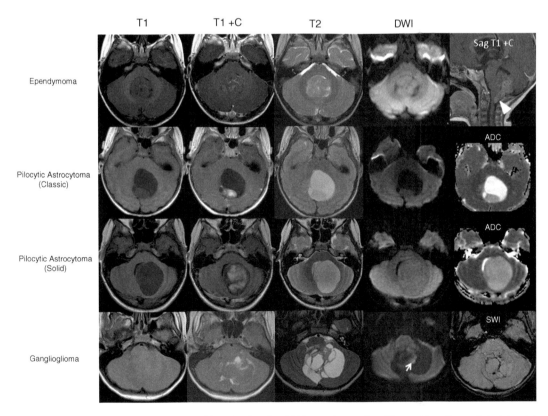

Fig. 4.5 Other posterior fossa tumors. Though signal characteristics of ependymomas are nonspecific, most do not have restricted diffusion (increased signal on DWI, decreased on ADC); protrusion through the foramina of Luschka and the foramen magnum (arrow head) are highly suggestive. Pilocytic astrocytomas (PA) may be cystic with an enhancing nodule (classic) or solid; the solid portions are T2 hyperintense without restricted diffusion. Gangliogliomas may look similar to PAs but are more likely to have foci of restricted diffusion (arrow); hemorrhage (dark on SWI) is variably present

4.5.2 Pineal, Sellar, and Suprasellar Tumors

4.5.2.1 Pineal Region Tumors

Pineal region neoplasms account for up to 8% of intracranial tumors in children. Germ cell tumors (GCTs) are most common (approximately 40%), followed by pineal parenchymal tumors (up to 27% of pineal region tumors) (Smith et al. 2010). Because the pineal gland also contains glial and connective tissue, gliomas, ependymomas, ATRTs, and other tumor types may also arise from the pineal gland (Dhall et al. 2010). Dermoid/epidermoid cysts, arachnoid cysts, lipomas, and meningiomas may also arise in the pineal region. Signs and symptoms associated with regional mass effect include Parinaud syndrome, precocious puberty, and hydrocephalus.

Germ cell tumors (GCTs) are classified as germinomas or non-germinomatous GCTs (teratoma, yolk sac tumor, choriocarcinoma, embryonal carcinoma, mixed), and are more common in males. Among pineal GCTs, germinomas are the most common and occur 10 times more frequently in males. Frequent metastasis necessitates spinal surveillance, but germinomas are very responsive to radiation therapy and have an excellent prognosis. Calcifications tend to be focal, either displaced or engulfed, compared to "blasted" calcifications in pineal parenchymal tumors; otherwise, they appear very similar to pineal parenchymal tumors on imaging—iso- to hyperdense on CT, iso- to hyperintense on T1 and T2, and avid enhancement (which tends to be homogeneous). Restricted diffusion may be present (Fig. 4.6). This appearance does not readily differentiate germinomas

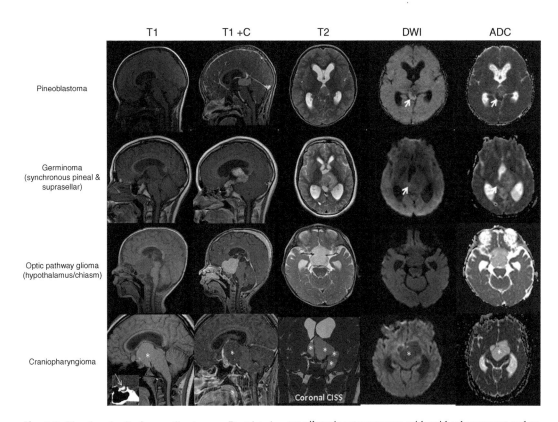

Fig. 4.6 Pineal and sellar/suprasellar tumors. Restricted diffusion (arrows) in a pineal tumor suggests pineoblastoma, but may be seen in other pineal parenchymal tumors or in germ cell tumors. Synchronous pineal and suprasellar masses suggest germinoma. Most optic pathway gliomas are pilocytic astrocytomas, with avid enhancement and no restricted diffusion. Craniopharyngiomas are typically calcified on CT (inset). Cysts (*) are well differentiated from surrounding CSF on CISS/FIESTA images, which are heavily T2-weighted images insensitive to CSF pulsation

from non-germinomatous GCTs, either, with the exception of mature teratomas which may be identified by the presence of fat.

Of the pineal parenchymal tumors, pineoblastoma, a WHO grade IV embryonal tumor, is the most common in children, and occurs both sporadically and in up to 9% of children with bilateral retinoblastoma around 2 years after diagnosis (Brennan et al. 2012; Chung et al. 2007; Borja et al. 2013). Pineocytoma (WHO grade I) and pineal parenchymal tumor of intermediate differentiation (PPTID, WHO grade II or III) may also occur in children but are more common in adults. There is significant overlap in imaging appearance of pineal parenchymal tumors, but infiltration of regional structures and the presence of necrosis are suggestive of pineoblastoma; restricted diffusion may be present in the latter, but is not a consistent finding (Fig. 4.6). Cystic pineocytomas may be differentiated from simple pineal cysts by internal or nodular enhancement. Leptomeningeal metastasis is common in pineoblastoma; therefore spine imaging should also be performed (Smith et al. 2010). Though not pathognomonic, calcifications in pineal parenchymal tumors tend to be scattered or peripheral, in contrast to the focal, "displaced" or "engulfed" calcifications seen in germ cell tumors (Awa et al. 2014). Pineal or habenular calcifications may be seen in healthy young children and are not, by themselves, diagnostic of tumor (Whitehead et al. 2015).

4.5.2.2 Sellar and Suprasellar Tumors

Up to 50% of pediatric suprasellar tumors are adamantinomatous craniopharyngiomas, which are typically calcified, have a sellar component and have solid and large cystic components, unlike adult-type papillary craniopharyngioma, which are solid and suprasellar. Symptoms are due to mass effect; metastasis is rare (Schroeder and Vezina 2011). Coronal CISS/FIESTA images are useful for resolving tiny tumor cysts and nodules, and evaluating the relationship to surrounding structures (Fig. 4.6).

The most common tumor of the hypothalamus/optic chiasm is the pilocytic astrocytoma; pilomyxoid histology predicts more aggressive behavior. Seventy-five percent is present in the first decade. About one-third are associated with neurofibroma-

tosis type 1 (NF-1); involvement of the intracranial and intraorbital optic nerves is more common in these cases. In NF-1, tumors are generally indolent and minimally symptomatic, with occasional spontaneous regression, thus are observed until clinically or radiographically progressive. For patients with orbital involvement, MRI should include thin (≤3 mm) axial and coronal T1WI, fat-saturated T2WI, and post-contrast fat-saturated T1W images of the orbits. To prevent image blurring related to ocular motion, anesthesia is generally required. Older patients should be reminded not to wear eye makeup, which can cause significant artifact on MRI. Surveillance in patients with NF-1-related optic pathway tumors should include whole-brain pre- and post-contrast T1WI to evaluate for additional enhancing low-grade astrocytomas, to which they are predisposed. Sporadic optic pathway gliomas are typically limited to the optic chiasm, hypothalamus and optic tracts, are partially cystic, and behave more aggressively; leptomeningeal metastasis may occur (Fig. 4.6). Though they may appear well-circumscribed on imaging, infiltration is common. Otherwise, imaging characteristics are similar to supratentorial and infratentorial pilocytic astrocytomas (Chung et al. 2007; Koeller and Rushing 2004; Czyzyk et al. 2003). Gangliogliomas rarely involve the hypothalamus/optic chiasm and have an appearance similar to pilocytic astrocytomas (Saleem et al. 2007).

Germinomas are the most common suprasellar GCT; 25–35% are suprasellar and do not have a gender bias. Pineal and suprasellar tumors occur simultaneously in 15% (Fig. 4.6). Small germinomas are typically homogeneous and confined to the infundibulum, but larger tumors may involve the basal ganglia (Schroeder and Vezina 2011). Though germinomas frequently metastasize via the CSF, they are very responsive to radiation therapy and have an excellent prognosis (Smith et al. 2010). Though non-germinomatous GCTs may have cystic components, solid components are typically of lower signal intensity than pilocytic astrocytomas, assisting in differentiation (Schroeder and Vezina 2011). Langerhans cell histiocytosis (LCH) may also involve the pituitary stalk; mild thickening of the stalk (>2.7 mm) and loss of the usual neurohypophyseal T1 hyperintensity may be the earliest sign, but imaging may be negative early in disease.

Hamartomas of the tuber cinereum are small, solid non-enhancing lesions which are isointense to gray matter on T1WI and T2WI with rare cysts.

Pituitary microadenomas are <10 mm in size and show delayed enhancement on dynamic imaging. Macroadenomas are slightly more common, usually solid and may extend outside the sella or have cystic foci (Schroeder and Vezina 2011).

4.5.3 Brainstem Tumors

Approximately 10–20% of pediatric brain tumors occur in the brainstem, most frequently the pons. Most (60–80%) of these have an appearance known as diffuse intrinsic pontine glioma (DIPG), which is an imaging-based diagnosis applied when a central, poorly marginated/infil-

trating, T2 hyperintense, T1 hypointense tumor with minimal if any enhancement and no cystic or exophytic components occupies >50% of the axial diameter of the pons (Hankinson et al. 2011) (Fig. 4.7). Historically, tumors meeting these radiographic criteria have been treated without biopsy, whereas those exhibiting atypical features suggesting an alternative diagnosis (well-circumscribed, off-midline, avidly enhancing, cystic/necrotic prior to treatment) are biopsied. However, recent efforts toward development of targeted chemotherapies have driven an increase in the rate of biopsy of even typical-appearing DIPGs, revealing the underlying diagnoses to be a fairly equal distribution of grade II, III, and IV astrocytomas (Puget et al. 2015). The 2016 WHO classification includes DIPGs in the new entity termed "diffuse midline

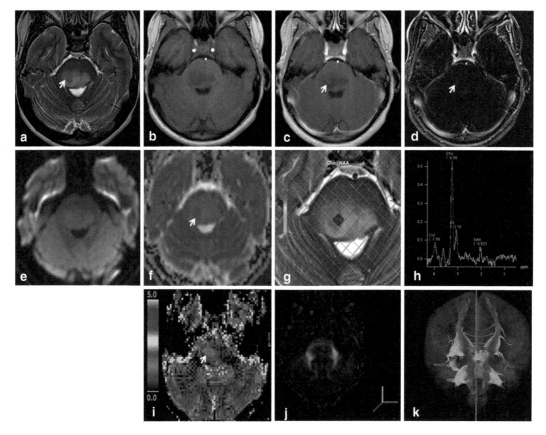

Fig. 4.7 Diffuse infiltrating pontine glioma. Infiltrating tumor involving predominantly the dorsal pons shows a (**a**) focal T2 hypointense area (arrow) with faint enhancement between the pre-contrast T1 (**b**) and post-contrast T1WI (**c**), best seen on T1 subtraction images (**d**). This focus also shows restricted diffusion (**e**-DWI, **f**-ADC), elevated choline:NAA ratio (**g**, **h**) and elevated cerebral blood volume (CBV) (**i**) consistent with focally higher-grade tumor. Diffusion tensor imaging (**j**) and tractography (**k**) show that the tumor infiltrates, rather than displaces, the white matter tracts

glioma, H3 K27M-mutant" (Louis et al. 2016). Tumors fitting imaging criteria for DIPG are generally diagnosed from 5 to 10 years of age, without gender bias. Although overall survival remains poor at a median of 9 months regardless of tumor grade, tumors with mesenchymal rather than proliferative gene expression seem to have a better prognosis (Puget et al. 2015). Rarely, even typical-appearing "DIPGs" may have an alternative diagnosis, such as embryonal tumor (Buczkowicz et al. 2014).

Tumors not meeting radiographic criteria for DIPG represent the range of pathologies occurring elsewhere in white matter. Outside the cerebellum, pilocytic astrocytomas have a predilection for midline structures such as the brainstem; a well-circumscribed, cystic/solid mass with avidly enhancing solid component without restricted diffusion is highly suggestive of the diagnosis (Koeller and Rushing 2004). Gangliogliomas and embryonal tumors, as well as rarer tumor types, may also occur in the brainstem (Fig. 4.8). Because focal tumors may be partially or entirely resected, these have a better prognosis, particularly avidly enhancing, partially cystic and/or exophytic tumors, which are most frequently low-grade pilocytic astrocy-

tomas or less commonly gangliogliomas (Ramos et al. 2013). Therefore, radiographic differentiation between focal and diffuse tumors may have a significant impact on management and prognosis of brainstem tumors. In cases where significant edema may obscure the margins of an otherwise focal brainstem tumor, DTI may be helpful for differentiating focal from infiltrating midline tumors (Figs. 4.7 and 4.8) and identify candidates for biopsy and/or resection.

Patients with NF-1 have an increased risk for astrocytomas of the brainstem, most commonly pilocytic or low-grade, which occur most frequently in the medulla or midbrain. These are most frequently asymptomatic and have an indolent course, and are therefore typically observed unless they progress. Non-enhancing tumor may be difficult to differentiate from neurofibromatosis-related T2 hyperintensities, which occur not only in the brainstem but also in the cerebellar white matter, basal ganglia, and thalami and appear somewhat expansile. However, these lesions, which are likely caused by intramyelinic edema/vacuolization (Billiet et al. 2014), do not enhance and should not be frankly exophytic, features more suggestive of tumor. Spectroscopy and degree of brainstem enlargement may be helpful in differentiating NF-related

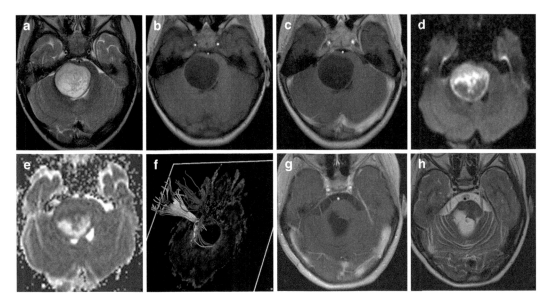

Fig. 4.8 Focal pontine tumor (embryonal tumor, NOS). A well-circumscribed, T2-hyperintense (**a**) pontine mass show little enhancement between pre-contrast (**b**) and post-contrast (**c**) T1WI, restricted diffusion consistent with hypercellularity on DWI (**d**) and ADC map (**e**). DTI

tractography (**f**) shows displacement, rather than infiltration, of white matter tracts, suggesting at least partial resectability. 4.8 years later, post-contrast T1WI (**g**) and T2WI (**h**) show a postoperative defect with no evidence of recurrent tumor

white matter lesions from non-enhancing tumor (Broniscer et al. 1997).

Tectal gliomas are rare (<5% of brainstem tumors), typically low grade (WHO grade I–II) and have a benign course, though they may cause hydrocephalus requiring shunt placement or third ventriculostomy if they obstruct the cerebral aqueduct. Typically they are T1 hypo- or isointense to brain, T2 hyperintense and do not enhance. Like brainstem gliomas in NF-1, they are typically observed unless they are progressive or large or enhance prior to therapy (Ramos et al. 2013).

4.5.4 Supratentorial Brain Tumors

Brain tumors are more commonly supratentorial in children under age 2 and over age 10 (Rickert and Paulus 2001; Ostrom et al. 2015). Astrocytomas are most common in all ages. Though teratomas account for the majority of brain tumors diagnosed in utero, their prognosis is poor with only about 10% survival (Milani et al. 2015), and in infants <1 year of age gliomas are therefore most common, followed by ATRT, choroid plexus tumors, and tumors previously known

as PNET (recently re categorized in the 2016 WHO classification scheme as embryonal tumor, NOS) (Ostrom et al. 2015; Louis et al. 2016).

Desmoplastic infantile tumors (DIT), which may be gangliogliomas (DIG) or astrocytomas (DIA), are rare WHO grade I tumors occurring exclusively in infants <18 months of age, distinguished only by the presence of neuronal elements in DIG. On MRI, a large, supratentorial mixed cystic/solid mass involving more than one lobe with dural attachment in an infant is suggestive. Hemorrhage is uncommon but may occur. They may be suprasellar. Solid components enhance and may show restricted diffusion, despite the benign nature of the lesion (Jurkiewicz et al. 2015). The absence of fat or calcification differentiates DIT from teratoma. Differential considerations include ATRT, ependymoma, embryonal tumor, NOS, and glioblastoma multiforme (GBM) (Bader et al. 2015) (Fig. 4.9).

Forty percent of ependymomas are supratentorial. In contrast to infratentorial ependymomas, which are intraventricular, supratentorial ependymomas are largely (if not all) parenchymal tumors, and tend to occur in older children/adolescents, though they may occur at any age

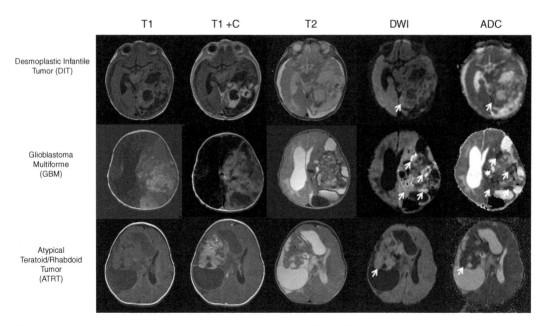

Fig. 4.9 Large supratentorial tumors in infants. Restricted diffusion (arrows) (high signal on DWI, low signal on ADC) is more common in the solid components of GBMs and ATRTs, which are also more likely to hemorrhage (arrows) than DITs

(Mermuys et al. 2005). The appearance is quite variable; although most are fairly large at diagnosis and have a cystic and/or necrotic component, small, homogeneous cerebral ependymomas occur and may mimic astrocytoma. The solid components have variable signal on T1WI and T2WI, but tend to be isointense to brain on both sequences, with heterogeneous enhancement. At our institution, a large proportion of supratentorial ependymomas are anaplastic, which may account for the presence of restricted diffusion within the solid components of some tumors. Edema is common. Most seem to occur in a peritrigonal location, and large tumor cysts may protrude into the ventricle, mimicking an intraventricular location (Fig. 4.10).

As described above, ATRT is a highly malignant tumor of very young children, rarely occurring in children >4 years of age, and is the most common embryonal tumor in infants <1 year of age (Ostrom et al. 2015). About half are supratentorial, where they tend to be quite large at presentation (Figs. 4.9 and 4.10). The appearance and location are variable; though most are parenchymal, they may be intraventricular or appear extra-axial. They are most frequently both solid and cystic/necrotic, with frequent hemorrhage and/or calcification. Compared to gray matter, the solid components are usually T1 hypointense and heterogeneously T2 hyperintense, hyperdense on CT, and enhance (Meyers et al. 2006; Parmar et al. 2006). Restricted diffusion is variably present. ATRT should be included in the differential diagnosis of a large, heterogeneous supratentorial mass in a young child, along with other embryonal tumors, ependymoma, and DIT.

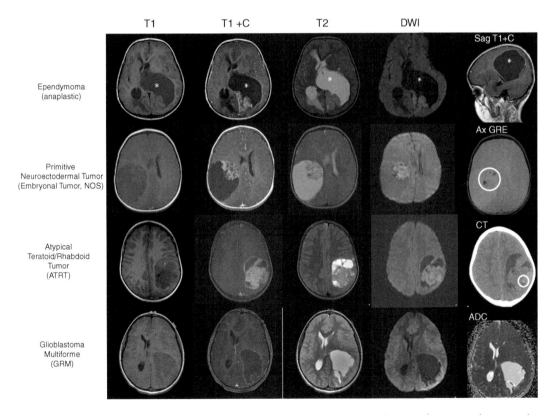

Fig. 4.10 Supratentorial tumors in older children. Ependymomas, ATRTs, and GBMs may be indistinguishable on imaging; all may appear solid ±cysts, with restricted diffusion (high signal on DWI, low signal on ADC) in the solid components. A peritrigonal location is common in ependymoma, but not pathognomonic; large cysts (*) may mimic the adjacent ventricle. Calcifications (dark on GRE, bright on CT, circled) are common in and ATRT and may also be present in ependymomas

Supratentorial embryonal tumors are rare (<1% of pediatric brain tumors) and molecularly heterogeneous. Tumors previously known as primitive neuroectodermal tumors (PNETs) have been reclassified into embryonal tumors with rhabdoid features; embryonal tumors with multilayered rosettes with and without C19MC alteration; medulloepithelioma; and embryonal tumor, NOS (Louis et al. 2016). Historically, this group of tumors have a 30–40% likelihood of leptomeningeal metastasis at diagnosis, necessitating meticulous screening of brain and spine at diagnosis for accurate staging (Borja et al. 2013; Picard et al. 2012). Overall prognosis is poor and closely linked to extent of resection (Jakacki et al. 2015; Picard et al. 2012; Borja et al. 2013). Though they may occur in children of any age, supratentorial embryonal tumors are most common in children under the age of 5 (Jakacki et al. 2015). Like other embryonal tumors, solid components are typically hyperdense to gray matter on CT, isointense to gray matter on FLAIR and T2WI, and show restricted diffusion (low ADC) due to their high nucleus-to-cytoplasm ratio. rCBV is elevated. Though supratentorial embryonal tumors frequently appear well-circumscribed, many are infiltrative. Cysts/necrosis, hemorrhage, and calcifications are common (Borja et al. 2013; Jakacki et al. 2015) (Fig. 4.10).

4.5.4.1 Astrocytomas

As in the posterior fossa, astrocytoma is the most common tumor of the cerebral hemisphere. Though anaplastic astrocytomas (WHO grade III) and glioblastoma multiforme (GBM (WHO grade IV) occur, most cerebral astrocytomas are low-grade (WHO grades I–II) and diffuse; only about 10% of supratentorial astrocytomas are pilocytic, compared to 85% in the posterior fossa (Koeller and Rushing 2004).

WHO grade of astrocytomas may be approximated by their degree of enhancement, restricted diffusion, T2 signal intensity, or application of advanced imaging techniques such as perfusion imaging and spectroscopy (Treister et al. 2014; Borja et al. 2013). Low-grade cerebral astrocytomas generally appear ill-defined and hypointense to gray matter on T1WI, hyperintense on T2WI and FLAIR, and show no restricted diffusion or enhancement. Although enhancement suggests higher tumor grade, there is significant overlap; the solid components of pilocytic astrocytomas may avidly enhance. Restricted diffusion (low ADC) suggests increased cellularity and higher tumor grade. Low-grade astrocytomas tend to have very high signal on T2WI, whereas more cellular (higher-grade) regions appear of lower T2 signal intensity due to decreased water content. Finally, higher-grade tumors, including GBMs (WHO grade IV) (Figs. 4.9 and 4.10), have a greater tendency toward hemorrhage and necrosis, and frequently have elevated rCBV reflecting increased angiogenesis, a hallmark of transition from lower to higher-grade glioma. Cho:NAA and Cho:Cr ratios are also elevated, as further described below. Imaging features of GBM may suggest underlying genetic alterations; enhancement corresponds to angiogenesis, and to EGFR overexpression, which may inform treatment with EGFR inhibitors. Infiltrating tumor is generally present beyond the enhancing or bulky tumor components, tends to increase with anti-angiogenic therapy, and portends a worse prognosis (Belden et al. 2011).

Pleomorphic xanthoastrocytomas are rare WHO grade II cortical/subcortical neoplasms occurring most frequently in the temporal lobes of adolescents and young adults. They appear as well-circumscribed, cystic/solid masses with heterogeneous enhancement and no restricted diffusion. Ganglioglioma, oligodendroglioma, and pilocytic astrocytoma are in the differential diagnosis (Borja et al. 2013).

Oligodendrogliomas occur very rarely in children, most frequently in the frontal and temporal lobes. In children, <40% calcify and they are otherwise nonspecific in appearance—T1 hypointense, T2 hyperintense, and without restricted diffusion. Enhancement is infrequent (Borja et al. 2013).

4.5.4.2 Mixed Glioneuronal Tumors

Subependymal giant cell astrocytomas (SEGAs) are intraventricular mixed glioneuronal tumors arising almost exclusively in children and young adults with tuberous sclerosis complex (TSC), possibly from the subependymal nodules (SEN) typical of the disorder, though this is controversial. Both SEGA and SEN may avidly enhance; therefore, diagnosis of SEGA depends on documentation of serial growth of a subependymal nodule, or a nodule ≥1 cm in any dimension located at the caudothalamic groove/foramen of Monro. SEGA are slow-growing, but may result in hydrocephalus due to obstruction of the foramen of Monro, necessitating screening by MRI (Roth et al. 2013). Signal is variable on T1WI, and hyperintense to gray matter on T2 and FLAIR. Restricted diffusion is absent, but rCBV and Cho:NAA ratios may be elevated (Borja et al. 2013). Identification of SEN or SEGA should prompt evaluation for other CNS manifestations of TSC, including cortical tubers and retinal hamartomas.

Gangliogliomas/gangliocytomas are rare tumors composed of neoplastic glial elements and either mature (gangliocytoma, WHO grade I) or neoplastic (ganglioglioma, WHO grade I-II) neuronal elements. Accounting for <5% of pediatric CNS tumors overall, >80% occur in the cerebral hemispheres; more than half of these occur in the temporal lobe (Dudley et al. 2015). They are indistinguishable from one another on imaging and may appear as a well-circumscribed cyst with mural nodule, solid mass, or mixed cystic/solid mass, similar to pilocytic astrocytoma (Adesina and Rauch 2010). Edema is unusual and, like many slow-growing, low-grade tumors, may be associated with scalloping of the overlying calvarium. Solid components are iso- to hypointense to gray matter on T1WI, hyperintense on T2, enhance, and show no restricted diffusion.

Dysembryoplastic neuroepithelial tumors (DNET) are WHO grade I mixed glioneuronal tumors associated with epilepsy, occurring in older children and young adults. The typical appearance is that of a bubbly-appearing cortical mass with little or no enhancement, hypodense on CT, hypointense on T1WI, and hyperintense on T2WI. Rare edema, calcifications, and hemorrhage have been noted. They may be multiple and recur, necessitating imaging follow-up (Daghistani et al. 2013).

4.5.5 Extra-Axial Tumors

Though they are the most common intracranial tumor in adults, meningiomas are very rare in children (2–4% of all CNS tumors); the incidence increases with age (Ostrom et al. 2014, 2015; Poretti et al. 2012). Meningiomas are typically associated with the dura or are intraventricular, are iso- to hypointense to gray matter on both T1 and T2-weighted MR images, avidly enhance, and may show restricted diffusion on DWI. Cranial nerve schwannomas are also rare in children and are usually seen in the setting of neurofibromatosis type 2 (NF-2); they tend to be T1 isointense, T2 hyperintense, and avidly enhance, and most commonly involve the eighth cranial nerve in the internal auditory canal (acoustic schwannoma). Because of the rarity of these tumors in children, alternative diagnoses should be entertained in children with extra-axial tumors, even those fitting these signal characteristics, without additional imaging or clinical evidence of NF-2. Meningiomas may also occur following craniospinal irradiation, particularly in patients with predisposition syndromes like Gorlin (basal cell nevus) syndrome (Bree and Shah 2011).

Choroid plexus papillomas and carcinomas occur in all age groups, though more frequently in young children, accounting for 10–20% of intracranial neoplasms in infants <1 year of age. In children, the most common location is the lateral ventricle; the fourth ventricle is less common, though more common in adults. Patients usually present with hydrocephalus. The imaging appearance of papillomas and carcinomas is similar; both appear as lobulated intraventricular enhancing masses, iso- to hyperdense on CT, T1 iso- to hyperintense and T2 hyperintense on MRI. In solid portions, diffusion may be mildly restricted, and calcifications may be present (Fig. 4.11). Features suggesting carcinoma over papilloma include a greater degree of invasion of regional structures, necrosis, hemorrhage, and elevated myoinositol on MR spectroscopy (Jaiswal et al. 2013; Borja et al. 2013; Ogiwara et al. 2012).

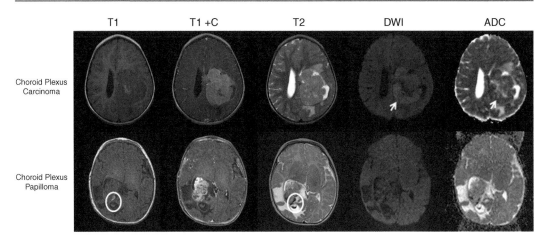

Fig. 4.11 Choroid plexus papillomas and carcinomas are undistinguishable by imaging. Though invasion of surrounding structures and hemorrhage (circled) are usually suggestive of carcinoma, this is not always the case, as demonstrated here. Either may show restricted diffusion (arrows)

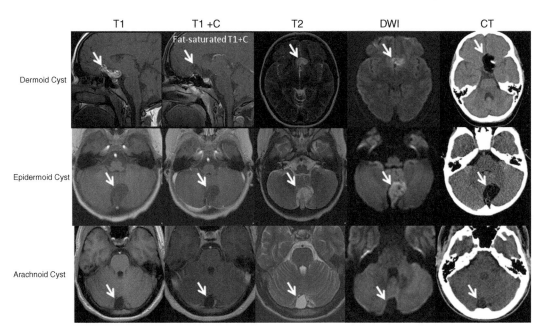

Fig. 4.12 Benign extra-axial cystic lesions (arrows). Dermoid cysts appear fat-laden, with suppression on fat-saturation and very low density on CT. Epidermoid cysts have an appearance more suggestive of "dirty CSF" and may be distinguishable from arachnoid cysts only by increased signal on DWI

Dermoid and epidermoid cysts are benign, slow-growing congenital lesions with ectodermal elements. Dermoid cysts tend to occur in the midline, are most frequently sellar/suprasellar and appear heterogeneously T1 hyperintense, and may rupture. Epidermoid cysts tend to occur off-midline and appear similar to CSF on T1WI, T2WI, and FLAIR, but appear hyperintense to CSF on DWI, differentiating them from arachnoid cysts (Fig. 4.12).

4.5.6 Spinal and Cervicomedullary Tumors

Sixty percent of intramedullary spinal cord neoplasms in children are grade I–II (pilocytic and fibrillary) astrocytomas, followed by epen-dymomas (30%) and gangliogliomas (15%). Intramedullary cord tumors typically feature a non-neoplastic polar cyst, which is a non-enhancing cyst at the upper and/or lower margin of the tumor (Fig. 4.13). Tumor cysts, on the other hand, peripherally enhance (Fig. 4.14).

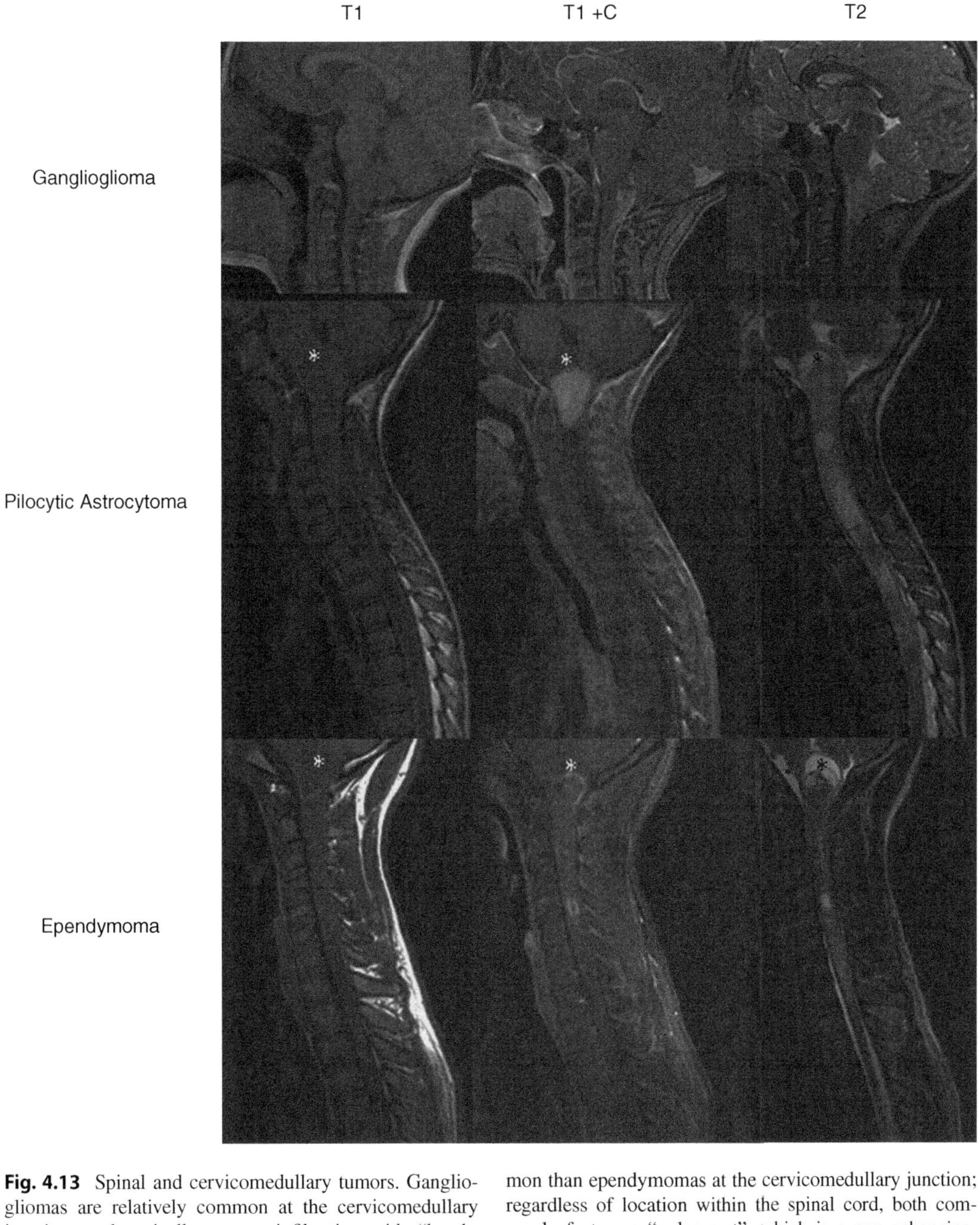

Fig. 4.13 Spinal and cervicomedullary tumors. Ganglio-gliomas are relatively common at the cervicomedullary junction, and typically appear infiltrative with "brush-like" enhancement. Pilocytic astrocytomas are more com-mon than ependymomas at the cervicomedullary junction; regardless of location within the spinal cord, both com-monly feature a "polar cyst", which is a non-enhancing, non-neoplastic cyst at the upper and/or lower margin (*)

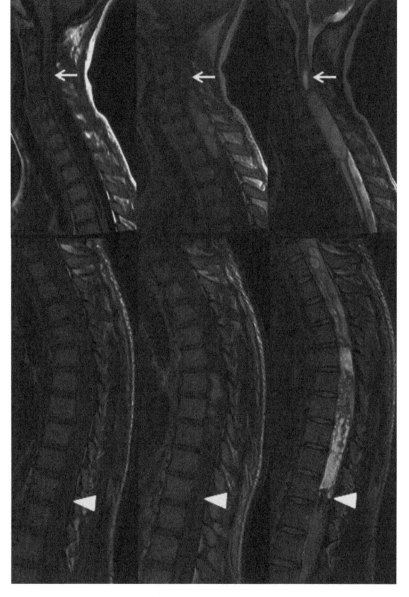

Fig. 4.14 Pilocytic astrocytoma vs. ganglioglioma. This focal, enhancing cervicothoracic pilocytic astrocytoma features a hemorrhagic, peripherally enhancing tumor cyst (arrow) within its superior portion. Spinal cord gan- gliogliomas are more likely to cover >8 vertebral body segments, like this mixed cystic and solid holocord gan- glioglioma with hemorrhage (arrow head)

Though definitive differentiation of spinal cord tumors is not possible by MRI, certain features suggest different diagnoses. Ependymomas tend to occur centrally within the cord and are more likely to hemorrhage, but less likely to have intra- tumoral cysts than astrocytomas. Astrocytomas and gangliogliomas tend to be eccentric, and though holocord involvement may occur in astro- cytoma, gangliogliomas are more likely to cover a large number (>8) of vertebral segments, with cysts/necrosis and hemorrhage common (Koeller et al. 2000; Smith et al. 2012; Gupta et al. 2014).

Ependymomas are more frequent in patients with NF-2, and astrocytomas are more frequent in patients with NF-1. Enhancement of astrocytomas and gangliogliomas is usually heterogeneous; avid, homogeneous enhancement is suggestive of ependymoma. A cleavage plane or "cap sign," or a low T2 signal rim (hemosiderin) are also suggestive of ependymoma. Rarer intramedullary tumor types include ATRT, GBM, and PNET/embryonal tumor; hemangioblastomas of the spinal cord are exceedingly rare in the absence of von Hippel-Lindau syndrome (Smith et al. 2012).

At the cervicomedullary junction, most (approximately 85%) intramedullary tumors in children are low-grade (WHO grades I–II), with pilocytic astrocytoma (approximately 40%) and ganglioglioma (approximately 25%) being most common; high-grade gliomas and ependymomas are much less common in this location (McAbee et al. 2015) (Fig. 4.13). Though pilocytic astrocytomas and gangliogliomas are not readily differentiated on imaging, foci of restricted diffusion or hemorrhage may be present in gangliogliomas, but are uncommon in pilocytic astrocytomas (Gupta et al. 2014; Koeller and Rushing 2004). Otherwise, elevated rCBV, restricted diffusion, and elevated choline:NAA ratios are suggestive of rare, high-grade tumors.

Leptomeningeal metastases of primary brain tumors are the most common intradural extramedullary spinal tumor in children. Myxopapillary ependymomas (WHO grade I), which are much rarer in children than in adults, occur at the conus medullaris or from the filum terminale, or rarely in extraspinal locations near the sacrum. They may be iso- or hyperintense on T1WI, are hyperintense on T2WI, may hemorrhage and have heterogeneous enhancement. Because of their potential for leptomeningeal dissemination and high (>50%) recurrence rate in children even after gross total resection, long-term spinal imaging surveillance is recommended (Koeller et al. 2000; Soderlund et al. 2012; Stephen et al. 2012). Schwannomas are focal benign neoplasms of peripheral nerves that occur most frequently, and may be multiple, in NF-2. Neurofibromas are infiltrative nerve sheath tumors that rarely occur outside of NF-1 in children; some may appear as poorly defined masses comprised of serpiginous-appearing signal, termed plexiform neurofibroma. Both neurofibromas and schwannomas may scallop bone and widen neural foramina, are isointense on T1WI and hyperintense on T2WI and enhance. Central low signal, known as the "target sign," is suggestive of neurofibroma, whereas cysts or fat suggest schwannoma. Malignant transformation of neurofibromas to malignant peripheral nerve sheath tumors is heralded by rapid growth. Meningiomas are also rare in the spinal canal of children outside of NF2, but are most commonly the clear cell variant, which is more aggressive due to its infiltrative growth pattern and potential for metastasis (Soderlund et al. 2012).

4.6 Future Directions in Pediatric CNS Tumor Imaging

Continued advances in technological imaging promise to improve the noninvasive detection and specific characterization of pediatric CNS tumors. High-field MR spectroscopy can resolve previously "MR invisible" metabolites such as 2-hydroxyglutarate, which is associated with mutated isocitrate dehydrogenases 1 and 2 in grade II and III gliomas (Choi et al. 2012), improving imaging-based specificity in assessing tumor grade. Combined PET/MRI scanners improve both spatial and temporal resolution for brain tumor metabolic imaging, with the potential for nearly simultaneous, complementary measures of tumor and brain physiologic function/markers (Stanescu et al. 2013). Targeted MRI and PET contrast agents currently under investigation may, in the future, enable detection of specific molecular markers for diagnosis and evaluation of efficacy of treatment, and permit early change to alternative therapeutic agents without the long wait to document lack of response (Gulyas and Halldin 2012; Iqbal et al. 2011; Abakumov et al. 2015). Finally, the development of quiet, motion-insensitive MR sequences promises to reduce our reliance on anesthesia to acquire high-resolution diagnostic images without compromise by motion (Heismann et al. 2014; Ida et al. 2014; Idiyatullin et al. 2006; Pierre et al. 2014), and improve the patient's imaging experience.

References

Abakumov MA, Nukolova NV, Sokolsky-Papkov M, Shein SA, Sandalova TO, Vishwasrao HM, Grinenko NF, Gubsky IL, Abakumov AM, Kabanov AV, Chekhonin VP (2015) VEGF-targeted magnetic nanoparticles for MRI visualization of brain tumor. Nanomedicine 11(4):825–833. https://doi.org/10.1016/j.nano.2014.12.011

Adesina AM, Rauch RA (2010) Ganglioglioma and Gangliocytoma. In: Adesina AM, Tihan T, Fuller CE, Poussaint TY (eds) Atlas of pediatric brain tumors. Springer Science+Business Media, LLC, pp 181–192. https://doi.org/10.1007/978-1-4419-1062-2_18

Awa R, Campos F, Arita K, Sugiyama K, Tominaga A, Kurisu K, Yamasaki F, Karki P, Tokimura H, Fukukura Y, Fujii Y, Hanaya R, Oyoshi T, Hirano H (2014) Neuroimaging diagnosis of pineal region tumors-quest for pathognomonic finding of germinoma. Neuroradiology 56(7):525–534. https://doi.org/10.1007/s00234-014-1369-4

Bader A, Heran M, Dunham C, Steinbok P (2015) Radiological features of infantile glioblastoma and desmoplastic infantile tumors: British Columbia's Children's Hospital experience. J Neurosurg Pediatr 16(2):119–125. https://doi.org/10.3171/2014.10.PEDS13634

Bartels U, Shroff M, Sung L, Dag-Ellams U, Laperriere N, Rutka J, Bouffet E (2006) Role of spinal MRI in the follow-up of children treated for medulloblastoma. Cancer 107(6):1340–1347. https://doi.org/10.1002/cncr.22129

Belden CJ, Valdes PA, Ran C, Pastel DA, Harris BT, Fadul CE, Israel MA, Paulsen K, Roberts DW (2011) Genetics of glioblastoma: a window into its imaging and histopathologic variability. Radiographics 31(6):1717–1740. https://doi.org/10.1148/rg.316115512

Billiet T, Madler B, D'Arco F, Peeters R, Deprez S, Plasschaert E, Leemans A, Zhang H, den Bergh BV, Vandenbulcke M, Legius E, Sunaert S, Emsell L (2014) Characterizing the microstructural basis of "unidentified bright objects" in neurofibromatosis type 1: a combined in vivo multicomponent T2 relaxation and multi-shell diffusion MRI analysis. Neuroimage Clin 4:649–658. https://doi.org/10.1016/j.nicl.2014.04.005

Borja MJ, Plaza MJ, Altman N, Saigal G (2013) Conventional and advanced MRI features of pediatric intracranial tumors: supratentorial tumors. AJR Am J Roentgenol 200(5):W483–W503. https://doi.org/10.2214/AJR.12.9724

Brandao LA, Shiroishi MS, Law M (2013) Brain tumors: a multimodality approach with diffusion-weighted imaging, diffusion tensor imaging, magnetic resonance spectroscopy, dynamic susceptibility contrast and dynamic contrast-enhanced magnetic resonance imaging. Magn Reson Imaging Clin N Am 21(2):199–239. https://doi.org/10.1016/j.mric.2013.02.003

Bree AF, Shah MR (2011) Consensus statement from the first international colloquium on basal cell nevus syndrome (BCNS). Am J Med Genet A 155A(9):2091–2097. https://doi.org/10.1002/ajmg.a.34128

Brennan RC, Wilson MW, Kaste S, Helton KJ, McCarville MB (2012) US and MRI of pediatric ocular masses with histopathological correlation. Pediatr Radiol 42(6):738–749. https://doi.org/10.1007/s00247-012-2374-6

Broniscer A, Gajjar A, Bhargava R, Langston JW, Heideman R, Jones D, Kun LE, Taylor J (1997) Brain stem involvement in children with neurofibromatosis type 1: role of magnetic resonance imaging and spectroscopy in the distinction from diffuse pontine glioma. Neurosurgery 40(2):331–337; discussion 337-338

Buczkowicz P, Bartels U, Bouffet E, Becher O, Hawkins C (2014) Histopathological spectrum of paediatric diffuse intrinsic pontine glioma: diagnostic and therapeutic implications. Acta Neuropathol 128(4):573–581. https://doi.org/10.1007/s00401-014-1319-6

Buxton RB (2010) Interpreting oxygenation-based neuroimaging signals: the importance and the challenge of understanding brain oxygen metabolism. Front Neuroenerg 2:8. https://doi.org/10.3389/fnene.2010.00008

Cho HH, Choi YH, Cheon JE et al (2016) Free-breathing radial 3D fat-suppressed T1-weighted gradient-Echo sequence for contrast-enhanced pediatric spinal imaging: comparison with T1-weighted Turbo spin-Echo sequence. AJR Am J Roentgenol 207:177–182

Choi C, Ganji SK, DeBerardinis RJ, Hatanpaa KJ, Rakheja D, Kovacs Z, Yang XL, Mashimo T, Raisanen JM, Marin-Valencia I, Pascual JM, Madden CJ, Mickey BE, Malloy CR, Bachoo RM, Maher EA (2012) 2-hydroxyglutarate detection by magnetic resonance spectroscopy in IDH-mutated patients with gliomas. Nat Med 18(4):624–629. https://doi.org/10.1038/nm.2682

Chung EM, Specht CS, Schroeder JW (2007) From the archives of the AFIP: pediatric orbit tumors and tumorlike lesions: neuroepithelial lesions of the ocular globe and optic nerve. Radiographics 27(4):1159–1186. https://doi.org/10.1148/rg.274075014

Czyzyk E, Jozwiak S, Roszkowski M, Schwartz RA (2003) Optic pathway gliomas in children with and without neurofibromatosis 1. J Child Neurol 18(7):471–478

Daghistani R, Miller E, Kulkarni AV, Widjaja E (2013) Atypical characteristics and behavior of dysembryoplastic neuroepithelial tumors. Neuroradiology 55(2):217–224. https://doi.org/10.1007/s00234-013-1135-z

Dhall G, Khatua S, Finlay JL (2010) Pineal region tumors in children. Curr Opin Neurol 23(6):576–582. https://doi.org/10.1097/WCO.0b013e3283404ef1

Dudley RW, Torok MR, Gallegos DR, Mulcahy-Levy JM, Hoffman LM, Liu AK, Handler MH, Hankinson TC (2015) Pediatric low-grade ganglioglioma: epidemiology, treatments, and outcome analysis on 348 children from the surveillance, epidemiology, and end results database. Neurosurgery 76(3):313–319.; discussion 319; quiz 319–320. https://doi.org/10.1227/NEU.0000000000000619

Ellingson BM, Bendszus M, Sorensen AG, Pope WB (2014) Emerging techniques and technologies in brain tumor imaging. Neuro-Oncology 16(Suppl 7):vii12–vii23. https://doi.org/10.1093/neuonc/nou221

Engelhard HH, Corsten LA (2005) Leptomeningeal metastasis of primary central nervous system (CNS) neoplasms. Cancer Treat Res 125:71–85

Fish DE, Kim A, Ornelas C, Song S, Pangarkar S (2011) The risk of radiation exposure to the eyes of the interventional pain physician. Radiol Res Pract 2011:609537. https://doi.org/10.1155/2011/609537

Fukuoka H, Hirai T, Okuda T, Shigematsu Y, Sasao A, Kimura E, Hirano T, Yano S, Murakami R, Yamashita Y (2010) Comparison of the added value of contrast-enhanced 3D fluid-attenuated inversion recovery and magnetization-prepared rapid acquisition of gradient echo sequences in relation to conventional postcontrast T1-weighted images for the evaluation of leptomeningeal diseases at 3T. AJNR Am J Neuroradiol 31(5):868–873. https://doi.org/10.3174/ajnr.A1937

Gajjar AJ, Robinson GW (2014) Medulloblastoma-translating discoveries from the bench to the bedside. Nat Rev Clin Oncol 11(12):714–722. https://doi.org/10.1038/nrclinonc.2014.181

Gibson P, Tong Y, Robinson G, Thompson MC, Currle DS, Eden C, Kranenburg TA, Hogg T, Poppleton H, Martin J, Finkelstein D, Pounds S, Weiss A, Patay Z, Scoggins M, Ogg R, Pei Y, Yang ZJ, Brun S, Lee Y, Zindy F, Lindsey JC, Taketo MM, Boop FA, Sanford RA, Gajjar A, Clifford SC, Roussel MF, McKinnon PJ, Gutmann DH, Ellison DW, Wechsler-Reya R, Gilbertson RJ (2010) Subtypes of medulloblastoma have distinct developmental origins. Nature 468(7327):1095–1099. https://doi.org/10.1038/nature09587

Griffiths PD, Coley SC, Romanowski CA, Hodgson T, Wilkinson ID (2003) Contrast-enhanced fluid-attenuated inversion recovery imaging for leptomeningeal disease in children. AJNR Am J Neuroradiol 24(4):719–723

Gulyas B, Halldin C (2012) New PET radiopharmaceuticals beyond FDG for brain tumor imaging. Q J Nucl Med Mol Imaging 56(2):173–190

Gupta K, Orisme W, Harreld JH, Qaddoumi I, Dalton JD, Punchihewa C, Collins-Underwood R, Robertson T, Tatevossian RG, Ellison DW (2014) Posterior fossa and spinal gangliogliomas form two distinct clinico-pathologic and molecular subgroups. Acta Neuropathol Commun 2(1):18. https://doi.org/10.1186/2051-5960-2-18

Hakyemez B, Erdogan C, Ercan I, Ergin N, Uysal S, Atahan S (2005) High-grade and low-grade gliomas: differentiation by using perfusion MR imaging. Clin Radiol 60(4):493–502. https://doi.org/10.1016/j.crad.2004.09.009

Hankinson TC, Campagna EJ, Foreman NK, Handler MH (2011) Interpretation of magnetic resonance images in diffuse intrinsic pontine glioma: a survey of pediatric neurosurgeons. J Neurosurg Pediatr 8(1):97–102. https://doi.org/10.3171/2011.4.PEDS1180

Harreld JH, Sabin ND, Rossi MG, Awwad R, Reddick WE, Yuan Y, Glass JO, Ji Q, Gajjar A, Patay Z (2014) Elevated cerebral blood volume contributes to increased FLAIR signal in the cerebral sulci of Propofol-sedated children. AJNR Am J Neuroradiol 35(8):1574–1579. https://doi.org/10.3174/ajnr.A3911

Harreld JH, Mohammed N, Goldsberry G, Li X, Li Y, Boop F, Patay Z (2015) Postoperative Intraspinal subdural collections after pediatric posterior Fossa tumor resection: incidence, imaging, and clinical features. AJNR Am J Neuroradiol 36:993. https://doi.org/10.3174/ajnr.A4221

Heismann B, Ott M, Grodzki D (2014) Sequence-based acoustic noise reduction of clinical MRI scans. Magn Reson Med 73:1104. https://doi.org/10.1002/mrm.25229

Hwang JH, Egnaczyk GF, Ballard E, Dunn RS, Holland SK, Ball WS Jr (1998) Proton MR spectroscopic characteristics of pediatric pilocytic astrocytomas. AJNR Am J Neuroradiol 19(3):535–540

Ida M, Wakayama T, Nielsen ML, Abe T, Grodzki DM (2014) Quiet T1-weighted imaging using PETRA: initial clinical evaluation in intracranial tumor patients. J Magn Reson Imaging 41:447. https://doi.org/10.1002/jmri.24575

Idiyatullin D, Corum C, Park JY, Garwood M (2006) Fast and quiet MRI using a swept radiofrequency. J Magn Reson 181(2):342–349. https://doi.org/10.1016/j.jmr.2006.05.014

Iqbal U, Albaghdadi H, Nieh MP, Tuor UI, Mester Z, Stanimirovic D, Katsaras J, Abulrob A (2011) Small unilamellar vesicles: a platform technology for molecular imaging of brain tumors. Nanotechnology 22(19):195102. https://doi.org/10.1088/0957-4484/22/19/195102

Jaiswal S, Vij M, Mehrotra A, Kumar B, Nair A, Jaiswal AK, Behari S, Jain VK (2013) Choroid plexus tumors: a clinico-pathological and neuro-radiological study of 23 cases. Asian J Neurosurg 8(1):29–35. https://doi.org/10.4103/1793-5482.110277

Jakacki RI, Burger PC, Kocak M, Boyett JM, Goldwein J, Mehta M, Packer RJ, Tarbell NJ, Pollack IF (2015) Outcome and prognostic factors for children with supratentorial primitive neuroectodermal tumors treated with carboplatin during radiotherapy: a report from the Children's Oncology Group. Pediatr Blood Cancer 62(5):776–783. https://doi.org/10.1002/pbc.25405

Jurkiewicz E, Grajkowska W, Nowak K, Kowalczyk P, Walecka A, Dembowska-Baginska B (2015) MR imaging, apparent diffusion coefficient and histopathological features of desmoplastic infantile tumors-own experience and review of the literature. Childs Nerv Syst 31(2):251–259. https://doi.org/10.1007/s00381-014-2593-2

Kimonis VE, Goldstein AM, Pastakia B, Yang ML, Kase R, DiGiovanna JJ, Bale AE, Bale SJ (1997) Clinical manifestations in 105 persons with nevoid basal cell carcinoma syndrome. Am J Med Genet 69(3):299–308

Koeller KK, Rushing EJ (2004) From the archives of the AFIP: pilocytic astrocytoma: radiologic-pathologic correlation. Radiographics 24(6):1693–1708. https://doi.org/10.1148/rg.246045146

Koeller KK, Rosenblum RS, Morrison AL (2000) Neoplasms of the spinal cord and filum terminale: radiologic-pathologic correlation. Radiographics 20(6):1721–1749. https://doi.org/10.1148/radiographics.20.6.g00nv151721

Koral K, Alford R, Choudhury N, Mossa-Basha M, Gargan L, Gimi B, Gao A, Zhang S, Bowers DC, Koral KM, Izbudak I (2014) Applicability of apparent diffusion coefficient ratios in preoperative diagnosis of common pediatric cerebellar tumors across two institutions. Neuroradiology 56(9):781–788. https://doi.org/10.1007/s00234-014-1398-z

Kremer S, Abu Eid M, Bierry G, Bogorin A, Koob M, Dietemann JL, Fruehlich S (2006) Accuracy of delayed post-contrast FLAIR MR imaging for the diagnosis of leptomeningeal infectious or tumoral diseases. J Neuroradiol 33(5):285–291

Larsen DW, Teitelbaum GP, Norman D (1996) Cerebrospinal fluid flow artifact. A possible pitfall on fast-spin-echo MR imaging of the spine simulating intradural pathology. Clin Imaging 20(2):140–142

Law M, Young RJ, Babb JS, Peccerelli N, Chheang S, Gruber ML, Miller DC, Golfinos JG, Zagzag D, Johnson G (2008) Gliomas: predicting time to progression or survival with cerebral blood volume measurements at dynamic susceptibility-weighted contrast-enhanced perfusion MR imaging. Radiology 247(2):490–498. https://doi.org/10.1148/radiol.2472070898

Liang D, Bhatta S, Gerzanich V, Simard JM (2007) Cytotoxic edema: mechanisms of pathological cell swelling. Neurosurg Focus 22(5):E2

Lisanti C, Carlin C, Banks KP, Wang D (2007) Normal MRI appearance and motion-related phenomena of CSF. AJR Am J Roentgenol 188(3):716–725

Louis DN, Perry A, Reifenberger G, von Deimling A, Figarella-Branger D, Cavenee WK, Ohgaki H, Wiestler OD, Kleihues P, Ellison DW (2016) The 2016 World Health Organization classification of tumors if the central nervous system: a summary. Acta Neuropathol 131:803. https://doi.org/10.1007/s00401-016-1545-1

Maroldi R, Ambrosi C, Farina D (2005) Metastatic disease of the brain: extra-axial metastases (skull, dura, leptomeningeal) and tumour spread. Eur Radiol 15(3):617–626. https://doi.org/10.1007/s00330-004-2617-5

Mathews VP, Caldemeyer KS, Lowe MJ, Greenspan SL, Weber DM, Ulmer JL (1999) Brain: gadolinium-enhanced fast fluid-attenuated inversion-recovery MR imaging. Radiology 211(1):257–263

McAbee JH, Modica J, Thompson CJ, Broniscer A, Orr B, Choudhri AF, Boop FA, Klimo P Jr (2015) Cervicomedullary tumors in children. J Neurosurg Pediatr 16(4):357–366. https://doi.org/10.3171/2015.5.PEDS14638

McRobbie DW (2007) MRI from picture to proton, 2nd edn. Cambridge University Press, Cambridge, New York

McRobbie DW, Moore EA, Graves MJ, Prince MR (2007) MRI from picture to proton, 2nd edn. Cambridge University Press, New York

Mermuys K, Jeuris W, Vanhoenacker PK, Van Hoe L, D'Haenens P (2005) Best cases from the AFIP: supratentorial ependymoma. Radiographics 25(2):486–490. https://doi.org/10.1148/rg.252045095

Meyers SP, Khademian ZP, Biegel JA, Chuang SH, Korones DN, Zimmerman RA (2006) Primary intracranial atypical teratoid/rhabdoid tumors of infancy and childhood: MRI features and patient outcomes. AJNR Am J Neuroradiol 27(5):962–971

Miglioretti DL, Johnson E, Williams A, Greenlee RT, Weinmann S, Solberg LI, Feigelson HS, Roblin D, Flynn MJ, Vanneman N, Smith-Bindman R (2013) The use of computed tomography in pediatrics and the associated radiation exposure and estimated cancer risk. JAMA Pediatr 167(8):700–707. https://doi.org/10.1001/jamapediatrics.2013.311

Milani HJ, Araujo Junior E, Cavalheiro S, Oliveira PS, Hisaba WJ, Barreto EQ, Barbosa MM, Nardozza LM, Moron AF (2015) Fetal brain tumors: prenatal diagnosis by ultrasound and magnetic resonance imaging. World J Radiol 7(1):17–21. https://doi.org/10.4329/wjr.v7.i1.17

Mitsuya K, Nakasu Y, Horiguchi S, Harada H, Nishimura T, Bando E, Okawa H, Furukawa Y, Hirai T, Endo M (2010) Perfusion weighted magnetic resonance imaging to distinguish the recurrence of metastatic brain tumors from radiation necrosis after stereotactic radiosurgery. J Neuro-Oncol 99(1):81–88. https://doi.org/10.1007/s11060-009-0106-z

Mukherjee P, Berman JI, Chung SW, Hess CP, Henry RG (2008) Diffusion tensor MR imaging and fiber tractography: theoretic underpinnings. AJNR Am J Neuroradiol 29(4):632–641. https://doi.org/10.3174/ajnr.A1051

Ogiwara H, Dipatri AJ Jr, Alden TD, Bowman RM, Tomita T (2012) Choroid plexus tumors in pediatric patients. Br J Neurosurg 26(1):32–37. https://doi.org/10.3109/02688697.2011.601820

Ostrom QT, Gittleman H, Liao P, Rouse C, Chen Y, Dowling J, Wolinsky Y, Kruchko C, Barnholtz-Sloan J (2014) CBTRUS statistical report: primary brain and central nervous system tumors diagnosed in the United States in 2007–2011. Neuro-Oncology 16(suppl 4):iv1–iv63. https://doi.org/10.1093/neuonc/nou223

Ostrom QT, de Blank PM, Kruchko C, Petersen CM, Liao P, Finlay JL, Stearns DS, Wolff JE, Wolinsky Y, Letterio JJ, Barnholtz-Sloan JS (2015) Alex's lemonade stand foundation infant and childhood primary brain and central nervous system tumors diagnosed in the United States in 2007–2011. Neuro-Oncology 16(suppl 10):x1–x36. https://doi.org/10.1093/neuonc/nou327

Pajtler KW, Witt H, Sill M, Jones DT, Hovestadt V, Kratochwil F, Wani K, Tatevossian R, Punchihewa C, Johann P, Reimand J, Warnatz HJ, Ryzhova M, Mack S, Ramaswamy V, Capper D, Schweizer L, Sieber L, Wittmann A, Huang Z, van Sluis P, Volckmann R, Koster J, Versteeg R, Fults D, Toledano H, Avigad S, Hoffman LM, Donson AM, Foreman N, Hewer E, Zitterbart K, Gilbert M, Armstrong TS, Gupta N, Allen JC, Karajannis MA, Zagzag D, Hasselblatt M, Kulozik AE, Witt O, Collins VP, von Hoff K, Rutkowski S, Pietsch T, Bader G, Yaspo ML, von Deimling A, Lichter P, Taylor MD, Gilbertson R, Ellison DW, Aldape K, Korshunov A, Kool M, Pfister SM (2015) Molecular classification of ependymal tumors across all CNS compartments, histopathological grades, and age groups. Cancer Cell 27(5):728–743. https://doi.org/10.1016/j.ccell.2015.04.002

Pang J, Banerjee A, Tihan T (2008) The value of tandem CSF/MRI evaluation for predicting disseminated disease in childhood central nervous system neoplasms. J Neuro-Oncol 87(1):97–102. https://doi.org/10.1007/s11060-007-9493-1

Parmar H, Hawkins C, Bouffet E, Rutka J, Shroff M (2006) Imaging findings in primary intracranial atypical teratoid/rhabdoid tumors. Pediatr Radiol 36(2):126–132. https://doi.org/10.1007/s00247-005-0037-6

Patay Z, DeSain LA, Hwang SN, Coan A, Li Y, Ellison DW (2015) MR imaging characteristics of wingless-type-subgroup pediatric Medulloblastoma. AJNR Am J Neuroradiol 36:2386. https://doi.org/10.3174/ajnr.A4495

Perreault S, Ramaswamy V, Achrol AS et al (2014) MRI surrogates for molecular subgroups of medulloblastoma. AJNR Am J Neuroradiol 35:1263–1269

Picard D, Miller S, Hawkins CE, Bouffet E, Rogers HA, Chan TS, Kim SK, Ra YS, Fangusaro J, Korshunov A, Toledano H, Nakamura H, Hayden JT, Chan J, Lafay-Cousin L, Hu P, Fan X, Muraszko KM, Pomeroy SL, Lau CC, Ng HK, Jones C, Van Meter T, Clifford SC, Eberhart C, Gajjar A, Pfister SM, Grundy RG, Huang A (2012) Markers of survival and metastatic potential in childhood CNS primitive neuro-ectodermal brain tumours: an integrative genomic analysis. Lancet Oncol 13(8):838–848. https://doi.org/10.1016/S1470-2045(12)70257-7

Pierce TT, Provenzale JM (2014) Evaluation of apparent diffusion coefficient thresholds for diagnosis of medulloblastoma using diffusion-weighted imaging. Neuroradiol J 27(1):63–74

Pierce T, Kranz PG, Roth C, Leong D, Wei P, Provenzale JM (2014) Use of apparent diffusion coefficient values for diagnosis of pediatric posterior fossa tumors. Neuroradiol J 27(2):233–244. https://doi.org/10.15274/NRJ-2014-10027

Pierre EY, Grodzki D, Aandal G, Heismann B, Badve C, Gulani V, Sunshine JL, Schluchter M, Liu K, Griswold MA (2014) Parallel imaging-based reduction of acoustic noise for clinical magnetic resonance imaging. Investig Radiol 49:620. https://doi.org/10.1097/RLI.0000000000000062

Poltinnikov IM, Merchant TE (2006) CSF cytology has limited value in the evaluation of patients with ependymoma who have MRI evidence of metastasis. Pediatr Blood Cancer 47(2):169–173. https://doi.org/10.1002/pbc.20587

Poretti A, Meoded A, Huisman TA (2012) Neuroimaging of pediatric posterior fossa tumors including review of the literature. J Magn Reson Imaging 35(1):32–47. https://doi.org/10.1002/jmri.22722

Puget S, Beccaria K, Blauwblomme T, Roujeau T, James S, Grill J, Zerah M, Varlet P, Sainte-Rose C (2015) Biopsy in a series of 130 pediatric diffuse intrinsic pontine gliomas. Childs Nerv Syst 31(10):1773–1780. https://doi.org/10.1007/s00381-015-2832-1

Ramaswamy V, Remke M, Bouffet E, Faria CC, Perreault S, Cho YJ, Shih DJ, Luu B, Dubuc AM, Northcott PA, Schuller U, Gururangan S, McLendon R, Bigner D, Fouladi M, Ligon KL, Pomeroy SL, Dunn S, Triscott J, Jabado N, Fontebasso A, Jones DT, Kool M, Karajannis MA, Gardner SL, Zagzag D, Nunes S, Pimentel J, Mora J, Lipp E, Walter AW, Ryzhova M, Zheludkova O, Kumirova E, Alshami J, Croul SE, Rutka JT, Hawkins C, Tabori U, Codispoti KE, Packer RJ, Pfister SM, Korshunov A, Taylor MD (2013) Recurrence patterns across medulloblastoma subgroups: an integrated clinical and molecular analysis. Lancet Oncol 14(12):1200–1207. https://doi.org/10.1016/S1470-2045(13)70449-2

Ramos A, Hilario A, Lagares A, Salvador E, Perez-Nunez A, Sepulveda J (2013) Brainstem gliomas. Semin Ultrasound CT MR 34(2):104–112. https://doi.org/10.1053/j.sult.2013.01.001

Rickert CH, Paulus W (2001) Epidemiology of central nervous system tumors in childhood and adolescence based on the new WHO classification. Childs Nerv Syst 17(9):503–511. https://doi.org/10.1007/s003810100496

Roth J, Roach ES, Bartels U, Jozwiak S, Koenig MK, Weiner HL, Franz DN, Wang HZ (2013) Subependymal giant cell astrocytoma: diagnosis, screening, and treatment. Recommendations from the international tuberous sclerosis complex consensus conference 2012. Pediatr Neurol 49(6):439–444. https://doi.org/10.1016/j.pediatrneurol.2013.08.017

Saleem SN, Said AH, Lee DH (2007) Lesions of the hypothalamus: MR imaging diagnostic features. Radiographics 27(4):1087–1108. https://doi.org/10.1148/rg.274065123

Schroeder JW, Vezina LG (2011) Pediatric sellar and suprasellar lesions. Pediatr Radiol 41(3):287–298.; quiz 404-285. https://doi.org/10.1007/s00247-010-1968-0

Shah KB, Guha-Thakurta N, Schellingerhout D, Madewell JE, Kumar AJ, Costelloe CM (2011) Comparison of gadolinium-enhanced fat-saturated T1-weighted FLAIR and fast spin-echo MRI of the spine at 3 T for evaluation of extradural lesions. AJR Am J Roentgenol 197(3):697–703

Smith AB, Rushing EJ, Smirniotopoulos JG (2010) From the archives of the AFIP: lesions of the pineal region: radiologic-pathologic correlation. Radiographics 30(7):2001–2020. https://doi.org/10.1148/rg.307105131

Smith AB, Soderlund KA, Rushing EJ, Smirniotopolous JG (2012) Radiologic-pathologic correlation of pediatric and adolescent spinal neoplasms: part 1, intramedullary spinal neoplasms. AJR Am J Roentgenol 198(1):34–43. https://doi.org/10.2214/AJR.10.7311

Soderlund KA, Smith AB, Rushing EJ, Smirniotopolous JG (2012) Radiologic-pathologic correlation of pediatric and adolescent spinal neoplasms: part 2, Intradural extramedullary spinal neoplasms. AJR Am J Roentgenol 198(1):44–51. https://doi.org/10.2214/AJR.11.7121

Stanescu L, Ishak GE, Khanna PC, Biyyam DR, Shaw DW, Parisi MT (2013) FDG PET of the brain in pediatric patients: imaging spectrum with MR imaging correlation. Radiographics 33(5):1279–1303. https://doi.org/10.1148/rg.335125152

Stephen JH, Sievert AJ, Madsen PJ, Judkins AR, Resnick AC, Storm PB, Rushing EJ, Santi M (2012) Spinal cord ependymomas and myxopapillary ependymomas in the first 2 decades of life: a clinicopathological and immunohistochemical characterization of 19 cases. J Neurosurg Pediatr 9(6):646–653. https://doi.org/10.3171/2012.2.PEDS11285

Sun L (2010) Early childhood general anaesthesia exposure and neurocognitive development. Br J Anaesth 105(Suppl 1):i61–i68. https://doi.org/10.1093/bja/aeq302

Terterov S, Krieger MD, Bowen I, McComb JG (2010) Evaluation of intracranial cerebrospinal fluid cytology in staging pediatric medulloblastomas, supratentorial primitive neuroectodermal tumors, and ependymomas. J Neurosurg Pediatr 6(2):131–136. https://doi.org/10.3171/2010.5.PEDS09333

Treister D, Kingston S, Hoque KE, Law M, Shiroishi MS (2014) Multimodal magnetic resonance imaging evaluation of primary brain tumors. Semin Oncol 41(4):478–495. https://doi.org/10.1053/j.seminoncol.2014.06.006

Warmuth-Metz M, Kuhl J, Krauss J, Solymosi L (2004) Subdural enhancement on postoperative spinal MRI after resection of posterior cranial fossa tumours. Neuroradiology 46(3):219–223. https://doi.org/10.1007/s00234-003-1158-y

Whitehead MT, Oh C, Raju A, Choudhri AF (2015) Physiologic pineal region, choroid plexus, and dural calcifications in the first decade of life. AJNR Am J Neuroradiol 36(3):575–580. https://doi.org/10.3174/ajnr.A4153

Yamashita Y, Kumabe T, Higano S, Watanabe M, Tominaga T (2009) Minimum apparent diffusion coefficient is significantly correlated with cellularity in medulloblastomas. Neurol Res 31(9):940–946. https://doi.org/10.1179/174313209X382520

Zeng Q, Liu H, Zhang K, Li C, Zhou G (2011) Noninvasive evaluation of cerebral glioma grade by using multivoxel 3D proton MR spectroscopy. Magn Reson Imaging 29(1):25–31. https://doi.org/10.1016/j.mri.2010.07.017

Zukotynski K, Fahey F, Kocak M, Kun L, Boyett J, Fouladi M, Vajapeyam S, Treves T, Poussaint TY (2014) 18F-FDG PET and MR imaging associations across a spectrum of pediatric brain tumors: a report from the pediatric brain tumor consortium. J Nucl Med 55(9):1473–1480. https://doi.org/10.2967/jnumed.114.139626

Predisposition Syndromes to Central Nervous System Cancers

5

Alberto Broniscer and Kim Nichols

5.1 Introduction

Recent genome-wide studies have unveiled the molecular characteristics of several pediatric central nervous system (CNS) cancers (Gajjar et al. 2014). Despite this tremendous progress, very little is known about primary risk factor(s) for the development of CNS cancers in children, including previous exposure to ionizing irradiation and genetic predisposition syndromes (Ron et al. 1988; Spector et al. 2015).

Despite their rare occurrence, genetic predisposition syndromes play a disproportionately important role in the management of children with CNS cancers due to their influence on therapeutic strategies, treatment-related toxicities, and long-term prognosis, and the need for genetic counseling of families and screening of affected individuals (Listernick et al. 1994; Tabori et al. 2010; Teplick et al. 2011; Alderfer et al. 2015). Likewise, the unveiling of mechanisms involved in rare CNS cancer predisposition syndromes has greatly increased our understanding of the somatic molecular abnormalities that occur in sporadic tumors (Vortmeyer et al. 1999; Lin and Gutmann 2013; Cowan et al. 1997).

In this chapter, we highlight important clinical, genetic, and therapeutic aspects associated with several genetic predisposition syndromes that are relevant for medical professionals taking care of children with CNS cancers, from the ones commonly encountered in clinical practice (e.g., Neurofibromatosis type 1) to extremely rare conditions that have improved the understanding of the biology of some of these devastating tumors. One of our main goals was to provide a comprehensive review of data in an easily accessible manner to help clinicians with the practical management of these complex patients.

5.2 Neurofibromatosis Type 1 (NF-1)

Online Mendelian Inheritance in Man (OMIM): #162200; *NF1* is located at 17q11.2

- Common autosomal dominant syndrome with high penetrance and variable clinical expression even among family members
- Incidence of approximately 1 in 3000
- Approximately half of affected patients do not have a family history of NF-1
- Syndromic features consist of skin, soft tissue, and neurologic manifestations, but may also include bone involvement and abnormalities in the eyes

A. Broniscer, M.D., M.S. (✉) · K. Nichols
Department of Oncology, St. Jude Children's
Research Hospital, Memphis, TN, USA
e-mail: Alberto.broniscer@stjude.org;
kim.nichols@stjude.org

5.2.1 Background and Genetics

Although presumptive cases of NF-1 had already been described as early as the thirteenth century (Ahn et al. 1996), von Recklinghausen was the first to recognize that some NF-1-associated non-CNS tumors originated from nervous tissue (Ahn et al. 1996).

NF1 is a tumor suppressor gene. Individuals with NF-1 carry one mutated allele in all body cells (except for very rare individuals with mosaicism) and an additional abnormality is gained in the second allele in cancer cells (Lin and Gutmann 2013). *NF1* encodes neurofibromin, a protein that functions as a negative regulator of the signaling protein RAS, which plays a key role in cell proliferation, differentiation, migration, and apoptosis (Lin and Gutmann 2013). Consequently, loss of neurofibromin expression and/or function secondary to biallelic *NF1* abnormalities leads to activation of RAS and other downstream pathways (e.g., mitogen activated kinase kinase [MEK] and mammalian target of rapamycin [mTOR] pathways) and is directly associated with the predisposition of patients with NF-1 to develop several cancers (Lin and Gutmann 2013).

5.2.2 Clinical Aspects

Clinical criteria to diagnose NF-1 were developed in 1987 (Table 5.1) (National Institutes of Health Consensus Development Conference Statement: neurofibromatosis. Bethesda, Md., USA, July 13–15, 1987 1988). Children with NF-1 are at an increased risk of developing several different types of cancer, including malignant peripheral nerve sheath tumor (MPNST), leukemia, and CNS cancers (Lin and Gutmann 2013). Optic pathway glioma (OPG; pilocytic astrocytoma [World Health Organization (WHO) grade 1]) is the most common CNS cancer in children with NF-1, affecting between 15 and 20% of patients (Listernick et al. 1994). Optic nerve involvement is seen in most patients with OPG, 50% of which are bilateral (Listernick et al. 1994; Thiagalingam et al. 2004). While

Table 5.1 National Institutes of Health (NIH) criteria for neurofibromatosis type 1 (NF-1) (National Institutes of Health Consensus Development Conference Statement: neurofibromatosis. Bethesda, Md., USA, July 13–15, 1987 1988)

Patients should have two or more of the following criteria:
1. Six or more café-au-lait spots >0.5 cm in prepubertal individuals or >1.5 cm in postpubertal individuals
2. Two or more neurofibromas of any type or at least one plexiform neurofibroma
3. Freckling in the axillary and inguinal regions
4. Optic glioma
5. Two or more Lisch nodules (benign iris hamartomas)
6. A distinctive osseous lesion such as sphenoid dysplasia or thinning of long bone cortex, with or without pseudarthrosis
7. A first-degree relative with NF1 by the above criteria

approximately half to two-thirds of cases affect the optic chiasm, isolated chiasmatic involvement is less common (Listernick et al. 1994; Thiagalingam et al. 2004). The median age at the time of diagnosis of OPG is around 4 years, with symptomatic patients presenting at a younger age (Listernick et al. 1994). However, symptomatic OPG can also be diagnosed in older children, and occasionally even in the second and third decades of life (Thiagalingam et al. 2004; King et al. 2003; Listernick et al. 2004). Children with NF-1 who develop OPGs generally have a more indolent course compared to those without NF-1. Half to two-thirds of children with NF-1 and OPG do not require therapy for tumor growth and/or progressive clinical problems such as vision loss during their follow-up (Listernick et al. 1994; Thiagalingam et al. 2004; King et al. 2003). Patients with chiasmatic tumors have a higher risk of vision loss and precocious puberty (Listernick et al. 1994). Likewise, children younger than 6 years seem to be at higher risk of vision loss secondary to OPGs (Listernick et al. 1994).

Children with NF-1 have an increased risk of developing pilocytic and other low-grade astrocytomas outside the optic pathway, including synchronous and metachronous tumors involving the brainstem and cerebellum (Bilaniuk et al. 1997; Dunn et al. 2007). Brainstem gliomas can affect up to 10% of children with NF-1 and they occur in association with OPG in 40% of patients (Bilaniuk et al. 1997; Pollack et al. 1996). Three types of brainstem gliomas are observed in children with NF-1: (1) tectal plate tumors, which are very indolent and commonly cause hydrocephalus; (2) focal enhancing low-grade tumors; and (3) diffuse tumors, which may affect multiple brainstem segments. Unlike patients without NF-1, the latter tumors more commonly arise from the medulla and not from the pons (Pollack et al. 1996; Molloy et al. 1995; Bilaniuk et al. 1997). The presence of NF-1 has long been recognized as a potentially favorable prognostic factor in children with diffuse brainstem gliomas (Milstein et al. 1989; Raffel et al. 1989). Children with NF-1 and focal or diffuse brainstem gliomas have an increased risk of hydrocephalus compared to those without NF-1 (Bilaniuk et al. 1997; Molloy et al. 1995; Pollack et al. 1996). Children with NF-1 and brainstem gliomas may present with symptomatology attributable to brainstem involvement, often with a protracted course, or may be asymptomatic (Pollack et al. 1996; Molloy et al. 1995).

High-grade gliomas are also seen in children with NF-1 (Rosenfeld et al. 2010; Huttner et al. 2010), although the risk is substantially lower than that of low-grade tumors, and their development may be associated with previous use of irradiation (Rosenfeld et al. 2010). Finally, children with NF-1 are at increased risk of developing intradural, extramedullary spinal tumors, particularly intraneural and less commonly plexiform neurofibromas (Khong et al. 2003; Nguyen et al. 2015). Although spinal neurofibromas were observed upon screening in 13% of 53 asymptomatic children with NF-1 (Khong et al. 2003), their occurrence was more common in patients with symptoms attributable to spinal involvement (up to 70–80%) (Nguyen et al. 2015). Spinal neurofibromas also more commonly affect adolescents and adults than children with NF-1, which could be related to the natural history of these tumors and/or the development of symptoms over time (Nguyen et al. 2015).

5.2.3   Relevant Therapeutic Issues

The review of treatment for low- and high-grade gliomas in children with NF-1 is beyond the scope of this chapter. However, important differences in therapy between patients with and without NF-1 need to be emphasized. Children with NF-1 have an increased risk of developing second cancers after irradiation, particularly other gliomas and MPNSTs, when compared to nonirradiated NF-1 patients (Sharif et al. 2006). Cerebral vascular malformations, including arterial stenosis and occlusion, and moyamoya syndrome have been described in 2.5% of children with NF-1 who were screened by magnetic resonance imaging (MRI) for intracranial complications (Rosser et al. 2005). Another study demonstrated a significantly increased risk of symptomatic cerebral vasculopathy in children with NF-1 treated with irradiation for an OPG compared to similar patients without NF-1 (risk of 30% vs. 6%, respectively) (Grill et al. 1999). Children with NF-1 are known to be at increased risk of learning disabilities as well (North et al. 1997). Therefore, patients with NF-1 and low-grade gliomas, particularly OPGs, are preferentially treated with chemotherapy irrespective of age (Fisher et al. 2012). Upfront treatment with chemotherapy in children with NF-1 and OPGs, particularly with carboplatin-based regimens, has produced objective radiologic responses (complete, partial, and minor responses), disease stabilization, and improved visual acuity in 32%, 59%, and 32% of cases, respectively (Fisher et al. 2012). However, careful follow-up of visual function in these children is mandatory since worsening visual acuity was observed even in patients who experienced objective radiologic responses to chemotherapy (Fisher et al. 2012). Irradiation is reserved for tumors that do not respond to chemotherapy, particularly when there is concern for visual loss. Based on the importance of the activation of downstream cellular pathways in the genesis of NF-1-related tumors, clinical trials using MEK and mTOR inhibitors are underway for children with NF-1 and low-grade gliomas.

Due to their generally more favorable prognosis, anticancer therapy is usually recommended only upon documentation of overt clinical and radiologic progression in patients with NF-1 and brainstem gliomas (Pollack et al. 1996; Molloy et al. 1995). Although a minority of patients with NF-1 and brainstem glioma may have a deadly course (Molloy et al. 1995), the majority of these patients fare well even without any anticancer therapy (Molloy et al. 1995; Pollack et al. 1996). The treatment and prognosis of children with NF-1 and high-grade gliomas does not differ from that of patients without NF-1.

5.2.4　Screening

Screening of asymptomatic children with NF-1 by brain MRI is not recommended since it does not predict tumor behavior and normal results do not exclude the subsequent development of OPGs (Listernick et al. 1994, 2007). Furthermore, asymptomatic OPGs detected by MRI rarely cause clinical repercussion and may occasionally regress spontaneously (Listernick et al. 1994; Thiagalingam et al. 2004; King et al. 2003; Perilongo et al. 1999). Yearly ophthalmological evaluations, including visual acuity testing and fundoscopy, have been recommended as screening tools for children with NF-1, at least up to 7 years of age (Listernick et al. 2007; Ferner et al. 2007). Young children with NF-1 and known OPG should have their vision monitored at shorter intervals, particularly in the first 2 years after diagnosis (Fisher et al. 2012). However, the yield of visual acuity testing may be limited in children with NF-1 due to patients' young age, lack of cooperation, and presence of learning disabilities (Pilling and Taylor 2010). New experimental modalities assessing the integrity of the anterior visual pathway, including the evaluation of the peripapillary retinal nerve fiber and the ganglion cell-inner plexiform layers by optical coherence tomography, have shown promising results as screening tools to detect early vision loss in children with and without NF-1 and OPG (Chang et al. 2010; Gu et al. 2014). However, these and other methods still require validation in larger patient cohorts.

Recent studies analyzing the correlations between genotype and phenotype in patients with NF-1 have shown an association between mutations clustering in the 5′ portion of *NF1* (exons 1 through 16) and an increased risk for development of OPG (Ars et al. 2003; Sharif et al. 2011; Bolcekova et al. 2013). If this finding is confirmed in larger studies, it is possible that this high-risk population may benefit from alternative screening recommendations for OPG.

5.3　Neurofibromatosis Type 2 (NF-2)

OMIM: #101000; *NF2* is located at 22q12.2

- Autosomal dominant syndrome with nearly 100% penetrance and variable clinical expression based on genotype characteristics
- Incidence varies between 1 in 25,000 and 1 in 200,000
- Approximately half of the cases are de novo mutations with an unusually high rate of somatic mosaicism (between 25 and 60%) depending on the severity of involvement
- Multitude of syndromic features consisting of involvement of skin and eyes and predisposition to peripheral neuropathies and CNS cancers

5.3.1　Background and Genetics

J. H. Wishart first described a patient with bilateral vestibular schwannomas, a hallmark of NF-2, in the first half of the nineteenth century (Ahn et al. 1996). However, it was not until 1987 that the distinct characteristics of NF-1 and NF-2 were clearly defined (National Institutes of Health Consensus Development Conference Statement: neurofibromatosis. Bethesda, Md., USA, July 13–15, 1987 1988).

NF2, a tumor suppressor gene, was first identified in 1993 (Rouleau et al. 1993). Its product, merlin (also known as schwannomin) interacts with multiple proteins in the cell membrane and cytoskeleton (Asthagiri et al. 2009). This interaction affects the regulation of various cellular signaling pathways including the phosphoinositide-3 kinase (PI3K) and MEK pathways by mechanisms not completely understood that lead to cell growth and proliferation (Asthagiri et al. 2009).

5.3.2 Clinical Aspects

Patients with NF-2 have a predisposition to develop multiple CNS cancers including schwannomas, meningiomas, spinal ependymomas, and more rarely astrocytomas and neurofibromas (Asthagiri et al. 2009). Although bilateral vestibular schwannomas are a hallmark of NF-2, unilateral tumors or involvement of other cranial or peripheral nerves or spinal roots may occur (Asthagiri et al. 2009). Multiple clinical criteria to diagnose NF-2 have been described (Table 5.2) (Evans et al. 1992; Gutmann et al. 1997; Baser et al. 2011). However, recently proposed criteria that take into account additional parameters, including age of recognition of each clinical sign as well as genetic confirmation, seem to confer increased sensitivity in diagnosing NF-2, including mosaic cases (Table 5.3) (Baser et al. 2011).

Only about 20% of patients with NF-2 are diagnosed at less than 15 years of age (Evans et al. 1999). The presentation of children with NF-2 is, in general, distinct from that of adults

Table 5.2 Diagnostic criteria for neurofibromatosis type 2 (NF-2)

1987 NIH criteria (National Institutes of Health consensus development conference statement: Neurofibromatosis. Bethesda, Md., USA, July 13–15, 1987 1988)
A patient who meets either condition A or B has NF-2.
A. Bilateral vestibular schwannomas (VS)
B. First-degree family relative with NF-2 and unilateral VS or any two of neurofibroma, meningioma, glioma, schwannoma, or juvenile posterior subcapsular lenticular opacity
1992 Manchester criteria (Evans et al. 1992)
A patient who meets condition A, B, C, or D has NF-2.
A. Bilateral VS
B. First-degree family relative with NF-2 and unilateral VS or any two of neurofibroma, meningioma, glioma, schwannoma, or posterior subcapsular lenticular opacities
C. Unilateral VS and any two of neurofibroma, meningioma, glioma, schwannoma, or posterior subcapsular lenticular opacities
D. Multiple meningiomas (two or more) and unilateral VS or any two of neurofibroma, glioma, schwannoma, or cataract
1997 National Neurofibromatosis Foundation Criteria (Gutmann et al. 1997)
Confirmed (definite) NF-2
A patient who meets either condition A or B has NF-2.
A. Bilateral VS
B. First-degree family relative with NF-2 and unilateral VS <30 years or any two of meningioma, glioma, schwannoma, or juvenile posterior subcapsular lenticular opacity/juvenile cortical cataract
Presumptive or probable NF-2
A patient who meets either condition C or D has presumptive or probable NF-2.
C. Unilateral VS <30 years and at least one of meningioma, glioma, schwannoma, or juvenile posterior subcapsular lenticular opacity/juvenile cortical cataract
D. Multiple meningiomas (two or more) and unilateral VS <30 years or at least one of glioma, schwannoma, or juvenile posterior subcapsular lenticular opacity/juvenile cortical cataract

Note: In the Manchester criteria, "any two of" refers to two individual tumors or cataract, whereas in the other sets of criteria, it refers to two tumor types or cataract

Reprinted by permission from Macmillan Publishers Ltd.: Genet Med 13:576–581, copyright (2011)

Table 5.3 The Baser criteria for neurofibromatosis type 2 (NF-2) (Baser et al. 2011)

Feature	If present at or before the age of 30 years	If present after the age of 30 years
First-degree relative with NF-2 diagnosed by these criteria	2	2
Unilateral vestibular schwannoma	2	1[a]
Second vestibular schwannoma	4	3[a]
One meningioma	2	1
Second meningioma (no additional points for more than two meningiomas)	2	1
Cutaneous schwannoma (one or more)	2	1
Cranial nerve tumor (excluding vestibular schwannoma) (one or more)	2	1
Mononeuropathy	2	1
Cataract (one or more)	2	0

The patient is given points as shown in the table

[a]Points are not given for unilateral or second vestibular schwannoma if age at diagnosis is more than 70 years

- A diagnosis of definite NF2 is established if the total number of points is 6 or more
- NF2 mutation testing is indicated if the total number of points is 4 or 5
- A diagnosis of definite NF2 is established if a constitutional pathogenic NF2 mutation is found on mutation testing
- If no constitutional pathogenic NF2 mutation is found on mutation testing:
- A diagnosis of mosaic NF2 is established if mosaicism for a pathogenic NF2 mutation is found in the blood or no detectable pathogenic NF2 mutation is found in the blood but the same pathogenic NF2 mutation is found in two separate NF2-associated tumors
- Otherwise, a temporary diagnosis of possible NF2 is made, pending further clarification. Clarification may occur if the patient is established to have a different condition (e.g., schwannomatosis or multiple meningiomas) by standard diagnostic criteria or if evolution of the patient's disease over time permits establishing a diagnosis of definite NF2 or mosaic NF2 according to the criteria given above

Reprinted by permission from Macmillan Publishers Ltd.: Genet Med 13:576–581, copyright (2011)

(Asthagiri et al. 2009) (Evans et al. 1999). For example, hearing loss, tinnitus, and facial palsies, which are common diagnostic findings in adults, are seen at presentation in only 30–40% of children with NF-2 (Asthagiri et al. 2009; Evans et al. 1999). Approximately one-third of children with NF-2 present with symptoms associated with a meningioma and 10% with symptoms from a spinal tumor (Evans et al. 1999). Children also present with mononeuropathy more commonly than adults (Evans et al. 1999). One of the main differences between children and adults applies to familial cases since screening of suspected cases, including genetic testing, can lead to early detection and management of asymptomatic tumors (Evans et al. 1999).

Vestibular schwannoma is one of the main sources of morbidity in patients with NF-2 (Asthagiri et al. 2009). Little is known about the natural history and growth rate of these tumors in children since the data are scant and the majority of studies combined data from adult and pediatric patients (Plotkin et al. 2014). However, at least one study reported a potentially slower growth rate in the pediatric age group (Choi et al. 2014). Approximately 10–18% of children with a meningioma are eventually diagnosed with NF-2 (Evans et al. 1999; Kotecha et al. 2011). Patients with NF-2 have an increased risk of developing multifocal meningiomas and of experiencing tumor progression independent of other prognostic factors (Kotecha et al. 2011). Based on this association, some studies have recommended ruling out NF-2 in all children diagnosed with a meningioma (Baumgartner and Sorenson 1996). Ependymomas are the most common intramedullary spinal tumors in patients with NF-2 (Aguilera et al. 2011; Hagel et al. 2012). Multiple spinal ependymomas are present in up to 60% of patients with NF-2 (Plotkin et al. 2011). Most of these tumors are WHO grade 2 and predominantly involve the cervical spine or cervicomedullary junction (Hagel et al. 2012; Plotkin et al. 2011).

5.3.3   Relevant Therapeutic Issues

The principles of management of NF-2-related CNS cancers in children are similar to those used for adults and are based on maintenance of quality of life and preservation of function (e.g., hearing and facial function in patients with vestibular schwannomas) (Evans et al. 2005). The therapeutic approach for children with vestibular schwannomas is still controversial but most studies recommend observation for asymptomatic cases (Choi et al. 2014). Until recently, surgery or local irradiation, particularly radiosurgery, had been the only treatment modalities available for patients with vestibular schwannomas and NF-2. More recently, anticancer agents have been tested in such patients, particularly based on some of the biologic aspects of NF-2-induced tumorigenesis (Karajannis and Ferner 2015). Among these agents, bevacizumab (Avastin; Genentech, South San Francisco, USA; F. Hoffmann-La Roche, Switzerland), a humanized IgG1 monoclonal antibody that binds vascular endothelial growth factor (VEGF), has shown activity against progressive vestibular schwannomas and the potential to improve hearing in some patients with NF-2 (Plotkin et al. 2009). However, these patients may require long-term administration of bevacizumab since treatment interruption precipitates regrowth of tumors (Mautner et al. 2010). Although irradiation may be required for children with NF-2, there is a concern that patients may be at higher risk for developing subsequent malignant neoplasms in irradiated areas, including MPNSTs and other brain cancers (Baser et al. 2000). NF-2-associated spinal cord ependymomas have an indolent behavior and surgical intervention is only required in patients with progressive symptoms (Hagel et al. 2012; Aguilera et al. 2011). Patients with NF-2 and grade 2 ependymomas can be cured if complete surgical resection is attained (Asthagiri et al. 2009).

5.3.4   Screening

Presymptomatic genetic testing of individuals at risk and/or suspected of having NF-2 is critical for early diagnosis and improved medical care (Asthagiri et al. 2009). However, the sensitivity of genetic testing for germline *NF2* mutations is limited by the high rate of de novo cases and the existence of somatic mosaicism and is variable dependent on the clinical context (e.g., familial versus nonfamilial cases) (Evans et al. 2012). The recommendations regarding the appropriate age at which to obtain genetic testing in children at risk for NF-2 vary among different countries (Asthagiri et al. 2009).

Although hearing testing, particularly auditory brainstem response, continues to be used as a screen for hearing loss in patients at risk for NF-2 (Evans et al. 2000), thin-slice brain MRI with and without contrast is the standard to screen for vestibular schwannomas and other intracranial neoplasms (Evans et al. 2000). Spine MRIs are also recommended for at-risk children to rule out spinal involvement (Evans et al. 2012). Although recommendations regarding the age at which to start imaging vary, most studies agree that the first brain MRI could be obtained at 10–12 years of age (Evans et al. 2005), except for severely affected families where it is commonly recommended to begin screening 5–10 years before the earliest age of onset. Detailed recommendations for screening studies dependent on individual risk for NF-2 were recently published but are beyond the scope of this chapter (Evans et al. 2012).

5.4   Tuberous Sclerosis Complex (TSC)

OMIM: #191100; *TSC1* is located at 9q34.13.
OMIM: #613254; *TSC2* is located at 16p13.3

- Autosomal dominant syndrome with high penetrance but variable clinical expression
- Incidence varies with age, race, and mode of ascertainment ranging from 1 in 6000 to 1 in 95,000
- Multitude of syndromic features affecting skin, mucous membranes, CNS, eyes, kidneys, heart, lungs, gastrointestinal tract, and endocrine system

5.4.1 Background and Genetics

TSC was first recognized in the nineteenth century (Morgan and Wolfort 1979). In 1880, Bourneville reported the association of multiple brain tumors with seizures and mental retardation in a child with TSC (Morgan and Wolfort 1979). *TSC1* and *TSC2* were identified as the genes responsible for TSC in the early 1990s (Haines et al. 1991; European Chromosome 16 Tuberous Sclerosis 1993). Hamartin and tuberin, the respective products of *TSC1* and *TSC2*, interact with each other and inhibit mTOR complex 1 signaling by their direct effect on Rheb (Inoki and Guan 2009). mTOR complex 1 signaling, a cellular pathway associated with key cellular functions including protein synthesis, cell growth, and proliferation, is activated by abnormalities in *TSC1* and *TSC2* (Inoki and Guan 2009).

5.4.2 Clinical Aspects

TSC is characterized by the involvement of multiple organ systems with variable degrees of clinical expression, even among close family members as much as possible (Northrup et al. 1993). Table 5.4 provides updated clinical, radiologic, and molecular criteria for the diagnosis of TSC (Northrup et al. 2013). Some of the most significant medical problems associated with

Table 5.4 Diagnostic criteria for tuberous sclerosis complex (TSC) (Northrup et al. 2013)

A.   Genetic diagnostic criteria
The identification of *TSC1* or *TSC2* pathogenic mutation in DNA from normal tissue is sufficient to make a definite diagnosis of tuberous sclerosis complex (TSC). Pathogenic mutation clearly inactivate or impact the function of the TSC1 or TSC2 proteins or prevents protein synthesis. Other *TSC1* or *TSC2* variants whose effect on function are less certain do not meet these criteria, and are not sufficient to make a definite diagnosis of TSC. Note that 10–25% of TSC patients have no mutation identified by conventional genetic testing, and a normal result does not exclude TSC, or have any effect on the use of clinical diagnostic criteria to diagnose TSC.
B.   Clinical diagnostic criteria
Major features
1. Hypomelanotic macules ($\geq$3, at least 5-mm diameter)
2. Angiofibromas ($\geq$3) or fibrous cephalic plaque
3. Ungual fibromas ($\geq$2)
4. Shagreen patch
5. Multiple retinal hamartomas
6. Cortical dysplasias, including tuber and cerebral white matter radial migration lines
7. Subependymal nodules
8. Subependymal giant cell astrocytoma
9. Cardiac rhabdomyoma
10. Lymphangioleiomyomatosis (LAM)[a]
11. Angiomyolipomas ($\geq$2)[a]
Minor features
1. "Confetti" skin lesions
2. Dental enamel pits (>3)
3. Intraoral fibromas ($\geq$2)
4. Retinal achromic patch
5. Multiple renal cysts
6. Nonrenal hamartomas

Definite diagnosis: Two major features or one major feature with $\geq$ 2 minor features
Possible diagnosis: Either one major feature or $\geq$ minor features
[a]A combination of the two major clinical features (LAM and angiomyolipomas) without other features does not meet criteria for a definite diagnosis
Reprinted from Pediatr Neurol 49 (4), Northrup H, Krueger DA; International Tuberous Sclerosis Complex Consensus Group, Tuberous sclerosis complex diagnostic criteria update: recommendations of the 2012 International Tuberous Sclerosis Complex Consensus Conference, 243–254, Copyright (2013) with permission from Elsevier

TSC are related to brain involvement and include epilepsy, learning disability, and the risk of developing subependymal giant cell astrocytoma (SEGA) (Northrup et al. 2013). SEGA is radiologically detected in 6–20% of patients with TSC (Adriaensen et al. 2009).

5.4.3 Relevant Therapeutic Issues

Until recently, surgical resection had been the only available therapeutic option for patients with SEGA, particularly those with symptoms associated with hydrocephalus or enlarging tumors (Roth et al. 2013). Everolimus (Afinitor; Novartis Pharma Stein AG, Stein, Switzerland), an oral mTOR inhibitor approved by the FDA for the treatment of SEGA in patients with TSC, has produced durable objective responses in the majority of patients (Franz et al. 2013, 2014). The choice of therapy between surgery and the use of mTOR inhibitors depends on multiple factors, including the patient's clinical condition, tumor site, and available expertise at each institution (Roth et al. 2013).

5.4.4 Screening

It is recommended that patients with TSC be screened for SEGAs with brain MRIs every 1–3 years until the age of 25 years (Roth et al. 2013). These recommendations, however, can vary based on the clinical condition and tumor growth pattern for each patient. The recommended follow-up beyond 25 years of age is not clear since the pattern of growth of SEGA in this age group is limited.

5.5 Gorlin Syndrome (Also Known as Nevoid Basal-Cell Carcinoma Syndrome)

OMIM: #1109400; *PTCH2* is located at 1p34.1; *PTCH1* is located at 9q22.32; *SUFU* is located at 10q24.32

- Autosomal dominant syndrome with complete penetrance and variable expression
- Incidence ranges from 1 in 30,000 to 1 in 235,000
- Approximately 20–30% of cases are due to de novo mutations
- Multiple syndromic features including macrocephaly, as well as skeletal and dermatologic abnormalities

5.5.1 Background and Genetics

Although evidence of the existence of Gorlin syndrome dates back to 1000 B.C. (Satinoff and Wells 1969), this syndrome was first reported in 1960 (Gorlin and Goltz 1960). In 1996, it was discovered that Gorlin syndrome is caused by heterozygous germline loss-of-function mutations in *PTCH1*, which encodes a receptor for the Sonic Hedgehog (SHH) protein (Hahn et al. 1996; Johnson et al. 1996). In vertebrates, SHH binds to PTCH1 (Stone et al. 1996), and thereby prevents PTCH1-mediated inhibition of the transmembrane protein Smoothened (SMO). No longer restrained, SMO then activates the GLI family transcription factors, which translocate to the nucleus and induce expression of downstream genes (i.e., *GLI1, GLI2, PTCH1, CCND1, BCL2,* and *MYCN*). Through this mechanism, Hedgehog signaling regulates cell growth and differentiation and is instrumental during cerebellar patterning (Ingham and McMahon 2001; Roussel and Hatten 2011). It is thus not surprising that deregulation of this pathway results in the developmental defects and tumors typical of Gorlin syndrome.

Heterozygous germline *PTCH1* mutations represent 40–85% of individuals with typical Gorlin syndrome (Wicking et al. 1997; Soufir et al. 2006), and mutations in *SUFU* and in *PTCH2,* which encodes a protein highly homologous to *PTCH1*, account for the remaining cases (Taylor et al. 2002; Smith et al. 2014b; Fan et al. 2008; Fujii et al. 2013). Recent reports describe rare individuals with 9q22.3 microdeletion syndrome who harbor large chromosomal deletions encompassing *PTCH1* (Muller et al. 2012). In addition to the typical features of

Gorlin syndrome, these patients may present with craniosynostosis, obstructive hydrocephalus, and macrosomia (Muller et al. 2012).

5.5.2　Clinical Aspects

Gorlin syndrome is usually diagnosed based on physical examination and imaging findings according to established criteria (Table 5.5) (Kimonis et al. 1997). Molecular testing is used to confirm the diagnosis in individuals with atypical manifestations or to identify asymptomatic carriers when other relatives are known to be affected.

Medulloblastoma and meningioma are the two predominant CNS cancers in patients with Gorlin syndrome (Kimonis et al. 1997, 2004; Evans et al. 1993). Approximately 5% of patients

Table 5.5 Diagnostic criteria for Gorlin syndrome (Kimonis et al. 1997)

A. Major criteria
1. More than two basal-cell carcinomas, or one in a patient less than 20 years old
2. Odontogenic keratocysts of the jaw, proven by histopathology
3. Three or more palmar or plantar pits
4. Bilamellar calcification of the falx cerebri
5. Bifid, fused or markedly splayed ribs
6. First-degree relative(s) with Gorlin syndrome
B. Minor criteria
1. Macrocephaly determined after adjustment for height
2. Congenital malformations: cleft lip or palate, frontal bossing, "coarse" face, moderate or severe hypertelorism
3. Other skeletal abnormalities: Sprengel deformity[b], marked pectus deformity, marked syndactyly of the digits
4. Radiological abnormalities: Bridging of the sella turcica, vertebral anomalies such as hemivertibrae, fusion or elongation of the vertebral bodies, modeling defects of the hands and feet, or flame-shaped lucencies of the hands or feet.
5. Ovarian fibroma
6. Medulloblastoma

[a]A clinical diagnosis of Gorlin syndrome is made based on the presence of two major or one major and two minor criteria
[b]Congenital skeletal abnormality where one scapula sits higher than the other

with Gorlin syndrome develop a medulloblastoma (Evans et al. 1993). The risk of developing medulloblastoma in patients with Gorlin syndrome and germline *SUFU* mutations seems to be strikingly higher compared to those with *PTCH1* mutations (Smith et al. 2014b). Medulloblastoma is usually diagnosed before 3 years of age in patients with Gorlin syndrome (Smith et al. 2014b; Amlashi et al. 2003; Garre et al. 2009; Brugieres et al. 2012). Nodular/desmoplastic and medulloblastoma with extensive nodularity are by far the most prevalent histologic variants seen in these patients (Smith et al. 2014b; Amlashi et al. 2003; Garre et al. 2009; Brugieres et al. 2012). In addition to medulloblastoma and meningioma, other brain tumors have been reported sporadically in patients with Gorlin syndrome (Smith et al. 2014b; Evans et al. 1991; Choudry et al. 2007). However, it is not clear whether some of these CNS tumors result from the underlying genetic defect or are instead secondary to the irradiation used to treat medulloblastoma. Non-CNS cancers have been rarely described in patients with Gorlin syndrome (Cajaiba et al. 2006).

5.5.3　Relevant Therapeutic Issues

Several clinical trials have demonstrated that young children (less than 3 years) with nodular/desmoplastic and medulloblastoma with extensive nodularity have an excellent prognosis when treated with radical tumor resection followed by intensive combination chemotherapy without irradiation (Rutkowski et al. 2005; Leary et al. 2011). Therefore, it is expected that nowadays most children with Gorlin syndrome and medulloblastoma will receive therapy without irradiation. Still, early recognition of features suspicious for Gorlin syndrome is critical to avoid as much as possible the use of irradiation in such patients. The risk of secondary neoplasms after the use of irradiation, particularly basal-cell carcinomas and meningiomas, is extremely high in patients with Gorlin syndrome (Smith et al. 2014b; Amlashi et al. 2003; Garre et al. 2009; Brugieres et al. 2012; Choudry et al. 2007; Walter et al.

1997). Although meningiomas and basal-cell carcinomas are low-grade cancers, they may cause significant morbidity and may even lead to late deaths in these patients (Smith et al. 2014b; Amlashi et al. 2003; Garre et al. 2009; Brugieres et al. 2012; Choudry et al. 2007; Walter et al. 1997).

Vismodegib, a small-molecule inhibitor of SMO, a proximal component of the SHH pathway, has been successfully used in adults with advanced basal-cell carcinoma, a cancer commonly driven by somatic abnormalities in this pathway (Von Hoff et al. 2009). Vismodegib has also been tested in children and adults with medulloblastoma (Rudin et al. 2009; Gajjar et al. 2013; Robinson et al. 2015). Activity of vismodegib was observed only in patients with SHH medulloblastoma that harbored proximal (e.g., *PTCH1* or SMO mutations) but not distal abnormalities (e.g., *SUFU* mutations) in this pathway (Robinson et al. 2015; Kool et al. 2014). Although SMO inhibitors have already been used with some success in patients with Gorlin syndrome and basal-cell carcinomas (Tang et al. 2012), no information is available about their role in the treatment of CNS cancers in this same population.

5.5.4 Screening

Protocols for surveillance of children and adults with Gorlin syndrome have been developed (Bree et al. 2011). It is recommended that children with Gorlin syndrome undergo baseline clinical and genetic evaluation with annual follow-ups thereafter. Dermatologic, cardiac, dental, and ophthalmologic evaluations are also recommended at regular intervals (Bree et al. 2011). It is critical that imaging protocols avoid radiation exposure in such patients. Therefore, brain MRI is the preferred method to screen for medulloblastoma starting at baseline and then followed by yearly exams until the age of 8 years (Bree et al. 2011). Children with Gorlin syndrome and germline *SUFU* mutations may benefit from a more intense surveillance regimen with intervals between MRIs of 3 to 6 months at younger ages (Smith et al. 2014b). Brain MRIs are only recommended if symptoms develop in older children and adults (Bree et al. 2011). The recommendation for imaging surveillance for patients previously treated for medulloblastoma, particularly those who received irradiation, is obviously different than the ones described before.

Screening for Gorlin syndrome has been recommended for all children diagnosed with medulloblastoma with extensive nodularity (Garre et al. 2009). Screening for Gorlin syndrome is also recommended for children with nodular/desmoplastic medulloblastoma who harbor any other major or minor criteria (Bree et al. 2011).

5.6 Li-Fraumeni Syndrome (LFS)

OMIM: #151623; *TP53* is located at 17p13.1

- Autosomal dominant syndrome with high penetrance and variable expression
- Incidence is approximately 1 in 5000
- Between 7 and 20% of affected individuals have de novo mutations
- No known associated syndromic features

5.6.1 Background and Genetics

LFS was first described in 1969 in four families with soft tissue sarcomas and early onset breast cancer (Li and Fraumeni 1969). To date, over 500 families have been reported, but it is proposed that many more may exist (Testa et al. 2013). The association between *TP53* and LFS was described in 1990 (Malkin et al. 1990). Also commonly referred to as "guardian of the genome," *TP53* encodes the critical DNA binding protein p53, which plays essential roles in mediating cellular stress responses and initiating cell-cycle arrest, senescence, and apoptosis in response to DNA damage (Zilfou and Lowe 2009).

5.6.2 Clinical Aspects

Several classification systems have been developed to help determine those to whom *TP53* genetic testing should be offered (Table 5.6) (Li et al. 1988; Tinat et al. 2009). Germline *TP53* mutations are generally identified in more than 70% of patients who meet classic LFS diagnostic criteria (Ruijs et al. 2010). In contrast, the mutation detection rate drops to 20% in individuals classified as "Li-Fraumeni-like," who exhibit some but not all of the features associated with LFS (Ruijs et al. 2010). The lifetime cancer risk in individuals with LFS is extraordinarily high, approximately 68% in men and 93% in women, with nearly half of cancers presenting in individuals under 30 years of age (Testa et al. 2013; Bougeard et al. 2015). Patients with LFS are at greatest risk to develop six core "component" cancers, including CNS tumors, breast cancer, soft tissue sarcomas, osteosarcomas, adrenocortical carcinomas, and leukemias (Testa et al. 2013; Gonzalez et al. 2009; Olivier et al. 2003).

Table 5.6 Diagnostic criteria for Li Fraumeni syndrome (LFS)

A. Classic criteria: (Li et al. 1988) LFS is defined by the presence of all of the following:
1. Proband diagnosed with a sarcoma before 45 years
2. A first-degree relative with any cancer before 45 years
3. A first- or second-degree relative, along the same lineage, with any cancer before 45 years or a sarcoma at any age
B. 2009 Revised Chompret criteria: (Tinat et al. 2009)
1. Proband with a tumor belonging to the LFS spectrum (i.e. soft tissue sarcoma, osteosarcoma, brain tumor, premenopausal breast cancer, adrenocortical carcinoma, leukemia, lung bronchoalveolar cancer) before 46 years, AND
2. One or more first- or second-degree relatives with an LFS tumor (except breast cancer if the proband has breast cancer) before 56 years or with multiple tumors, OR
3. Proband with multiple tumors (except multiple breast tumors), two of which belong to the LFS spectrum and the first of which occurred before 46 years, OR
4. Proband with adrenocortical carcinoma or choroid plexus tumor, regardless of family history

CNS tumors, including glioblastoma and other astrocytomas, medulloblastomas, ependymomas, and choroid plexus carcinomas, are observed in approximately 25% of patients with LFS (Ruijs et al. 2010; Bougeard et al. 2015; Farrell and Plotkin 2007). Infiltrative astrocytomas are the most common CNS cancers in patients with LFS (Ruijs et al. 2010). Whereas *TP53* germline mutations are observed in 45–100% of children with choroid plexus carcinoma depending on geographical variations (Gonzalez et al. 2009; Custodio et al. 2011; Seidinger et al. 2011; Tabori et al. 2010), this abnormality is hardly ever observed in patients with choroid plexus papillomas (Tabori et al. 2010). Somatic *TP53* mutations are seen in 16% and 21% of wingless (WNT) and SHH medulloblastomas, respectively (Zhukova et al. 2013). While concomitant *TP53* germline mutations were documented in approximately half of patients with somatically mutated SHH medulloblastomas, none of the patients with WNT tumors harbored this abnormality (Zhukova et al. 2013). There appears to be a biphasic age distribution of CNS cancers in patients with LFS, with the highest prevalence rates before age 10 and after 20 years of age (Olivier et al. 2003).

5.6.3 Relevant Therapeutic Issues

Cancers identified in patients with LFS are treated similarly to identical tumors in patients without LFS. Although it is preferential to avoid DNA-damaging agents (such as ionizing radiation) due to the increased risk for second malignancies in patients with LFS (Hisada et al. 1998), this is not an option for patients with high-grade CNS neoplasms. SHH medulloblastomas with *TP53* mutations, which commonly harbor other molecular abnormalities including *NMYC* amplification, are associated with a very poor prognosis (Seidinger et al. 2011; Kool et al. 2014). Likewise, children with LFS and medulloblastoma fare poorly despite treatment with craniospinal irradiation and intensive combination chemotherapy (Zhukova et al. 2013). The presence of somatic *TP53* mutations is also a poor prognostic factor in patients with choroid plexus carcinoma compared to those without this abnormality (Tabori et al. 2010). Similar to medulloblastoma, children with LFS and choroid plexus carcinoma also seem to have a worse outcome compared to nonaffected patients (Tabori et al. 2010).

5.6.4 Screening

The recommendations for screening in patients with LFS are emerging but no formal guidelines exist. For *TP53* germline mutation carriers, annual physical examination with attention to the neurological examination is recommended. Studies are ongoing to determine whether newer radiologic approaches that avoid ionizing radiation, alone or in combination with other screening measures, are effective in detecting tumors in patients with LFS. One study of rapid whole-body MRI with dedicated brain MRI reported increased survival in patients with LFS (Villani et al. 2011). Several larger prospective studies are ongoing in an effort to confirm these positive results.

5.7 Constitutional (or Biallelic) Mismatch-Repair Deficiency (CMMRD) Syndrome

OMIM: #276300.*MSH2* is located at 2p21; *MSH6* is located at 2p16.3; *MLH1* is located at 3p22.2; *PMS2* is located at 7p22.1

- Autosomal recessive syndrome with very high penetrance
- Extremely rare but incidence not yet established
- Syndromic features include the presence of cutaneous stigmata, mostly reminiscent of NF-1, and occasionally organ malformations

5.7.1 Background and Genetics

Although CMMRD syndrome was only formally recognized in 1999 (Ricciardone et al. 1999; Wang et al. 1999), its characteristics overlap with those of Turcot syndrome, which is the association of CNS cancers and colonic polyposis and/or carcinomas (Turcot et al. 1959). The mismatch-repair (MMR) system is a complex pathway involved in important cellular functions, including the repair of small insertions and single base-pair mismatches in DNA, immunoglobulin class-switch recombination, apoptosis, and signaling of DNA damage (Jiricny 2006). Monoallelic germline mutations in *MSH2*, *MSH6*, *MLH1*, or *PMS2*, which are important components of the MMR system, cause Lynch syndrome, the most common form of hereditary colorectal cancer (Lynch and de la Chapelle 2003). Biallelic (homozygous or compound heterozygous) germline mutations of the same genes cause CMMRD syndrome.

5.7.2 Clinical Aspects

CMMRD syndrome is characterized primarily by a predisposition to hematologic, CNS, colorectal and other cancers in the spectrum of Lynch syndrome, café au lait spots and other skin abnormalities, defects in the synthesis of immunoglobulin subclasses, and more rarely congenital malformations (Wimmer et al. 2014). The dermatologic and gastrointestinal involvement associated with CMMRD is highly variable, making the diagnosis more difficult (Wimmer et al. 2014; Durno et al. 2015). Due to the autosomal recessive pattern of transmission, consanguinity should raise the suspicion of this diagnosis although family history is commonly not striking for the presence of Lynch syndrome-associated cancers (Durno et al. 2015).

CNS cancers account for 36–48% of all malignancies associated with CMMRD syndrome (Wimmer et al. 2014; Bakry et al. 2014). High-grade gliomas comprise approximately three-quarters of CNS cancers, followed by low-grade gliomas (up to 16%), and primitive neuroectodermal tumors/medulloblastoma (10–18%) (Wimmer et al. 2014; Bakry et al. 2014). *PMS2* and *MSH6* germline mutations are observed in approximately 60% and 21–33%, respectively, of patients with CNS cancers and CMMRD syndrome (Wimmer et al. 2014; Bakry et al. 2014). The histologic characteristics of CMMRD syndrome-associated CNS cancers appear indistinguishable from those of non-syndromic patients. Unlike Lynch syndrome-associated cancers (Lynch and de la Chapelle 2003), microsatellite instability is an unreliable tool to screen for CMMRD syndrome in patients with CNS cancers (Bakry et al. 2014). There is evidence, however, that loss of expression of the respective MMR protein in tumor and/or normal tissue by immunohistochemistry may be sensitive in detecting patients with CMMRD syndrome (Bakry et al. 2014). However, normal expression of the respective MMR protein occurs in some patients with CMMRD syndrome and thus genetic testing remains the gold standard for confirming this diagnosis. The prognosis of patients with CNS cancer and CMMRD syndrome, particularly those with high-grade tumors, is unclear but some long-term survivors have been described, suggesting that their outcome may not be that poor (Turcot et al. 1959; Hamilton et al. 1995).

5.7.3 Relevant Therapeutic Issues

To date, there are no special treatment recommendations for patients with CNS cancers and CMMRD syndrome. Children with CMMRD and high-grade CNS neoplasms commonly undergo irradiation depending on their age, despite the sparse data about the sensitivity of MMR-deficient cancers to this treatment modality (Martin et al. 2010). Likewise, no unique chemotherapy regimens have been applied to such patients; however, temozolomide and other medications that depend on an intact MMR system for their cytotoxic activity are believed to have no role in the treatment of patients with CMMRD syndrome (Jiricny 2006).

5.7.4 Screening

Screening protocols have been developed for patients with CMMRD syndrome (Table 5.7) (Bakry et al. 2014; Vasen et al. 2014). Current recommendations include brain MRIs at regular intervals to detect brain tumors. The recommended age to start specific screening procedures varied between the two published studies (Bakry et al. 2014; Vasen et al. 2014). Early detection and resection of asymptomatic CNS cancers is a rational approach in this patient population based on the extremely high risk of cancer development and malignant transformation over time (Bakry et al. 2014; Shlien et al. 2015).

Table 5.7 Screening recommendations for patients with constitutional mismatch-repair deficiency syndrome (Bakry et al. 2014)

Cancer	Surveillance strategy
Children	
Colon	Colonoscopy annually[a]
Upper GI tract and small bowel	EGD annually[a], Video capsule endoscopy annually[a]
Brain[b]	Ultrasound at birth and then brain MRI every 6 months
Leukemia, lymphoma[b]	Complete blood count, erythrocyte sedimentation rate, lactate dehydrogenase every 4 months
Adults	
Colon	Colonoscopy annually[a]
Upper GI tract and small bowel	EGD annually[a], Video capsule endoscopy annually[a]
Brain[b]	Brain MRI every 6 months
Leukemia, lymphoma[b]	Complete blood count, erythrocyte sedimentation rate, lactate dehydrogenase every 4 months
Uterus	Ultrasound annually
Upper urinary tract	Ultrasound and urine cytology annually

Abbreviations: *EGD* esophagogastroduodenoscopy, *GI* gastrointestinal, *MRI* magnetic resonance imaging
[a]To start at 3 years of age or at diagnosis
[b]Brain and leukemia/lymphoma screening should commence at birth if diagnosed prenatally
Reprinted from Eur J Cancer 50 (5), Bakry D, Aronson M, Durno C et al., Genetic and clinical determinants of constitutional mismatch repair deficiency syndrome: report from the constitutional mismatch repair deficiency consortium, 987–996, Copyright 2014 with permission from Elsevier

5.8 Rhabdoid Tumor Predisposition Syndrome (RTPS) 1

OMIM: #609322; *SMARCB1* is located at 22q11.23

- Autosomal dominant syndrome with high penetrance
- Extremely rare but incidence not yet established
- The majority of patients have no associated syndromic features, except for rare individuals with distal 22q11 deletions who may have multiple congenital malformations, including cardiac defects, preauricular tags, and cleft lip and palate

5.8.1 Background and Genetics

Biallelic alterations of *SMARCB1* are observed in the majority of atypical teratoid/rhabdoid tumors (AT/RTs) and extra-CNS malignant rhabdoid tumors (Versteege et al. 1998; Biegel et al. 1999). This finding, combined with the description of patients harboring germline *SMARCB1* abnormalities and the occurrence of multifocal and/or familial cases of rhabdoid tumors, led to the recognition of RTPS1 in 1998 (Biegel et al. 1999; Sevenet et al. 1999). *SMARCB1* is a core member of the SWI/SNF chromatin-remodeling complex that regulates gene expression and plays a key role in proliferation and differentiation (Kim and Roberts 2014). Currently, the mechanisms by which *SMARCB1* abnormalities lead to tumorigenesis are not well understood, but seem to result from global disruptions in gene transcription due to alterations in chromatin remodeling.

5.8.2 Clinical Aspects

Although somatic *SMARCB1* abnormalities have been described in multiple CNS and extra-CNS cancers (Wilson and Roberts 2011), RTPS1 has so far been mostly associated with the development of AT/RTs and extra-CNS rhabdoid tumors (Kordes et al. 2010; Bourdeaut et al. 2011). Germline *SMARCB1* abnormalities are predominantly found in younger patients (less than 2 years) with AT/RT (Bourdeaut et al. 2011; Kordes et al. 2010), with a peak incidence of 60% in infants less than 6 months of age (Bourdeaut et al. 2011). The incidence of RTPS1 varies between 24 and 42% in unselected cases of AT/RT (Bourdeaut et al. 2011; Kordes et al. 2010; Eaton et al. 2011). Despite preferentially affecting younger patients, *SMARCB1* germline mutations have been described in older children with AT/RT as well (Bourdeaut et al. 2011; Eaton et al. 2011). Therefore, germline *SMARCB1* testing is recommended for all patients with AT/RT. Although transmission of germline *SMARCB1* mutations through multiple generations has been described (Taylor et al. 2000), this is an uncommon occurrence and most mutations arise de novo. For unclear reasons, the risk of developing AT/RT and extra-CNS rhabdoid tumors in patients with RTPS1 is limited to early infancy (Kordes et al. 2010).

Several case reports have described patients with heterozygous germline 22q11.2 distal deletion encompassing *SMARCB1* who developed AT/RTs or extra-CNS rhabdoid tumors (Jackson et al. 2007; Sathyamoorthi et al. 2009; Lafay-Cousin et al. 2009; Toth et al. 2011; Beddow et al. 2011). Some of these cases displayed syndromic features that are for the most part distinct from those found in DiGeorge (DGS) or velo-cardio-facial syndrome (VCFS) (Ben-Shachar et al. 2008). Since the majority of patients with 22q11.2 harbor deletions that are proximal to *SMARCB1* and affect genes involved in DGS/VCFS (Ben-Shachar et al. 2008), their distinct phenotype is not surprising.

SMARCB1 germline mutations have also been described in a subset of patients with familial schwannomatosis, which is characterized by the development of multiple schwannomas without vestibular involvement (MacCollin et al. 2005; Hulsebos et al. 2007; Hadfield et al. 2008). Exceptional cases of other cancers, including multiple meningiomas and rare soft tissue cancers, have also been associated with *SMARCB1* germline mutations (Hulsebos et al. 2007, 2014a; Carter et al. 2012; Forest et al. 2012; van den Munckhof et al. 2012). Interestingly, only rare families with germline *SMARCB1* abnormalities have been described to have individuals affected with either schwannomatosis or AT/RTs (Eaton et al. 2011; Swensen et al. 2009). Genetic analysis of *SMARCB1* abnormalities in patients with schwannomatosis and AT/RT showed mostly distinct patterns (Smith et al. 2014a). Germline abnormalities consisting of missense, splice site, or in-frame deletions affecting the 5′ and 3′ portions of the gene, which cause alterations in function and/or expression of SMARCB1, predominated in patients with schwannomatosis (Smith et al. 2014a; Hulsebos et al. 2014b). On the other hand, patients with AT/RT were more likely to have nonsense mutations, whole gene or multiple exon deletions or duplications, which lead to complete loss of SMARCB1 expression (Smith et al. 2014a; Hulsebos et al. 2014b).

5.8.3 Relevant Therapeutic Issues

Although children with AT/RT and RTPS1 are presumed to have a worse prognosis than those without this syndrome mostly because of younger age, a higher incidence of multifocal disease, and inability to undergo irradiation (Bourdeaut et al. 2011), long-term survivors have been reported (Kordes et al. 2014).

5.8.4 Screening

No established recommendations currently exist for the surveillance of patients with RTPS1. However, it is intuitive that children who harbor *SMARCB1* germline abnormalities warrant regular monitoring for CNS and non-CNS tumors, particularly at young ages. Furthermore, although the incidence of rhabdoid tumors among patients with 22q11.2 distal deletion syndrome is unknown, it is clear that this high-risk cohort deserves to be screened (Beddow et al. 2011).

5.9 Rhabdoid Tumor Predisposition Syndrome (RTPS) 2

OMIM: #613325; *SMARCA4* is located at 19p13.2

- Autosomal dominant syndrome with incomplete penetrance
- Extremely rare accounting for less than 5% of all inherited cases of rhabdoid tumors
- No known associated syndromic features

5.9.1 Background and Genetics

Monoallelic germline and biallelic somatic abnormalities of *SMARCA4* were first recognized in rare patients with histologically typical AT/RT and rhabdoid tumors that did not harbor *SMARCB1* abnormalities (Schneppenheim et al. 2010; Hasselblatt et al. 2011; Witkowski et al. 2013). This condition is now known as RTPS2. *SMARCA4*, another member of the SWI/SNF complex, is also believed to function as a tumor suppressor gene (Medina and Sanchez-Cespedes 2008).

5.9.2 Clinical Aspects

Unlike RTPS1 (Kordes et al. 2010; Bourdeaut et al. 2011; Eaton et al. 2011), there is evidence that RTPS2 occurs in the majority of young children with AT/RT that harbor somatic *SMARCA4* mutations (Hasselblatt et al. 2014). Several asymptomatic adult carriers of germline *SMARCA4* abnormalities have been reported suggesting an incomplete penetrance (Hasselblatt et al. 2014). The only other type of cancer clearly associated with RTPS2 is small cell carcinoma of the ovary, hypercalcemic type (SCCOHT), a very rare undifferentiated cancer that mostly affects adolescents and young adults (mean age at diagnosis in the third decade of life) (Witkowski et al. 2014). Based on its histologic and genetic characteristics, SCCOHT is now considered a form of rhabdoid tumor. *SMARCA4*-mutated AT/RTs are aggressive tumors and no survivors have been reported to date. It is peculiar that the two cancers associated with RTPS2, rhabdoid tumors and SCCOHT, affect patients at distinct age groups. This difference in presentation may be related to unique characteristics of precancerous progenitor cells in the ovary and CNS, distinct *SMARCA4* mutations found in each type of cancer, and/or local environmental factors at the tumor site.

5.9.3 Relevant Therapeutic Issues

So far, patients with RTPS2 have received the same aggressive therapeutic approach used for other young children with AT/RT.

5.9.4 Screening

No recommendations exist for surveillance of children with *SMARCA4*-mutated AT/RT.

5.10 DICER1 Syndrome

OMIM: #601200; *DICER1* is located at chromosome 14q32.13

- Autosomal dominant syndrome with incomplete penetrance
- Rare but incidence not yet established
- No known associated syndromic features

5.10.1 Background and Genetics

The association of heterozygous germline *DICER1* mutations and pleuropulmonary blastoma, a rare cancer of early childhood, was first described in 2009 (Hill et al. 2009). DICER1 plays a key role in processing small RNAs,

including microRNAs, and thereby is involved in the modulation of messenger RNA expression (Foulkes et al. 2014).

5.10.2 Clinical Aspects

Germline *DICER1* mutations have been observed in patients with several types of rare pediatric cancers, including pleuropulmonary blastoma, cystic nephroma, multinodular goiter and thyroid cancers, and Sertoly-Leydig cell tumors of the ovary (Foulkes et al. 2014). So far, four patients with pineoblastoma who harbored a germline heterozygous *DICER1* mutation have been reported (Sabbaghian et al. 2012; de Kock et al. 2014b). In the largest series to date, three of 18 selected children with pineoblastoma (patients' ages at diagnosis of 3, 3.3, and 17.1 years) harbored germline truncating mutations with concomitant lack of expression of DICER1 by immunohistochemistry in the tumor (de Kock et al. 2014b).

Pituitary blastoma is a very rare pituitary gland cancer of young children that was first described in 2008 (Scheithauer et al. 2008). In a recent study, 9 of 13 children with pituitary blastoma were found to have heterozygous germline *DICER1* mutations (de Kock et al. 2014a).

Although other brain tumors, including medulloblastoma and cerebral medulloepithelioma, have been rarely observed in families with germline *DICER1* mutations, no clear association has been established between these cancers and DICER1 syndrome (Slade et al. 2011).

5.10.3 Relevant Therapeutic Issues

No information is available about any aspects of therapy that might be different in children with DICER1 syndrome compared to nonaffected patients. Interestingly, a recent study described the sequential variation of serum levels of specific microRNAs in a child with a germline *DICER1* mutation treated for a pleuropulmonary blastoma and suggested that this strategy could be used as a biomarker of response to therapy

(Murray et al. 2014). Sequential assessment of specific microRNAs in serum and cerebrospinal fluid may also have utility in children with brain tumors and DICER1 syndrome.

5.10.4 Screening

Genetic testing has been recommended for all patients who present with rare cancers associated with DICER1 syndrome, including pineoblastoma and pituitary blastoma, particularly when there is a positive family history of similar tumors and/or multinodular goiter (Foulkes et al. 2014; de Kock et al. 2014b). The need for screening in patients with DICER1 syndrome is undeniable, particularly because of the risk of developing multiple neoplasms (Schultz et al. 2014). Although no formal guidelines have been established to date to screen for cancers in patients with germline *DICER1* mutation, one study recommended a baseline and annual physical examination with targeted review of systems. Depending on age, symptoms, and clinical findings, the recommended tests include chest CT, renal or pelvic ultrasound, thyroid ultrasound, and brain MRI to rule out brain tumors.

References

Adriaensen ME, Schaefer-Prokop CM, Stijnen T, Duyndam DA, Zonnenberg BA, Prokop M (2009) Prevalence of subependymal giant cell tumors in patients with tuberous sclerosis and a review of the literature. Eur J Neurol 16(6):691–696. https://doi.org/10.1111/j.1468-1331.2009.02567.x

Aguilera DG, Mazewski C, Schniederjan MJ, Leong T, Boydston W, Macdonald TJ (2011) Neurofibromatosis-2 and spinal cord ependymomas: report of two cases and review of the literature. Childs Nerv Syst 27(5):757–764. https://doi.org/10.1007/s00381-010-1351-3

Ahn MS, Jackler RK, Lustig LR (1996) The early history of the neurofibromatosis. Evolution of the concept of neurofibromatosis type 2. Arch Otolaryngol Head Neck Surg 122(11):1240–1249

Alderfer MA, Zelley K, Lindell RB, Novokmet A, Mai PL, Garber JE, Nathan D, Scollon S, Chun NM, Patenaude AF, Ford JM, Plon SE, Schiffman JD, Diller LR, Savage SA, Malkin D, Ford CA, Nichols KE (2015) Parent decision-making around the genetic testing of children for germline TP53 mutations. Cancer 121(2):286–293. https://doi.org/10.1002/cncr.29027

Amlashi SF, Riffaud L, Brassier G, Morandi X (2003) Nevoid basal cell carcinoma syndrome: relation with desmoplastic medulloblastoma in infancy. A population-based study and review of the literature. Cancer 98(3):618–624. https://doi.org/10.1002/cncr.11537

Ars E, Kruyer H, Morell M, Pros E, Serra E, Ravella A, Estivill X, Lazaro C (2003) Recurrent mutations in the NF1 gene are common among neurofibromatosis type 1 patients. J Med Genet 40(6):e82

Asthagiri AR, Parry DM, Butman JA, Kim HJ, Tsilou ET, Zhuang Z, Lonser RR (2009) Neurofibromatosis type 2. Lancet 373(9679):1974–1986. https://doi.org/10.1016/S0140-6736(09)60259-2

Bakry D, Aronson M, Durno C, Rimawi H, Farah R, Alharbi QK, Alharbi M, Shamvil A, Ben-Shachar S, Mistry M, Constantini S, Dvir R, Qaddoumi I, Gallinger S, Lerner-Ellis J, Pollett A, Stephens D, Kelies S, Chao E, Malkin D, Bouffet E, Hawkins C, Tabori U (2014) Genetic and clinical determinants of constitutional mismatch repair deficiency syndrome: report from the constitutional mismatch repair deficiency consortium. Eur J Cancer 50(5):987–996. https://doi.org/10.1016/j.ejca.2013.12.005

Baser ME, Evans DG, Jackler RK, Sujansky E, Rubenstein A (2000) Neurofibromatosis 2, radiosurgery and malignant nervous system tumours. Br J Cancer 82(4):998. https://doi.org/10.1054/bjoc.1999.1030

Baser ME, Friedman JM, Joe H, Shenton A, Wallace AJ, Ramsden RT, Evans DG (2011) Empirical development of improved diagnostic criteria for neurofibromatosis 2. Genet Med 13(6):576–581. https://doi.org/10.1097/GIM.0b013e318211faa9

Baumgartner JE, Sorenson JM (1996) Meningioma in the pediatric population. J Neuro-Oncol 29(3):223–228

Beddow RA, Smith M, Kidd A, Corbett R, Hunter AG (2011) Diagnosis of distal 22q11.2 deletion syndrome in a patient with a teratoid/rhabdoid tumour. Eur J Med Genet 54(3):295–298. https://doi.org/10.1016/j.ejmg.2010.12.007

Ben-Shachar S, Ou Z, Shaw CA, Belmont JW, Patel MS, Hummel M, Amato S, Tartaglia N, Berg J, Sutton VR, Lalani SR, Chinault AC, Cheung SW, Lupski JR, Patel A (2008) 22q11.2 distal deletion: a recurrent genomic disorder distinct from DiGeorge syndrome and velocardiofacial syndrome. Am J Hum Genet 82(1):214–221. https://doi.org/10.1016/j.ajhg.2007.09.014

Biegel JA, Zhou JY, Rorke LB, Stenstrom C, Wainwright LM, Fogelgren B (1999) Germ-line and acquired mutations of INI1 in atypical teratoid and rhabdoid tumors. Cancer Res 59(1):74–79

Bilaniuk LT, Molloy PT, Zimmerman RA, Phillips PC, Vaughan SN, Liu GT, Sutton LN, Needle M (1997) Neurofibromatosis type 1: brain stem tumours. Neuroradiology 39(9):642–653

Bolcekova A, Nemethova M, Zatkova A, Hlinkova K, Pozgayova S, Hlavata A, Kadasi L, Durovcikova D, Gerinec A, Husakova K, Pavlovicova Z, Holobrada M,

Kovacs L, Ilencikova D (2013) Clustering of mutations in the 5′ tertile of the NF1 gene in Slovakia patients with optic pathway glioma. Neoplasma 60(6):655–665. https://doi.org/10.4149/neo_2013_084

Bougeard G, Renaux-Petel M, Flaman JM, Charbonnier C, Fermey P, Belotti M, Gauthier-Villars M, Stoppa-Lyonnet D, Consolino E, Brugieres L, Caron O, Benusiglio PR, Bressac-de Paillerets B, Bonadona V, Bonaiti-Pellie C, Tinat J, Baert-Desurmont S, Frebourg T (2015) Revisiting Li-Fraumeni syndrome from TP53 mutation carriers. J Clin Oncol 33(21):2345–2352. https://doi.org/10.1200/JCO.2014.59.5728

Bourdeaut F, Lequin D, Brugieres L, Reynaud S, Dufour C, Doz F, Andre N, Stephan JL, Perel Y, Oberlin O, Orbach D, Bergeron C, Rialland X, Freneaux P, Ranchere D, Figarella-Branger D, Audry G, Puget S, Evans DG, Pinas JC, Capra V, Mosseri V, Coupier I, Gauthier-Villars M, Pierron G, Delattre O (2011) Frequent hSNF5/INI1 germline mutations in patients with rhabdoid tumor. Clin Cancer Res 17(1):31–38. https://doi.org/10.1158/1078-0432.CCR-10-1795

Bree AF, Shah MR, Group BC (2011) Consensus statement from the first international colloquium on basal cell nevus syndrome (BCNS). Am J Med Genet A 155A(9):2091–2097. https://doi.org/10.1002/ajmg.a.34128

Brugieres L, Remenieras A, Pierron G, Varlet P, Forget S, Byrde V, Bombled J, Puget S, Caron O, Dufour C, Delattre O, Bressac-de Paillerets B, Grill J (2012) High frequency of germline SUFU mutations in children with desmoplastic/nodular medulloblastoma younger than 3 years of age. J Clin Oncol 30(17):2087–2093. https://doi.org/10.1200/JCO.2011.38.7258

Cajaiba MM, Bale AE, Alvarez-Franco M, McNamara J, Reyes-Mugica M (2006) Rhabdomyosarcoma, Wilms tumor, and deletion of the patched gene in Gorlin syndrome. Nat Clin Pract Oncol 3(10):575–580. https://doi.org/10.1038/ncponc0608

Carter JM, O'Hara C, Dundas G, Gilchrist D, Collins MS, Eaton K, Judkins AR, Biegel JA, Folpe AL (2012) Epithelioid malignant peripheral nerve sheath tumor arising in a schwannoma, in a patient with "neuroblastoma-like" schwannomatosis and a novel germline SMARCB1 mutation. Am J Surg Pathol 36(1):154–160. https://doi.org/10.1097/PAS.0b013e3182380802

Chang L, El-Dairi MA, Frempong TA, Burner EL, Bhatti MT, Young TL, Leigh F (2010) Optical coherence tomography in the evaluation of neurofibromatosis type-1 subjects with optic pathway gliomas. J AAPOS 14(6):511–517. https://doi.org/10.1016/j.jaapos.2010.08.014

Choi JW, Lee JY, Phi JH, Wang KC, Chung HT, Paek SH, Kim DG, Park SH, Kim SK (2014) Clinical course of vestibular schwannoma in pediatric neurofibromatosis type 2. J Neurosurg Pediatr 13(6):650–657. https://doi.org/10.3171/2014.3.PEDS13455

Choudry Q, Patel HC, Gurusinghe NT, Evans DG (2007) Radiation-induced brain tumours in nevoid basal cell carcinoma syndrome: implications for treatment and surveillance. Childs Nerv Syst 23(1):133–136. https://doi.org/10.1007/s00381-006-0178-4

Cowan R, Hoban P, Kelsey A, Birch JM, Gattamaneni R, Evans DG (1997) The gene for the naevoid basal cell carcinoma syndrome acts as a tumour-suppressor gene in medulloblastoma. Br J Cancer 76(2):141–145

Custodio G, Taques GR, Figueiredo BC, Gugelmin ES, Oliveira Figueiredo MM, Watanabe F, Pontarolo R, Lalli E, Torres LF (2011) Increased incidence of choroid plexus carcinoma due to the germline TP53 R337H mutation in southern Brazil. PLoS One 6(3):e18015. https://doi.org/10.1371/journal.pone.0018015

de Kock L, Sabbaghian N, Druker H, Weber E, Hamel N, Miller S, Choong CS, Gottardo NG, Kees UR, Rednam SP, van Hest LP, Jongmans MC, Jhangiani S, Lupski JR, Zacharin M, Bouron-Dal Soglio D, Huang A, Priest JR, Perry A, Mueller S, Albrecht S, Malkin D, Grundy RG, Foulkes WD (2014b) Germ-line and somatic DICER1 mutations in pineoblastoma. Acta Neuropathol 128(4):583–595. https://doi.org/10.1007/s00401-014-1318-7

de Kock L, Sabbaghian N, Plourde F, Srivastava A, Weber E, Bouron-Dal Soglio D, Hamel N, Choi JH, Park SH, Deal CL, Kelsey MM, Dishop MK, Esbenshade A, Kuttesch JF, Jacques TS, Perry A, Leichter H, Maeder P, Brundler MA, Warner J, Neal J, Zacharin M, Korbonits M, Cole T, Traunecker H, McLean TW, Rotondo F, Lepage P, Albrecht S, Horvath E, Kovacs K, Priest JR, Foulkes WD (2014a) Pituitary blastoma: a pathognomonic feature of germ-line DICER1 mutations. Acta Neuropathol 128(1):111–122. https://doi.org/10.1007/s00401-014-1285-z

Dunn IF, Agarwalla PK, Papanastassiou AM, Butler WE, Smith ER (2007) Multiple pilocytic astrocytomas of the cerebellum in a 17-year-old patient with neurofibromatosis type I. Childs Nerv Syst 23(10):1191–1194. https://doi.org/10.1007/s00381-007-0343-4

Durno CA, Sherman PM, Aronson M, Malkin D, Hawkins C, Bakry D, Bouffet E, Gallinger S, Pollett A, Campbell B, Tabori U, International BC (2015) Phenotypic and genotypic characterisation of biallelic mismatch repair deficiency (BMMR-D) syndrome. Eur J Cancer 51(8):977–983. https://doi.org/10.1016/j.ejca.2015.02.008

Eaton KW, Tooke LS, Wainwright LM, Judkins AR, Biegel JA (2011) Spectrum of SMARCB1/INI1 mutations in familial and sporadic rhabdoid tumors. Pediatr Blood Cancer 56(1):7–15. https://doi.org/10.1002/pbc.22831

European Chromosome 16 Tuberous Sclerosis C (1993) Identification and characterization of the tuberous sclerosis gene on chromosome 16. Cell 75(7):1305–1315

Evans DG, Baser ME, O'Reilly B, Rowe J, Gleeson M, Saeed S, King A, Huson SM, Kerr R, Thomas N, Irving R, MacFarlane R, Ferner R, McLeod R, Moffat D, Ramsden R (2005) Management of the patient and family with neurofibromatosis 2: a consensus conference statement. Br J Neurosurg 19(1):5–12. https://doi.org/10.1080/02688690500081206

Evans DG, Birch JM, Orton CI (1991) Brain tumours and the occurrence of severe invasive basal cell carcinoma in first degree relatives with Gorlin syndrome. Br J Neurosurg 5(6):643–646

Evans DG, Birch JM, Ramsden RT (1999) Paediatric presentation of type 2 neurofibromatosis. Arch Dis Child 81(6):496–499

Evans DG, Huson SM, Donnai D, Neary W, Blair V, Newton V, Harris R (1992) A clinical study of type 2 neurofibromatosis. Q J Med 84(304):603–618

Evans DG, Ladusans EJ, Rimmer S, Burnell LD, Thakker N, Farndon PA (1993) Complications of the naevoid basal cell carcinoma syndrome: results of a population based study. J Med Genet 30(6):460–464

Evans DG, Newton V, Neary W, Baser ME, Wallace A, Macleod R, Jenkins JP, Gillespie J, Ramsden RT (2000) Use of MRI and audiological tests in presymptomatic diagnosis of type 2 neurofibromatosis (NF2). J Med Genet 37(12):944–947

Evans DG, Raymond FL, Barwell JG, Halliday D (2012) Genetic testing and screening of individuals at risk of NF2. Clin Genet 82(5):416–424. https://doi.org/10.1111/j.1399-0004.2011.01816.x

Fan Z, Li J, Du J, Zhang H, Shen Y, Wang CY, Wang S (2008) A missense mutation in PTCH2 underlies dominantly inherited NBCCS in a Chinese family. J Med Genet 45(5):303–308. https://doi.org/10.1136/jmg.2007.055343

Farrell CJ, Plotkin SR (2007) Genetic causes of brain tumors: neurofibromatosis, tuberous sclerosis, von Hippel-Lindau, and other syndromes. Neurol Clin 25(4):925–946., viii. https://doi.org/10.1016/j.ncl.2007.07.008

Ferner RE, Huson SM, Thomas N, Moss C, Willshaw H, Evans DG, Upadhyaya M, Towers R, Gleeson M, Steiger C, Kirby A (2007) Guidelines for the diagnosis and management of individuals with neurofibromatosis 1. J Med Genet 44(2):81–88. https://doi.org/10.1136/jmg.2006.045906

Fisher MJ, Loguidice M, Gutmann DH, Listernick R, Ferner RE, Ullrich NJ, Packer RJ, Tabori U, Hoffman RO, Ardern-Holmes SL, Hummel TR, Hargrave DR, Bouffet E, Charrow J, Bilaniuk LT, Balcer LJ, Liu GT (2012) Visual outcomes in children with neurofibromatosis type 1-associated optic pathway glioma following chemotherapy: a multicenter retrospective analysis. Neuro-Oncology 14(6):790–797. https://doi.org/10.1093/neuonc/nos076

Forest F, David A, Arrufat S, Pierron G, Ranchere-Vince D, Stephan JL, Clemenson A, Delattre O, Bourdeaut F (2012) Conventional chondrosarcoma in a survivor of rhabdoid tumor: enlarging the spectrum of tumors associated with SMARCB1 germline mutations. Am J Surg Pathol 36(12):1892–1896. https://doi.org/10.1097/PAS.0b013e31826cbe7a

Foulkes WD, Priest JR, Duchaine TF (2014) DICER1: mutations, microRNAs and mechanisms. Nat Rev Cancer 14(10):662–672. https://doi.org/10.1038/nrc3802

Franz DN, Belousova E, Sparagana S, Bebin EM, Frost M, Kuperman R, Witt O, Kohrman MH, Flamini JR, Wu JY, Curatolo P, de Vries PJ, Berkowitz N, Anak O, Niolat J, Jozwiak S (2014) Everolimus for subependymal giant cell astrocytoma in patients with tuberous sclerosis complex: 2-year open-label extension of the randomised EXIST-1 study. Lancet Oncol 15(13):1513–1520. https://doi.org/10.1016/S1470-2045(14)70489-9

Franz DN, Belousova E, Sparagana S, Bebin EM, Frost M, Kuperman R, Witt O, Kohrman MH, Flamini JR, Wu JY, Curatolo P, de Vries PJ, Whittemore VH, Thiele EA, Ford JP, Shah G, Cauwel H, Lebwohl D, Sahmoud T, Jozwiak S (2013) Efficacy and safety of everolimus for subependymal giant cell astrocytomas associated with tuberous sclerosis complex (EXIST-1): a multicentre, randomised, placebo-controlled phase 3 trial. Lancet 381(9861):125–132. https://doi.org/10.1016/S0140-6736(12)61134-9

Fujii K, Ohashi H, Suzuki M, Hatsuse H, Shiohama T, Uchikawa H, Miyashita T (2013) Frameshift mutation in the PTCH2 gene can cause nevoid basal cell carcinoma syndrome. Familial Cancer 12(4):611–614. https://doi.org/10.1007/s10689-013-9623-1

Gajjar A, Pfister SM, Taylor MD, Gilbertson RJ (2014) Molecular insights into pediatric brain tumors have the potential to transform therapy. Clin Cancer Res 20(22):5630–5640. https://doi.org/10.1158/1078-0432.CCR-14-0833

Gajjar A, Stewart CF, Ellison DW, Kaste S, Kun LE, Packer RJ, Goldman S, Chintagumpala M, Wallace D, Takebe N, Boyett JM, Gilbertson RJ, Curran T (2013) Phase I study of vismodegib in children with recurrent or refractory medulloblastoma: a pediatric brain tumor consortium study. Clin Cancer Res 19(22):6305–6312. https://doi.org/10.1158/1078-0432.CCR-13-1425

Garre ML, Cama A, Bagnasco F, Morana G, Giangaspero F, Brisigotti M, Gambini C, Forni M, Rossi A, Haupt R, Nozza P, Barra S, Piatelli G, Viglizzo G, Capra V, Bruno W, Pastorino L, Massimino M, Tumolo M, Fidani P, Dallorso S, Schumacher RF, Milanaccio C, Pietsch T (2009) Medulloblastoma variants: age-dependent occurrence and relation to Gorlin syndrome--a new clinical perspective. Clin Cancer Res 15(7):2463–2471. https://doi.org/10.1158/1078-0432.CCR-08-2023

Gonzalez KD, Noltner KA, Buzin CH, Gu D, Wen-Fong CY, Nguyen VQ, Han JH, Lowstuter K, Longmate J, Sommer SS, Weitzel JN (2009) Beyond Li Fraumeni syndrome: clinical characteristics of families with p53 germline mutations. J Clin Oncol 27(8):1250–1256. https://doi.org/10.1200/JCO.2008.16.6959

Gorlin RJ, Goltz RW (1960) Multiple nevoid basal-cell epithelioma, jaw cysts and bifid rib. A syndrome. N Engl J Med 262:908–912. https://doi.org/10.1056/NEJM196005052621803

Grill J, Couanet D, Cappelli C, Habrand JL, Rodriguez D, Sainte-Rose C, Kalifa C (1999) Radiation-induced cerebral vasculopathy in children with neurofibromatosis and optic pathway glioma. Ann Neurol 45(3):393–396

Gu S, Glaug N, Cnaan A, Packer RJ, Avery RA (2014) Ganglion cell layer-inner plexiform layer thickness and vision loss in young children with optic pathway gliomas. Invest Ophthalmol Vis Sci 55(3):1402–1408. https://doi.org/10.1167/iovs.13-13119

Gutmann DH, Aylsworth A, Carey JC, Korf B, Marks J, Pyeritz RE, Rubenstein A, Viskochil D (1997) The diagnostic evaluation and multidisciplinary management of neurofibromatosis 1 and neurofibromatosis 2. JAMA 278(1):51–57

Hadfield KD, Newman WG, Bowers NL, Wallace A, Bolger C, Colley A, McCann E, Trump D, Prescott T, Evans DG (2008) Molecular characterisation of SMARCB1 and NF2 in familial and sporadic schwannomatosis. J Med Genet 45(6):332–339. https://doi.org/10.1136/jmg.2007.056499

Hagel C, Stemmer-Rachamimov AO, Bornemann A, Schuhmann M, Nagel C, Huson S, Evans DG, Plotkin S, Matthies C, Kluwe L, Mautner VF (2012) Clinical presentation, immunohistochemistry and electron microscopy indicate neurofibromatosis type 2-associated gliomas to be spinal ependymomas. Neuropathology 32(6):611–616. https://doi.org/10.1111/j.1440-1789.2012.01306.x

Hahn H, Wicking C, Zaphiropoulous PG, Gailani MR, Shanley S, Chidambaram A, Vorechovsky I, Holmberg E, Unden AB, Gillies S, Negus K, Smyth I, Pressman C, Leffell DJ, Gerrard B, Goldstein AM, Dean M, Toftgard R, Chenevix-Trench G, Wainwright B, Bale AE (1996) Mutations of the human homolog of drosophila patched in the nevoid basal cell carcinoma syndrome. Cell 85(6):841–851

Haines JL, Short MP, Kwiatkowski DJ, Jewell A, Andermann E, Bejjani B, Yang CH, Gusella JF, Amos JA (1991) Localization of one gene for tuberous sclerosis within 9q32-9q34, and further evidence for heterogeneity. Am J Hum Genet 49(4):764–772

Hamilton SR, Liu B, Parsons RE, Papadopoulos N, Jen J, Powell SM, Krush AJ, Berk T, Cohen Z, Tetu B et al (1995) The molecular basis of Turcot's syndrome. N Engl J Med 332(13):839–847. https://doi.org/10.1056/NEJM199503303321302

Hasselblatt M, Gesk S, Oyen F, Rossi S, Viscardi E, Giangaspero F, Giannini C, Judkins AR, Fruhwald MC, Obser T, Schneppenheim R, Siebert R, Paulus W (2011) Nonsense mutation and inactivation of SMARCA4 (BRG1) in an atypical teratoid/rhabdoid tumor showing retained SMARCB1 (INI1) expression. Am J Surg Pathol 35(6):933–935. https://doi.org/10.1097/PAS.0b013e3182196a39

Hasselblatt M, Nagel I, Oyen F, Bartelheim K, Russell RB, Schuller U, Junckerstorff R, Rosenblum M, Alassiri AH, Rossi S, Schmid I, Gottardo NG, Toledano H, Viscardi E, Balbin M, Witkowski L, Lu Q, Betts MJ, Foulkes WD, Siebert R, Fruhwald MC, Schneppenheim R (2014) SMARCA4-mutated atypical teratoid/rhabdoid tumors are associated with inherited germline alterations and poor prognosis. Acta Neuropathol 128(3):453–456. https://doi.org/10.1007/s00401-014-1323-x

Hill DA, Ivanovich J, Priest JR, Gurnett CA, Dehner LP, Desruisseau D, Jarzembowski JA, Wikenheiser-Brokamp KA, Suarez BK, Whelan AJ, Williams G, Bracamontes D, Messinger Y, Goodfellow PJ (2009) DICER1 mutations in familial pleuropulmonary blastoma. Science 325(5943):965. https://doi.org/10.1126/science.1174334

Hisada M, Garber JE, Fung CY, Fraumeni JF Jr, Li FP (1998) Multiple primary cancers in families with Li-Fraumeni syndrome. J Natl Cancer Inst 90(8):606–611

Hulsebos TJ, Kenter S, Siebers-Renelt U, Hans V, Wesseling P, Flucke U (2014a) SMARCB1 involvement in the development of leiomyoma in a patient with schwannomatosis. Am J Surg Pathol 38(3):421–425. https://doi.org/10.1097/PAS.0000000000000110

Hulsebos TJ, Kenter S, Verhagen WI, Baas F, Flucke U, Wesseling P (2014b) Premature termination of SMARCB1 translation may be followed by reinitiation in schwannomatosis-associated schwannomas, but results in absence of SMARCB1 expression in rhabdoid tumors. Acta Neuropathol 128(3):439–448. https://doi.org/10.1007/s00401-014-1281-3

Hulsebos TJ, Plomp AS, Wolterman RA, Robanus-Maandag EC, Baas F, Wesseling P (2007) Germline mutation of INI1/SMARCB1 in familial schwannomatosis. Am J Hum Genet 80(4):805–810. https://doi.org/10.1086/513207

Huttner AJ, Kieran MW, Yao X, Cruz L, Ladner J, Quayle K, Goumnerova LC, Irons MB, Ullrich NJ (2010) Clinicopathologic study of glioblastoma in children with neurofibromatosis type 1. Pediatr Blood Cancer 54(7):890–896. https://doi.org/10.1002/pbc.22462

Ingham PW, McMahon AP (2001) Hedgehog signaling in animal development: paradigms and principles. Genes Dev 15(23):3059–3087. https://doi.org/10.1101/gad.938601

Inoki K, Guan KL (2009) Tuberous sclerosis complex, implication from a rare genetic disease to common cancer treatment. Hum Mol Genet 18(R1):R94–R100. https://doi.org/10.1093/hmg/ddp032

Jackson EM, Shaikh TH, Gururangan S, Jones MC, Malkin D, Nikkel SM, Zuppan CW, Wainright LM, Zhang F, Biegel JA (2007) High-density single nucleotide polymorphism array analysis in patients with germline deletions of 22q11.2 and malignant rhabdoid tumor. Hum Genet 122(2):117–127. https://doi.org/10.1007/s00439-007-0386-3

Jiricny J (2006) The multifaceted mismatch-repair system. Nat Rev Mol Cell Biol 7(5):335–346. https://doi.org/10.1038/nrm1907

Johnson RL, Rothman AL, Xie J, Goodrich LV, Bare JW, Bonifas JM, Quinn AG, Myers RM, Cox DR, Epstein EH Jr, Scott MP (1996) Human homolog of patched, a candidate gene for the basal cell nevus syndrome. Science 272(5268):1668–1671

Karajannis MA, Ferner RE (2015) Neurofibromatosis-related tumors: emerging biology and therapies. Curr Opin Pediatr 27(1):26–33. https://doi.org/10.1097/MOP.0000000000000169

Khong PL, Goh WH, Wong VC, Fung CW, Ooi GC (2003) MR imaging of spinal tumors in children with neurofibromatosis 1. AJR Am J Roentgenol 180(2):413–417. https://doi.org/10.2214/ajr.180.2.1800413

Kim KH, Roberts CW (2014) Mechanisms by which SMARCB1 loss drives rhabdoid tumor growth. Cancer Genet 207(9):365–372. https://doi.org/10.1016/j.cancergen.2014.04.004

Kimonis VE, Goldstein AM, Pastakia B, Yang ML, Kase R, DiGiovanna JJ, Bale AE, Bale SJ (1997) Clinical manifestations in 105 persons with nevoid basal cell carcinoma syndrome. Am J Med Genet 69(3):299–308

Kimonis VE, Mehta SG, Digiovanna JJ, Bale SJ, Pastakia B (2004) Radiological features in 82 patients with nevoid basal cell carcinoma (NBCC or Gorlin) syndrome. Genet Med 6 (6):495–502. doi:10.109701. GIM.0000145045.17711.1C

King A, Listernick R, Charrow J, Piersall L, Gutmann DH (2003) Optic pathway gliomas in neurofibromatosis type 1: the effect of presenting symptoms on outcome. Am J Med Genet A 122A(2):95–99. https://doi.org/10.1002/ajmg.a.20211

Kool M, Jones DT, Jager N, Northcott PA, Pugh TJ, Hovestadt V, Piro RM, Esparza LA, Markant SL, Remke M, Milde T, Bourdeaut F, Ryzhova M, Sturm D, Pfaff E, Stark S, Hutter S, Seker-Cin H, Johann P, Bender S, Schmidt C, Rausch T, Shih D, Reimand J, Sieber L, Wittmann A, Linke L, Witt H, Weber UD, Zapatka M, Konig R, Beroukhim R, Bergthold G, van Sluis P, Volckmann R, Koster J, Versteeg R, Schmidt S, Wolf S, Lawerenz C, Bartholomae CC, von Kalle C, Unterberg A, Herold-Mende C, Hofer S, Kulozik AE, von Deimling A, Scheurlen W, Felsberg J, Reifenberger G, Hasselblatt M, Crawford JR, Grant GA, Jabado N, Perry A, Cowdrey C, Croul S, Zadeh G, Korbel JO, Doz F, Delattre O, Bader GD, McCabe MG, Collins VP, Kieran MW, Cho YJ, Pomeroy SL, Witt O, Brors B, Taylor MD, Schuller U, Korshunov A, Eils R, Wechsler-Reya RJ, Lichter P, Pfister SM, Project IPT (2014) Genome sequencing of SHH medulloblastoma predicts genotype-related response to smoothened inhibition. Cancer Cell 25(3):393–405. https://doi.org/10.1016/j.ccr.2014.02.004

Kordes U, Bartelheim K, Modena P, Massimino M, Biassoni V, Reinhard H, Hasselblatt M, Schneppenheim R, Fruhwald MC (2014) Favorable outcome of patients affected by rhabdoid tumors due to rhabdoid tumor predisposition syndrome (RTPS). Pediatr Blood Cancer 61(5):919–921. https://doi.org/10.1002/pbc.24793

Kordes U, Gesk S, Fruhwald MC, Graf N, Leuschner I, Hasselblatt M, Jeibmann A, Oyen F, Peters O, Pietsch T, Siebert R, Schneppenheim R (2010) Clinical and molecular features in patients with atypical teratoid rhabdoid tumor or malignant rhabdoid tumor. Genes Chromosomes Cancer 49(2):176–181. https://doi.org/10.1002/gcc.20729

Kotecha RS, Pascoe EM, Rushing EJ, Rorke-Adams LB, Zwerdling T, Gao X, Li X, Greene S, Amirjamshidi A, Kim SK, Lima MA, Hung PC, Lakhdar F, Mehta N, Liu Y, Devi BI, Sudhir BJ, Lund-Johansen M, Gjerris F, Cole CH, Gottardo NG (2011) Meningiomas in children and adolescents: a meta-analysis of individual patient data. Lancet Oncol 12(13):1229–1239. https://doi.org/10.1016/S1470-2045(11)70275-3

Lafay-Cousin L, Payne E, Strother D, Chernos J, Chan M, Bernier FP (2009) Goldenhar phenotype in a child with distal 22q11.2 deletion and intracranial atypical teratoid

rhabdoid tumor. Am J Med Genet A 149A(12):2855–2859. https://doi.org/10.1002/ajmg.a.33119

Leary SE, Zhou T, Holmes E, Geyer JR, Miller DC (2011) Histology predicts a favorable outcome in young children with desmoplastic medulloblastoma: a report from the Children's Oncology Group. Cancer 117(14):3262–3267. https://doi.org/10.1002/cncr.25856

Li FP, Fraumeni JF Jr, Mulvihill JJ, Blattner WA, Dreyfus MG, Tucker MA, Miller RW (1988) A cancer family syndrome in twenty-four kindreds. Cancer Res 48(18):5358–5362

Li FP, Fraumeni JF Jr (1969) Rhabdomyosarcoma in children: epidemiologic study and identification of a familial cancer syndrome. J Natl Cancer Inst 43(6):1365–1373

Lin AL, Gutmann DH (2013) Advances in the treatment of neurofibromatosis-associated tumours. Nat Rev Clin Oncol 10(11):616–624. https://doi.org/10.1038/nrclinonc.2013.144

Listernick R, Charrow J, Greenwald M, Mets M (1994) Natural history of optic pathway tumors in children with neurofibromatosis type 1: a longitudinal study. J Pediatr 125(1):63–66

Listernick R, Ferner RE, Liu GT, Gutmann DH (2007) Optic pathway gliomas in neurofibromatosis-1: controversies and recommendations. Ann Neurol 61(3):189–198. https://doi.org/10.1002/ana.21107

Listernick R, Ferner RE, Piersall L, Sharif S, Gutmann DH, Charrow J (2004) Late-onset optic pathway tumors in children with neurofibromatosis 1. Neurology 63(10):1944–1946

Lynch HT, de la Chapelle A (2003) Hereditary colorectal cancer. N Engl J Med 348(10):919–932. https://doi.org/10.1056/NEJMra012242

MacCollin M, Chiocca EA, Evans DG, Friedman JM, Horvitz R, Jaramillo D, Lev M, Mautner VF, Niimura M, Plotkin SR, Sang CN, Stemmer-Rachamimov A, Roach ES (2005) Diagnostic criteria for schwannomatosis. Neurology 64(11):1838–1845. https://doi.org/10.1212/01.WNL.0000163982.78900.AD

Malkin D, Li FP, Strong LC, Fraumeni JF Jr, Nelson CE, Kim DH, Kassel J, Gryka MA, Bischoff FZ, Tainsky MA et al (1990) Germ line p53 mutations in a familial syndrome of breast cancer, sarcomas, and other neoplasms. Science 250(4985):1233–1238

Martin LM, Marples B, Coffey M, Lawler M, Lynch TH, Hollywood D, Marignol L (2010) DNA mismatch repair and the DNA damage response to ionizing radiation: making sense of apparently conflicting data. Cancer Treat Rev 36(7):518–527. https://doi.org/10.1016/j.ctrv.2010.03.008

Mautner VF, Nguyen R, Knecht R, Bokemeyer C (2010) Radiographic regression of vestibular schwannomas induced by bevacizumab treatment: sustain under continuous drug application and rebound after drug discontinuation. Ann Oncol 21(11):2294–2295. https://doi.org/10.1093/annonc/mdq566

Medina PP, Sanchez-Cespedes M (2008) Involvement of the chromatin-remodeling factor BRG1/SMARCA4 in human cancer. Epigenetics 3(2):64–68

Milstein JM, Geyer JR, Berger MS, Bleyer WA (1989) Favorable prognosis for brainstem gliomas in neurofibromatosis. J Neuro-Oncol 7(4):367–371

Molloy PT, Bilaniuk LT, Vaughan SN, Needle MN, Liu GT, Zackai EH, Phillips PC (1995) Brainstem tumors in patients with neurofibromatosis type 1: a distinct clinical entity. Neurology 45(10):1897–1902

Morgan JE, Wolfort F (1979) The early history of tuberous sclerosis. Arch Dermatol 115(11):1317–1319

Muller EA, Aradhya S, Atkin JF, Carmany EP, Elliott AM, Chudley AE, Clark RD, Everman DB, Garner S, Hall BD, Herman GE, Kivuva E, Ramanathan S, Stevenson DA, Stockton DW, Hudgins L (2012) Microdeletion 9q22.3 syndrome includes metopic craniosynostosis, hydrocephalus, macrosomia, and developmental delay. Am J Med Genet A 158A(2):391–399. https://doi.org/10.1002/ajmg.a.34216

Murray MJ, Bailey S, Raby KL, Saini HK, de Kock L, Burke GA, Foulkes WD, Enright AJ, Coleman N, Tischkowitz M (2014) Serum levels of mature microRNAs in DICER1-mutated pleuropulmonary blastoma. Oncogene 3:e87. https://doi.org/10.1038/oncsis.2014.1

National Institutes of Health Consensus Development Conference Statement: neurofibromatosis (1988) Neurofibromatosis, vol 1(3). Bethesda, MD, USA, July 13–15, 1987. p 172–178

Nguyen R, Dombi E, Akshintala S, Baldwin A, Widemann BC (2015) Characterization of spinal findings in children and adults with neurofibromatosis type 1 enrolled in a natural history study using magnetic resonance imaging. J Neuro-Oncol 121(1):209–215. https://doi.org/10.1007/s11060-014-1629-5

North KN, Riccardi V, Samango-Sprouse C, Ferner R, Moore B, Legius E, Ratner N, Denckla MB (1997) Cognitive function and academic performance in neurofibromatosis. 1: consensus statement from the NF1 cognitive disorders task force. Neurology 48(4):1121–1127

Northrup H, Krueger DA, International Tuberous Sclerosis Complex Consensus G (2013) Tuberous sclerosis complex diagnostic criteria update: recommendations of the 2012 International Tuberous Sclerosis Complex Consensus Conference. Pediatr Neurol 49(4):243–254. https://doi.org/10.1016/j.pediatrneurol.2013.08.001

Northrup H, Wheless JW, Bertin TK, Lewis RA (1993) Variability of expression in tuberous sclerosis. J Med Genet 30(1):41–43

Olivier M, Goldgar DE, Sodha N, Ohgaki H, Kleihues P, Hainaut P, Eeles RA (2003) Li-Fraumeni and related syndromes: correlation between tumor type, family structure, and TP53 genotype. Cancer Res 63(20):6643–6650

Perilongo G, Moras P, Carollo C, Battistella A, Clementi M, Laverda A, Murgia A (1999) Spontaneous partial regression of low-grade glioma in children with neurofibromatosis-1: a real possibility. J Child Neurol 14(6):352–356

Pilling RF, Taylor RH (2010) Screening children with NF1 for optic pathway glioma--no. Eye 24(9):1432–1434. https://doi.org/10.1038/eye.2010.94

Plotkin SR, Merker VL, Muzikansky A, Barker FG 2nd, Slattery W 3rd (2014) Natural history of vestibular schwannoma growth and hearing decline in newly diagnosed neurofibromatosis type 2 patients. Otol Neurotol 35(1):e50–e56. https://doi.org/10.1097/MAO.0000000000000239

Plotkin SR, O'Donnell CC, Curry WT, Bove CM, MacCollin M, Nunes FP (2011) Spinal ependymomas in neurofibromatosis type 2: a retrospective analysis of 55 patients. J Neurosurg Spine 14(4):543–547. https://doi.org/10.3171/2010.11.SPINE10350

Plotkin SR, Stemmer-Rachamimov AO, Barker FG 2nd, Halpin C, Padera TP, Tyrrell A, Sorensen AG, Jain RK, di Tomaso E (2009) Hearing improvement after bevacizumab in patients with neurofibromatosis type 2. N Engl J Med 361(4):358–367. https://doi.org/10.1056/NEJMoa0902579

Pollack IF, Shultz B, Mulvihill JJ (1996) The management of brainstem gliomas in patients with neurofibromatosis 1. Neurology 46(6):1652–1660

Raffel C, McComb JG, Bodner S, Gilles FE (1989) Benign brain stem lesions in pediatric patients with neurofibromatosis: case reports. Neurosurgery 25(6):959–964

Ricciardone MD, Ozcelik T, Cevher B, Ozdag H, Tuncer M, Gurgey A, Uzunalimoglu O, Cetinkaya H, Tanyeli A, Erken E, Ozturk M (1999) Human MLH1 deficiency predisposes to hematological malignancy and neurofibromatosis type 1. Cancer Res 59(2):290–293

Robinson GW, Orr BA, Wu G, Gururangan S, Lin T, Qaddoumi I, Packer RJ, Goldman S, Prados MD, Desjardins A, Chintagumpala M, Takebe N, Kaste SC, Rusch M, Allen SJ, Onar-Thomas A, Stewart CF, Fouladi M, Boyett JM, Gilbertson RJ, Curran T, Ellison DW, Gajjar A (2015) Vismodegib exerts targeted efficacy against recurrent sonic hedgehog-subgroup Medulloblastoma: results from phase II Pediatric brain tumor consortium studies PBTC-025B and PBTC-032. J Clin Oncol 33(24):2646–2654. https://doi.org/10.1200/JCO.2014.60.1591

Ron E, Modan B, Boice JD Jr, Alfandary E, Stovall M, Chetrit A, Katz L (1988) Tumors of the brain and nervous system after radiotherapy in childhood. N Engl J Med 319(16):1033–1039. https://doi.org/10.1056/NEJM198810203191601

Rosenfeld A, Listernick R, Charrow J, Goldman S (2010) Neurofibromatosis type 1 and high-grade tumors of the central nervous system. Childs Nerv Syst 26(5):663–667. https://doi.org/10.1007/s00381-009-1024-2

Rosser TL, Vezina G, Packer RJ (2005) Cerebrovascular abnormalities in a population of children with neurofibromatosis type 1. Neurology 64(3):553–555. https://doi.org/10.1212/01.WNL.0000150544.00016.69

Roth J, Roach ES, Bartels U, Jozwiak S, Koenig MK, Weiner HL, Franz DN, Wang HZ (2013) Subependymal giant cell astrocytoma: diagnosis, screening, and treatment. Recommendations from the international tuberous sclerosis complex consensus conference 2012. Pediatr Neurol 49(6):439–444. https://doi.org/10.1016/j.pediatrneurol.2013.08.017

Rouleau GA, Merel P, Lutchman M, Sanson M, Zucman J, Marineau C, Hoang-Xuan K, Demczuk S, Desmaze C, Plougastel B et al (1993) Alteration in a new gene encoding a putative membrane-organizing protein causes neuro-fibromatosis type 2. Nature 363(6429):515–521. https://doi.org/10.1038/363515a0

Roussel MF, Hatten ME (2011) Cerebellum development and medulloblastoma. Curr Top Dev Biol 94:235–282. https://doi.org/10.1016/B978-0-12-380916-2.00008-5

Rudin CM, Hann CL, Laterra J, Yauch RL, Callahan CA, Fu L, Holcomb T, Stinson J, Gould SE, Coleman B, LoRusso PM, Von Hoff DD, de Sauvage FJ, Low JA (2009) Treatment of medulloblastoma with hedgehog pathway inhibitor GDC-0449. N Engl J Med 361(12):1173–1178. https://doi.org/10.1056/NEJMoa0902903

Ruijs MW, Verhoef S, Rookus MA, Pruntel R, van der Hout AH, Hogervorst FB, Kluijt I, Sijmons RH, Aalfs CM, Wagner A, Ausems MG, Hoogerbrugge N, van Asperen CJ, Gomez Garcia EB, Meijers-Heijboer H, Ten Kate LP, Menko FH, van't Veer LJ (2010) TP53 germline mutation testing in 180 families suspected of Li-Fraumeni syndrome: mutation detection rate and relative frequency of cancers in different familial phenotypes. J Med Genet 47(6):421–428. https://doi.org/10.1136/jmg.2009.073429

Rutkowski S, Bode U, Deinlein F, Ottensmeier H, Warmuth-Metz M, Soerensen N, Graf N, Emser A, Pietsch T, Wolff JE, Kortmann RD, Kuehl J (2005) Treatment of early childhood medulloblastoma by postoperative chemotherapy alone. N Engl J Med 352(10):978–986. https://doi.org/10.1056/NEJMoa042176

Sabbaghian N, Hamel N, Srivastava A, Albrecht S, Priest JR, Foulkes WD (2012) Germline DICER1 mutation and associated loss of heterozygosity in a pineoblastoma. J Med Genet 49(7):417–419. https://doi.org/10.1136/jmedgenet-2012-100898

Sathyamoorthi S, Morales J, Bermudez J, McBride L, Luquette M, McGoey R, Oates N, Hales S, Biegel JA, Lacassie Y (2009) Array analysis and molecular studies of INI1 in an infant with deletion 22q13 (Phelan-McDermid syndrome) and atypical teratoid/rhabdoid tumor. Am J Med Genet A 149A(5):1067–1069. https://doi.org/10.1002/ajmg.a.32775

Satinoff MI, Wells C (1969) Multiple basal cell naevus syndrome in ancient Egypt. Med Hist 13(3):294–297

Scheithauer BW, Kovacs K, Horvath E, Kim DS, Osamura RY, Ketterling RP, Lloyd RV, Kim OL (2008) Pituitary blastoma. Acta Neuropathol 116(6):657–666. https://doi.org/10.1007/s00401-008-0388-9

Schneppenheim R, Fruhwald MC, Gesk S, Hasselblatt M, Jeibmann A, Kordes U, Kreuz M, Leuschner I, Martin Subero JI, Obser T, Oyen F, Vater I, Siebert R (2010) Germline nonsense mutation and somatic inactivation of SMARCA4/BRG1 in a family with rhabdoid tumor predisposition syndrome. Am J Hum Genet 86(2):279–284. https://doi.org/10.1016/j.ajhg.2010.01.013

Schultz KA, Yang J, Doros L, Williams GM, Harris A, Stewart DR, Messinger Y, Field A, Dehner LP, Hill DA (2014) Pleuropulmonary blastoma familial tumor predisposition syndrome: a unique constellation of neoplastic conditions. Pathol Case Rev 19(2):90–100. https://doi.org/10.1097/PCR.0000000000000027

Seidinger AL, Mastellaro MJ, Paschoal Fortes F, Godoy Assumpcao J, Aparecida Cardinalli I, Aparecida Ganazza M, Correa Ribeiro R, Brandalise SR, Dos Santos Aguiar S, Yunes JA (2011) Association of the highly prevalent TP53 R337H mutation with pediatric choroid plexus carcinoma and osteosarcoma in Southeast Brazil. Cancer 117(10):2228–2235. https://doi.org/10.1002/cncr.25826

Sevenet N, Sheridan E, Amram D, Schneider P, Handgretinger R, Delattre O (1999) Constitutional mutations of the hSNF5/INI1 gene predispose to a variety of cancers. Am J Hum Genet 65(5):1342–1348. https://doi.org/10.1086/302639

Sharif S, Ferner R, Birch JM, Gillespie JE, Gattamaneni HR, Baser ME, Evans DG (2006) Second primary tumors in neurofibromatosis 1 patients treated for optic glioma: substantial risks after radiotherapy. J Clin Oncol 24(16):2570–2575. https://doi.org/10.1200/JCO.2005.03.8349

Sharif S, Upadhyaya M, Ferner R, Majounie E, Shenton A, Baser M, Thakker N, Evans DG (2011) A molecular analysis of individuals with neurofibromatosis type 1 (NF1) and optic pathway gliomas (OPGs), and an assessment of genotype-phenotype correlations. J Med Genet 48(4):256–260. https://doi.org/10.1136/jmg.2010.081760

Shlien A, Campbell BB, de Borja R, Alexandrov LB, Merico D, Wedge D, Van Loo P, Tarpey PS, Coupland P, Behjati S, Pollett A, Lipman T, Heidari A, Deshmukh S, Avitzur N, Meier B, Gerstung M, Hong Y, Merino DM, Ramakrishna M, Remke M, Arnold R, Panigrahi GB, Thakkar NP, Hodel KP, Henninger EE, Goksenin AY, Bakry D, Charames GS, Druker H, Lerner-Ellis J, Mistry M, Dvir R, Grant R, Elhasid R, Farah R, Taylor GP, Nathan PC, Alexander S, Ben-Shachar S, Ling SC, Gallinger S, Constantini S, Dirks P, Huang A, Scherer SW, Grundy RG, Durno C, Aronson M, Gartner A, Meyn MS, Taylor MD, Pursell ZF, Pearson CE, Malkin D, Futreal PA, Stratton MR, Bouffet E, Hawkins C, Campbell PJ, Tabori U, Biallelic Mismatch Repair Deficiency C (2015) Combined hereditary and somatic mutations of replication error repair genes result in rapid onset of ultra-hypermutated cancers. Nat Genet 47 (3):257–262. doi:https://doi.org/10.1038/ng.3202

Slade I, Bacchelli C, Davies H, Murray A, Abbaszadeh F, Hanks S, Barfoot R, Burke A, Chisholm J, Hewitt M, Jenkinson H, King D, Morland B, Pizer B, Prescott K, Saggar A, Side L, Traunecker H, Vaidya S, Ward P, Futreal PA, Vujanic G, Nicholson AG, Sebire N, Turnbull C, Priest JR, Pritchard-Jones K, Houlston R, Stiller C, Stratton MR, Douglas J, Rahman N (2011) DICER1 syndrome: clarifying the diagnosis, clinical features and management implications of a pleiotropic tumour predisposition syndrome. J Med Genet 48(4):273–278. https://doi.org/10.1136/jmg.2010.083790

Smith MJ, Beetz C, Williams SG, Bhaskar SS, O'Sullivan J, Anderson B, Daly SB, Urquhart JE, Bholah Z, Oudit D, Cheesman E, Kelsey A, McCabe MG, Newman WG, Evans DG (2014b) Germline mutations in SUFU cause Gorlin syndrome-associated childhood medulloblastoma and redefine the risk associated with PTCH1 mutations. J Clin Oncol 32(36):4155–4161. https://doi.org/10.1200/JCO.2014.58.2569

Smith MJ, Wallace AJ, Bowers NL, Eaton H, Evans DG (2014a) SMARCB1 mutations in schwannomatosis and genotype correlations with rhabdoid tumors. Cancer Genet 207(9):373–378. https://doi.org/10.1016/j.cancergen.2014.04.001

Soufir N, Gerard B, Portela M, Brice A, Liboutet M, Saiag P, Descamps V, Kerob D, Wolkenstein P, Gorin I, Lebbe C, Dupin N, Crickx B, Basset-Seguin N, Grandchamp B (2006) PTCH mutations and deletions in patients with typical nevoid basal cell carcinoma syndrome and in patients with a suspected genetic predisposition to basal cell carcinoma: a French study. Br J Cancer 95(4):548–553. https://doi.org/10.1038/sj.bjc.6603303

Spector LG, Pankratz N, Marcotte EL (2015) Genetic and nongenetic risk factors for childhood cancer. Pediatr Clin N Am 62(1):11–25. https://doi.org/10.1016/j.pcl.2014.09.013

Stone DM, Hynes M, Armanini M, Swanson TA, Gu Q, Johnson RL, Scott MP, Pennica D, Goddard A, Phillips H, Noll M, Hooper JE, de Sauvage F, Rosenthal A (1996) The tumour-suppressor gene patched encodes a candidate receptor for sonic hedgehog. Nature 384(6605):129–134. https://doi.org/10.1038/384129a0

Swensen JJ, Keyser J, Coffin CM, Biegel JA, Viskochil DH, Williams MS (2009) Familial occurrence of schwannomas and malignant rhabdoid tumour associated with a duplication in SMARCB1. J Med Genet 46(1):68–72. https://doi.org/10.1136/jmg.2008.060152

Tabori U, Shlien A, Baskin B, Levitt S, Ray P, Alon N, Hawkins C, Bouffet E, Pienkowska M, Lafay-Cousin L, Gozali A, Zhukova N, Shane L, Gonzalez I, Finlay J, Malkin D (2010) TP53 alterations determine clinical subgroups and survival of patients with choroid plexus tumors. J Clin Oncol 28(12):1995–2001. https://doi.org/10.1200/JCO.2009.26.8169

Tang JY, Mackay-Wiggan JM, Aszterbaum M, Yauch RL, Lindgren J, Chang K, Coppola C, Chanana AM, Marji J, Bickers DR, Epstein EH Jr (2012) Inhibiting the hedgehog pathway in patients with the basal-cell nevus syndrome. N Engl J Med 366(23):2180–2188. https://doi.org/10.1056/NEJMoa1113538

Taylor MD, Gokgoz N, Andrulis IL, Mainprize TG, Drake JM, Rutka JT (2000) Familial posterior fossa brain tumors of infancy secondary to germline mutation of the hSNF5 gene. Am J Hum Genet 66(4):1403–1406. https://doi.org/10.1086/302833

Taylor MD, Liu L, Raffel C, Hui CC, Mainprize TG, Zhang X, Agatep R, Chiappa S, Gao L, Lowrance A, Hao A, Goldstein AM, Stavrou T, Scherer SW, Dura WT, Wainwright B, Squire JA, Rutka JT, Hogg D (2002) Mutations in SUFU predispose to medulloblastoma. Nat Genet 31(3):306–310. https://doi.org/10.1038/ng916

Teplick A, Kowalski M, Biegel JA, Nichols KE (2011) Educational paper: screening in cancer predisposition syndromes: guidelines for the general pediatrician. Eur J Pediatr 170(3):285–294. https://doi.org/10.1007/s00431-010-1377-2

Testa JR, Malkin D, Schiffman JD (2013) Connecting molecular pathways to hereditary cancer risk syndromes. Am Soc Clin Oncol Educ Book 33:81–90. https://doi.org/10.1200/EdBook_AM.2013.33.81

Thiagalingam S, Flaherty M, Billson F, North K (2004) Neurofibromatosis type 1 and optic pathway gliomas: follow-up of 54 patients. Ophthalmology 111(3):568–577. https://doi.org/10.1016/j.ophtha.2003.06.008

Tinat J, Bougeard G, Baert-Desurmont S, Vasseur S, Martin C, Bouvignies E, Caron O, Bressac-de Paillerets B, Berthet P, Dugast C, Bonaiti-Pellie C, Stoppa-Lyonnet D, Frebourg T (2009) 2009 version of the Chompret criteria for Li Fraumeni syndrome. J Clin Oncol 27(26):e108–e109.; author reply e110. https://doi.org/10.1200/JCO.2009.22.7967

Toth G, Zraly CB, Thomson TL, Jones C, Lapetino S, Muraskas J, Zhang J, Dingwall AK (2011) Congenital anomalies and rhabdoid tumor associated with 22q11 germline deletion and somatic inactivation of the SMARCB1 tumor suppressor. Genes Chromosomes Cancer 50(6):379–388. https://doi.org/10.1002/gcc.20862

Turcot J, Despres JP, St Pierre F (1959) Malignant tumors of the central nervous system associated with familial polyposis of the colon: report of two cases. Dis Colon Rectum 2:465–468

van den Munckhof P, Christiaans I, Kenter SB, Baas F, Hulsebos TJ (2012) Germline SMARCB1 mutation predisposes to multiple meningiomas and schwannomas with preferential location of cranial meningiomas at the falx cerebri. Neurogenetics 13(1):1–7. https://doi.org/10.1007/s10048-011-0300-y

Vasen HF, Ghorbanoghli Z, Bourdeaut F, Cabaret O, Caron O, Duval A, Entz-Werle N, Goldberg Y, Ilencikova D, Kratz CP, Lavoine N, Loeffen J, Menko FH, Muleris M, Sebille G, Colas C, Burkhardt B, Brugieres L, Wimmer K, CMMR-D EU-CCf (2014) Guidelines for surveillance of individuals with constitutional mismatch repair-deficiency proposed by the European consortium "care for CMMR-D" (C4CMMR-D). J Med Genet 51(5):283–293. https://doi.org/10.1136/jmedgenet-2013-102238

Versteege I, Sevenet N, Lange J, Rousseau-Merck MF, Ambros P, Handgretinger R, Aurias A, Delattre O (1998) Truncating mutations of hSNF5/INI1 in aggressive paediatric cancer. Nature 394(6689):203–206. https://doi.org/10.1038/28212

Villani A, Tabori U, Schiffman J, Shlien A, Beyene J, Druker H, Novokmet A, Finlay J, Malkin D (2011) Biochemical and imaging surveillance in germline TP53 mutation carriers with Li-Fraumeni syndrome: a prospective observational study. Lancet Oncol 12(6):559–567. https://doi.org/10.1016/S1470-2045(11)70119-X

Von Hoff DD, LoRusso PM, Rudin CM, Reddy JC, Yauch RL, Tibes R, Weiss GJ, Borad MJ, Hann CL, Brahmer JR, Mackey HM, Lum BL, Darbonne WC, Marsters JC Jr, de Sauvage FJ, Low JA (2009) Inhibition of the hedgehog pathway in advanced basal-cell carcinoma. N Engl J Med 361(12):1164–1172. https://doi.org/10.1056/NEJMoa0905360

Vortmeyer AO, Stavrou T, Selby D, Li G, Weil RJ, Park WS, Moon YW, Chandra R, Goldstein AM, Zhuang Z (1999) Deletion analysis of the adenomatous polyposis coli and PTCH gene loci in patients with sporadic and nevoid basal cell carcinoma syndrome-associated medulloblastoma. Cancer 85(12):2662–2667

Walter AW, Pivnick EK, Bale AE, Kun LE (1997) Complications of the nevoid basal cell carcinoma syndrome: a case report. J Pediatr Hematol Oncol 19(3):258–262

Wang Q, Lasset C, Desseigne F, Frappaz D, Bergeron C, Navarro C, Ruano E, Puisieux A (1999) Neurofibromatosis and early onset of cancers in hMLH1-deficient children. Cancer Res 59(2):294–297

Wicking C, Shanley S, Smyth I, Gillies S, Negus K, Graham S, Suthers G, Haites N, Edwards M, Wainwright B, Chenevix-Trench G (1997) Most germ-line mutations in the nevoid basal cell carcinoma syndrome lead to a premature termination of the PATCHED protein, and no genotype-phenotype correlations are evident. Am J Hum Genet 60(1):21–26

Wilson BG, Roberts CW (2011) SWI/SNF nucleosome remodellers and cancer. Nat Rev Cancer 11(7):481–492. https://doi.org/10.1038/nrc3068

Wimmer K, Kratz CP, Vasen HF, Caron O, Colas C, Entz-Werle N, Gerdes AM, Goldberg Y, Ilencikova D, Muleris M, Duval A, Lavoine N, Ruiz-Ponte C, Slavc I, Burkhardt B, Brugieres L, CMMRD EU-CCf (2014) Diagnostic criteria for constitutional mismatch repair deficiency syndrome: suggestions of the European consortium 'care for CMMRD' (C4CMMRD). J Med Genet 51(6):355–365. https://doi.org/10.1136/jmedgenet-2014-102284

Witkowski L, Carrot-Zhang J, Albrecht S, Fahiminiya S, Hamel N, Tomiak E, Grynspan D, Saloustros E, Nadaf J, Rivera B, Gilpin C, Castellsague E, Silva-Smith R, Plourde F, Wu M, Saskin A, Arseneault M, Karabakhtsian RG, Reilly EA, Ueland FR, Margiolaki A, Pavlakis K, Castellino SM, Lamovec J, Mackay HJ, Roth LM, Ulbright TM, Bender TA, Georgoulias V, Longy M, Berchuck A, Tischkowitz M, Nagel I, Siebert R, Stewart CJ, Arseneau J, McCluggage WG, Clarke BA, Riazalhosseini Y, Hasselblatt M, Majewski J, Foulkes WD (2014) Germline and somatic SMARCA4 mutations characterize small cell carcinoma of the ovary, hypercalcemic type. Nat Genet 46(5):438–443. https://doi.org/10.1038/ng.2931

Witkowski L, Lalonde E, Zhang J, Albrecht S, Hamel N, Cavallone L, May ST, Nicholson JC, Coleman N, Murray MJ, Tauber PF, Huntsman DG, Schonberger S, Yandell D, Hasselblatt M, Tischkowitz MD, Majewski J, Foulkes WD (2013) Familial rhabdoid tumour 'avant la lettre'--from pathology review to exome sequencing and back again. J Pathol 231(1):35–43. https://doi.org/10.1002/path.4225

Zhukova N, Ramaswamy V, Remke M, Pfaff E, Shih DJ, Martin DC, Castelo-Branco P, Baskin B, Ray PN, Bouffet E, von Bueren AO, Jones DT, Northcott PA, Kool M, Sturm D, Pugh TJ, Pomeroy SL, Cho YJ, Pietsch T, Gessi M, Rutkowski S, Bognar L, Klekner A, Cho BK, Kim SK, Wang KC, Eberhart CG, Fevre-Montange M, Fouladi M, French PJ, Kros M, Grajkowska WA, Gupta N, Weiss WA, Hauser P, Jabado N, Jouvet A, Jung S, Kumabe T, Lach B, Leonard JR, Rubin JB, Liau LM, Massimi L, Pollack IF, Shin Ra Y, Van Meir EG, Zitterbart K, Schuller U, Hill RM, Lindsey JC, Schwalbe EC, Bailey S, Ellison DW, Hawkins C, Malkin D, Clifford SC, Korshunov A, Pfister S, Taylor MD, Tabori U (2013) Subgroup-specific prognostic implications of TP53 mutation in medulloblastoma. J Clin Oncol 31(23):2927–2935. https://doi.org/10.1200/JCO.2012.48.5052

Zilfou JT, Lowe SW (2009) Tumor suppressive functions of p53. Cold Spring Harb Perspect Biol 1(5):a001883. https://doi.org/10.1101/cshperspect.a001883

Modern Principles of CNS Tumor Classification

6

Stefan M. Pfister, David Capper,
and David T. W. Jones

6.1 Introduction

Childhood brain tumors remain a major clinical challenge, and one that is further complicated by the fact that histologically similar or even indistinguishable tumors can show significant molecular heterogeneity—something that is still under intense investigation. Recent advances in genome and epigenome research have revealed extensive clinically useful features of distinct molecular entities, or subgroups thereof, which will help in the classification of these tumors, as well as in treatment stratification and therapeutic target identification.

This chapter aims at summarizing these recent advances in a systematic way, with a basic distinction between glial/glioneuronal and non-glial brain tumors (Fig. 6.1).

6.2 Molecular Classification of Brain Tumors

Among the non-glial brain tumors, embryonal tumors are by far the most common and clinically relevant category in pediatric neuro-oncology. Pineal tumors, craniopharyngioma, choroid plexus tumors, meningiomas, and other representatives (e.g., central nervous system (CNS) lymphomas, germ cell tumors or brain metastases) are less well studied in terms of molecular classification to date, although the field here is starting to develop as well (Holsken et al. 2016; Brastianos et al. 2014; Thomas et al. 2016; Wang et al. 2014; Ichimura et al. 2016).

S. M. Pfister (✉)
Hopp Children's Cancer Center at the NCT Heidelberg (KiTZ), Heidelberg, Germany

Division of Pediatric Neurooncology, German Cancer Consortium (DKTK), German Cancer Research Center (DKFZ), Heidelberg, Germany

Department of Pediatric Oncology, Hematology and Immunology, University Hospital Heidelberg, Heidelberg, Germany
e-mail: s.pfister@dkfz-heidelberg.de

D. Capper
Department of Neuropathology, Berlin Institute of Health, Charité-Universitätsmedizin Berlin, Berlin, Germany

German Cancer Consortium (DKTK), Partner Site Berlin, German Cancer Research Center (DKFZ), Heidelberg, Germany

D. T. W. Jones
Hopp Children's Cancer Center at the NCT Heidelberg (KiTZ), Heidelberg, Germany

Division of Pediatric Neurooncology, German Cancer Consortium (DKTK), German Cancer Research Center (DKFZ), Heidelberg, Germany

© Springer International Publishing AG, part of Springer Nature 2018
A. Gajjar et al. (eds.), *Brain Tumors in Children*, https://doi.org/10.1007/978-3-319-43205-2_6

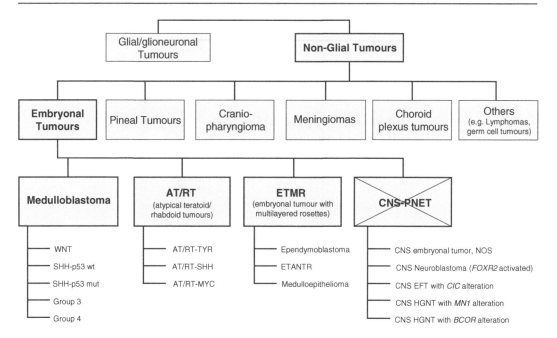

Fig. 6.1 Molecular classification of embryonal brain tumors. The term "CNS-PNET" was discarded in the update of the fourth edition of the WHO classification based on the fact that it was previously used for a weakly defined mixture of not otherwise specified embryonal tumors

6.3   Medulloblastoma

The first histopathological brain tumor entity for which consistent molecular subgroups were identified was medulloblastoma. Based on several independent studies (Cho et al. 2011; Milde et al. 2010; Kool et al. 2008; Northcott et al. 2011; Thompson et al. 2006; Remke et al. 2011), a consensus was reached that this heterogeneous entity consists of four distinct molecular subgroups designated Wnt/Wingless (WNT), Sonic Hedgehog (SHH), Group 3 and Group 4 (Taylor et al. 2012, Fig. 6.2). These subgroups have also been recognized in the update of the fourth edition of the World Health Organization (WHO) classification for CNS tumors (published in 2016) in accordance with the previously published guidelines for multilayered diagnoses (Louis et al. 2014). Additionally, SHH medulloblastomas were split into two distinct subentities based on TP53 status (SHH-TP53 wild type and SHH-TP53 mutant). Several methods have been proposed to identify these groups, including sets of immunohistochemistry-based tests (Ellison et al. 2011a), transcriptome analysis (either genome-wide or using a subset of lineage genes), and array-based DNA methylation analysis. The latter turned out to be the most robust method to date, and can also reliably be performed from very small amounts of formalin-fixed, paraffin-embedded (FFPE) tissue (Hovestadt et al. 2013; Schwalbe et al. 2013).

WNT medulloblastomas typically harbor a somatic activating *CTNNB1* mutation in exon 3, which is never found in other medulloblastoma subgroups, and are often associated with a loss of one copy of chromosome 6 (Clifford et al. 2006). Frequent somatic *TP53* mutations do not seem to confer an inferior prognosis within this molecular subgroup (Zhukova et al. 2013). They typically show classic medulloblastoma morphology.

SHH medulloblastomas show a bimodal age distribution with peak incidence rates in infancy and adulthood. The vast majority of SHH medulloblastomas harbor germline or somatic altera-

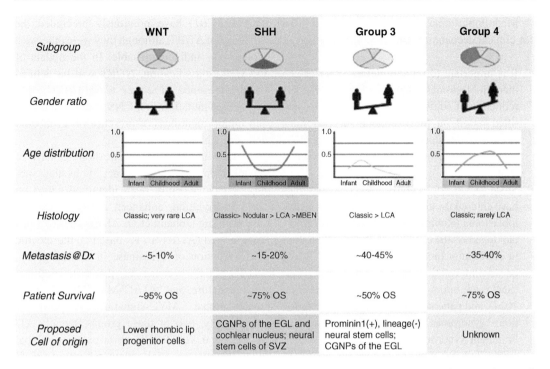

Fig. 6.2 Molecular classification of medulloblastoma. The histopathological spectrum of medulloblastoma comprises a very heterogeneous collection of four core molecular entities, which display extensive heterogeneity in terms of demographics, frequency of metastatic spread, survival, cell of origin, and accompanying genetic events. Source: Nat Rev Cancer. 2012 Dec;12(12):818–34. doi: https://doi.org/10.1038/nrc3410

tions in SHH pathway genes, including *PTCH1, SMO, SUFU, MYCN, GLI2,* and *SHH* itself (Kool et al. 2014). In children between 5 and 16 years of age (in whom SHH medulloblastomas generally occur less commonly), these tumors are often associated with anaplastic histology, germline *TP53* mutations and extensive chromosome shattering (chromothripsis) in the tumor, as well as with inferior prognosis (Zhukova et al. 2013; Kool et al. 2014; Rausch et al. 2012). The histological spectrum of SHH medulloblastomas includes desmoplastic tumors and medulloblastoma with extensive nodularity (these two histological variants comprising almost exclusively SHH tumors), as well as classic and anaplastic medulloblastoma.

Group 3 medulloblastomas represent the most aggressive subgroup in clinical trial series, with the highest incidence of metastatic dissemination and worst prognosis (Pietsch et al. 2014). In addition to *MYC* amplification, which has been recognized as a molecular driver for decades (Scheurlen et al. 1998), more recent discoveries included the presence of *MYC-PVT1* fusion genes (Northcott et al. 2012a) in a relevant subset of MYC-driven Group 3 tumors, and the activation of the *GFI1/GFI1B* oncogenes by enhancer hijacking (Northcott et al. 2014). Moreover, genome duplication was identified as a frequent early event in this group (Jones et al. 2012). Group 3 medulloblastomas most commonly show classic, anaplastic, or large cell morphology.

Group 4 is less well characterized in terms of single genetic drivers, but is very frequently associated with the formation of an isochromosome 17q. *GFI1/GFI1B* activation and genome duplication are also observed in subsets of Group 4 tumors, and *KDM6A* appears to be the single most commonly mutated gene (Jones et al. 2012; Robinson et al. 2012; Pugh et al. 2012; Northcott et al. 2012b).

Medulloblastoma subgrouping is already used for clinical decision-making in multiple ways:

- It is important to reliably detect WNT-driven medulloblastomas; the question of whether reduction of adjuvant therapy intensity is justified based on the excellent survival rates achieved with standard treatment protocols is currently being explored in large clinical trials.
- Since novel molecularly targeted therapies have entered the clinical stage for SHH medulloblastoma (Robinson et al. 2015), it is important to assess the exact SHH pathway mutation in each tumor (and matched germline). Based on this information, response to Smoothened (SMO) inhibitors can be predicted (Kool et al. 2014), and patients with hereditary predisposition syndromes (Gorlin Syndrome, Li Fraumeni Syndrome) and their families can be counselled and stratified to separate treatment protocols (e.g., omission of radiotherapy).
- MYC-amplified Group 3 tumors are considered very-high risk, and clinical trials stratifying these patients to novel treatment approaches (e.g., upfront phase II window) are currently under consideration.

6.4 Atypical Teratoid Rhabdoid Tumors

It has long been known that the hallmark molecular feature of atypical teratoid/rhabdoid tumor (AT/RT) is somatic or germline inactivation of members of the SWI/SNF chromatin remodeling complex. *SMARCB1* is altered in about 95% of cases (Versteege et al. 1998; Biegel et al. 1999), and is also frequently mutated in the germline, especially in young children (Sredni and Tomita 2015). In the remaining 5% of cases, a mutation in *SMARCA4* can typically be detected (Schneppenheim et al. 2010; Hasselblatt et al. 2014). Biallelic disruption of either of these two genes in the tumor results in complete loss of protein expression, which can be detected by loss of nuclear staining using immunohistochemistry. Tumors that lack the typical histological rhabdoid features, but show loss of INI1 (the gene product

of *SMARCB1*) have previously precluded the diagnosis of AT/RT, although they were otherwise biologically indistinguishable. In the update of the WHO classification, AT/RT will be defined by the presence of either a *SMARCB1* or a *SMARCA4* mutation in a CNS small round blue cell tumor, regardless of presence of a rhabdoid cell component.

Despite the relative genetic homogeneity of AT/RTs, three highly distinct molecular subgroups have recently been identified based on DNA methylation, enhancer, and gene expression profiling (Johann et al. 2016). These groups were termed "AT/RT-TYR" based on the specific overexpression of Tyrosinase in this subgroup, "AT/RT-SHH" because of the transcriptional SHH signature, and "AT/RT-MYC" based on the transcriptional MYC-signature, respectively. Interestingly, two of these groups, namely AT/RT-TYR and AT/RT-SHH, show extensive global hypermethylation—only comparable to the CpG Island Methylator Phenotype (CIMP) observed in IDH-mutated glioma. This phenotype might comprise a rationale for epigenetic treatment approaches. Also noteworthy is that the type of *SMARCB1* mutation is strikingly different between the subgroups: AT/RT-TYR typically harbor large deletions of chromosome 22q accompanied by mutation of the second allele, AT/RT-SHH are characterized by biallelic point mutations in *SMARCB1*, and AT/RT-MYC often show focal homozygous deletions (Fig. 6.3). The clinical and therapeutic impact of these molecular subgroups is yet to be assessed.

6.5 Embryonal Tumors with Multilayered Rosettes

Embryonal tumors with (true) multilayered rosettes (ETMR) have been recognized in previous versions of the WHO classification of CNS tumors as ependymoblastoma, embryonal tumor with abundant neuropil and true rosettes (ETANTR), and medulloepithelioma (Louis et al. 2007). With the discovery of the specific high-level amplification of a micro-RNA cluster on chromosome 19q13.41 (C19MC) (Li et al. 2009; Korshunov et al. 2010), which is detectable in

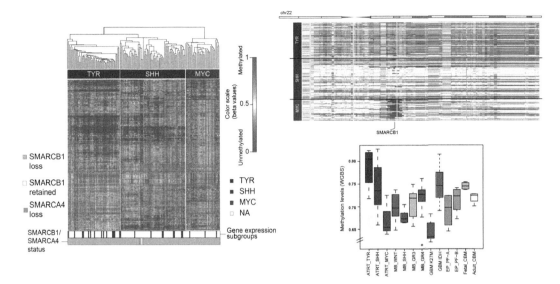

Fig. 6.3 Molecular classification of AT/RT. Molecular subgroups can be readily identified by DNA methylation analysis, enhancer profiling, or gene-expression profiling. The subgroups show distinctively different patterns of *SMARCB1* mutation. AT/RT-TYR and AT/RT-SHH are characterized by extensive global hypermethylation of the tumor genome. Source: Cancer Cell. 2016 Mar 14;29(3):379–93. doi: https://doi.org/10.1016/j.ccell.2016.02.001. Epub 2016 Feb 25

about 95% of cases in all of the aforementioned histopathological variants (Korshunov et al. 2014), ETMR have now become a single molecularly defined entity. This amplicon also gives rise to a fusion between *TTYH1* and C19MC, with the promoter of the former driving expression of the micro-RNAs (Kleinman et al. 2014). If the amplicon is not detectable in a tumor within the morphological spectrum of ETMR or the testing is not available, it is termed embryonal tumor with multilayered rosettes, NOS. As another unifying feature, the vast majority of ETMRs show significant expression of LIN28A, which is typically not observed in other brain tumors (apart from some cases of AT/RT with weaker, patchy expression) (Korshunov et al. 2012).

6.6   Other Primitive Neuroectodermal Tumors of the CNS

Originally, embryonal tumors of the CNS were all called "primitive neuroectodermal tumors" (PNETs) (Rorke 1983). After the distinction of medulloblastoma and then AT/RT as separate entities, the term PNET still remained and was used as a term for embryonal CNS tumors (typically supratentorially located) that would not fall into any of the other categories. The diagnostic gray zone, e.g., between "PNET," anaplastic ependymoma, and small cell glioblastoma (among others), has long been recognized. In the latest update of the WHO classification, the term "CNS-PNET" has disappeared, and provisionally been replaced by "CNS embryonal tumor, NOS."

Based on very recent molecular studies, institutionally diagnosed "CNS PNETs" can, in the majority of cases, be molecularly re-classified into a known brain tumor entity. However, at least four previously unrecognized molecular entities remain, all of which are characterized by a highly specific genetic event in the respective subgroup (Fig. 6.4) (Sturm et al. 2016). These novel molecular entities include: (1) CNS neuroblastoma with frequent FOXR2 activation, which show the most prototypic neuroblastic morphology and would probably be diagnosed as "PNET" by a vast majority of pathologists; (2) CNS Ewing family tumors with recurrent CIC fusions, which probably represent a CNS counterpart of Ewing-like sarcomas (also showing CIC fusions); (3) CNS high-grade neuroepithelial tumors with MN1 alteration, which often, but not always, show morphological features

Fig. 6.4 Molecular classification of CNS-PNET. In an unbiased international cohort of cases diagnosed as CNS-PNET institutionally, about 75–80% of cases fall into well-defined molecular categories using DNA methylation analysis. The remaining four groups highly enriched for "CNS-PNETs" likely comprise four previously unrecognized disease entities, each characterized by a highly specific genetic event occurring in the majority of cases. Source: Sturm et al. Cell. 2016 Feb 25;164(5):1060–72. doi: https://doi.org/10.1016/j.cell.2016.01.015

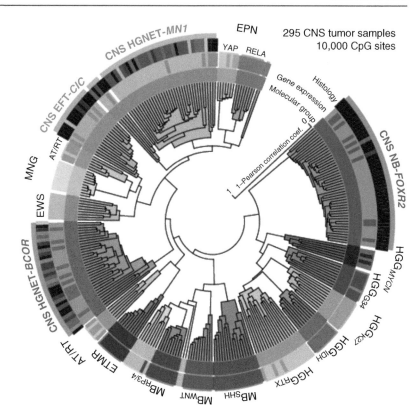

of astroblastoma, and (4) CNS high-grade neuroepithelial tumors with BCOR alteration. The clinical features of these novel entities, their response to adjuvant therapy, their prognosis, and additional genetic hits have yet to be assessed. Based on their unique molecular makeup, however, it is expected that these (and maybe additional) molecularly defined entities will be recognized in the 5th full edition of the WHO classification for CNS tumors.

6.7 Molecular Classification of Pediatric Gliomas and Glioneuronal Tumors

6.7.1 Low-Grade Glioma and Glioneuronal Tumors

Low-grade glioma (LGG) and low-grade glioneuronal tumors (LGNT) together comprise the most common brain tumor group in children (Fig. 6.5). Recent molecular insights into their tumor biology have, however, revealed striking differences in

terms of the underlying driver events in different histopathological or molecular subgroups. Thus, in the very near future, summarizing everything into these two broad categories will no longer be appropriate. A characteristic unifying feature of these low-grade, slow-growing, typically non-metastasizing entities is that they are assumed to very often be driven by a single oncogenic insult, e.g., BRAF duplication in pilocytic astrocytoma (Jones et al. 2008; Pfister et al. 2008), FGFR mutation, kinase duplication or fusion in dysembryonic neuroepithelial tumors (DNET) (Rivera et al. 2016; Qaddoumi et al. 2016), or MYB/MYBL1 aberrations in angiocentric and diffuse glioma (Qaddoumi et al. 2016; Tatevossian et al. 2010; Ramkissoon et al. 2013; Bandopadhayay et al. 2016).

For pilocytic astrocytoma (PA), it was convincingly shown in different studies that almost all tumors harbor mutually exclusive mutations in the MAPK pathway leading to constitutive activation (Fig. 6.6a) (Jones et al. 2013; Zhang et al. 2013). Of note, PA is molecularly indistinguishable from pilomyxoid astrocytoma, so that in the update of the

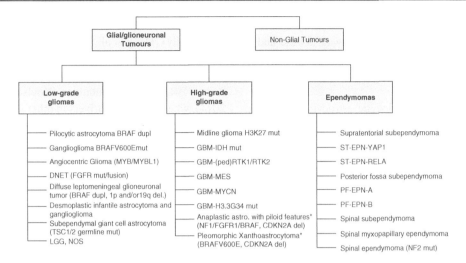

Fig. 6.5 Molecular classification of pediatric gliomas/glioneuronal tumors. Entities marked with an asterisk are considered intermediate prognosis. Molecular categories are provisional based on the authors' experience, and are subject to change in future

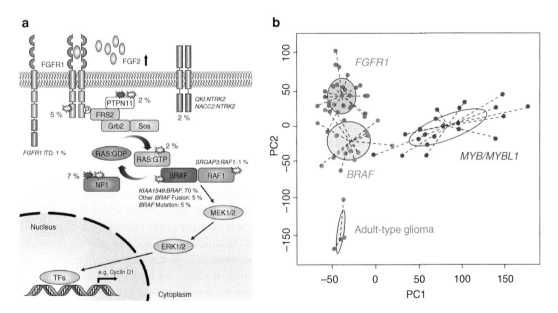

Fig. 6.6 Molecular features of low-grade glioma/glioneuronal tumors in children. (**a**) Mutually exclusive aberrations in the MAPK pathway characterize pilocytic astrocytoma, the most common pediatric brain tumor. (**b**) Prototypic genetic changes in DNET (red), ganglioglioma (green), and angiocentric glioma (blue), with grouping based on DNA methylation data. Source: Nat Genet. 2013 Aug;45(8):927–32. doi: https://doi.org/10.1038/ng.2682. Epub 2013 Jun 30. and Qaddoumi et al. Acta Neuropathol. 2016 Jan 25. [Epub ahead of print]

WHO classification this was defined a histological variant of PA rather than a separate entity. The most common single aberration in pilocytic astrocytoma, occurring in about 70% of cases, is a truncating fusion of *BRAF* (*KIAA1549-BRAF* gene fusion). A highly relevant fraction of PAs, particularly those arising in the optic nerve, chiasms, and optic tract, is driven by underlying germline mutations in NF1 (a negative regulator of RAS genes in the MAPK pathway). Conversely, patients with neurofibromatosis type 1 have an approximate risk of 10% of developing an optic pathway glioma before age 15.

Collectively, these findings make pilocytic astrocytoma a prototypic single pathway disease and an excellent candidate entity for the therapeutic use of molecularly targeted therapies, such as inhibitors of MEK1/2.

In contrast to pilocytic astrocytoma, gangliogliomas are much more commonly defined by point mutations in BRAF (V600E) instead of truncating fusions (Schindler et al. 2011). This again comprises a very attractive drug target for future clinical trials with a variety of drugs available to directly target this aberration.

Overexpression and complex rearrangements involving *MYB* or *MYBL1*, often in conjunction with *QKI*, have been identified in subsets of LGGs for some years already (Tatevossian et al. 2010). When more recently larger cohorts were examined and correlated with morphology, it became apparent that tumors with the histopathological picture of an angiocentric glioma regularly show aberrations in MYB family genes—indicating that these aberrations might indeed define this entity (Qaddoumi et al. 2016; Ramkissoon et al. 2013). Finally, the mechanism of the tumorigenic potential of MYB-QKI rearrangements was recently elucidated (Bandopadhayay et al. 2016).

A recent paper investigating a large number of dysembryoplastic neuroepithelial tumors (DNETs) (Rivera et al. 2016) confirmed data from smaller series (Qaddoumi et al. 2016) that different genetic aberrations in *FGFR1* are of central importance for these tumors. In the majority of cases, hotspot mutations (N546K or K656E) were identified, whereas internal duplications occurred in a smaller subset of cases. Additionally, germline *FGFR1* mutations appear to predispose to familial cases of DNET. As with BRAF, FGFR1 comprises a very attractive drug target with several highly potent inhibitors on the market or in development.

Diffuse leptomeningeal glioneuronal tumors (Gardiman et al. 2010), also referred to as disseminated oligodendroglial-like leptomeningeal tumor of childhood (DOLN) (Rodriguez et al. 2012), were recently shown to be characterized by concurrent *KIAA1549-BRAF* gene fusion and 1p deletion (sometimes also 1p/19q co-deletion as observed in adult type oligodendroglioma, but

without the ubiquitous *IDH1* mutation in the latter entity) (Deng et al. 2018).

Subsets of rare, but pediatric-specific, desmoplastic infantile astrocytomas/gangliogliomas harbor BRAFV600E mutations (Koelsche et al. 2014), whereas genetic drivers in other subsets of this entity remain to be determined.

Subependymal giant-cell astrocytoma comprises another prototypic single-hit disease, which occurs in patients with tuberous sclerosis, who harbor germline mutations in *TSC1* or *TSC2*. As expected based on their biology, these tumors show an excellent response to targeted inhibition of mTOR (Franz et al. 2013).

In summary, several of these molecular entities will, in case of non-resectability, in the future most likely be subjected to molecularly targeted therapies rather than conventional radio- or chemotherapy. Therefore, assessment of prototypic genetic events for molecular stratification of these tumors should be considered standard-of-care diagnostics from now on.

6.7.2 High-Grade Glioma

High-grade gliomas in children by definition comprise gliomas of WHO grades III and IV. With advanced molecular classification, this paradigm is partially challenged, since entities like pleomorphic xanthoastrocytoma, which can be grade III when showing signs of anaplasia or grade II when these features are missing, show a homogeneous molecular picture across different grades; therefore, it might not be justified that a fraction of them is currently treated as "LGG" and another, yet molecularly identical fraction, is treated as "HGG." Thus, two "intermediate risk" entities, namely pleomorphic xanthoastrocytoma and anaplastic astrocytoma with piloid features (Reinhardt et al. 2018), are listed with an asterisk in Fig. 6.5.

In children, an additional caveat with seemingly high-grade gliomas according to the histopathological pattern is that a proportion of these tumors that look like HGGs show features of true low-grade gliomas at a molecular level and share the excellent prognosis of LGGs (Korshunov et al. 2015). When accounting for these, the "intermediate risk" tumors, and the small number of IDH1-mutant pediatric glioblastomas, the survival of the remaining "true glioblastomas" is as bad as for adult glioblastoma.

Recent genomic discoveries in pediatric HGGs have revealed highly specific mutations in two residues of the H3.3 and H3.1 histone genes (Schwartzentruber et al. 2012), with mutations at K27 occurring both in H3.3 and H3.1, specifically in midline HGGs (Schwartzentruber et al. 2012; Buczkowicz et al. 2014; Taylor et al. 2014; Wu et al. 2014; Fontebasso et al. 2014), and G34 in H3.3 in hemispheric HGGs in slightly older patients (Schwartzentruber et al. 2012). The mutation in K27, which is replaced by a methionine, mimics monomethylation of K27, in turn leading to entrapping of EZH2 (the enzyme catalyzing the methylation of K27) (Bender et al. 2013; Lewis et al. 2013). This dominant functional inactivation of EZH2 is associated with genome-wide loss of H3K27 trimethylation, which can be detected as a surrogate marker for the K27M mutation (Venneti et al. 2013). The specificity of K27M mutations to pediatric HGGs of the midline and the striking epigenetic phenotype led to the recognition of this as a separate molecular entity in the update of the WHO classification, designated diffuse midline glioma with H3K27 mutation. This also includes diffuse intrinsic pontine gliomas (DIPGs), often associated with mutations in *ACVR1* and amplification of *PDGFRA*, but also tumors in the thalamus (where H3 K27M mutations are typically associated with *TP53* mutations), and throughout the spinal cord.

As previously mentioned, H3.3 G34 mutations occur almost exclusively in hemispheric tumors, and in slightly older patients, almost always in conjunction with mutations in *TP53* and *ATRX*. Interestingly, it was also shown that tumors occur that show a "PNET-like" morphology harboring a G34 mutation. However, these tumors are molecularly indistinguishable from G34-mutant tumors demonstrating a typical HGG morphology, indicating that these likely belong to a single entity with a wide spectrum of morphological phenotypes (Korshunov et al. 2016).

Additional molecular subgroups of HGGs in children as assessed by DNA methylation analysis include the RTK1 group with frequent amplification of *PDGFRA*, the RTK2 subgroup, and a small subgroup characterized by co-amplification of *MYCN* and *ID2*, which was first described in Buczkowicz et al. (2014) and now confirmed in independent larger cohorts (Korshunov et al. 2017; Sturm et al. 2016) (Fig. 6.7).

IDH1-mutated HGGs are exceedingly rare in younger children, but start to occur with a somewhat higher incidence in adolescence, with an age-peak in young adults.

6.7.3 Ependymoma

For ependymoma, one of the major challenges in classification is the poor reproducibility of grading, which was until very recently used for risk stratification (Ellison et al. 2011b). Thus, a more reliable classification system is urgently needed (Fig. 6.8).

The existence of two distinct subgroups of posterior fossa ependymomas (PF-A and PF-B) has long been established (Witt et al. 2011; Mack et al. 2014; Wani et al. 2012). However, it is noteworthy that a genetic driver for the clinically highly aggressive PF-A tumors has yet to be identified. The fact these two highly distinct groups can only be reliably separated by array-based DNA methylation or gene expression analysis has hindered their introduction into the update of the WHO classification.

In the supratentorial region, a highly prevalent fusion gene was identified, namely fusions of *RELA*, a downstream NFκB effector, with *C11orf95* (Parker et al. 2014). Interestingly, these fusions, which might comprise a meaningful drug target but certainly an important diagnostic aid, exclusively occur in one molecular subgroup of supratentorial ependymoma, designated ST-EPN-RELA.

In a large and comprehensive international analysis of 500 primary ependymoma samples from all anatomic locations and across all grades, an additional subgroup of supratentorial ependymomas with a specific recurrent fusion gene was identified, namely fusions of *YAP1* with different partners (Pajtler et al. 2015). Additionally, a distinct molecular group of subependymomas was identified in all three com-

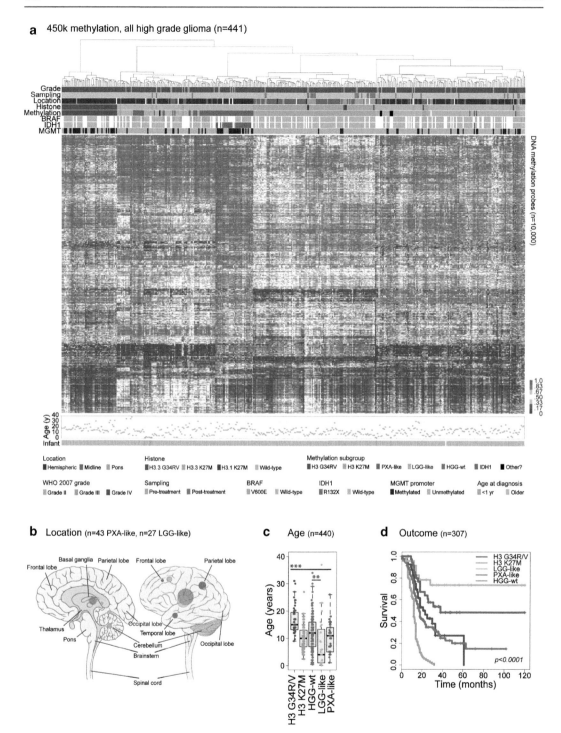

Fig. 6.7 Heatmap representation of DNA methylation-based subgroups of pediatric HGG. Clear groups can be seen for Histone 3 K27 and G34-mutant tumors and IDH-mutant tumors, while H3/IDH wildtype tumors are more heterogeneous, and display evidence for possible PXA-like or low-grade-like tumors amongst the 'true' molecular HGGs

Fig. 6.8 Molecular classification of ependymoma. Using DNA methylation profiling, ependymomas of all grades and anatomic locations can be segregated into nine biologically and clinically meaningful subgroups. Source: Cancer Cell. 2015 May 11;27(5):728–43. doi: https://doi.org/10.1016/j.ccell.2015.04.002

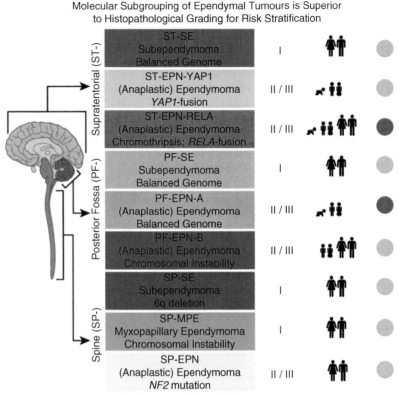

Molecular Subgrouping of Ependymal Tumours is Superior to Histopathological Grading for Risk Stratification

WHO grade Age Group Outcome

partments (including the spine), as well as molecular subgroups highly enriched for tumors that were diagnosed as myxopapillary ependymomas or classic ependymomas of the spine (frequently occurring in patients with neurofibromatosis type 2).

In conclusion, the advent of next-generation molecular tools has revolutionized the classification of childhood brain tumors, and appreciation of the immediate clinical benefits of the integration of molecular data into the diagnostic process has only started. The power of cutting-edge molecular profiling tools to ever more precisely characterize biological tumor subsets holds enormous potential for the future.

References

Bandopadhayay P et al (2016) MYB-QKI rearrangements in angiocentric glioma drive tumorigenicity through a tripartite mechanism. Nat Genet 48(3):273–282

Bender S et al (2013) Reduced H3K27me3 and DNA hypomethylation are major drivers of gene expression in K27M mutant pediatric high-grade gliomas. Cancer Cell 24(5):660–672

Biegel JA et al (1999) Germ-line and acquired mutations of INI1 in atypical teratoid and rhabdoid tumors. Cancer Res 59(1):74–79

Brastianos PK et al (2014) Exome sequencing identifies BRAF mutations in papillary craniopharyngiomas. Nat Genet 46(2):161–165

Buczkowicz P et al (2014) Genomic analysis of diffuse intrinsic pontine gliomas identifies three molecular subgroups and recurrent activating ACVR1 mutations. Nat Genet 46(5):451–456

Cho Y-J et al (2011) Integrative genomic analysis of medulloblastoma identifies a molecular subgroup that drives poor clinical outcome. J Clin Oncol 29(11):1424–1430

Clifford S et al (2006) Wnt/wingless pathway activation and chromosome 6 loss characterize a distinct molecular sub-group of medulloblastomas associated with a favorable prognosis. Cell Cycle 5(22):2666–2670

Deng MY et al (2018) Molecularly defined diffuse leptomeningeal glioneuronal tumor (DLGNT) comprises two subgroups with distinct clinical and genetic features. Acta Neuropathol. https://doi.org/10.1007/s00401-018-1865-4 [Epub ahead of print]

Ellison DW et al (2011a) Medulloblastoma: clinicopathological correlates of SHH, WNT, and non-SHH/WNT molecular subgroups. Acta Neuropathol 121(3):381–396

Ellison DW et al (2011b) Histopathological grading of pediatric ependymoma: reproducibility and clinical relevance in European trial cohorts. J Negat Results Biomed 10:7–7

Fontebasso AM et al (2014) Recurrent somatic mutations in ACVR1 in pediatric midline high-grade astrocytoma. Nat Genet 46(5):462–466

Franz DN et al (2013) Efficacy and safety of everolimus for subependymal giant cell astrocytomas associated with tuberous sclerosis complex (EXIST-1): a multicentre, randomised, placebo-controlled phase 3 trial. Lancet 381(9861):125–132

Gardiman MP et al (2010) Diffuse leptomeningeal glioneuronal tumors: a new entity? Brain Pathol 20(2):361–366

Hasselblatt M et al (2014) SMARCA4-mutated atypical teratoid/rhabdoid tumors are associated with inherited germline alterations and poor prognosis. Acta Neuropathol 128(3):453–456

Holsken A et al (2016) Adamantinomatous and papillary craniopharyngiomas are characterized by distinct epigenomic as well as mutational and transcriptomic profiles. Acta Neuropathol Commun 4(1):20

Hovestadt V et al (2013) Robust molecular subgrouping and copy-number profiling of medulloblastoma from small amounts of archival tumour material using high-density DNA methylation arrays. Acta Neuropathol 125(6):913–916

Ichimura K et al (2016) Recurrent neomorphic mutations of MTOR in central nervous system and testicular germ cell tumors may be targeted for therapy. Acta Neuropathol:1–13

Johann PD et al (2016) Atypical teratoid/rhabdoid tumors are comprised of three epigenetic subgroups with distinct enhancer landscapes. Cancer Cell 29(3):379–393

Jones DTW et al (2008) Tandem duplication producing a novel oncogenic BRAF fusion gene defines the majority of pilocytic astrocytomas. Cancer Res 68(21):8673–8677

Jones DT et al (2012) Dissecting the genomic complexity underlying medulloblastoma. Nature 488(7409):100–105

Jones DT et al (2013) Recurrent somatic alterations of FGFR1 and NTRK2 in pilocytic astrocytoma. Nat Genet 45(8):927–932

Kleinman CL et al (2014) Fusion of TTYH1 with the C19MC microRNA cluster drives expression of a brain-specific DNMT3B isoform in the embryonal brain tumor ETMR. Nat Genet 46(1):39–44

Koelsche C et al (2014) BRAF V600E expression and distribution in desmoplastic infantile astrocytoma/ganglioglioma. Neuropathol Appl Neurobiol 40(3):337–344

Kool M et al (2008) Integrated genomics identifies five medulloblastoma subtypes with distinct genetic profiles, pathway signatures and clinicopathological features. PLoS One 3(8):e3088

Kool M et al (2014) Genome sequencing of SHH medulloblastoma predicts genotype-related response to smoothened inhibition. Cancer Cell 25(3):393–405

Korshunov A et al (2010) Focal genomic amplification at 19q13.42 comprises a powerful diagnostic marker for embryonal tumors with ependymoblastic rosettes. Acta Neuropathol 120(2):253–260

Korshunov A et al (2012) LIN28A immunoreactivity is a potent diagnostic marker of embryonal tumor with multilayered rosettes (ETMR). Acta Neuropathol 124(6):875–881

Korshunov A et al (2014) Embryonal tumor with abundant neuropil and true rosettes (ETANTR), ependymoblastoma, and medulloepithelioma share molecular similarity and comprise a single clinicopathological entity. Acta Neuropathol 128(2):279–289

Korshunov A et al (2015) Integrated analysis of pediatric glioblastoma reveals a subset of biologically favorable tumors with associated molecular prognostic markers. Acta Neuropathol 129(5):669–678

Korshunov A et al (2016) Histologically distinct neuroepithelial tumors with histone 3 G34 mutation are molecularly similar and comprise a single nosologic entity. Acta Neuropathol 131(1):137–146

Korshunov A et al (2017) H3-/IDH-wild type pediatric glioblastoma is comprised of molecularly and prognostically distinct subtypes with associated oncogenic drivers. Acta Neuropathol. 134(3):507–516. https://doi.org/10.1007/s00401-017-1710-1 [Epub 2017 Apr 11]

Lewis PW et al (2013) Inhibition of PRC2 activity by a gain-of-function H3 mutation found in pediatric glioblastoma. Science 340(6134):857–861

Li M et al (2009) Frequent amplification of a chr19q13.41 microRNA polycistron (C19MC) in aggressive primitive neuro-ectodermal brain tumors. Cancer Cell 16(6):533–546

Louis DN et al (2007) The 2007 WHO classification of tumours of the central nervous system. Acta Neuropathol 114(2):97–109

Louis DN et al (2014) International Society of Neuropathology-Haarlem Consensus Guidelines for nervous system tumor classification and grading. Brain Pathol 24(5):429–435

Mack SC et al (2014) Epigenomic alterations define lethal CIMP-positive ependymomas of infancy. Nature 506(7489):445–450

Milde T et al (2010) HDAC5 and HDAC9 in medulloblastoma: novel markers for risk stratification and role in tumor cell growth. Clin Cancer Res 16(12):3240–3252

Northcott PA et al (2011) Medulloblastoma comprises four distinct molecular variants. J Clin Oncol 29(11):1408–1414. https://doi.org/10.1200/JCO.2009.27.4324 [Epub 2010 Sep 7]

Northcott PA et al (2012a) Subgroup specific structural variation across 1,000 medulloblastoma genomes. Nature 488(7409):49–56

Northcott PA et al (2012b) Medulloblastomics: the end of the beginning. Nat Rev Cancer 12(12):818–834

Northcott PA et al (2014) Enhancer hijacking activates GFI1 family oncogenes in medulloblastoma. Nature 511(7510):428–434

Pajtler KW et al (2015) Molecular classification of ependymal tumors across all CNS compartments, histopathological grades, and age groups. Cancer Cell 27(5):728–743

Parker M et al (2014) C11orf95-RELA fusions drive oncogenic NF-κB signaling in ependymoma. Nature 506(7489):451–455

Pfister S et al (2008) BRAF gene duplication constitutes a mechanism of MAPK pathway activation in low-grade astrocytomas. J Clin Invest 118(5):1739–1749

Pietsch T et al (2014) Prognostic significance of clinical, histopathological, and molecular characteristics of medulloblastomas in the prospective HIT2000 multicenter clinical trial cohort. Acta Neuropathol 128(1):137–149

Pugh TJ et al (2012) Medulloblastoma exome sequencing uncovers subtype-specific somatic mutations. Nature 488(7409):106–110

Qaddoumi I et al (2016) Genetic alterations in uncommon low-grade neuroepithelial tumors: BRAF, FGFR1, and MYB mutations occur at high frequency and align with morphology. Acta Neuropathol:1–13

Ramkissoon LA et al (2013) Genomic analysis of diffuse pediatric low-grade gliomas identifies recurrent oncogenic truncating rearrangements in the transcription factor MYBL1. Proc Natl Acad Sci U S A 110(20):8188–8193

Rausch T et al (2012) Genome sequencing of pediatric medulloblastoma links catastrophic DNA rearrangements with TP53 mutations. Cell 148(1–2):59–71

Reinhardt A et al (2018) Anaplastic astrocytoma with piloid features, a novel molecular class of IDH wildtype glioma with recurrent MAPK pathway, CDKN2A/B and ATRX alterations. Acta Neuropathol. https://doi.org/10.1007/s00401-018-1837-8 [Epub ahead of print]

Remke M et al (2011) FSTL5 is a marker of poor prognosis in non-WNT/non-SHH medulloblastoma. J Clin Oncol 29(29):3852–3861

Rivera B et al (2016) Germline and somatic FGFR1 abnormalities in dysembryoplastic neuroepithelial tumors. Acta Neuropathol:1–17

Robinson G et al (2012) Novel mutations target distinct subgroups of medulloblastoma. Nature 488(7409):43–48

Robinson GW et al (2015) Vismodegib exerts targeted efficacy against recurrent sonic hedgehog–subgroup Medulloblastoma: results from phase II pediatric brain tumor consortium studies PBTC-025B and PBTC-032. J Clin Oncol 33(24):2646–2654

Rodriguez FJ et al (2012) Disseminated oligodendroglial-like leptomeningeal tumor of childhood: a distinctive clinicopathologic entity. Acta Neuropathol 124(5):627–641

Rorke L (1983) The cerebellar medulloblastoma and its relationship to primitive neuroectodermal tumors. J Neuropathol Exp Neurol 42(1):1–15

Scheurlen WG et al (1998) Molecular analysis of childhood primitive neuroectodermal tumors defines markers associated with poor outcome. J Clin Oncol 16(7):2478–2485

Schindler G et al (2011) Analysis of BRAF V600E mutation in 1,320 nervous system tumors reveals high mutation frequencies in pleomorphic xanthoastrocytoma, ganglioglioma and extra-cerebellar pilocytic astrocytoma. Acta Neuropathol 121(3):397–405

Schneppenheim R et al (2010) Germline nonsense mutation and somatic inactivation of SMARCA4/BRG1 in a family with rhabdoid tumor predisposition syndrome. Am J Hum Genet 86(2):279–284

Schwalbe EC et al (2013) DNA methylation profiling of medulloblastoma allows robust subclassification and improved outcome prediction using formalin-fixed biopsies. Acta Neuropathol 125(3):359–371

Schwartzentruber J et al (2012) Driver mutations in histone H3.3 and chromatin remodelling genes in paediatric glioblastoma. Nature 482(7384):226–231

Sredni ST, Tomita T (2015) Rhabdoid tumor predisposition syndrome. Pediatr Dev Pathol 18(1):49–58

Sturm D et al (2016) New brain tumor entities emerge from molecular classification of CNS-PNETs. Cell 164(5):1060–1072

Tatevossian RG et al (2010) MYB upregulation and genetic aberrations in a subset of pediatric low-grade gliomas. Acta Neuropathol 120(6):731–743

Taylor MD et al (2012) Molecular subgroups of medulloblastoma: the current consensus. Acta Neuropathol 123(4):465–472

Taylor KR et al (2014) Recurrent activating ACVR1 mutations in diffuse intrinsic pontine glioma. Nat Genet 46(5):457–461

Thomas C et al (2016) Methylation profiling of choroid plexus tumors reveals 3 clinically distinct subgroups. Neuro-Oncology 18:790

Thompson MC et al (2006) Genomics identifies medulloblastoma subgroups that are enriched for specific genetic alterations. J Clin Oncol 24(12):1924–1931

Venneti S et al (2013) Evaluation of Histone 3 lysine 27 trimethylation (H3K27me3) and enhancer of zest 2 (EZH2) in pediatric glial and glioneuronal tumors shows decreased H3K27me3 in H3F3A K27M mutant glioblastomas. Brain Pathol 23(5):558–564. https://doi.org/10.1111/bpa.12042

Versteege I et al (1998) Truncating mutations of hSNF5/INI1 in aggressive paediatric cancer. Nature 394(6689):203–206

Wang L et al (2014) Novel somatic and germline mutations in intracranial germ cell tumors. Nature 511(7508):241–245

Wani K et al (2012) A prognostic gene expression signature in infratentorial ependymoma. Acta Neuropathol 123(5):727–738

Witt H et al (2011) Delineation of two clinically and molecularly distinct subgroups of posterior fossa ependymoma. Cancer Cell 20(2):143–157

Wu G et al (2014) The genomic landscape of diffuse intrinsic pontine glioma and pediatric non-brainstem high-grade glioma. Nat Genet 46(5):444–450

Zhang J et al (2013) Whole-genome sequencing identifies genetic alterations in pediatric low-grade gliomas. Nat Genet 45(6):602–612

Zhukova N et al (2013) Subgroup-specific prognostic implications of TP53 mutation in medulloblastoma. J Clin Oncol 31(23):2927–2935

Medulloblastoma

7

Nicholas G. Gottardo and Christopher I. Howell

7.1 Introduction

Medulloblastoma is a highly malignant small round blue cell tumor of the posterior fossa. It accounts for approximately 20% of all brain tumors in children (Pizer and Clifford 2009), is the most common malignant brain tumor of childhood and, with greater advances against other common cancers in children, such as acute leukemias, is currently responsible for about 10% of all childhood cancer deaths (Pizer and Clifford 2009). Around 30% of patients present with metastatic disease, which is essentially restricted to the central nervous system (CNS), with metastasis outside the brain and spinal cord reported in less than 1% of cases at diagnosis in large series (Zeltzer et al. 1999). Since the 1970s the application of multimodal therapy including maximal resection followed by craniospinal irradiation (CSI) and chemotherapy have transformed a disease that was invariably fatal when treated with surgery alone to one which can be cured for approximately 70% of all patients. The stratification of patients based on age, amount of residual tumor, and the presence of metastatic disease has traditionally classified patients into three distinct clinical groups: average-risk medulloblastoma,

high-risk medulloblastoma, and infant medulloblastoma. while high-risk disease occurs in children ≥3 years old with <1.5 cm^2 of residual tumor and/or metastatic disease, while high-risk disease occurs in children ≥3 years old with ≥1.5 cm^2 of residual tumor or metastatic disease.

Historically, very young children (typically under 3 years of age) have by convention tended to be referred to as "infants." Because the term infant elsewhere in pediatric practice has the specific meaning of under 1 year of age, we consider very young children to be the preferred term. Using the most common definition of <3 years of age, very young children account for around 25% of medulloblastoma patients. These patients represent a particular challenge, as they have high-risk disease and yet the particular susceptibility of the developing brain preclude the use of radiotherapy; the exact contributions to poor outcome of restricted treatment options, association with known high-risk features, and/or novel biological features unique to this age group (Pizer and Clifford 2008) are now under investigation.

Over the past two decades studies conducted for children with average-risk medulloblastoma have focused on reducing the dose of CSI in order to reduce the incidence and severity of the most damaging side effects, particularly neurocognitive morbidity (Mulhern et al. 1998, 2005; Ris et al. 2001). This strategy has resulted in the successful reduction of CSI from 36 to 23.4 Gy without adversely affecting efficacy. This group has an

N. G. Gottardo (✉)
Perth Children's Hospital, Perth, WA, Australia
e-mail: nick.gottardo@health.wa.gov.au

C. I. Howell
Great North Children's Hospital, Royal Victoria Infirmary, Newcastle upon Tyne, UK

© Springer International Publishing AG, part of Springer Nature 2018
A. Gajjar et al. (eds.), *Brain Tumors in Children*, https://doi.org/10.1007/978-3-319-43205-2_7

overall 5-year survival rate of around 80–85% following 23.4 Gy CSI, with a posterior fossa boost to 55.8 Gy in conjunction with platinum-based chemotherapy (Packer et al. 2006; Lannering et al. 2012; Gajjar et al. 2006). The recently closed Children's Oncology Group (COG) average-risk medulloblastoma trial (ACNS0331) investigated a further reduction in CSI dose to 18 Gy for children 3–7 years, the age group most vulnerable to neurocognitive sequelae (Michalski 2016). In contrast, high-risk patients have survival rates approaching 70% using a variety of intensified treatments centered on increased radiotherapy doses (Gajjar et al. 2006; Tarbell et al. 2013; von Bueren et al. 2011) [von B 2016]. This progress has not come about through the use of novel therapies, but through the improved use of existing ones. It is recognized however that such cures come at a significant cost in terms of treatment-related morbidity, particularly with regard to neurodevelopment and endocrine dysfunction; moreover improvements obtained from optimizing current treatment modalities have plateaued as maximal doses of radiotherapy and chemotherapy as well as the limits of stratification based on clinical parameters alone have been reached. New therapeutic options are therefore urgently required. Recent advances in our understanding of medulloblastoma biology have revealed four core distinct molecular medulloblastoma subtypes with characteristic patterns of genetic abnormality, demographics and clinical behavior, and evidence of discrete tumor origins, and offer the promise of improved treatment stratification and novel, targeted therapies. Current clinical trials (NCT01878617 2013; SIOPE Medulloblastoma/PNET working group 2015) [COG ACNS 1422] designate patients with WNT pathway activation and no other adverse features as good risk, while *MYC* family amplification and large-cell/anaplastic histology have been added to the list of features that define high-risk disease (NCT01878617 2013; SIOPE Medulloblastoma/PNET working group 2015). Future trials will need to incorporate rapid, up-front subgroup assignment to identify patients who may benefit from specific targeted therapies and to allow accurate assessment of such treatments.

7.2 Epidemiology

Medulloblastoma is primarily a disease of childhood, with a median age at diagnosis of 6 years, however all ages are affected—from infants to adults, with the incidence decreasing with age. Of the 16,044 primary CNS tumors included in the Central Brain Tumor Registry of the United States (CBTRUS) statistical report for children aged 0–14 years between 2007 and 2011, 1494 (9.3%) were classified as medulloblastoma, corresponding to 0.49 cases per 100,000 person-years in the USA (Ostrom et al. 2015a, b). The incidence is up to 20 times less common in adults compared to childhood. Overall medulloblastoma is more common in males, with a male-to-female ratio of 1.6:1 (Ostrom et al. 2015a, b).

7.3 Clinical Presentation

Clinical presentation in medulloblastoma is variable and age-dependent. Since medulloblastomas arise in the posterior fossa, classically, patients present with symptoms suggestive of progressively increasing intracranial pressure (ICP) reflecting obstructed cerebrospinal fluid (CSF) flow due to mass-effects: early morning headache; vomiting and visual disturbances, associated with papilloedema on fundoscopy; and signs of cerebellar dysfunction such as slurred speech, ataxia and nystagmus (Ramaswamy et al. 2014). False-localizing signs such as cranial nerve palsies due to raised ICP rather than direct involvement of cranial nerve nuclei can also occur. A retrospective review of pediatric medulloblastoma patients (Brasme et al. 2012) found that 91% of older children had vomiting and 87% had complained of headache prior to diagnosis, although 35% did not have morning headache (Fig. 7.1). Fourteen percent had at least one sign of life-threatening intracranial hypertension at the time of diagnosis. In practice, diagnosis of possible brain tumors in children represents a significant clinical challenge (Ramaswamy et al. 2014; Wilne et al. 2006). The French study found a significant delay (91 vs. 60 days from onset of first symptom) in diagnosis in children in whom

Fig. 7.1 Incidence of medulloblastoma by age

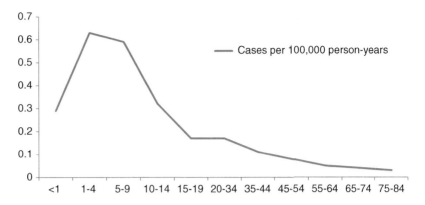

First reported symptom, over 3 yr   **First reported symptom, under 3 yr**

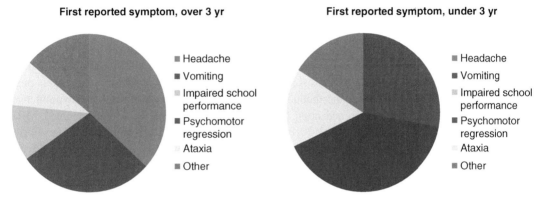

- Headache
- Vomiting
- Impaired school performance
- Psychomotor regression
- Ataxia
- Other

Fig. 7.2 First reported symptom in 191 childhood medulloblastoma, by age. Data from Brasme et al. (2012)

psychological explanations were ascribed to behavioral symptoms, such as impaired school performance, behavioral problems, depression, or anxiety; especially where headache and vomiting occurred late in the development of the illness, or did not fit the classic pattern of progressive and inexorable deterioration; and where neurological examination or fundoscopy was normal. Failure to match the "classic" clinical picture therefore appears to provide false reassurance.

A more recent retrospective study demonstrated that individual medulloblastoma subgroups (see section below) had different symptom intervals, with WNT and Group 4 tumors having a median interval of 8 weeks compared to 2 weeks for SHH tumors and 4 weeks for Group 3 tumors (Ramaswamy et al. 2014).

The clinical picture is further complicated in very young children, where features can be obscured by the child's stage of anatomical and neurological development. In particular, raised

ICP can be mitigated by widening of cranial sutures leading to increase in head circumference, while ataxia, clumsiness, and speech problems may be interpreted as (and may still lie within) normal variation in acquisition of developmental milestones. Younger children are also more commonly affected by more benign causes of vomiting, such as gastroenteritis and gastroesophageal reflux, and may be less able to report symptoms such as headache even when language skills are well developed. Medulloblastoma in very young children has a longer symptom interval than in older children (Ramaswamy et al. 2014). Features suggestive of an intracranial lesion in younger children include behavioral change, developmental delay, and, in particular, developmental regression (Brasme et al. 2012). The most commonly reported first symptom in very young children was psychomotor regression (loss of developmental milestones) in 40%, followed by vomiting in 28% (Fig. 7.2). By the time of diagnosis, 72% of patients had vomiting, 60% psychomotor regression, and 60% also exhibited ataxia. Approximately half were reported to have macrocrania. Notably, however, 28% of these patients had neither headache nor vomiting. Approximately one-third of under 3 s had at least one sign of life-threatening intracranial hypertension at the time of diagnosis (Brasme et al. 2012).

7.4   Diagnosis

All children with a history and clinical examination suggestive of an intracranial space-occupying lesion require urgent investigation (Wilne et al. 2010; Hamilton et al. 2015). While the imaging investigation of choice is a contrast-enhanced MRI of the brain and spinal cord, this takes some time and is likely to require general anesthetic in younger children who cannot be relied upon to stay still during the procedure (Wilne et al. 2010). This may not be immediately possible in children presenting to nonspecialist centers, or in those with signs of life-threatening intracranial hypertension. Many children therefore undergo an initial CT scan which demonstrates the presence of an intracranial mass, with subsequent MRI imaging of brain and spinal cord once the patient is stable and a general anesthetic is available. MR imaging allows the assessment of tumor size and the presence of metastases, permitting staging of the disease, and allowing planning of surgical resection (Fig. 7.3).

Non-contrast CT in medulloblastoma typically shows a hyper-attenuating (or dense) lesion surrounded by vasogenic edema, compared with normal cerebellar parenchyma, which corresponds to cell density. Punctate foci of calcification, also seen in other posterior fossa tumors such as ependymoma, can be seen in approximately 20% of medulloblastoma cases and is not a particularly useful discriminator (Fig. 7.4). The degree of hyper-attenuation is variable. Contrast enhancement is usually homogeneous. Medulloblastoma appears iso- or hypointense relative to white matter on T1-weighted MRI images (Fig. 7.4a–c), and is often heterogeneous, varying between hyper- and hypointense, with respect to gray matter on T2-weighted imaging (Fig. 7.4c, d). Diffusion-weighted imaging (DWI) shows increased signal with associated decreased apparent diffusion coefficient due to cell-dense

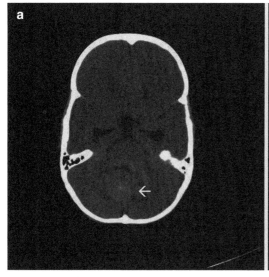
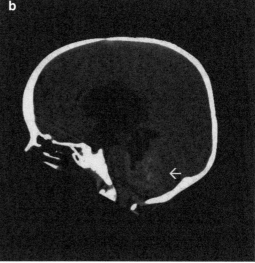
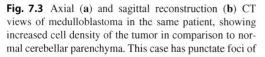

Fig. 7.3 Axial (**a**) and sagittal reconstruction (**b**) CT views of medulloblastoma in the same patient, showing increased cell density of the tumor in comparison to normal cerebellar parenchyma. This case has punctate foci of calcification (arrows), which occur in around 20% of medulloblastoma cases and is not a useful discriminator in radiological diagnosis in these tumors. Images courtesy of Dr. Andrew Thomson (Perth Children's Hospital)

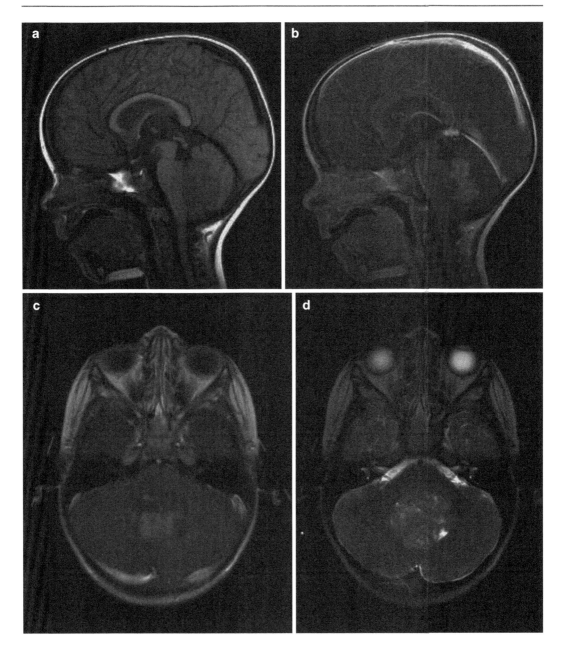

Fig. 7.4 Sagittal T1 MRI images, pre- (**a**) and post-gadolinium (**b**), showing mass arising from the superior medullary velum and filling the forth ventricle, and demonstrating heterogeneous contrast enhancement within the tumor. The corresponding post-contrast Axial T1 image is shown in (**c**). T2-weighted image of the same lesion (**d**) again shows a midline mass with a heterogeneous signal; with dark hypointense areas of increased cell density within the tumor. Diffusion-weighted (DWI) image (**e**) and corresponding apparent diffusion coeffi-cient map (**f**), respectively, showing restricted diffusion (bright DWI) and reduced apparent diffusion coefficient (dark ADC) due to cell-dense tumor stroma and relatively few free protons (i.e., little free water) in the extracellular interstitial space. Metastatic disease shown in (**g**) sagittal T1 image showing "drop" metastases within spinal cord, appearing as high intensity (bright) signal; (**h**) axial T1 image demonstrating nodular metastasis within the right parietal region. Images courtesy of Dr. Andrew Thomson (Perth Children's Hospital)

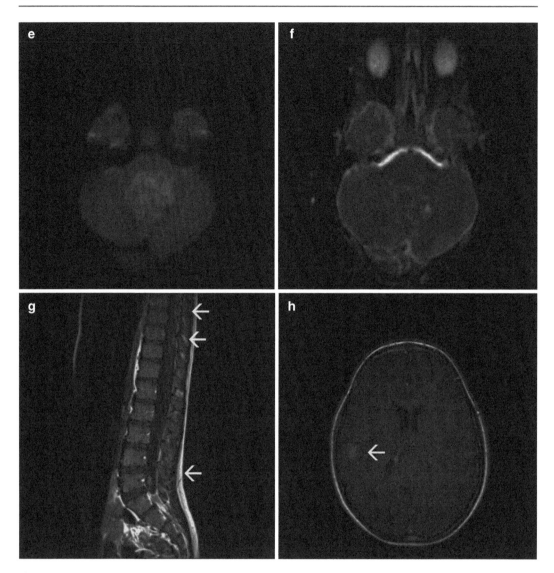

Fig. 7.4 (continued)

tumor stroma and relatively few free protons (i.e., little free water) in the extracellular interstitial space (Eran et al. 2010) (Fig. 7.4e, f).

Advances in MR imaging, including diffusion weighting and MR spectroscopy, allow increasingly confident differentiation of medulloblastoma from other posterior fossa tumors (e.g., ependymoma, pilocytic astrocytoma) by radiological appearance alone (Schneider et al. 2007; Bull et al. 2012; Rasalkar et al. 2013), and indeed recent research indicates that MR spectroscopy may be able to distinguish between histological (Fruehwald-Pallamar et al. 2011) and molecular (Bluml et al. 2016) subtypes of medulloblastoma. At present and for the foreseeable future, however, formal diagnosis is made histologically on tissue samples obtained surgically.

In addition to identifying the presence of a posterior fossa mass, and raising the possible diagnosis of medulloblastoma, initial diagnostic imaging, along with postsurgical MRI (and increasingly intraoperative MRI (Lam et al. 2001; Avula et al. 2015)) also forms part of the baseline for subsequent monitoring and follow-up of disease. Radiological response to treatment is a valuable interim marker of treatment efficacy. In this context, standardized approaches to imaging, with respect to anatomical coverage, contrast, and sequences obtained, are increasingly being mandated as a precondition for entry into clinical trials (Ellingson et al. 2015), to allow for standardized assessment of response to treatment across centers. It is important that standardized imaging be achievable for all treatment centers, and that its requirements do not have the effect of restricting trial entry to centers with state-of-the-art MRI scanners.

7.5   Staging

As tumor size is not prognostic and medulloblastoma does not metastasize via the lymphatic system, M-stage, as defined by Chang (Chang et al. 1969) is the only component of TNM staging currently used in this disease (Table 7.1).

In the absence of radiologically detectable metastatic disease (M2 or above), postoperative CSF sampling via lumbar puncture is required to differentiate between M0 and M1 disease. Optimum timing of this procedure is debated, with pragmatic considerations (recovery from surgery, "sharing" an anesthetic with central line insertion or postoperative imaging) often being important. A degree of controversy exists regarding whether M3 disease is in fact more advanced than M2 disease, based on the direction of physiological CSF circulation (Phi et al. 2011). The presence of extensive M3 disease or clinical features suggestive of spread beyond the CNS (pain,

Table 7.1 Chang classification of metastatic disease in medulloblastoma

Metastatic (M) stage	Definition
M0	No metastasis
M1	Tumor cells present on CSF microscopy
M2	Intracranial metastases
M3	Spinal metastases
M4	Metastasis beyond the CNS

elevated liver, or bone enzymes) indicates a need for further investigation such as bone scan or bone marrow aspiration to confirm or refute the presence of M4 disease, which occurs in approximately 1% of patients (Zeltzer et al. 1999).

7.6   Surgery

Many patients with medulloblastoma present with severe intracranial hypertension as a consequence of hydrocephalus (Fig. 7.5), requiring emergent/urgent insertion of an external ventricular drain (EVD) or definitive tumor surgery to re-establish CSF flow (Due-Tonnessen and Helseth 2007).

Surgical removal of posterior fossa tumors is usually performed by posterior craniotomy, via the occiput, with the patient in a face-down position. Surgery and postsurgical management requires specialist pediatric neurosurgical, neuroanesthetic expertise, and intensive care facilities. Frozen section histology can give an indication of pathology while the surgical procedure is ongoing. While diagnosis can be achieved from tissue biopsy alone, current management of all posterior fossa tumors indicates total or near-total surgical excision and thus primary resection is performed at this stage, using Cavitron Ultrasonic Surgical Aspiration (CUSA) equipment which preferentially fragments tumor tissue and allows simultaneous irrigation and aspiration, under visualization via an operating microscope (Nejat et al. 2008). Further postoperative MRI scanning is required to assess residual tumor volume. As with lumbar puncture, optimum timing of this investigation is currently a subject for debate. Recent protocols have aimed to reimage within 72 h of surgery (von Bueren et al. 2011), with a recent trend towards MRI being performed intraoperatively or immediately postoperatively (before waking the patient from anesthesia) where this is available (Choudhri et al. 2014). Postoperatively, up to 40% of children will require permanent CSF diversion; either via an endoscopic third ventriculostomy or insertion of ventriculoperitoneal shunt (Due-Tonnessen and Helseth 2007).

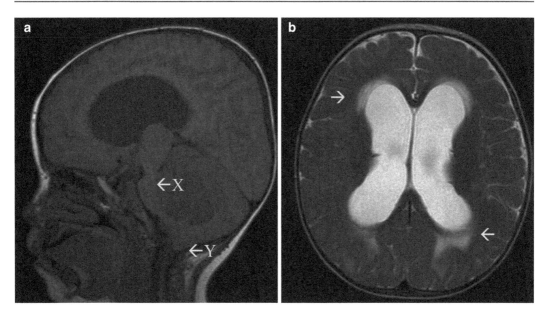

Fig. 7.5 MRI images of medulloblastoma in a very young child. (**a**) Sagittal T1-weighted MRI image, showing a large, heterogeneous mass in the cerebellum. Forward pressure at X results in hydrocephalus, seen as an enlarged third ventricle (dark area above X). Note also incipient "coning"-herniation of the brainstem and cerebellar tonsils at Y: a life-threatening neurosurgical emergency. (**b**) T2-weighted axial MRI image of same patient, showing enlarged lateral ventricles and periventricular transudate (arrows) due to hydrocephalus. Images kindly provided by Dr. James Hayden (Alder Hey Children's NHS Foundation Trust)

7.7   Posterior Fossa Syndrome (Also Known as Cerebellar Mutism)

Posterior fossa syndrome is a recognized consequence of injury to the cerebellum in children, that usually commences in the early (1 or 2 days postoperatively) (Robertson et al. 2006), but classically not immediately after posterior fossa tumor resection. Initially termed cerebellar mutism, due to the prominent symptom of inability to speak, the term posterior fossa syndrome is more apt given the constellation of other signs and symptoms, including pseudobulbar palsy, truncal hypotonia, ataxia, irritability which can be severe, and altered mental status (Mulhern et al. 2005; Pollack et al. 1995; Gudrunardottir et al. 2011). The incidence varies from 8 to 38% of patients, depending on the reported severity (Mulhern et al. 2005; Pollack et al. 1995; Gudrunardottir et al. 2011), with younger patients with high-risk disease at greater risk for development of posterior fossa syndrome (Mulhern et al. 2005). Posterior fossa surgery for medulloblastoma has been reported to be more commonly associated with the development of posterior fossa syndrome, compared with posterior fossa surgery for other indications (Robertson et al. 2006). The exact underlying cause remains unknown but has been hypothesized to involve disruption of dentate-thalamic-cortical tracts, possibly as a result of vermian splitting (Gudrunardottir et al. 2011), which results in cerebello-cerebral diaschisis with consequent decreased functionality of the frontal areas of the cerebrum involved in language and higher cognition (Marien et al. 2013; Miller et al. 2010). Consequently, avoidance of vermian splitting by the use of alternative surgical approaches such as the telovelar approach, as well as more gentle cerebellar retraction have been proposed to decrease the risk for developing posterior fossa syndrome (Gudrunardottir et al. 2011). No treatment currently exists. Though most patients recover over weeks to months, some patients are left with significant residual life-long deficits including dysarthria, and motor dysfunction (Huber et al. 2006; Puget et al. 2009).

7.8 Histology

Histologically, medulloblastoma is an embryonal tumor that may express markers of both neuronal and glial lineage (Gilbertson and Ellison 2008). In the past high-grade tumors that did not show signs of differentiation along either a neuronal or glial path were classified as primitive neuroectodermal tumors (PNET), with medulloblastomas also being termed posterior fossa PNETs (Rorke 1983). However, since PNETs elsewhere in the CNS have been shown to be biologically and clinically distinct to medulloblastoma (Pizer and Clifford 2008; Gilbertson and Ellison 2008; Pomeroy et al. 2002), this terminology is now redundant. Atypical teratoid rhabdoid tumors (ATRT) have in the past been mistaken for medulloblastoma, especially in very young children, but can now be distinguished by their characteristic negative staining for the protein INI1 (Biegel 2006).

The recently updated 2016 World Health Organization (WHO 2016) classification of CNS tumors identifies four different histopathological variants (Louis et al. 2016):

- Classic medulloblastoma
- Large cell/anaplastic medulloblastoma.
- Desmoplastic/nodular medulloblastoma.
- Medulloblastoma with extensive nodularity (MBEN).

Classic medulloblastoma consists of sheets of "small round blue cells": cells with a high nuclear:cytoplasmic ratio and little morphological evidence of differentiation. Arrangement of cells into "rosettes" (Fig. 7.6a) and "palisades" may be present. Individual classic tumors may show some signs of anaplasia or desmoplasia, without meeting criteria for these classifications; in particular, they may contain nodules with neurocytic differentiation (Fig. 7.6b), but without internodular desmoplasia. This "biphasic" phenotype is classified as classic histology. Classic medulloblastoma is coded by the International Classification of Disease—Oncology as ICD-O 9470/3. The rare melanotic and medullomyoblastic types, previously considered to be separate entities, are classified as medulloblastoma not otherwise specified (also coded as 9470/3) in this classification (Louis et al. 2016; Ellison 2010; Pfister et al. 2009).

Desmoplastic/nodular (DN) tumors are named for their nodules of cells that show signs of neurocyte differentiation (expression of proteins such as synaptophysin and Neu-N, detectable by immunohistochemistry), with areas of internodular fibrous connective (desmoplastic) tissue, which stains positive for reticulin (Fig. 7.6c). In *medulloblastoma with extensive nodularity (MBEN)*, as the name suggests, nodular features predominate (Fig. 7.6d). Internodular desmoplasia is sparse (but demonstrably present). MBEN is only found in under 3 s, in whom DN histology is also more common; both are covered by the ICD-O code 9471/3 (Louis et al. 2007, 2016; Ellison 2010; Giangaspero et al. 2007; McManamy et al. 2007). MBEN is often associated with Gorlin syndrome, also known as nevoid basal cell carcinoma syndrome (see Table 7.2). Due to the occurrence of nevoid basal cell carcinomas following radiotherapy in these patients, radiotherapy should be avoided (Garre et al. 2009).

Large cell/anaplastic (LCA) medulloblastoma. Anaplastic tumors are characterized by marked cellular (i.e., nuclear) pleomorphism, with cell molding and wrapping, resulting in a crazy-paving appearance (Fig. 7.6e). Pure large-cell tumors, where large cells with round nuclei, open chromatin, and single nucleoli predominate, are rare, and such cells in the vast majority of cases occur in conjunction with anaplasia. High rates of mitosis and apoptosis feature in both anaplastic and large-cell tumors, reflecting their lack of differentiation. The overlap between large-cell and anaplastic tumors is reflected by the fact that they are frequently grouped together in studies taking histology into account, and that they are assigned the same (ICD-O code 9474/3) by the 2007 WHO Classification (Ellison 2010; Louis et al. 2007; Giangaspero et al. 2007), consequently the anaplastic and large cell variants have been combined in the 2016 updated WHO classification (Louis et al. 2016).

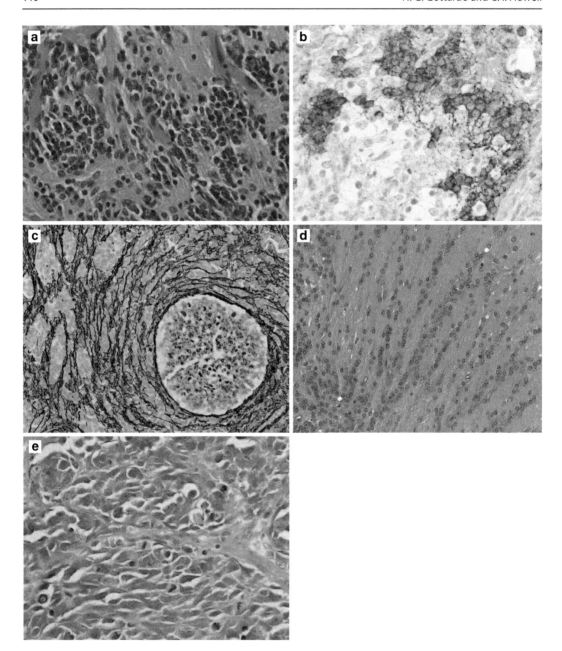

Fig. 7.6 (**a**) *Classic medulloblastoma* with the typical cytological features of sheets of cells with large nuclei in comparison to overall size (high nuclear/cytoplasmic ratio), and rosettes (circular arrangement of cells). (**b**) synaptophysin immunostain revealing that medulloblastomas usually express, in at least some cells, this marker of neuronal differentiation. (**c**) Desmoplastic/nodular medulloblastoma demonstrating the typical reticulin-positive boundary staining of nodules (black). (**d**) The medulloblastoma with extensive nodularity (MBEN) variant over-laps with the D/N medulloblastoma but in MBEN nodular areas are larger and become elongated and rich in neuropil-like tissue. These areas contain populations of small round cells which exhibit a linear "streaming" pattern. (**e**) Large cell/anaplastic medulloblastoma. Nuclei in anaplastic disease show marked variability in size, shape, and staining intensity (pleomorphism), giving a "crazy-paving" appearance; Large cell histology shows groups of large, round cells. Images courtersy of Dr. David Ellison (St Jude Children's Research Hospital)

Table 7.2 Familial cancer predisposition syndromes associated with medulloblastoma

Familial cancer predisposition syndromes (Alternative name)	Germline gene(s) mutated	Other features	Subgroup association
Turcot syndrome (Turcot et al. 1959; Online Mendelian Inheritance in Man 2015a)	Adenomatous Polyposis Coli (*APC*)	Multiple adenomatous colon polyps, increased risk of colorectal cancer and CNS tumors (medulloblastoma and glioblastoma). May be associated with familial adenomatous polyposis (FAP) or lynch syndrome (hereditary non-polyposis colorectal carcinoma (HNPCC))	WNT
Gorlin syndrome (basal cell nevus syndrome) (Gorlin and Chaudhary 1960; Online Mendelian Inheritance in Man 2013; Smith et al. 2014)	*PTCH1, SUFU*	Developmental abnormalities, bone cysts. Increased incidence of both basal cell carcinoma and medulloblastoma	SHH
Li Fraumeni syndrome (Zhukova et al. 2013; Li and Fraumeni Jr. 1969)	*TP53*	Cancer predisposition syndrome. Characterized by young age of onset of malignancy and multiple cancer types and primary sites particularly breast, sarcomas (rhabdomyosarcoma and osteogenic sarcoma), brain (particularly glioblastoma and medulloblastoma) adrenocortical carcinoma	SHH
Rubinstein Taybi syndrome (Miller and Rubinstein 1995; Online Mendelian Inheritance in Man 2015b)	*CREBBP*	Mental retardation, postnatal growth deficiency, microcephaly, dysmorphic facies. Broadened thumbs and halluces Increased incidence of neoplasia with CNS disease, especially medulloblastoma	
Fanconi anemia (Dewire et al. 2009; Online Mendelian Inheritance in Man 2012) Complementation group D1	*BRCA2*	Developmental abnormalities in a number of organ systems, early-onset bone marrow failure Predisposition to medulloblastoma; hypersensitivity to DNA crosslinking agents; chromosomal abnormalities	

The different medulloblastoma histological subtypes exhibit distinct clinical behavior and outcomes. Most notably, the large cell/anaplastic (LCA) subtype is an independent predictor of poor prognosis (Gajjar et al. 2006; Eberhart et al. 2002; McManamy et al. 2003) (Ryan et al. 2012; Ellison et al. 2011a) and is treated as high-risk disease in the current COG, SIOP-Europe and St Jude's protocols (NCT01878617 2013; SIOPE Medulloblastoma/PNET working group 2015; Children's Oncology Group 2016a). By contrast, MBEN histology is associated with good outcome despite being confined to very young children (Rutkowski et al. 2010), while DN histology has better outcome than classic histology in very young children (Rutkowski et al. 2010; Leary et al. 2011; Dhall et al. 2008).

The different histological subtypes have distinct age distributions, with MBEN found only in very young children and DN histology also more common in this group (McManamy et al. 2007; Rutkowski et al. 2010). In addition, there are strong associations between molecular medulloblastoma subgroups (see below) and particular histological classifications; however subgroup does not define histology.

7.9 Familial Cancer Predisposition Syndromes

The link between medulloblastoma and familial cancer syndromes was first identified by investigation of two familial cancer syndromes: Turcot syndrome and Gorlin syndrome, now known to be associated with the Wnt/Wingless (WNT) signaling and Sonic Hedgehog (SHH) pathways, respectively. Although overall only a minority of patients with medulloblastoma have an underlying cancer predisposition syndrome,

medulloblastoma may occasionally be the initial manifestation of the presence of germline
mutations in these predisposition syndromes.
The mechanisms by which these syndromes
lead to increased risk of medulloblastoma are
increasingly being understood, and in some
cases have been pivotal to the emerging understanding of disease biology and subtypes.
Syndromes known to be associated with medulloblastoma are shown in Table 7.2.

7.10   Treatment of Medulloblastoma

7.10.1 The Past: Empiric Use of Radiotherapy and Chemotherapy

Medulloblastoma was first defined as a distinct
CNS tumor by Cushing and Bailey in 1925
(Bailey and Cushing 1925). Following even
apparent complete surgical resection alone, all
medulloblastomas recur, leading to death within
a median time of 4 months (range 2–21 months)
(Bailey and Cushing 1925). The introduction of
postoperative radiotherapy by these authors in
1919 demonstrated an increased duration of survival revealing the radio sensitivity of these
tumors (Bailey and Cushing 1925). A report by
Bloom and colleagues in 1969 and other similar
reports (Hughes et al. 1988) established radiotherapy as the backbone of medulloblastoma
therapy.

Encouraged by the success of chemotherapy in
acute lymphoblastic leukemia, chemotherapy was
empirically added as adjuvant therapy, initially
using vincristine, lomustine, and prednisone. A
randomized trial revealed the efficacy of chemotherapy for the treatment of medulloblastoma.
Patients with metastatic disease who received
adjuvant chemotherapy had a significantly better
5-year EFS compared with those who only
received radiotherapy (Evans et al. 1990). Similar
results were reported by the first International
Society of Pediatric Oncology (SIOP) trial (Tait
et al. 1990). Results from a phase II trial which
included children with relapsed medulloblastoma

demonstrated the platinum alkylator cisplatin to
be particularly effective against medulloblastoma
(Sexauer et al. 1985).

Once a significant number of long-term survivors were seen, several clinical risk factors
emerged as critically important for cure, some of
which had been noted decades earlier (Bloom
et al. 1969). These included the extent of surgical
resection (defined as <1.5 cm^2 of residual tumor),
the absence of metastatic disease and brainstem
invasion (Zeltzer et al. 1999; Tait et al. 1990),
such that children 3 years of age and over following gross total resection and no metastatic disease are classified as average-risk, the remainder
being categorized as high risk. Subsequent clinical trials stratified patients according to these
criteria.

However, disturbing data from randomized
trials conducted by the Pediatric Oncology Group
(POG) and the Children's Cancer Group (CCG)
revealed that survivors were left with significant,
often devastating neurocognitive consequences,
with an average of 15–20 intelligence quotient
(IQ) scores lost for patients treated with 36 Gy
CSI. The decline in IQ scores was most significant in children younger than 8.5 years (IQ 70 vs.
IQ 85) (Mulhern et al. 1998). In addition, other
significant late sequelae such as neuroendocrine
deficiencies have also been observed (Laughton
et al. 2008). More recently, the devastating
sequelae of second malignancies have been
increasingly appreciated (Packer et al. 2013).

7.10.1.1 Average-Risk Medulloblastoma
The concerns about the damaging effects of high-
dose CSI prompted clinicians to empirically
reduce the CSI dose for patients with average-
risk disease. Initial attempts to reduce radiotherapy alone resulted in inferior survival (Deutsch
et al. 1996; Thomas et al. 2000).

A seminal pilot study for children aged
between 3 and 10 years of age with average-risk
medulloblastoma delivered reduced-dose CSI
(23.4 Gy) followed by eight cycles of adjuvant
chemotherapy consisting of lomustine, cisplatin,
and vincristine (frequently termed Packer chemotherapy) revealed that the dose of CSI could

be reduced from 36 Gy if combined with effective adjuvant chemotherapy (Packer et al. 1999). This pilot study formed the basis for the COG A9961 trial for average-risk medulloblastoma, in which all patients received 23.4 Gy CSI and a posterior fossa boost to 55.8 Gy, with weekly vincristine during radiotherapy. After the completion of radiotherapy, patients were randomly assigned to either the standard regimen of lomustine, cisplatin, and vincristine or the cyclophosphamide containing regimen with cisplatin, and vincristine following the completion of radiotherapy. A total of 379 eligible patients were enrolled. The 5-year EFS was 81 ± 2%, with no difference in EFS in either arm of the study (Packer et al. 2006). This study established 23.4 Gy CSI as the standard dose of CSI for children over 3 years of age with average-risk medulloblastoma.

To decrease the significant toxicity associated with cisplatin and vincristine, a multicenter study led by St Jude Children's Research Hospital, called SJMB96, utilized a shortened schedule of four courses of high-dose cyclophosphamide (16 g/m^2 cumulative dose) with stem cell support enabling dose intensity, in combination with reduced doses of cisplatin and vincristine (Packer et al. 2006; Gajjar et al. 2006). Average-risk patients received 23.4 Gy CSI followed by a 3D boost to the posterior fossa (to 36 Gy) and tumor bed (total dose 55.8 Gy). The 5-year EFS and OS for the 86 enrolled patients were 83% (CI 73–93) and 85% (CI 75–94) confirming that dose reductions are feasible for CSI but also for vincristine and cisplatin, without adversely affecting survival.

Another strategy to reduce the late-toxicity associated with radiotherapy, especially damage to the cochlea, has been the adoption of conformal techniques limiting the boost volume to the tumor bed rather than the whole posterior fossa have been evaluated (Carrie et al. 2005, 2009; Merchant et al. 2008). These studies have revealed no increase in local tumor relapses compared with whole posterior fossa boosts. This strategy was investigated in the most recently concluded COG average-risk medulloblastoma trial (ACNS0331), which assessed reduction in

CSI dose to 18 Gy as well as a limited target volume boost to the tumor bed (termed involved field radiotherapy (IFRT)) (to a total of 54 Gy) in a randomized fashion for children 3–7 years old. Preliminary review of the data revealed no significant difference between those patients who received IFRT versus those who received posterior fossa radiotherapy (PFRT) (5-year EFS and OS of 82 ± 3% and 84%, respectively, for IFRT compared with 80.8 ± 3% and 85%, respectively, for PFRT) (Michalski 2016).

While the declines in IQ were less dramatic for children who received 23.4 Gy CSI compared with 36 Gy CSI, the worst declines were seen for those younger children (<8.5 years) at the time of radiotherapy, with a mean IQ loss of 4.3 points per year (Ris et al. 2001) revealing a significant impact on neurocognitive functioning of 24 Gy CSI. This data prompted the COG to undertake the most recently concluded average-risk medulloblastoma trial (ACNS0331), which investigated a further reduction in CSI dose to 18 Gy as well as a limited target volume boost to the tumor bed (to a total of 54 Gy), for children 3–7 years, the age group most vulnerable to neurocognitive sequelae. Preliminary review of the data revealed that empiric reduction of CSI to 18 Gy in average-risk medulloblastoma patients aged 3–7 years of age results in inferior survival (Michalski 2016). Analysis according to molecular subgroups is pending.

On the other hand, in order to exploit the chemosensitivity of medulloblastoma, European investigators focused on the timing of chemotherapy in relation to radiotherapy and pioneered the use of "sandwich chemotherapy" (pre- and post-radiotherapy chemotherapy). The SIOP II study randomized children identified as "low risk" to 35 Gy CSI versus 25 Gy CSI to receive or not receive pre-radiation chemotherapy. Children who received pre-radiotherapy chemotherapy and the lower-dose CSI had a particularly poor survival, with a 5-year EFS of only 41.7% (Bailey et al. 1995). The study revealed that delaying CSI was deleterious, resulting in reduced survival. Similarly, the German GPOH HIT '91 trial, which randomized patients to receive either two cycles of sandwich chemotherapy or immediate radiotherapy followed by maintenance chemotherapy, demonstrated that for average-risk medulloblastoma pre-radiation chemotherapy was inferior to immediate radiotherapy followed by maintenance chemotherapy (Kortmann et al. 2000; von Hoff et al. 2009).

The SIOP III study randomized children with average-risk medulloblastoma between radiotherapy alone (36 Gy CSI with a posterior fossa boost to 56 Gy) and pre-radiotherapy chemotherapy consisting of four cycles vincristine, carboplatin, cyclophosphamide, and etoposide, followed by the same radiotherapy dose. Of note, patients with M1 disease were also included in this study. The 5-year EFS for the 179 eligible patients was 74% for patients that received chemotherapy followed by radiotherapy, compared with 60% for the group that received radiotherapy alone. This study verified the effectiveness of postoperative radiotherapy alone at a dose of 36 Gy CSI with a posterior fossa boost to 56 Gy, as being able to cure approximately 60% of patients and also confirmed that the addition of chemotherapy significantly improved survival (Taylor et al. 2003), albeit not as much as when used post-radiotherapy (Packer et al. 2006; Gajjar et al. 2006).

Building upon the radiosensitivity and proven efficacy of radiotherapy in medulloblastoma, the successor SIOP study (SIOP-PNET 4) assessed hyperfractionated radiotherapy (HFRT) (Lannering et al. 2012). The premise behind hyperfractionation lies in the shorter tissue repair characteristics of normal tissue compared with tumors (Thames et al. 1982; Barton 1995).Thus in order to restrict toxicity to normal tissues while effecting greater tumor cell kill, hyperfractionation involves dividing the daily radiotherapy dose into two small parcels, typically into 1 Gy, separated by 6–8 h, compared with 1.8–2 Gy daily for conventional fractionation. A total of 340 patients which included patients with residual tumor >1.5 cm^2, were randomized between HFRT (36 Gy CSI, 60 Gy posterior fossa and 68 Gy tumor bed 2 × 1 Gy fractions/day) and standard fractionated radiotherapy (23.4 Gy CSI and 54 Gy to the whole posterior fossa). All patients received weekly vincristine during radiotherapy and the same post-radiotherapy chemotherapy. There was no significant difference in survival, in relapse site or incidence of severe hearing loss between the two treatment arms. Inferior survival was observed for the 32 patients with residual tumor >1.5 cm^2 central review and those patients in whom the commencement of radiotherapy was delayed more than 49 days. Inferior survival had previously been observed for delayed start of postoperative radiotherapy beyond 50 days (del Charco et al. 1998; Paulino et al. 2003). Consistent with the COG A9961 trial (Packer et al. 2006), survival was inferior for the small number of patients whose imaging was not centrally reviewed (Lannering et al. 2012) (Table 7.3).

Conclusions for Average-Risk Medulloblastoma

Overall, these studies reveal that the use of post-radiotherapy chemotherapy (most commonly lomustine, cisplatin, cyclophosphamide, and vincristine) has resulted in the successful reduction of CSI from 36 to 23.4 Gy without adversely affecting efficacy, yielding a 5-year survival rate of between 80 and 85% (Packer et al. 2006; Lannering et al. 2012; Gajjar et al. 2006). Pre-radiotherapy chemotherapy produces inferior survival compared to post-radiotherapy chemotherapy, possibly as a result of the delayed initiation of radiotherapy. The use of HFRT does not protect against local or leptomeningeal relapse or reduce the incidence of severe ototoxicity (Lannering et al. 2012). Real-time central radiology review of MRI scans should be adopted in future international cooperative group trials (Gottardo et al. 2014; Ramaswamy et al. 2016) to minimize the chances of inadvertently treating patients with excess residual disease or leptomeningeal dissemination as average-risk, with consequent decreased survival (Packer et al. 2006; Lannering et al. 2012). Delays in initiating radiotherapy beyond 7 weeks after surgical resection result in inferior survival.

The majority of patients relapse within the first 2 years and very rarely beyond 5 years. No effective therapeutic strategies exist for patients who relapse, with virtually no chance of cure, despite the use of very intensive salvage regimes including megatherapy with autologous stem cell rescue

Table 7.3 Summary of selected average-risk medulloblastoma trials from the 1980s onwards

Study Enrolment dates Published	Cases	Treatment	Outcome	Main conclusions
SIOP II 1984–89 Bailey et al. Med Pediatr Oncol 1995; 25: 166–178	153 M0–1, R0, no brainstem involvement	Randomization between 35 and 25 Gy CSI (total to PF 55 Gy in all cases), and to sandwich chemotherapy before RTx or not	Standard RTx alone: 5-year EFS 60.0 ± 7.8% Reduced-dose RTx alone: 5-year EFS 69.1 ± 7.8% Sandwich chemo and Std RTx: 5-year EFS 75.3 ± 7.2% Sandwich chemo and reduced RTx: 5-year EFS 41.7 ± 8.2%	No benefit to addition of sandwich chemotherapy overall, while in reduced-dose RTx group delay in starting RTx was detrimental. Discrepancies between local reporting of stage and central review.
CCG 9892 1990–94 Packer et al. JCO 1999;17:2127–2136	65 M0R0	23.4 Gy CSI (PF 55.8 Gy) with weekly vincristine, then vincristine, cisplatin and lomustine	5-year EFS 78 ± 5%	Reduced-dose CSI plus subsequent chemotherapy comparable to standard-dose RTx alone in previously reported studies
HIT-91 1991–97 Kortmann et al Int J Radiat Onc Biol phys 2000;46:269–279 Updated results von Hoff EJC 2009	118 M0–1, R±	35.2 Gy CSI (PF 55.2 Gy); either ifosfamide, ara-C, etoposide, HD-methotrexate and cisplatin *before* RTx (sandwich), or vincristine, cisplatin and lomustine following RTx (maintenance)	3-year EFS for post-radiotherapy chemotherapy 78 ± 6%; 65 ± 5% for pre-RTx chemotherapy group. 10-year EFS M0 83 ± 6% maintenance vs. 53 ± 6% sandwich chemotherapy ($p = 0.004$); M1 71 ± 11% maintenance vs. 36 ± 12% $p = (0.023)$	Results favor surgery-radiotherapy-chemotherapy sequence over surgery-chemotherapy-radiotherapy, despite giving additional post-radiotherapy chemotherapy to poor responders in the chemotherapy-first group. Presence of patients with M1 and R+ disease makes comparison with other studies difficult. At 10 years, significantly worse OS with "sandwich" chemotherapy for M0 and M1 patients
SIOP-PNET3 1992–2000 Taylor et al. JCO 2003; 21:1581–1591	179 M0R0	35 Gy CSI (PF 55 Gy) ± preceding vincristine, etoposide, carboplatin and cyclophosphamide	60% 5-year EFS for radiotherapy-only patients; 74% for chemotherapy plus radiotherapy	Addition of platinum-based chemotherapy improves survival compared to radiotherapy alone
A9961 1996–2000 Packer et al JCO 2006; 24: 4202–4208	383 M0R0	Weekly vincristine alongside 23.4 Gy CSI (PF 55.8 Gy), followed by either vincristine, cisplatin, lomustine; or vincristine, cisplatin, cyclophosphamide (1 year duration maintenance chemo)	5-year EFS 82 ± 3% vs. 80 ± 3%, respectively (not significant)	No difference between chemotherapy arms; standard risk patients can achieve 80% + EFS with radiotherapy followed by chemotherapy. >4% 10-year SMN incidence (Packer et al. 2013) (packer neuro Oncol 2013)

(continued)

Table 7.3 (continued)

Study Enrolment dates Published	Cases	Treatment	Outcome	Main conclusions
SJMB96 1996–2003 Gajjar Lancet Oncol 2006; 7: 813–820	86 M0R0	23.4 Gy CSI (PF 55.8 Gy) followed by four cycles high-dose chemotherapy (vincristine, cisplatin, cyclophosphamide) and autologous SCR (4 months duration maintenance chemo)	5-year EFS 83% (95% CI 73–93%)	Duration of maintenance chemotherapy can safely be reduced by increasing intensity
SIOP-PNET 4 2001–2006 Lannering JCO	340	HFRT vs. SFRT CCDP, CCNU, VCR	5-year EFS: 78 vs. 77% No difference between randomized arms < 1.5 cm^2 residual 82 vs. 64% 5-year EFS	Hyperfractionated chemotherapy not beneficial in terms of survival or ototoxicity; inferior survival for residual disease and for delay in radiotherapy beyond 49 days postoperatively
ACNS0331 2004–2014 Michalski	513	Randomization: XRT 18 vs. 23.4 CSI AND PF vs. tumor bed. Followed by either vincristine, cisplatin, lomustine; or vincristine, cisplatin, cyclophosphamide (1 year duration maintenance chemo)	83% 5 year (23.4 CSI vs. 72% for 18 CSI). No difference for PF vs. tumor bed boost	Inferior results for 18 vs. 23.4 Gy in children aged 3–7 years

CSI craniospinal irradiation, *PF* posterior fossa, *RTx* radiotherapy, *chemo* chemotherapy, *EFS* event-free survival, *M* Chang M-stage, *R* residual disease, *HD* high-dose, *SCR* stem cell rescue, *HFRT* hyperfractionated radiotherapy, *SFRT* standard fractionated radiotherapy

(Gajjar and Pizer 2010). Although late-effects are less than for those patients receiving 36 Gy CSI, they remain problematic and continue to negatively impact upon the quality of life of survivors. Results from the most recently closed COG average-risk medulloblastoma trial (ACNS0331), which investigated a further reduction in CSI dose to 18 Gy for children 3–7 years, as well as a limited target volume boost to the tumor bed (to a total of 54 Gy) reveal that empiric reductions in CSI to 18 Gy to average-risk patients based on age, rather than molecular subgrouping yield inferior survival (Michalski 2016).

7.10.1.2 High-Risk Medulloblastoma

The quest for improved survival has overshadowed the concerns about late effects for patients classified as high-risk. Given the historical poor outcomes for these patients, therapeutic strategies have focused on approaches to increase survival. Therapeutic approaches for patients with high-risk disease have revolved around the use of higher doses of neuraxis radiotherapy (36–44 Gy) combined with intensified chemotherapy regimens (Zeltzer et al. 1999; Gajjar et al. 2006; Tarbell et al. 2013; Kortmann et al. 2000; von Hoff et al. 2009; Allen et al. 2009; Taylor et al. 2005; Gandola et al. 2009; Jakacki et al. 2012).

The CCG921 phase III study (Zeltzer et al. 1999) randomized between pre-radiotherapy chemotherapy (using the "8 in 1" regimen) and postradiotherapy chemotherapy (using vincristine, lomustine, prednisolone). All patients received 36 Gy CSI with a posterior fossa boost to 54 Gy. The 5-year PFS was inferior for the preradiotherapy arm.

The subsequent CCG 9931 study intensified both pre-radiotherapy chemotherapy and radiotherapy by utilizing HFRT (Allen et al. 2009) for patients with high-risk medulloblastoma and CNS-PNETs, but found no significant survival advantage added morbidity. Of note, 17% of patients, which also included CNS-PNET patients, progressed during chemotherapy. Response to pre-radiotherapy chemotherapy was not associated with improved survival, with no significant difference in survival between patients who achieved a CR to chemotherapy compared to those achieving either a partial response or stable disease. A similar result was found for patients with M2–3 disease in the SIOP-PNET-3 trial, which utilized an intensified pre-radiotherapy chemotherapy strategy, followed by 35 Gy CSI (Taylor et al. 2005). The 5-year EFS was only 35% for the 68 patients enrolled, and at 18% the proportion of patients progressing during the pre-radiotherapy chemotherapy was almost identical to the CCG study.

Around the same time, the POG 9031 phase III study for high-risk medulloblastoma patients aged 3–18 years also addressed the question of timing of chemotherapy in relation to radiotherapy (Tarbell et al. 2013). Patients were randomized to pre-radiotherapy chemotherapy compared with the same chemotherapy given post-radiotherapy. Patients received between 35.2 and 44 Gy CSI with a posterior fossa boost between 53.2 and 54.4 Gy. The 5-year event-free survival was 68.1 ± 3% and in contrast with the CCG-921, no difference between the two arms was observed. Survival was particularly good for patients with macrometastatic disease, with 5-year EFS of 69.2 ± 7.7% for M2 patients and 61.6 ± 8.4% for M3 patients. Patients with M4 disease had a dismal prognosis, with a 5-year EFS of 22.2 ± 13.9%. The outcome for patients with >1.5 cm^2 residual disease and without metastatic disease also did not differ significantly between patients who received pre-radiotherapy chemotherapy and immediate radiotherapy. Similar results were achieved for patients with >1.5 cm^2 residual disease and metastatic disease. The objective response rate was significantly higher for patients who received pre-radiotherapy chemotherapy compared to those who received immediate radiotherapy. Progressive disease was observed in 11% (12/112) of patients who received pre-radiotherapy chemotherapy. In contrast, no patient progressed during immediate radiotherapy. Again, response to chemotherapy was not associated with a statistically significant improvement in survival.

As with average-risk disease, European trials also investigated "sandwich" chemotherapy for high-risk medulloblastoma patients. In the SIOP II study, high-risk medulloblastoma patients received post-resection chemotherapy followed by 36 Gy CSI with a boost to 55 Gy to areas of gross disease followed by lomustine, cisplatin, and vincristine maintenance chemotherapy. High-risk patients did not benefit from the addition of sandwich chemotherapy (Bailey et al. 1995).

The German HIT 91 phase III trial (Kortmann et al. 2000; von Hoff et al. 2009) in which patients with metastatic medulloblastoma received the same chemotherapy regimen as average-risk patients, but with higher doses of CSI, yielded a mixed result. Patients with M1 disease had a 10-year OS of 70 ± 12% for immediate radiotherapy compared with 34 ± 12% for sandwich therapy ($p = 0.02$). In contrast, for patients with M2/3 disease the 10-year OS was almost identical between the two treatment groups (45 ± 12% compared with 42 ± 11% ($p = 0.99$)), akin to the POG9031 study, albeit with significantly inferior results.

The successor study HIT-SKK 2000, which enrolled 123 eligible patients with metastatic medulloblastoma also utilized sandwich chemotherapy but intensified the induction chemotherapy, including the addition of intrathecal methotrexate (von Bueren et al. 2016). For patients without progression, this was followed by 40 Gy CSI hyperfractionated non-accelerated radiotherapy (HART) followed by four cycles of maintenance with cisplatin, lomustine, and vincristine. Progressive disease was observed in 11% (14/123) of patients. The 5-year EFS and OS for the whole cohort were 62 and 74%, respectively, revealing an improvement from the HIT 91 trial. Poor prognostic factors included

LCA histology and nonresponse after the first cycle of chemotherapy.

In the St Jude Children's Research Hospital SJMB96 trial, high-risk medulloblastoma patients received post-resection radiotherapy consisting of 36 Gy CSI for M0/1 high-risk disease and 36 to 39.6 Gy for M2/M3 high-risk disease, with boosts to sites of gross disease (Packer et al. 2006; Gajjar et al. 2006). Post-radiotherapy chemotherapy was the same as average-risk patients, consisting of four cycles of high-dose cyclophosphamide (16 g/m^2 cumulative dose) combined with cisplatinum and vincristine with autologous stem cell support to enable administration of the intensified cyclophosphamide. The 5-year EFS and OS for the 44 enrolled patients were 70% (CI 55–85%) and 70% (CI 54–84%), respectively. For the 42 patients with M+ disease the 5-year EFS was 66% (CI 48–83).

An alternative therapeutic approach for patients with metastatic disease was used by the Milan group (Gandola et al. 2009) who utilized a sequence of high-dose chemotherapy followed by HART radiotherapy (two 1.3 Gy fractions/day for a total of 39 Gy in patients older than 10 years and 31.2 Gy for children under 10 years). Patients who achieved a CR prior to radiotherapy were to have maintenance therapy with vincristine and lomustine, while those without a CR to initial chemotherapy were to receive two cycles of high-dose (HD) chemotherapy with thiotepa (900 mg/m^2) with autologous stem cell rescue. A total of 33 consecutive patients were enrolled, one of whom died of a shunt infection during initial chemotherapy. Four (12%) further patients did not complete pre-radiotherapy chemotherapy and started radiotherapy early because of disease progression on chemotherapy ($n = 2$), infection delaying chemotherapy components ($n = 1$), or both ($n = 1$). Twelve patients were judged to be in CR after initial chemotherapy. HART was delivered largely as planned, although there were some modifications due to extent of metastatic disease. Only 14 children received HD thiotepa. While the 5-year PFS and OS was 70% and 73%, respectively, there are significant concerns regarding the neurotoxicity of high-dose alkylator agent therapy in patients who have previously been exposed to CSI. Half of children had neurological signs or symptoms ascribed to radiotherapy at a median follow-up of 82 months, while 6 of the 14 who had received HD thiotepa had MRI changes including leukodystrophy and volume loss.

The CCG 99702 (Nazemi et al. 2016) study intensified post radiotherapy therapy by utilizing three cycles of high-dose chemotherapy (cycles 1 and 3: carboplatin, vincristine, thiotepa; cycle 2: carboplatin, vincristine, cyclophosphamide) was stopped early after recruiting 24 eligible patients due to unacceptably high rates of veno-occlusive disease (VOD) (6/24 cases overall, with a seventh case diagnosed with VOD at post-mortem after death from treatment-related sepsis). This high rate of VOD was postulated to be due to the short interval (4–6 weeks) between prior radiotherapy with concurrent vincristine chemotherapy, compared to results of similar high-dose regimes not preceded by radiotherapy (HeadStart), or with longer intervals, no concurrent vincristine and incorporating cyclophosphamide rather than thiotepa (SJMB96). The optimum means of intensifying postsurgical therapy to improve survival, without unacceptable treatment-related morbidity, remains elusive (Nazemi et al. 2016).

A phase I/II study conducted by the COG, called ACNS99701 assessed the feasibility of including carboplatin during 36 Gy CSI with weekly vincristine, as a radiosensitizer for high-risk medulloblastoma patients (Jakacki et al. 2012). Chemo-radiotherapy was followed by a comparison of maintenance chemotherapy (lomustine and vincristine) with or without cisplatin. The study enrolled a total of 81 patients between March 1998 and November 2004. The 5-year PFS and OS for the whole cohort were 71 ± 6% and 78 ± 6%, respectively. Patients with M2 disease had a 5-year PFS and OS of 50 ± 16% and 70 ± 16%, while patients with and M3 disease had a 5-year PFS and OS of 67.7 ± 7% and 73 ± 6%. In this study patients with centrally reviewed LCA medulloblastoma had inferior survival.

The current COG high-risk medulloblastoma study (ACNS0332) (Children's Oncology Group 2006) is attempting to replicate the results of the

COG ACNS99701 pilot trial, in a phase III randomized fashion. In addition, patients are also randomized to retinoic acid, following preclinical data revealing it was a potent proapoptotic agent in medulloblastoma (Spiller et al. 2008) (Table 7.4).

Table 7.4 Summary of selected high-risk medulloblastoma trials from the 1980s onwards

Study Enrolment dates Published	Cases	Treatment	Outcome	Main conclusions
CHOP 1983–91 Packer et al. J Neurosurg 1994; 81:690–698	15 M1–M3	Weekly vincristine during radiotherapy (36 Gy CSI; 55.8 Gy to PF), followed by lomustine, cisplatin, and vincristine	5-year EFS 67 ± 15%	Definite role for chemotherapy in the management of medulloblastoma
SIOP II 1984–89 Bailey et al Med Pediatr Oncol 1995; 25: 166–178	135 M2+/R+ or with brainstem involvement	35 Gy CSI (PF 55 Gy); randomization to sandwich chemotherapy (procarbazine, vincristine, 2 mg/m^2 methotrexate) before RTx or not	Sandwich chemotherapy: 5-year EFS 56.3 ± 6.5% vs. 52.8 ± 6.1%.	No benefit to addition of sandwich therapy between surgery and radiotherapy
CCG 921 1986–92 Zeltzer et al JCO 1999: 17:832–45	188 HR	Two cycles 8-drugs-in-1-day chemotherapy prior to 36 Gy CSI plus boost, followed by 6 8-in-1 cycles vs. RTx followed by lomustine, vincristine, and prednisolone	5-year PFS 54.5 ± 5% for 8-in-1, 63 ± 5% for standard arm	Inferior results for "8-in-1" chemotherapy, attributed partly to the 28-day delay in starting RTx in this arm, despite expected optimization of timing of chemotherapy before RTx-related reduced perfusion, and previous good results with multidrug chemotherapy in phase II trials in recurrent disease
POG 9031 1990–96 Tarbell et al, JCO 2013. 31 (23) 2936–41	224 HR MB (108 M+, includes 76 M0 with totally resected T3b/ T4 tumors)	Three cycles cisplatin and etoposide either before or after radiotherapy (M1: 35.2 Gy; M2–3 40 Gy CSI; PF 53.2–54.4 Gy), followed by eight cycles cyclophosphamide and vincristine	5-year EFS: All patients: Chemo first 66 ± 4.5%; RTx first 70 ± 4.4% 5-year EFS: M0/ R+: Chemo first 59.6 ± 7.0%; RTx first 65.1 ± 6.8% ($p = 0.4$) 5-year EFS: M+/ R+: Chemo first 51.2 ± 9.2%; RTx first 64.0 ± 9.3% ($p = 0.2$)	No difference in outcome between chemo first and RTx first groups; good response for M0R0 patients with T3b/T4 disease, who would currently be classified as standard rather than high-risk disease. Good results for M2+ disease achieved at the expense of using 40 Gy CSI dose. Response to chemotherapy was not associated with a statistically significant improvement in survival (5-year EFS: 73 ± 7% vs. 56 ± 17%)

(continued)

Table 7.4 (continued)

Study Enrolment dates Published	Cases	Treatment	Outcome	Main conclusions
HIT-91 1991–97 Kortmann et al. Int J Radiat Onc Biol phys 2000;46:269–279 Updated results von Hoff EJC 2009	19 M2–M3	35.2 Gy CSI (PF 55.2 Gy) with either ifosfamide, ara-C, etoposide, HD-methotrexate, and cisplatin before radiotherapy (sandwich), or vincristine, cisplatin, and lomustine following radiotherapy (maintenance)	3-year EFS 30 ± 15% across both groups; 10-year EFS: Sandwich 40 ± 12% vs. 32 ± 11% ($p = 0.812$)	No benefit to sandwich chemotherapy in high-risk patients.
SIOP PNET3 1992–2000 Taylor et al EJC 2005; 41:727–734	68 M2–M3	Vincristine, etoposide, carboplatin, cyclophosphamide followed by 35.2 Gy CSI (PF 55.2 Gy)	5-year EFS 34.7% (95% CI 23.2–46.2%)	No apparent improvement in outcome for M2+ disease compared to previous studies with the addition of pre-RTx chemotherapy
SJMB96 1996–2003 Gajjar et al Lancet Oncol 2006; 7: 813–820	48 M1–M3	Topotecan pre-RTx, then 36–39.6 Gy CSI (PF 55.8 Gy), then four cycles high-dose chemotherapy (vincristine, cisplatin, cyclophosphamide) and autologous SCR	5-year EFS 70% (95% CI 55–85%) M+ disease 5-year EFS was 66% (CI 48–83).	Chemotherapy adds significantly to survival of high-risk patients; sequence of chemotherapy and choice of agent critical to success. LCA histology poor prognostic factor
COG 99701 1998–2004 Jakacki et al. JCO 2012; 30:2648–2653	161 M+, R+, or ST- PNET (81 M+)	Vincristine and daily carboplatin during radiotherapy (36 Gy plus boost to sites of disease), followed by maintenance chemotherapy—regimen A: Cyclophosphamide + vincristine regimen B: Same + cisplatin × six cycles	5-year PFS 71 + 11% in carboplatin dose-finding cohort (regimen A); 5-year PFS 59 + 10% for standardized carboplatin dose plus cisplatin cohort (regimen B) 5-year OS regimen A: 82% 5-year OS regimen B: 68% $p = 0.36$	Radiosensitization with carboplatin, followed by low-intensity maintenance chemotherapy is a promising strategy and is well tolerated. Importance of confirming new lesions by biopsy to exclude treatment-related effects noted
HIT 2000 2001–2007 von Bueren JCO 2016	123 (M+)	Cyclophosphamide, methotrexate, carboplatin, etoposide, vincristine, IT methotrexate × two cycles followed by CSI (40 Gy hyperfractionated or 35.2 Gy normofractionated) if no PD followed by maintenance with cisplatin, lomustine, vincristine × four cycles	5-year EFS 62% 5-year OS 74%	LCA histology and nonresponse after first HIT-SKK cycle were poor prognostic factors

CSI craniospinal irradiation, *PF* posterior fossa, *RTx* radiotherapy, *chemo* chemotherapy, *EFS* event-free survival, *M* Chang M-stage, *R* residual disease, *HD* high-dose, *SCR* stem cell rescue, *PD* progressive disease, *IT* intrathecal, *LCA* large cell/anaplastic

Conclusions for High-Risk Medulloblastoma

The outcome for patients with high-risk medulloblastoma has steadily improved with cure rates now approaching 70%, even for patients with macrometastatic disease (Gajjar et al. 2006; Tarbell et al. 2013; Jakacki et al. 2012; von Bueren et al. 2016). The common denominator among studies which have achieved these survival rates is the use of higher CSI doses (39–40 Gy) with boosts to sites of macrometastatic disease (Gajjar et al. 2006; Tarbell et al. 2013; von Bueren et al. 2016) or with carboplatin radiosensitization when lower doses of CSI (36 Gy) were utilized (Jakacki et al. 2012). However, such therapies are at the limits of their optimal therapeutic ratio with a fine balance between efficacy and toxicity (Gandola et al. 2009; Nazemi et al. 2016). In addition, late effects, especially neurocognitive are most marked with higher doses of CSI. The use of pre-radiotherapy chemotherapy either adds no survival benefit or is associated with inferior survival, where delays in prolonged radiotherapy delivery times ensue. Moreover, 11–18% of patients have been shown to progress during pre-radiotherapy chemotherapy. The sequence of postsurgical therapy intensification appears to be critical, as high-dose thiotepa-based megatherapy following CSI has been associated with significant morbidity including neurotoxicity (Valteau-Couanet et al. 2005) or hepatotoxicity (Nazemi et al. 2016).

7.10.1.3 Medulloblastoma in Very Young Children

Historical perspective: By the early 1980s it was apparent that very young children (i.e., those below the age of 3 years) with brain tumors had very poor outcomes with regard to both survival and severity of neurodevelopmental and neuroendocrine effects of treatment. As a result, there was considerable reluctance to embark on curative treatment despite the fact that it was well established that many brain tumors, including medulloblastoma, were radiosensitive (Bloom et al. 1969): in the largest population-based cohort of the era, 31% of 548 UK children

diagnosed before the age of 2 years between 1971 and 1985 (Lashford et al. 1996; Stiller and Bunch 1992) died either without any treatment, or within 1 month of neurosurgery as their only treatment. US-based population studies in the pre-chemotherapy era include a report of 54 cases over 40 years from 1935 in Connecticut (Farwell et al. 1978), and 91 cases recorded in the fledgling SEER registry between 1973 and 1980 (Duffner et al. 1986). The disparity between such figures suggests that significant numbers of very young children with brain tumors were not reaching specialist centers or embarking on treatment with curative intent.

Because many adverse effects of treatment were attributable to radiotherapy, attempts were made to investigate whether the addition of chemotherapy following surgery would permit the postponement of radiotherapy until beyond the most critical stages of neurological development. Early studies were performed as single-institution case series, and recruited primarily by patient age rather than by histological diagnosis. The principle of multidrug treatment protocols was relatively new at the time, and one of the earliest trials (van Eys et al. 1985) used a MOPP regimen adapted from that used in lymphoma. Although still only recruiting an average of two patients a year across all types of brain tumor, this study demonstrated that medulloblastoma was chemosensitive, and that complete responses could be achieved and in some cases sustained in medulloblastoma through the use of postoperative chemotherapy alone.

In subsequent studies multicenter studies (Geyer et al. 1994; Duffner et al. 1999), radiotherapy was successfully delayed for 1–2 years in some patients; furthermore, while the intention was that patients should receive radiotherapy according to local protocol at the end of chemotherapy, in practice it was common for treating centers not to proceed to radiotherapy in those children who showed no signs of active disease at this point. While phase 3 trials directly comparing different chemotherapy protocols were not performed in this era, comparison of trial outcomes suggested that, as with older children, the dose intensity achieved by using fewer drugs in higher doses gave a superior outcome to an eight drugs in 1-day approach (Geyer et al. 1994; Duffner et al. 1999). These trials also confirmed that completeness of initial resection (at this point in time generally assessed intraoperatively by the neurosurgeon rather than by cross-sectional imaging) was of independent prognostic significance in this age group. In Europe, both the UKCCSG/SIOP 9204 (Grundy et al. 2010) and the German HIT SKK87 studies found an excess of desmoplastic histology among very young children, with this subtype being an independent predictor of significantly better survival compared to classic histology (Rutkowski et al. 2005).

Early case series and collaborative trials had therefore provided proof of principle that chemotherapy could be used to postpone and in some cases omit radiotherapy in the treatment of medulloblastoma in very young children. Subsequent trials sought to improve on event-free survival by intensifying treatment with high-dose chemotherapy with autologous stem cell rescue or intraventricular chemotherapy.

The German-led HIT-SKK 92 trial showed excellent 5-year progression-free survival of $82 \pm 9\%$ for M0R0 patients using a 27-week chemotherapy program including 36 doses of intraventricular methotrexate administered via an implanted reservoir device (Rutkowski et al. 2005). Unfortunately neurodevelopmental outcome in patients treated with intraventricular methotrexate was inferior to that for systemic chemotherapy alone, though better than for radiotherapy in the HIT 87 cohort (Rutkowski et al. 2009). Follow-up MRI imaging demonstrated leukoencephalopathy associated with intraventricular methotrexate (Rutkowski et al. 2005).

The US Head-Start high dose chemotherapy/stem cell rescue program sought to intensify chemotherapy in very young children through the use of high dose chemotherapy part of radiation-sparing first-line therapy, while the French BBSFOP trial reserved high-dose chemotherapy until after disease progression. The French trial demonstrated less than 30% progression-free survival in M0R0 patients aged under 5 years with standard-dose chemotherapy alone (Grill et al.

2005), compared to 64% in the HeadStart cohort (Dhall et al. 2008). Recruitment of patients with metastatic or non-resected disease to the French trial was stopped early and earlier treatment intensification given. Both these trials had higher than anticipated treatment-related mortality associated with HDC/SCR, though the later HeadStart II trial had fewer problems (Dhall et al. 2008).

Meta-analysis of 270 cases of medulloblastoma in very young children (Rutkowski et al. 2010) confirmed the reasonable overall prognosis for very young children with fully resected, non-metastatic disease, with OR at 8 years of 77% for this group, compared to 50% for R+ and 27% for M2+. Very young children with desmoplastic or MBEN histology (40% of total cases) had 76% OS overall, and 85% for M0R0 cases. Most clinical subdivisions in this meta-analysis had significant disparity between progression-free survival and overall survival, representing a population of patients who survived following relapse or progression having subsequently received radiotherapy (over 20% of cases in the M0R0, M0R+ and Desmoplastic histology groups); this was not the case for those with metastatic disease, in whom OS was nearly identical to PFS (40 vs. 35% for M1; 27 vs. 26% for M2–3). This contrasts with the survival prospects of older children who relapse following radiotherapy, who subsequently do very poorly.

The last 30 years of trials have therefore shown that, as in older children, MB in very young children is chemosensitive, and can be cured by even standard-dose postoperative chemotherapy alone in a significant minority of cases. Increasing intensity of chemotherapy by intraventricular administration or using higher doses with stem cell support has improved this further, and encouragingly radiotherapy can still be successfully used as a rescue therapy in some patients in whom a radiation-sparing approach fails. Because of the different approach to medulloblastoma in this age group, very young children were not part of the larger medulloblastoma-specific trials that formed the initial basis for the explosion in our biological understanding of the disease, and the small medulloblastoma subsets of the baby brain cohorts did not initially receive much scientific attention. More recently, study of enlarged cohorts with greater representation of very young children has allowed new insights into the biology of the disease in very young children, and how they fit into the emerging overview of the disease landscape (Schwalbe et al. 2017; Cavalli et al. 2017).

Within the new paradigm of medulloblastoma subgroups, medulloblastoma in very young children is primarily a two-subgroup disease, with WNT cases absent in this age group, and Group 4 disease extremely rare (Schwalbe et al. 2017). In very young children, desmoplastic/nodular histology occurs almost exclusively in the SHH subgroup and is associated with better prognosis, and with survival with radiotherapy salvage following disease progression. There is emerging evidence that SHH medulloblastoma can be divided further into age-defined subgroups (Schwalbe et al. 2017; Cavalli et al. 2017), with an "Infant SHH" subtype characterized by mutations in *SUFU* rather than *PTCH*, and with resistance to inhibitors that act upstream in the SHH pathway. Group 3 disease is associated with rapid progression and treatment failure in association with *MYC* amplification and LCA histology. Again, in larger cohorts, subtypes within Group 3 particularly associated with very young children begin to emerge (Cavalli et al. 2017).

Future trials in the treatment of very young children with medulloblastoma face particular challenges: While there is an excess of SHH-activated tumors in this age group, pathway abnormalities are at a level that makes primary resistance to existing SHH pathway inhibitors likely. Inhibition of developmental pathways will also prove challenging: preclinical studies revealed premature fusion of growth plates resulting in permanent epiphyseal disruption in young mice (Kimura et al. 2008), which has since also been reported in a child treated with the SMO inhibitor Sonidegib (Kieran et al. 2017). In the current SJMB12 trial, use of the SMO inhibitor Vismodegib is restricted to patients who are skeletally mature (St Jude's Children's Research Hospital 2013).

As with older patients, the challenge of performing molecularly informed clinical trials that take into account the growing number of identifiable medulloblastoma subgroups requires international collaboration to recruit sufficient numbers; this problem is even more pressing for infants who make up a relatively small percentage of the total and have different biology and restricted treatment options (Table 7.5).

Summary of Clinical Trials in Medulloblastoma in Very Young Children

Much of our clinical understanding of medulloblastoma in very young children comes from small trials using a variety of different treatment regimens, often including large numbers of non-medulloblastoma patients. The demonstration that different tumor types had different responses to chemotherapy (Geyer et al. 1994; Duffner et al. 1993) resulted in disease-specific clinical trials for very young children with brain tumors. Subsequent follow-up of patients who did not receive trial-mandated radiotherapy demonstrated that some very young children with medulloblastoma could have long-term cure with surgery and chemotherapy alone (Geyer et al. 1994).

Later series of clinical trials for medulloblastoma in very young children revealed the prognostic importance of histology, metastatic disease, and subtotal resection (Leary et al. 2011). Nodular desmoplastic medulloblastoma portends a favorable prognosis, while metastatic disease and subtotal resection are associated with a poor prognosis. The best outcome is seen in patients with nonmetastatic nodular desmoplastic medulloblastoma, following a subtotal resection. The majority of these patients can be cured with intensive chemotherapy alone. In addition, it is clear that some very young children can be rescued following disease recurrence using radiotherapy, if radiotherapy was not used as part of up-front therapy (Rutkowski et al. 2010). To date no trials have been performed that take into account the increased understanding of disease biology (see sections below), particularly with regard to the molecular subgroups identified over the last decade.

Table 7.5 Summary of selected very young children medulloblastoma trials from the 1980s onwards

Study Enrolment dates (Reference)	Cases MB/of total	Treatment	Outcome	Main conclusions
MD Anderson 1976–1984 Van Eys et al. J Neurooncol 1985: 3(3)237–43	6/12	MOPP mechlorethamine, vincristine, procarbazine, prednisolone (single center cases series)	15/17 brain tumor patients had some response; 9 relapses after a median of 10.3 months	Confirmed feasibility of using chemotherapy to delay radiotherapy in children with brain tumors
MD Anderson 1976–1988 Ater et al. J Neurooncol 1997:32(3)243–52	12/17	Expanded van Eys cohort; restricted to MB and ependymoma	5/12 MB survive without relapse and thus without radiotherapy; 8/12 survive overall	IQ and growth status was preserved in those who did not receive radiotherapy
POG "Baby Brain" 1986–1990 Duffner et al. NEJM 1993:328 (24) 1725–31 Duffner et al. Neuro Oncol 1999: 1(2)152–61	62/192	Vincristine, cyclophosphamide, cisplatin, etoposide for 1 year (2–3 years old) or 2 years (<2 years old at diagnosis), then RTx	R+ disease: 13/27 CR or PR after 2 courses VCR/cyclo 5-year PFS 31.8 ± 8.3, OS 39.7 ± 6.9 5-year OS R0: 60 vs. 32% for R1; M0R0 69%; significant numbers did not proceed to RTx on completion of trial chemotherapy	No extra risk in delaying RTx by 2 years rather than 1 year. outcome for M0R0 comparable to contemporary trials for "standard risk" MB treated with RTx in older children Use of neoadjuvant chemotherapy could allow successful delay of radiation therapy in 40% of children under the age of 3 years. Cases of cure were seen with surgery and chemotherapy only.
CCG-921 1986–1992 Geyer et al. JCO 1994:12(4)1607–15	46/96	"8 in 1 day" for "infants" ≤ 18 months, intention for either local RTx after two cycles or CSI after 1 year	R+ disease: 6/14 CR or PR after two cycles 3-year PFS 22 ± 6%; M0R0 5/15 alive disease free at 5 years Only 9/96 patients received RTx as mandated prior to relapse	Ongoing reluctance to use radiotherapy; most relapses occurred during chemotherapy so decision to omit if disease free on completion reasonable
CCG-9921 1993–1997 Geyer et al JCO 2005: 23(30)7621–31 (Leary et al. 2011)	92/299	2 different 4-drug induction regimens, then maintenance; RTx according to R (post-induction) and M status	Regimen A 5-year EFS 37 ± 7%, regimen B 26 ± 7% M0R0: 5-year EFS 41 ± 8%; 5-year OS 54 ± 8% M0R+: 5-year EFS 26 ± 9%; 5-year OS 40 ± 11% M+:5-year EFS 25 ± 8%; 5-year OS 31 ± 9% DN: 5-year EFS 77 ± 9%; 5-year OS 85 ± 8% Classic: 5-year EFS 17 ± 5% 5-year OS 29 ± 6%	No difference between induction regimens; low concordance with trial-mandated RTx Retrospective review found better survival for desmoplastic disease and excluded 10/92 as non-MB

Table 7.5 (continued)

Study Enrolment dates (Reference)	Cases MB/of total	Treatment	Outcome	Main conclusions
COG P9934 2000–2006 Ashley et al. JCO 2012: 30(26)3181–6	74 (M0)	Four cycles induction chemotherapy followed by age and response adjusted conformal RTx	4-year EFS: 50 ± 6%; 4-year OS: 69 ± 5.5% DN: 4-year EFS: 58 ± 8% 4-year OS: 79 ± 7% Non-DN: EFS: 23 ± 12% 4-year OS: 31 ± 16%	High proportion of DN disease Impairment in cognition compared to healthy population but much of this present at diagnosis
Head start I, head start II 1992–1997, 1997–2002 Dhall et al. Pediatr Blood Cancer 2008:50(6)1169–75	21 (M0)	Five cycles induction then HDC/SCR; no radiotherapy until relapse	M0R0: CCR 13/14; M0R+: CR 7/7 after induction DN: 5-year EFS 67 ± 16%; OS 78 ± 14% Classic 5-year EFS 42 ± 14; OS 67 ± 14%	High rate of toxic death in head start I; 71% of survivors did not require radiotherapy; better outcomes for DN histology
Head start II 1997–2002 Chi et al. JCO 2004:22(24) 4881–7	9 (M+)	Five cycles induction including HD MTX then HDC/SCR; no radiotherapy until relapse	14/16 CR to induction, 1 PR, 1 stable disease 8 relapses; 5 received RTx and 2 were rescued	No toxic deaths; good response rates but not sustained; 60% of survivors did not need radiotherapy
UKCCSG 9204 1993–2003 Grundy et al. EJC 2010: 46(1) 120–133	31/97	Vincristine, carboplatin, HD methotrexate, cyclophosphamide and cisplatin	5 M0R0, 11 M0R+, 15 M+ 5-year OS DN/MBEN 52.9%, classic 33.3%	High proportion of desmoplastic and MBEN cases, with improved survival
BBSFOP 1990–2002 Grill et al. Lancet Oncol 2005:6(8) 573–80 Kalifa, Grill, J Neurooncol 2005: 75(3) 279–85	79	Standard-dose chemotherapy (carboplatin and procarbazine/etoposide and cisplatin/vincristine and cyclophosphamide; no radiotherapy until relapse	47/79 M0R0: 5-year PFS 29% (CI 18–44) 34/47 M0R0 & GTR: 5-year PFS: 41% (CI 26–58) 17/79 M0R+: 5-year PFS: 6% (CI 1–27) 15/79 M + RX: 5-year PFS: 13% (CI 4–38)	R0 cases with surgical subtotal resection had very poor survival Standard-dose chemotherapy insufficient to prevent relapse in R1 and M+ disease
HIT 87 1987–1992 Rutkowski et al Neuro Oncol 2009: 11(2) 201–20	29	M0R0: 3-drug maintenance including HD MTX R1M0, M+: 6-drug induction including HD MTX (two cycles) then maintenance; RTx at 3 years or at relapse	10-year PFS 48.5 ± 9.3%; 10-year OS 55.2 ± 9.3% M+ no survivors at 10 years DN/MBEN: 10-year PFS & 10-year OS: 88.9 ± 10.5% Cla 10-year PFS: 30.0 ± 10.3%; OS: 40.0 ± 11.0%	Long delay in publication; good survival overall and for M0R0 cases in particular; metastasis predict poor outcome Retrospective path review revealed desmoplasia to confer good prognosis
HIT 92 1992–1997 Rutkowski et al. NEJM 2005: 352(10) 978–86	43	Three cycles induction chemotherapy including intraventricular MTX	5-year PFS 58 ± 9%; 5-year OS: 66 ± 7% M0R0: 5-year PFS: 82 ± 9%; 5-year OS: 93 ± 6% M0R+: 5-year PFS: 50 ± 13%; 5-year OS: 56 ± 14% M+ RX: 5-year PFS: 33 ± 14%; 5-year OS: 38 ± 15%	High rates of survival with intraventricular MTX, particularly for M0R0 disease but even in high-risk cases; Evidence of developmental damage attributable to intraventricular MTX

(continued)

Table 7.5 (continued)

Study Enrolment dates (Reference)	Cases MB/of total	Treatment	Outcome	Main conclusions
HIT 2000 2000–2006 Von Bueren et al Neuro Oncol 2011: 13(6) 669–79	48 (M0)	Three cycles induction chemotherapy including intraventricular MTX, then two cycles consolidation if in CR	5-year survival without receiving CSI was 59 ± 7% DN: 5-year EFs 95 ± 5%; 5-year OS (100 ± 0%) Classic: 5-year EFS 30 ± 11%; 5-year OS 68 ± 10% LCA: 5-year EFS/OS: 33 ± 27% R0: 5-year EFS 60 ± 9%; 5-year OS 84 ± 6% R+: 5-year EFS 33 ± 19%; 5-year OS 50 ± 20%	Confirmed Desmoplasia and MBEN as a strong favorable prognostic factor; high proportion of classic disease relapsed without radiotherapy

CSI craniospinal irradiation, *PF* posterior fossa, *RTx* radiotherapy, *chemo* chemotherapy, *EFS* event-free survival, *M* Chang M-stage, *R* residual disease (R0: no residual disease; R+: residual disease; RX: any R status), *HD* high-dose, *SCR* stem cell rescue, *Cla* Classic histology, *DN* desmoplastic/nodular histology, *MBEN* medulloblastoma with extensive nodularity, *LCA* large cell/anaplastic histology, *GTR* gross total resection

7.11 Relapsed Medulloblastoma

With the exception of very young patients who relapse following radiation-sparing treatment and can subsequently be salvaged using radiotherapy, outcome in relapsed medulloblastoma is currently dismal (Pizer et al. 2011), with little prospect for cure. The biology of relapsed disease is poorly understood, as most biological studies, cell lines, and animal models have been based on primary tumor samples that are derived from material obtained at initial surgery, and re-biopsy at relapse has only rarely been performed. The importance of obtaining biological samples at relapse is increasingly being recognized, although there are competing considerations, notably the morbidity of surgery in what is still regarded as a palliative setting.

There is increasing evidence from paired diagnostic and relapse samples that significant changes in medulloblastoma biology occur during the course of treatment. In a cohort of 29 relapsed patients, a combination of *MYC*-family amplification and *TP53* pathway defects was acquired in 32% of cases, while such abnormalities were not

lost if present at initial biopsy (Hill et al. 2015). In a mouse model of relapsed SHH medulloblastoma (produced by partial resection followed by 18 Gy radiotherapy of tumors arising in mice with SHH pathway mutation) substantial genetic divergence was found between the original tumors and those recurring post treatment, possibly due to a clonal selection effect of radiotherapy (Morrissy et al. 2016). Driver *Trp53* mutations were not clonal at diagnosis but did become so at relapse. The same authors noted significant differences in somatic mutations in paired diagnostic and relapse samples from patients treated for medulloblastoma. Relapsed samples had increased prevalence of somatic mutations (a median fivefold increase in the majority of tumors), while many mutations found at diagnosis (60% of the total) were reduced or absent from relapse samples and many relapse samples had de novo mutations not seen in primary tumors. Almost 80% of recurrent SHH medulloblastomas were found to have *TP53* pathway mutations, *DYNC1H1* mutations, or chromosome 14 loss. Despite the acquisition of new driver mutations by the tumors in these studies, all cases studied remained in the same subgroup at relapse as at diagnosis, confirming the link between subgroups and fundamental and early changes in the development of the disease. Thus, evidence is emerging that tumor biology and behavior in patients who relapse is unlikely to be adequately represented or predicted by samples obtained at diagnosis. To ensure appropriate selection and assessment of targeted therapies at relapse, it will be important to confirm the presence of molecular targets in relapsed disease before embarking on treatment.

7.12 Late Effects of Medulloblastoma Therapy

Late effects in medulloblastoma survivors are complex and multifactorial, and affect a number of organ systems. Mechanical effects of the tumor itself, raised intracranial pressure, local damage to the cerebellum and its connections attributable to surgical resection, postoperative radiotherapy, and chemotherapy, as well as disruption of normal development because of prolonged periods of hospitalization all contribute to neurodevelopmental and cognitive problems, while cachexia and inadequate caloric intake due to treatment-related nausea are implicated in poor growth immediately following surgery and later complicated by effects of CSI: onset of growth hormone insufficiency and direct effects on growth of the bones of the axial skeleton, and dysfunction of the hypothalamo-gonadal axis affecting timing and control of pubertal growth (Meacham et al. 2004; Fouladi et al. 2005).

7.13 Impact of CSI on Neurological Development

CSI in particular is implicated in medulloblastoma late effects. It is a particular feature of medulloblastoma treatment compared to other pediatric malignancies, having been superseded by intrathecal and high-dose chemotherapy in the prophylaxis of CNS disease in leukemias. Other brain tumors can be adequately treated by sur-

gery alone in the case of low-grade tumors such as low-grade gliomas, or by localized radiotherapy without whole CNS coverage in the case of ependymomas.

A systematic review (Hanzlik et al. 2015) of papers published between 2000 and 2012 studying neuropsychological outcomes in a total of 456 children (age 0–18 years at diagnosis) treated for posterior fossa tumors and with a minimum follow-up of 3 years post-diagnosis found that medulloblastoma survivors consistently had significantly worse scores for IQ, memory, and attention/executive function than standardized population means, with medulloblastoma survivors tending to fare worse than survivors of both ependymoma and astrocytoma in studies where such comparisons were made. All 212 medulloblastoma patients in this review received CSI, despite 5 of 9 individual studies reporting the inclusion of children under the age of 3 years. Risk factors consistently associated with worse neuropsychological outcome included younger age at diagnosis, and whole brain rather than focal irradiation. While IQ scores in medulloblastoma patients are reported to be subject to ongoing decline (Ris et al. 2001; Palmer et al. 2007), reduction in IQ in ependymoma patients who had received posterior fossa radiation was static over a 5-year period following treatment (Netson et al. 2012).

A prospective longitudinal study compared the effects of risk-adapted CSI dose (23.4 vs. 36 Gy) on IQ and academic achievement (Mulhern et al. 1998). All patients were treated with the same adjuvant chemotherapy. Average-risk and high-risk patients revealed a decrease in mean IQ (0.99 vs. 3 IQ points/year), with the greatest decreases seen in younger (<7 years) patients (2.41 and 3.71 IQ points/year for average-risk and high-risk patients, respectively). These findings support the notion that CSI dose reductions for patients with average-risk disease result in increased preservation of neurocognitive function.

Ongoing loss of cognitive function long after radiotherapy in medulloblastoma is thought to be due to white matter loss. An MRI imaging study of 42 children with medulloblastoma CSI found that approximately 70% of the observed correlation between age at radiotherapy (and hence time since radiotherapy) and IQ was explained by differences in normally appearing white matter volume (Mulhern et al. 2001); later studies have shown correlations with individual components of cognitive function (Brinkman et al. 2012). Intrathecal methotrexate chemotherapy has also been implicated in white matter loss through long-term follow-up of twenty survivors of two consecutive historical cohorts, the first of which (1985–90) received intrathecal (IT) methotrexate in addition to postoperative chemo- and radiotherapy, while the second (1990–95) did not. The earlier cohort had worse cognitive outcomes, which correlated with extent of MRI findings of leukomalacia (Riva et al. 2002).

In recent years, prospective studies have looked at individual components of cognitive ability, with the aim of identifying which specific domains require intervention and rehabilitation. A study looking at processing speed, attention, and working memory in 126 childhood medulloblastoma survivors (Palmer et al. 2013) found that younger age at diagnosis was associated with a worse outcome for processing speed, while high-risk disease predicted worse outcome over all three domains. A different study used a standardized tool to investigate 12 different domains in a heterogeneous sample of eight children treated for medulloblastoma in childhood, at around 3 and 5 years posttreatment. This small study again found ongoing deterioration in cognitive function in most indices, with verbal comprehension, perceptual organization, social perception, and psychomotor skills particularly affected, and identified a need to plan for social as well as educational rehabilitation following treatment (Saury and Emanuelson 2011).

While increasingly complex psychometric testing, performed with progressively greater maturity of follow-up, is now being studied, there has been renewed interest in long-term "real-life" outcomes. An early, single-center case series of 37 very young medulloblastoma patients, all treated with radiotherapy between 1956 and 1988, found 13 still living and an additional 3 who survived for 10 years post treatment. Of

these 16 survivors, 9 had attended mainstream schools with support for learning difficulties and 6 had attended special schools. Of the 9 survivors who had reached school leaving age, 1 of the 2 who had obtained a job had managed to keep it until dying at the age of 22 from complications of chemotherapy. None of the survivors had married and only 1 was noted to be living independently (Kiltie et al. 1997). A more recent single-center series of 33 infants diagnosed with any brain tumor under the age of 1 year and treated between 1982 and 2005 found that of 20 survivors, 12 had a good outcome (defined as no or mild disability and leading an active life). Ten were either attending mainstream schooling or in skilled employment. Fourteen had some form of neurological deficit, including seizures, limb weakness, and cranial nerve dysfunction. One survivor still needed assisted ventilation and gastrostomy feeding. Again in this series, diagnosis of medulloblastoma ($n = 3$) was associated with worse outcome (Pillai et al. 2012).

7.14 Hearing Deficits

Audiologic toxicity is a major and frequently permanent side effect endured by medulloblastoma patients, mainly due to the use of cisplatin, but also secondary to the use of radiotherapy. Indeed, in the COG A9961 study, which utilized 23.40 Gy CSI and cisplatin-based chemotherapy, cumulative Grade 3 or 4 toxicity was seen in nearly one-quarter of the patients (Packer et al. 2006).

7.15 Endocrine Outcomes

Therapy for medulloblastoma involves radiation doses to the hypothalamic-pituitary axis resulting in significant endocrinologic toxicity, including growth hormone, thyroid hormone, adrenocorticotropic hormone (ACTH), and sex steroid deficiencies. Studies suggest that almost all children treated with radiation doses in excess of 35.00 Gy will develop growth hormone deficiency, which generally occurs within the first 5 years after treatment (Sklar and Constine 1995). Indeed, a prospective study for medulloblastoma, called SJMB96 (Laughton et al. 2008), where patients received risk-adapted CSI (23.4 Gy for average risk, 36.0 Gy for M0/1 high-risk disease and 36.0–39.6 Gy for M2/M3 high-risk disease), found that almost all patients (4-year cumulative incidence 93 ± 4% overall) experienced growth hormone failure which was associated with impaired linear growth. Of note while no significant difference was observed between the different treatment groups, the estimated decline in height z-scores was significantly greater in high-risk patients compared with average-risk patients, possibly due to the direct effects on bone in those receiving higher doses of CSI. Similarly, ACTH deficiency was not influenced by hypothalamic radiation dose, with a 36 ± 7% cumulative incidence for average-risk patients compared with 41 ± 10% cumulative incidence for high-risk patients. In contrast, TSH deficiency and primary hypothyroidism were both significantly more common in high-risk patients than average-risk patients (89 ± 13% vs. 54 ± 9%, and 44 ± 19% vs. 11 ± 8%, respectively). Consistent with these data a recent review of 109 children of all ages treated for medulloblastoma in a single center over a 20-year period from 1982 to 2002 described endocrine outcomes in 35 survivors for whom both treatment and late effects data was available (Uday et al. 2015). 34/35 patients (97%) developed complete or partial growth hormone deficiency. 16/35 survivors (46%) developed ACTH deficiency, and seven patients (20%) had precocious puberty, while one presented with delayed puberty. Eight survivors (23%) developed gonadal dysfunction as adults (7 males, 5 with primary hypogonadism (14%) of whom 3 (9%) had previously had either precocious or delayed puberty, and 2 with secondary hypogonadism (6%); 1 female (3%) with primary hypogonadism). Twenty (57%) survivors developed primary hypothyroidism, with six being symptomatic at presentation and the remainder diagnosed on routine follow-up screening. Reducing the CSI dose appears to improve endocrine outcomes. For example, in a small series (Xu et al. 2004) of seven survivors who had been treated

with 18 Gy CSI, although all seven patients required GH replacement, adult and sitting heights were significantly greater for the group that received 18 Gy compared to a historical cohort of 12 comparable children who received between 23 and 39 Gy CSI. Notably adult heights for the 18 Gy cohort were not different from mid-parental heights. In addition, hypothyroidism, hypoadrenalism, hypogonadism, and precocious puberty were all absent or less frequent in the 18 Gy group. The authors concluded that endocrine morbidity was significantly reduced with 18 Gy CSI (Xu et al. 2004).

In summary, a strong correlation between total radiation dose and the development of pituitary hormone deficiencies exists. Lower doses of CSI (18–24 Gy) are likely to cause isolated growth hormone deficiency, whereas higher doses (>60 Gy) frequently cause panhypopituitarism. A variable endocrine phenotype has been observed with intermediate doses. A high dose spread over a longer period of time in smaller fractions is likely to reduce the incidence of hypopituitarism (Uday et al. 2015). While survivors now undergo regular long-term follow-up, and the availability of hormone replacement means that deficiencies can be treated, the high prevalence of endocrine late-effects is still a significant contributor to treatment-related morbidity (Mostoufi-Moab and Grimberg 2010). Of note, growth hormone treatment has been shown not to be associated with an increased risk of medulloblastoma relapse, as was previously speculated (Rohrer et al. 2010; Darendeliler et al. 2006).

7.16 The Present: Molecular Stratification of Medulloblastoma

Over the past decade, the application of high-throughput array techniques to combined international cohorts totaling more than 1300 children with medulloblastoma has led to an avalanche of data and the dissection of the complex molecular biology of medulloblastoma. Whereas medulloblastoma was previously considered one disease, these studies have identified a compendium of at least four different diseases, defined by unique molecular profiles, clinical behavior, and outcomes.

The first transcriptomic analysis of a number of different malignant pediatric brain tumors in 2002 showed medulloblastoma, PNET, ATRT, and high-grade glioma to be distinct biological entities (Pomeroy et al. 2002). Subsequent cohorts, initially numbering a few dozen cases in the mid-2000s (Thompson et al. 2006; Kool et al. 2008) and building to nearly 200 patient samples in 2011 (Cho et al. 2011) demonstrated the existence of between 4 and 6 identifiable medulloblastoma subgroups. Common to all analyses were groups characterized by abnormalities in the WNT and SHH pathways, already identified due to their involvement in inherited cancer syndromes. The remaining Non-WNT, Non-SHH tumors were divided between 2 to 4 subgroups,

which while distinct from the SHH and WNT subgroups, showed a considerable degree of overlap between themselves. All studies found distinct subgroups within the non-WNT/SHH grouping, variously associated with isochromosome 17q and other chromosome 17 abnormalities, LCA histology, and *MYC* copy number abnormalities. The studies with the largest cohorts all identified subgroups associated with photoreceptor gene expression and neuronal activation, with a degree of overlap between the two (Kool et al. 2008; Cho et al. 2011). A consensus conference in Boston in late 2010 (Taylor et al. 2012) subsequently settled on four core subgroups comprising WNT, SHH, Group 3, and Group 4 medulloblastoma, with a recognition that future subdivisions within these subgroups was likely (Taylor et al. 2012; Northcott et al. 2011a; Kool et al. 2012) (Fig. 7.7). This molecular subgrouping

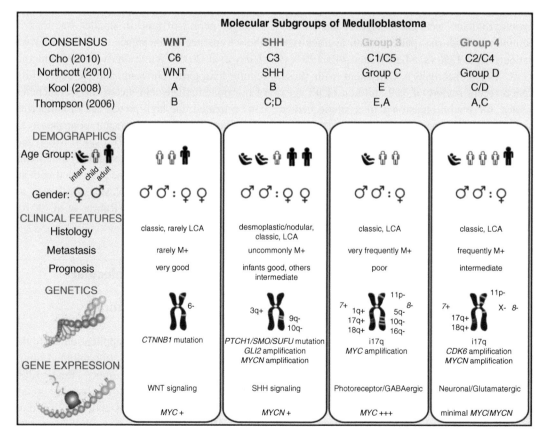

Fig. 7.7 Schematic diagram illustrating the four consensus subgroups identified in medulloblastoma, with their associated demographic, clinical, and biological features, and their relationships to previous attempts at subgrouping. Taken from Taylor et al. (2012)

has also been incorporated into the updated WHO classification of Tumors of the Central Nervous System, which utilizes a tiered approach to diagnosis (Louis et al. 2016).

Importantly, these subgroups are of immediate clinical value: the WNT subgroup, while the least common, identifies a group of childhood tumors with excellent prognosis (Ellison et al. 2005; Clifford et al. 2006), while small-molecule inhibitors of the SHH pathway are available for targeted therapy in the SHH subgroup (Rudin et al. 2009; Gajjar et al. 2013). Identification of medulloblastoma subgroups has also enabled resolution of previously inconclusive data regarding the prognostic significance of mutations and cytogenetic abnormalities found in medulloblastoma and allowed the development of subgroup-specific classifications combining with clinical and biological variables (Shih et al. 2014) (Table 7.6).

Although no unifying mutation has been identified and most of the mutations found in medulloblastoma were restricted to single cases, recurrent mutations in chromatin-regulating genes have been identified in up to 40% of medulloblastomas, many of which were subgroup specific (Jones et al. 2012, 2013), while a smaller proportion were seen across all four subgroups (e.g., mutations in *MLL2* and *MLL3* (Parsons et al. 2011)). Higher-level bioinformatic analysis of chromatin immunoprecipitation and sequencing (ChIP-seq) data has permitted the identification of networks of enhancers and superenhancers (large regions containing multiple enhancers) that map to the four major medulloblastoma subgroups, and in the case of Group 4, a superenhancer signature has indicated a possible cell of origin for this subgroup (Lin et al. 2016). Thus, epigenomic

dysregulation has emerged as a critical step in medulloblastoma pathogenesis.

The genetic landscape of medulloblastoma. Recurrent genetic aberrations identified in medulloblastoma (derived from Northcott et al. 2012a, b, Robinson et al. 2012, Pugh et al. 2012, Jones et al. 2012, and Northcott et al. 2014), averaged and displayed proportionally by height of terrain peaks. The figure reveals the unique subgroup-specific molecular aberration and highlights chromatin remodeling mutations as the unifying theme among all four medulloblastoma subgroups. Wingless (WNT) medulloblastoma (left; blue icy landscape), the most molecularly homogenous group, consists of *CTNNB1* mutations in 85%, monosomy 6 in 80%, *DDX3X* mutation in 50%, *TP53* mutation in 13%, and mutations in chromatin remodeling genes in 49.5% (composed of mutations in *SMARCA4* [25%], *MLL2* [12.5%], *CREBBP* [6%], *TRAPP* [3%], and *MED13* [3%]). For the chromatin remodeling peaks (darker colored shading), only the most commonly mutated gene is labeled. Sonic hedgehog (SHH) medulloblastoma (bottom; red volcanic landscape) consists of *PTCH1* mutation/deletion in 29%, *TP53* mutation in 18%, *DDX3X* mutation in 11%, *GLI2* amplification/mutation in 8%, *MYCN* amplification in 6%, *SUFU* mutation in 6%, *SMO* mutation in 3%, *PTEN* deletion in 2.5%, *MYCL1* amplification in 2%, *CDK6* amplification in 1%, *MYCC* amplification in 0.7%, and mutations in chromatin remodeling genes in 21% (composed of mutations in *MLL2* [12%], *BCOR* [3%], *LBD1* [3%], *NCOR2* [1.5%], and *SMARCA4* [1.5%]). Group 3 medulloblastoma (top; yellow desert rocky terrain) is characterized by *GFI1/1B* structural variants (e.g., inversions, duplications) in 41%, isochromosome (iso) 17q in 26%, transforming

Table 7.6 Proposed stratification algorithm based on molecular subgroup; M stage; GLI2 and MYC amplification status, and cytogenetic abnormalities in chromosomes 11, 14 and 17 (Shih et al. 2014)

	WNT	SHH	Group 3	Group 4
High risk		Either *GLI2* amp, OR both 14q loss and M+	Any one of *MYC* amp OR iso17q OR M+	Neither 11 loss nor 17 gain; M+
Standard risk		No *GLI2* amp; 14q loss OR M+;	None of the above	Neither 11 loss nor 17 gain; M-
Low risk	All low risk	None of the above		Either 11 loss or 17 gain

M+ metastatic disease at presentation, *amp* amplification, *iso17q* isochromosome 17q

growth factor (TGF)—signaling in 20%, *MYCC* amplification in 17%, *PVT1* alterations in 12%, *OTX2* amplification in 8%, *MYCN* amplification in 4%, *DDX3X* mutation in 3%, *CDK6* amplification in 1%, and mutations in chromatin remodeling genes in 28.5% (composed of mutations in *SMARCA4* [10.5%], other *KDM* family members [5%], *MLL2* [4%], *KDMA6A* [3%], *GPS2* [3%], *MLL3* [1%], *CREBBP* [1%], and *CHD7* [1%]). Group 4 medulloblastoma (right; green forest mountain terrain) is characterized by iso 17q in 80%, *GFI1/1B* structural variants in 10%, *SNCAIP* tandem duplications in 10%, *OTX2* amplification in 5.5%, *MYCN* amplification in 5%, *CDK6* amplification in 5%, *TP53* mutation in 1%, *MYCC* amplification in 1%, and mutations in chromatin remodeling genes in 30% (composed of mutations in *KDMA6A* [13%], other *KDM* family members [4%], *MLL3* [3%], *CHD7* [3%], *ZMYM3* [3%], *MLL2* [2%], *GPS2* [1%], and *BCOR* [1%])

7.16.1 WNT-Subgroup Medulloblastoma

The WNT subgroup is the best-characterized and least common subgroup, accounting for approximately 10% of medulloblastoma patients (Table 7.7). The association of Turcot syndrome with medulloblastoma (see Table 7.1) led to the identification of a subset of childhood medulloblastoma with aberrant WNT signaling, nuclear β catenin immunopositivity, and good prognosis prior to the era of expression analysis (Ellison et al. 2005; Clifford et al. 2006; Pomeroy and Sturla 2003).

WNT-subgroup medulloblastoma has a female preponderance and generally arises in older children, with a median age of 10 years; WNT tumors have not been reported in children under the age of 3 years. Almost all WNT subgroup medulloblastomas exhibit classic histology, though occasionally there are LCA. The nodular desmoplastic histological variant of medulloblastoma has not been reported in patients with WNT subgroup medulloblastoma (Ellison et al. 2011a, b). Most are non-metastatic at presentation (Kool et al. 2012). Animal studies suggest that they originate from cells located in the lower rhombic lip (Gibson et al. 2010) and occur as a result of aberrant cell migration; therefore, as a result they are most frequently located centrally and adherent to the brainstem (Fig. 7.9a). This location may have clinical implications at the time of surgical resection, in particular in relation to development of posterior fossa syndrome (see Sect. 7.7). Monosomy 6 is the hallmark cytogenetic abnormality of WNT subgroup and occurs in around 85% of cases (Gajjar et al. 2006; Ellison 2010; Ellison et al. 2011a, b; Fattet et al. 2009). Otherwise, WNT tumors are largely devoid of recurrent focal regions of deletion or gain (Northcott et al. 2012b).

MB_{WNT} is also very homogenous at a molecular level, and is defined by specific recurrent mutations (Jones et al. 2012; Northcott et al. 2012a; Robinson et al. 2012; Pugh et al. 2012) (Fig. 7.8). Mutations in exon 3 of the *CTNNB1* gene occur in 85% of cases, and result in reduced cytoplasmic degradation and nuclear accumulation of the WNT pathway transcription factor β-catenin. Mutations in *DDX3X*, which encodes

Table 7.7 Frequency of the four medulloblastoma subgroups

Reference	Total number of samples	WNT	SHH	Group 3	Group 4
Northcott et al. (2011b)	827	76 (9%)	266 (32%)	168 (20%)	317 (38%)
Robinson et al. (2015)	93	11 (12%)	13 (14%)	17 (18%)	38 (41%)
Pugh et al. (2012)	92	6 (6.5%)	23 (25%)	33 (36%)	30 (32.6%)
Jones et al. (2012)	125	15 (12%)	30 (24%)	26 (21%)	40 (32%)
Average	1137	10%	24%	24%	36%

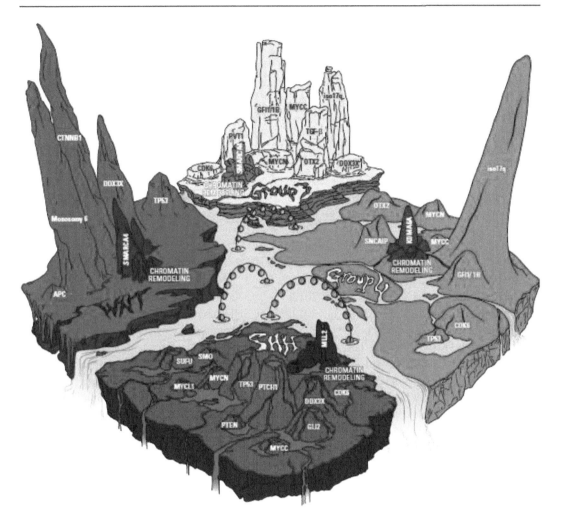

Fig. 7.8 The genetic landscape of medulloblastoma (taken from Gajjar et al. 2015). Recurrent genetic aberrations identified in medulloblastoma (derived from Northcott et al. 2012a, b; Robinson et al. 2012; Pugh et al. 2012; Jones et al. 2012; and Northcott et al. 2014), averaged and displayed proportionally by height of terrain peaks. The figure reveals the unique subgroup-specific molecular aberration and highlights chromatin remodeling mutations as the unifying theme among all four medulloblastoma subgroups. Wingless (WNT) medulloblastoma (left; blue icy landscape), the most molecularly homogenous group, consists of CTNNB1 mutations in 85%, monosomy 6 in 80%, DDX3X mutation in 50%, TP53 mutation in 13%, and mutations in chromatin remodeling genes in 49.5% (composed of mutations in SMARCA4 [25%], MLL2 [12.5%], CREBBP [6%], TRAPP [3%], and MED13 [3%]). For the chromatin remodeling peaks (darker colored shading), only the most commonly mutated gene is labeled. Sonic hedgehog (SHH) medulloblastoma (bottom; red volcanic landscape) consists of PTCH1 mutation/deletion in 29%, TP53 mutation in 18%, DDX3X mutation in 11%, GLI2 amplification/mutation in 8%, MYCN amplification in 6%, SUFU mutation in 6%, SMO mutation in 3%, PTEN deletion in 2.5%, MYCL1 amplification in 2%, CDK6 amplification in 1%, MYCC amplification in 0.7%, and mutations in chromatin remodeling genes in 21% (composed of mutations in MLL2 [12%], BCOR [3%], LBD1 [3%], NCOR2 [1.5%], and SMARCA4 [1.5%]). Group 3 medulloblastoma (top; yellow desert rocky terrain) is characterized by GFI1/1B structural variants (e.g., inversions, duplications) in 41%, isochromosome (iso) 17q in 26%, transforming growth factor (TGF)-signaling in 20%, MYCC amplification in 17%, PVT1 alterations in 12%, OTX2 amplification in 8%, MYCN amplification in 4%, DDX3X mutation in 3%, CDK6 amplification in 1%, and mutations in chromatin remodelling genes in 28.5% (composed of mutations in SMARCA4 [10.5%], other KDM family members [5%], MLL2 [4%], KDMA6A [3%], GPS2 [3%], MLL3 [1%], CREBBP [1%], and CHD7 [1%]). Group 4 medulloblastoma (right; green forest mountain terrain) is characterized by iso 17q in 80%, GFI1/1B structural variants in 10%, SNCAIP tandem duplications in 10%, OTX2 amplification in 5.5%, MYCN amplification in 5%, CDK6 amplification in 5%, TP53 mutation in 1%, MYCC amplification in 1%, and mutations in chromatin remodeling genes in 30% (composed of mutations in KDMA6A [13%], other KDM family members [4%], MLL3 [3%], CHD7 [3%], ZMYM3 [3%], MLL2 [2%], GPS2 [1%], and BCOR [1%])

for an RNA helicase required for chromosomal segregation, are enriched in MB$_{WNT}$, being present in 50% of cases compared to 11 and 3% of SHH and Group 3 tumors, respectively. Frequent coexistence of *DDX3X* and *CTNNB1* gene mutations suggests these may cooperate in the development of WNT subgroup medulloblastoma.

Of note, approximately 12–15% of WNT tumors are found to harbor *TP53* mutations; however, these are not associated with a poor prognosis or with underlying *TP53* germline mutations (Li Fraumeni syndrome) (Zhukova et al. 2013; Shih et al. 2014; Lindsey et al. 2011) in this subgroup. In WNT tumors, chromatin dysregulation occurs either through mutations in *MLL2* (13%) or the SWI/SNF chromatin remodeling complex member *SMARCA4* (25%) (Jones et al. 2012; Northcott et al. 2012a; Robinson et al. 2012; Pugh et al. 2012).

Most notably, MB$_{WNT}$ has the best prognosis of all subgroups. Patients with MB$_{WNT}$ have excellent survival using contemporary therapy, with 5-year EFS over 90% (Gajjar et al. 2006; Ellison et al. 2005, 2011b; Fattet et al. 2009). Preclinical studies suggest that the excellent prognosis associated with MB$_{WNT}$ is due to increased permeability of the blood brain barrier, secondary to paracrine signals driven by mutant β-catenin, which allows high levels of chemotherapy to build up within the tumor (Phoenix et al. 2016). While patients with MB$_{WNT}$ and LCA histology appear to retain a favorable outcome, the small number of cases reported (6% of MB$_{WNT}$ patients) makes the prognosis of this rare patient group uncertain (Ellison 2010; Ellison et al. 2011b). Given the extremely good prognosis of MB$_{WNT}$, the pressing clinical need in this group is to de-escalate treatment to reduce therapeutic toxicity while maintaining the excellent prospects for long-term overall survival. MB$_{WNT}$ tumors may be identified by using immunohistochemistry for nuclear β-catenin immunoreactivity on formalin-fixed paraffin embedded tissue, fluorescent in situ hybridization (FISH) to identify monosomy 6, or sequencing tumor DNA for mutations in *CTNNB1* (Ellison 2010; Ellison et al. 2011b). Combined β-catenin, YAP1 and filamin A immunoreactivity robustly confirms

the status of WNT-driven medulloblastomas (Ellison et al. 2011b), while Sanger sequencing of *CTNNB1* and methylation profiling may be even more reliable (Pietsch et al. 2014). For the purposes of clinical trials and treatment stratification, current international consensus suggests that WNT tumors should be identified using two diverse methods including nuclear β-catenin immunoreactivity, monosomy 6 by FISH or SNP array, or a *CTNNB1* mutation, WNT pattern by DNA methylation or by gene expression (Gottardo et al. 2014; Ramaswamy et al. 2016).

7.16.2 SHH Subgroup Medulloblastoma

The SHH subgroup is named for the sonic hedgehog signaling pathway, an important regulator of the growth and development of neural progenitor cells (Yang et al. 2008). SHH pathway activation is unique to MB$_{SHH}$, with around 87% of SHH tumors having identifiable mutations (e.g., *SUFU*, *PTCH*, *SMO*) or amplification (e.g., *GLI1*, *GLI2*) within the pathway (Kool et al. 2014). MB$_{SHH}$ accounts for approximately one-quarter of medulloblastoma cases (Table 7.7), most of which are of nodular desmoplastic histology (Kool et al. 2008; Cho et al. 2011), although classic and LCA histology also occur. The sex distribution is equal between males and females. Almost half of SHH cases and one-fifth of G3 cases harbor 9q loss. Animal studies suggest that SHH tumors arise from cerebellar granule neuron precursor cells (Gilbertson and Ellison 2008) and consequently these tumors are frequently located in the cerebellar hemispheres (Fig. 7.9b, c). MB$_{SHH}$ have a bimodal age distribution, occurring most commonly in very young children and adults, and are relatively rare during older childhood, while emerging evidence indicates the existence of biologically distinct subsets of MB$_{SHH}$ occurring at different ages (Schwalbe et al. 2017; Cavalli et al. 2017). Unlike MB$_{WNT}$, significant genomic heterogeneity is observed among the SHH subgroup (Fig. 7.8). Overall, around 20% of MB$_{SHH}$ patients have *TP53* mutations (Zhukova et al. 2013), often associated with

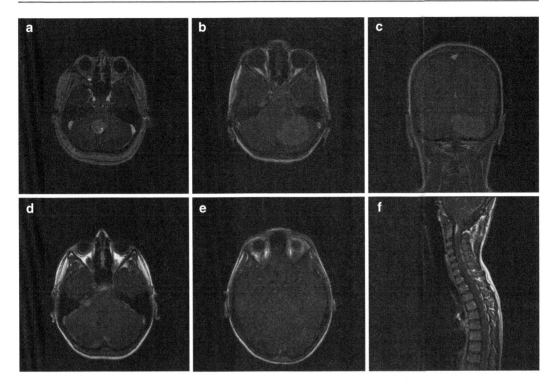

Fig. 7.9 Classic MRI characteristics for the different molecular subgroups. (**a**) WNT medulloblastoma: axial post-contrast T1 image demonstrating centrally located tumor adjacent to the brainstem. (**b**) and (**c**) SHH medulloblastoma: axial and coronal post-contrast T1 images revealing tumor in cerebellar hemisphere. (**d**), (**e**) and (**f**) Group 3 medulloblastoma: axial and spinal post-contrast T1 images showing widespread leptomeningeal dissemination, commonly seen in Group 3 disease. Images courtesy of Dr. Amar Gajjar (St Jude Children's Research Hospital)

LCA histology, 17p loss (25%) or *MYCN* (Jones et al. 2012; Pfaff et al. 2010), and *GLI2* amplifications (Kool et al. 2014). Copy number abnormalities of other p53 pathway components (*MDM4* and *PPM1D* amplifications, focal *TP53* deletions) occur exclusively in SHH tumors. Other notable pathways targeted in SHH subgroup medulloblastoma are IGF signaling (*IGF1R* and *IRS2* amplifications) and the PI3K pathway (*PI3KC2G* and *PI3KC2B* amplification; *PTEN* deletions). SHH tumors also contain mutations in chromatin remodeling genes in approximately 30% of cases; 14% of SHH tumors are characterized by mutations or amplifications targeting members of the nuclear receptor corepressor (N-CoR) complex, as well as *MLL2* (12%) and *SMARCA4* (1.5%) mutations.

Emerging evidence from sequencing (Kool et al. 2014) and methylation (Schwalbe et al. 2017) studies indicates age-dependent subdivisions within the SHH subgroup (Kool et al. 2012, 2014; Northcott et al. 2011b). *PTCH1* mutations occur commonly in all three age groups and are rarely associated with additional mutations; a third of these are germline mutations (Gorlin syndrome). In contrast, other mutations are age-dependent: *SUFU* mutations occur most commonly in under 3 s, while *TP53* mutation occurs predominantly in older children, with 80% having germline mutations (Li Fraumeni syndrome) (Kool et al. 2014). *MYCN* and *GLI2* amplifications often occur in *TP53*-mutated MB$_{SHH}$ tumors, often alongside multiple other abnormalities that indicate chromothripsis (Kool et al. 2014). Such mutations and events are rare or absent in very young children. *TP53* mutation is associated with poor outcome in MB$_{SHH}$ (Tabori et al. 2010), while in the absence of *TP53* mutation or clinical risk factors MB$_{SHH}$ has 5-year OS of 76% (Zhukova et al. 2013).

SFRP1, GLI1, and GAB1 have been proposed as subgroup-specific immunohistochemical markers for MB$_{SHH}$ (Taylor et al. 2012; Northcott et al. 2011a; Ellison et al. 2011b; Min et al. 2013), although at present an expression or methylation signature consistent with that of a SHH subgroup tumor is considered optimum (Gottardo et al. 2014).

7.16.3 Group 3 and Group 4 Tumors (Also Collectively Known as Non-SHH/Non-WNT Subgroup)

The current consensus considers two further subgroups, which in the absence of characteristic driving pathway aberrations are referred to as Group 3 and Group 4. Together these subgroups account for 60–65% of children with medulloblastoma. Group 3 and Group 4 represent a continuum with clear molecular separation at the extremes of the spectrum. *MYC* amplification is the dominant discriminatory driver in Group 3, whereas *MYCN* amplification is more commonly encountered in Group 4 (as well as the SHH subgroup) and tandem duplication of *SNCAIP* (α-synuclein-interacting protein) is seen exclusively in Group 4 medulloblastoma (Northcott et al. 2012b). Notably, Group 3 and Group 4 share significant molecular overlay representing an intermediate, difficult to classify subgroup. Clinical and molecular features common to Group 3 and Group 4 include male predominance (2:1 M:F ratio), the presence of isochromosome 17q, amplification or overexpression of the oncogene *OTX2* (66% prevalence in Group 4 compared with 26% in Group 3), more frequent occurrence of tetraploidy, identified as an early and common driver event (1/4 alleles affected) (Jones et al. 2012), and the infrequent existence of driver mutations. "Enhancer hijacking" has emerged as the hallmark molecular feature in Groups 3 and 4. This process results in recurrent structural variants (deletions, duplications and inversions) converging on a hotspot on chromosome 9q34, which results in the juxtaposition of the proto-oncogene *Growth Factor Independent 1* (*GFI1*) in approximately 40% of Group 3 and

of the related gene *GFI1B* in 10% of Group 4 tumors, next to active enhancer elements (Northcott et al. 2014). Thus, through the activation of diverse structural variants, *GFI1* and *GFI1B* are major drivers in Group 3 and Group 4 medulloblastoma.

7.16.3.1 Group 3 Tumors

MB$_{group3}$ tumors comprise around one-quarter of all medulloblastomas and occur predominantly in very young children and in older children. The LCA histology is enriched, particularly in very young children, although overall most MB$_{group3}$ cases have classic histology. Prevalence of metastasis, especially macrometastatic disease (M2+), is highest in these tumors, with between 30 and 50% of Group 3 patients presenting with disseminated disease (Taylor et al. 2012) (Fig. 7.9d–f). No single defining pathway or event unifies this subgroup, although photoreceptor gene programs are frequently upregulated. Although Group 3 medulloblastomas demonstrate a relative paucity of individual driver gene mutations, approximately one-third of cases exhibit deregulated histone methylation via a number of different gene mutations, including *SMARCA4*, *KDM6A* and other KDM family members, and *MLL2* (Fig. 7.8). In addition, Group 3 tumors appear to utilize alternate mechanisms to achieve the same functional result, since for tumors where no mutation was identified, increased expression of the polycomb gene *ENZ2*, replicated the consequences of chromatin modifying gene mutations. In addition, copy number profiling revealed dysregulation of genes which regulate the TGF-β signaling, either through gain (*ACVR2A*, *ACVR2B,* and *TGFBR1*) or deletion of pathway inhibitors *(CD109, FKBP1A,* and *SNX6)* in 20% of Group 3 tumors. *OTX2*, a known target of TGF-β signaling in the developing nervous system, is also amplified in approximately 8% of Group 3 patients. Notably, *MYC* amplification and *OTX2* amplification are mutually exclusive. Group 3 tumors have the worst outcome of the four subgroups, with relapse occurring early and an overall 5-year survival of 58% in children and 39% in those aged under 4 years (Kool et al. 2012). For patients with metastatic disease and *MYC* amplification, survival is dismal (Cho et al. 2011).

Currently, the best marker for identifying Group 3 is clustering with other Group 3 tumors, and although immunohistochemical positivity for NPR3 has been proposed as an alternative (Taylor et al. 2012; Northcott et al. 2011a), other studies have reported a lack of sensitivity (Min et al. 2013). This subgroup harbors the most promising candidate for a clinically and biologically distinct subordinate subtype, with *MYC* amplification identifying a putative "3α" group, which correlates with the C1 *MYC* subgroup reported by Cho and colleagues (2011). In contrast, non *MYC*-amplified 3b tumors correspond to Cho and colleagues' C5 photoreceptor group and share a similar outcome to Group 4 tumors. Given the very poor prognosis of Group 3, greater understanding of its pathogenesis and development of practical biomarkers and accurate experimental mouse models are research priorities (Taylor et al. 2012).

7.16.3.2 Group 4 Tumors

Group 4 is the largest subgroup, accounting for just over one-third of medulloblastoma cases (Table 7.7). Group 4 represents the prototypical medulloblastoma case, with onset in childhood rather than infancy or adulthood, classic histology, and the strongest association with isochromosome 17q (80% of cases). There is a strong male predominance, with a 2:1 ratio between the sexes, and interestingly 80% of MB_{group4} females have loss of an X chromosome (Taylor et al. 2012). Biologically, however, this subgroup is the least well-understood. The most common copy number aberration identified in Group 4 tumors was a single-copy gain of *SNCAIP* arising from a tandem duplication, which is present in around 10%. *SCNAIP* duplications were associated with isochromosome 17q, but mutually exclusive of copy number abnormalities, including *MYCN* and *CDK6* amplifications which are also commonly found in MB_{group4} (Fig. 7.8). Insights derived from the discovery of superenhancers have identified deep cerebellar neurons of the nuclear transitory zone, or possibly their precursors in the upper rhombic lip, as the putative cell of origin for Group 4 medulloblastoma (Lin et al. 2016).

The prognosis of Group 4 tumors is intermediate, with 5-year OS of approximately 60% for both children and the under 4 age group (Kool et al. 2012). In contrast, Group 4 patients with metastatic disease have a higher risk of relapse. Among Group 4 patients, those with either chromosome 11 loss or gain of chromosome 17 were found to be low risk, regardless of metastases; in cases lacking both these cytogenetic features, metastasis at presentation differentiated between high and intermediate risk. The few very young children within this subgroup (Shih et al. 2014) have a poor prognosis.

Like MB_{group3}, subgroup affiliation is currently best defined by clustering with other Group 4 tumors. KCNA1 immunopositivity has been proposed as a surrogate marker (Taylor et al. 2012; Northcott et al. 2011a), although this has been reported as lacking in specificity (Min et al. 2013). MB_{group4} tumors exhibit a relative paucity of mutations, but as with MB_{group3} deregulated histone methylation is a principal feature. Copy number profiling also reveals deregulated NF-Kappa B signaling, and infrequent homozygous deletions of *KDM6A* (Northcott et al. 2012b).

Further bioinformatic studies in larger cohorts (Schwalbe et al. 2017; Cavalli et al. 2017) have now provided the resolution to identify clinically relevant subdivisions of the four consensus subgroups from methylation and gene expression patterns. Unsurprisingly, the fault-lines within subgroups have occurred around events known to be enriched in but not universal to particular subgroups, such as *MYC* amplification in G3, and *MYCN* amplification in SHH and G4. Subtypes within the SHH subgroup are also defined by age, with MB-SHH in very young children identified as being distinct from SHH-activated disease in older children and adults.

7.17 The Future: Incorporation of Medulloblastoma Subgroup-Specific Therapies

The experience of the last four decades has shown that the successful treatment of medulloblastoma in children requires neurosurgery followed by radiotherapy and chemotherapy. To minimize the adverse effects of current treatments, improved stratification and new therapeutic options are required. Given the distinct clinical behavior and survival outcomes of the different molecular subgroups, a major feature of the next generation of medulloblastoma clinical trials will be the adoption of an integrated classification system based on clinical, histological, and molecular criteria in order to allow more precisely risk-stratified therapy. Thus, generic pan-medulloblastoma clinical trials will give way to subgroup-specific trials. Subgroup-based stratification will permit a decrease in therapy for patients with the best outcome to decrease morbidity, while introducing novel subgroup-specific therapies for the other subgroups. Current clinical trials from a number of collaborative groups have reached the stage where they have begun to stratify treatment on the basis of molecular subgroups. The St Jude Children's Research Hospital Trial SJMB12 incorporates WNT, SHH, and non-WNT/non-SHH subgroups into its stratification, investigating the effects of reducing therapy for WNT patients, while incorporating the SMO inhibitor, vismodegib, for older patients with SHH tumors, although a different target will be required in tumors driven by mutations downstream in the SHH pathway (Kool et al. 2014; Robinson et al. 2015). Novel cytotoxic chemotherapy is being utilized in high-risk patients with non-WNT/non-SHH subgroup medulloblastoma (St Jude's Children's Research Hospital 2013). Meanwhile, both the SIOP-Europe PNET 5 (SIOPE Medulloblastoma/PNET Working Group 2015) and COG ACNS1422 (Children's Oncology Group 2016b) medulloblastoma trials prospectively identify the WNT subgroup medulloblastoma and are also de-escalating both CSI dose and chemotherapy in these patients.

7.17.1 Mouse MB Models and Patient-Derived Xenografts

Novel subgroup-specific therapies for the other subgroups are also needed, but patient numbers limit the rate of new clinical trials. Preclinical testing using sophisticated animal models that better represent the human disease enables preliminary testing of many more drugs more rapidly than can be evaluated in the clinic. The increased understanding of the underlying biology and drivers of medulloblastoma has led to the development of a large number of genetically engineered mouse models representative of three of the different medulloblastoma subgroups, including a large number of SHH models, several Group 3 models (Kawauchi et al. 2012; Pei et al. 2012; Hanaford et al. 2016; Swartling et al. 2012) and one WNT model (Gibson et al. 2010).To date, no genetically engineered Group 4 models have been generated. The majority of these models have focused on mutations in SHH pathway genes (*Ptch1*, *Smo*, *Sufu*) in conjunction with *Trp53* knockout to increase the penetrance of the SHH pathway gene mutations, or on MYC-family (*Myc*, *Mycn*) stabilizing mutations or expression, again often in conjunction with *Trp53* knockdown or manipulation (Roussel and Robinson 2013). In analysis of gene expression in a representative cohort of over 400 MB cases and 140 tumors derived from 20 different mouse models of medulloblastoma found a single model corresponding to MB_{WNT}, 14 corresponding to MB_{SHH} (mostly driven by *Ptch1* or *Smo*) and 5 corresponding to MB_{Group3} (all containing Myc/Mycn amplification and/or *Trp53* abnormalities) (Poschl et al. 2014). This raises the concern that the increasingly recognized diversity within subgroups (Cavalli et al. 2017) is not adequately represented in traditional mouse models.

As an alternative to genetically engineered mouse models, patient-derived xenografts (PDX) are established by direct injection of medulloblastoma cells into the cerebellum of immune-deficient mice (Zhao et al. 2012). Because this approach avoids the selective, adaptive, and progressive changes associated with long-term in vitro culture, these are considered to better represent human medulloblastoma than traditional medulloblastoma cell lines that have been injected into the cerebellum of immune-deficient mice.

A number of promising therapies have been assessed using preclinical models. The novel cytotoxic agents gemcitabine and pemetrexed (Morfouace et al. 2014) showed activity against

MB in mouse models (Ramaswamy et al. 2014) and have subsequently been incorporated into a front-line clinical trial for medulloblastoma (St Jude's Children's Research Hospital 2013). Small-molecule inhibitors of bromodomain and extra terminal (BET)-containing proteins have been shown to be active against *MYC*-amplified medulloblastoma cell lines in vitro, and PDX models derived from children with Group 3 medulloblastoma and LCA histology tumors (Bandopadhayay et al. 2014). In addition, BET bromodomain inhibitors appear to overcome the primary (Kool et al. 2014) and secondary (Rudin et al. 2009) resistance associated with SMO inhibitors in SHH medulloblastomas, by modulating *GLI* transcription downstream of *SMO* and *SUFU* in a mouse model (Tang et al. 2014).

7.18 Summary

For very young children with medulloblastoma a greater understanding of the underlying disease biology is required. Historically, many such patients have been treated in clinical trials that have recruited patients with brain tumors of diverse pathological types, with the aim of evaluating the effects of treatment protocols that sought to minimize or delay the use of CSI and its attendant adverse effects on growth and development. Future trials should categorize primarily by diagnosis, rather than by age category, and very young children should be treated on appropriate medulloblastoma-specific trials to take advantage of innovations in subgroup-specific management of medulloblastoma. Such trials should also make age-specific provision to avoid or substitute radiotherapy as a first-line treatment.

With the increasing subdivision of medulloblastoma into subgroup-specific categories, large trial cohorts will be required, necessitating an even greater degree of international collaboration and cooperation than currently exists. Future trials should aim to recruit as close to 100% of eligible patients as possible, and to collect clinical data and biological data from all patients (Kotecha et al. 2015).

References

Allen J et al (2009) A phase II study of preradiotherapy chemotherapy followed by hyperfractionated radiotherapy for newly diagnosed high-risk medulloblastoma/primitive neuroectodermal tumor: a report from the Children's Oncology Group (CCG 9931). Int J Radiat Oncol Biol Phys 74(4):1006–1011

Ashley DM et al (2012) Induction chemotherapy and conformal radiation therapy for very young children with nonmetastatic medulloblastoma: Children's Oncology Group study P9934. J Clin Oncol 30(26):3181–3186

Ater JL et al (1997) MOPP chemotherapy without irradiation as primary postsurgical therapy for brain tumors in infants and young children. J Neuro-Oncol 32(3):243–252

Avula S et al (2015) Diffusion abnormalities on intraoperative magnetic resonance imaging as an early predictor for the risk of posterior fossa syndrome. Neuro-Oncology 17(4):614–622

Bailey P, Cushing H (1925) Medulloblastoma cerebelli: a common type of midcerebellar glioma of childhood. Arch NeurPsych 14(2):192–224

Bailey CC et al (1995) Prospective randomised trial of chemotherapy given before radiotherapy in childhood medulloblastoma. International Society of Paediatric Oncology (SIOP) and the (German) Society of Paediatric Oncology (GPO): SIOP II. Med Pediatr Oncol 25(3):166–178

Bandopadhayay P et al (2014) BET bromodomain inhibition of MYC-amplified medulloblastoma. Clin Cancer Res 20(4):912–925

Barton M (1995) Tables of equivalent dose in 2 Gy fractions: a simple application of the linear quadratic formula. Int J Radiat Oncol Biol Phys 31(2):371–378

Biegel JA (2006) Molecular genetics of atypical teratoid/rhabdoid tumor. Neurosurg Focus 20(1):E11

Bloom HJ, Wallace EN, Henk JM (1969) The treatment and prognosis of medulloblastoma in children. A study of 82 verified cases. Am J Roentgenol Radium Therapy, Nucl Med 105(1):43–62

Bluml S et al (2016) Molecular subgroups of medulloblastoma identification using noninvasive magnetic resonance spectroscopy. Neuro Oncol 18(1):126–131

Brasme JF et al (2012) Interval between onset of symptoms and diagnosis of medulloblastoma in children: distribution and determinants in a population-based study. Eur J Pediatr 171(1):25–32

Brinkman TM et al (2012) Cerebral white matter integrity and executive function in adult survivors of childhood medulloblastoma. Neuro-Oncology 14(Suppl 4): iv25–iv36

von Bueren AO et al (2011) Treatment of young children with localized medulloblastoma by chemotherapy alone: results of the prospective, multicenter trial HIT 2000 confirming the prognostic impact of histology. Neuro-Oncology 13(6):669–679

von Bueren AO et al (2016) Treatment of children and adolescents with metastatic medulloblastoma and prognostic relevance of clinical and biologic parameters. J Clin Oncol 34(34):4151–4160

Bull JG, Saunders DE, Clark CA (2012) Discrimination of paediatric brain tumours using apparent diffusion coefficient histograms. Eur Radiol 22(2):447–457

Carrie C et al (2005) Conformal radiotherapy, reduced boost volume, hyperfractionated radiotherapy, and online quality control in standard-risk medulloblastoma without chemotherapy: results of the French M-SFOP 98 protocol. Int J Radiat Oncol Biol Phys 63(3):711–716

Carrie C et al (2009) Online quality control, hyperfractionated radiotherapy alone and reduced boost volume for standard risk medulloblastoma: long-term results of MSFOP 98. J Clin Oncol 27(11):1879–1883

Cavalli FMG et al (2017) Intertumoral heterogeneity within medulloblastoma subgroups. Cancer Cell 31(6):737–754.e6

Chang CH, Housepian EM, Herbert C Jr (1969) An operative staging system and a megavoltage radiotherapeutic technic for cerebellar medulloblastomas. Radiology 93(6):1351–1359

del Charco JO et al (1998) Medulloblastoma: time-dose relationship based on a 30-year review. Int J Radiat Oncol Biol Phys 42(1):147–154

Chi SN et al (2004) Feasibility and response to induction chemotherapy intensified with high-dose methotrexate for young children with newly diagnosed high-risk disseminated medulloblastoma. J Clin Oncol 22(24):4881–4887

Children's Oncology Group (2016a) Chemotherapy and radiation therapy in treating young patients with newly diagnosed, previously untreated, high-risk medulloblastoma 2006 5 April 2016 [cited 2016 26/07/16]. https://clinicaltrials.gov/ct2/show/NCT00392327

Children's Oncology Group (2016b) Reduced craniospinal radiation therapy and chemotherapy in treating younger patients with newly diagnosed WNT-driven medulloblastoma. 25/7/2016 [cited 2016 25/7/2016]. https://clinicaltrials.gov/ct2/show/NCT02724579

Cho YJ et al (2011) Integrative genomic analysis of medulloblastoma identifies a molecular subgroup that drives poor clinical outcome. J Clin Oncol 29(11):1424–1430

Choudhri AF et al (2014) 3T intraoperative MRI for management of pediatric CNS neoplasms. AJNR Am J Neuroradiol 35(12):2382–2387

Clifford SC et al (2006) Wnt/Wingless pathway activation and chromosome 6 loss characterize a distinct molecular sub-group of medulloblastomas associated with a favorable prognosis. Cell Cycle 5(22):2666–2670

Darendeliler F et al (2006) Recurrence of brain tumours in patients treated with growth hormone: analysis of KIGS (Pfizer International Growth Database). Acta Paediatr 95(10):1284–1290

Deutsch M et al (1996) Results of a prospective randomized trial comparing standard dose neuraxis irradiation (3,600 cGy/20) with reduced neuraxis irradiation (2,340 cGy/13) in patients with low-stage medulloblastoma. A Combined Children's Cancer Group-Pediatric Oncology Group Study. Pediatr Neurosurg 24(4):167–176. discussion 176–7

Dewire MD et al (2009) Fanconi anemia and biallelic BRCA2 mutation diagnosed in a young child with an embryonal CNS tumor. Pediatr Blood Cancer 53(6):1140–1142

Dhall G et al (2008) Outcome of children less than three years old at diagnosis with non-metastatic medulloblastoma treated with chemotherapy on the "Head Start" I and II protocols. Pediatr Blood Cancer 50(6):1169–1175

Due-Tonnessen BJ, Helseth E (2007) Management of hydrocephalus in children with posterior fossa tumors: role of tumor surgery. Pediatr Neurosurg 43(2):92–96

Duffner PK et al (1986) Survival of children with brain tumors: SEER Program, 1973–1980. Neurology 36(5):597–601

Duffner PK et al (1993) Postoperative chemotherapy and delayed radiation in children less than three years of age with malignant brain tumors. N Engl J Med 328(24):1725–1731

Duffner PK et al (1999) The treatment of malignant brain tumors in infants and very young children: an update of the Pediatric Oncology Group experience. Neuro-Oncology 1(2):152–161

Eberhart CG et al (2002) Histopathologic grading of medulloblastomas: a Pediatric Oncology Group study. Cancer 94(2):552–560

Ellingson BM et al (2015) Consensus recommendations for a standardized brain tumor imaging protocol in clinical trials. Neuro-Oncology 17(9):1188–1198

Ellison DW (2010) Childhood medulloblastoma: novel approaches to the classification of a heterogeneous disease. Acta Neuropathol 120(3):305–316

Ellison DW et al (2005) β-catenin status predicts a favorable outcome in childhood medulloblastoma: the United Kingdom Children's Cancer Study Group Brain Tumour Committee. J Clin Oncol 23(31):7951–7957

Ellison DW et al (2011a) Definition of disease-risk stratification groups in childhood medulloblastoma using combined clinical, pathologic, and molecular variables. J Clin Oncol 29(11):1400–1407

Ellison DW et al (2011b) Medulloblastoma: clinico-pathological correlates of SHH, WNT, and non-SHH/WNT molecular subgroups. Acta Neuropathol 121(3):381–396

Eran A et al (2010) Medulloblastoma: atypical CT and MRI findings in children. Pediatr Radiol 40(7):1254–1262

Evans AE et al (1990) The treatment of medulloblastoma. Results of a prospective randomized trial of radiation therapy with and without CCNU, vincristine, and prednisone. J Neurosurg 72(4):572–582

van Eys J et al (1985) MOPP regimen as primary chemotherapy for brain tumors in infants. J Neuro-Oncol 3(3):237–243

Farwell JR, Dohrmann GJ, Flannery JT (1978) Intracranial neoplasms in infants. Arch Neurol 35(8):533–537

Fattet S et al (2009) Beta-catenin status in paediatric medulloblastomas: correlation of immuno-histochemical expression with mutational status, genetic profiles, and clinical characteristics. J Pathol 218(1):86–94

Fouladi M et al (2005) Intellectual and functional outcome of children 3 years old or younger who have CNS malignancies. J Clin Oncol 23(28): 7152–7160

Fruehwald-Pallamar J et al (2011) Magnetic resonance imaging spectrum of medulloblastoma. Neuroradiology 53(6):387–396

Gajjar A, Pizer B (2010) Role of high-dose chemotherapy for recurrent medulloblastoma and other CNS primitive neuroectodermal tumors. Pediatr Blood Cancer 54(4):649–651

Gajjar A, Bowers DC, Karajannis M, Leary S, Gottardo NG (2015) Pediatric brain tumors—innovative genomics information is transforming the diagnostic and clinical landscapape. J Clin Oncol 33(27):2986–2998. Epub 2015 Aug 24. Review.

Gajjar A et al (2006) Risk-adapted craniospinal radiotherapy followed by high-dose chemotherapy and stem-cell rescue in children with newly diagnosed medulloblastoma (St Jude Medulloblastoma-96): long-term results from a prospective, multicentre trial. Lancet Oncol 7(10):813–820

Gajjar A et al (2013) Phase I study of vismodegib in children with recurrent or refractory medulloblastoma: a pediatric brain tumor consortium study. Clin Cancer Res 19(22):6305–6312

Gandola L et al (2009) Hyperfractionated accelerated radiotherapy in the Milan strategy for metastatic medulloblastoma. J Clin Oncol 27(4):566–571

Garre ML et al (2009) Medulloblastoma variants: age-dependent occurrence and relation to Gorlin syndrome–a new clinical perspective. Clin Cancer Res 15(7):2463–2471

Geyer JR et al (1994) Survival of infants with primitive neuroectodermal tumors or malignant ependymomas of the CNS treated with eight drugs in 1 day: a report from the Children's Cancer Group. J Clin Oncol 12(8):1607–1615

Geyer JR et al (2005) Multiagent chemotherapy and deferred radiotherapy in infants with malignant brain tumors: a report from the Children's Cancer Group. J Clin Oncol 23(30):7621–7631

Giangaspero F, Eberhart C, Haapasalo H, Pietsch T, Wiestler OD, Ellison DW (2007) Medulloblastoma. In: Ohgaki H, Louis DN, Wiestler OD, Cavenee WK (eds) WHO classification of tumours of the central nervous system. IARC, Lyon, pp 132–140

Gibson P et al (2010) Subtypes of medulloblastoma have distinct developmental origins. Nature 468(7327): 1095–1099

Gilbertson RJ, Ellison DW (2008) The origins of medulloblastoma subtypes. Annu Rev Pathol 3: 341–365

Gorlin RJ, Chaudhary AP (1960) Multiple osteomatosis, fibromas, lipomas and fibrosarcomas of the skin and mesentery, epidermoid inclusion cysts of the skin, leiomyomas and multiple intestinal polyposis: a heritable disorder of connective tissue. N Engl J Med 263:1151–1158

Gottardo NG et al (2014) Medulloblastoma down under 2013: a report from the third annual meeting of the International Medulloblastoma Working Group. Acta Neuropathol 127(2):189–201

Grill J et al (2005) Treatment of medulloblastoma with postoperative chemotherapy alone: an SFOP prospective trial in young children. Lancet Oncol 6(8):573–580

Grundy RG et al (2010) Primary postoperative chemotherapy without radiotherapy for treatment of brain tumours other than ependymoma in children under 3 years: results of the first UKCCSG/SIOP CNS 9204 trial. Eur J Cancer 46(1):120–133

Gudrunardottir T et al (2011) Cerebellar mutism: review of the literature. Childs Nerv Syst 27(3):355–363

Hamilton W et al (2015) Suspected cancer (part 1–children and young adults): visual overview of updated NICE guidance. BMJ 350:h3036

Hanaford AR et al (2016) DiSCoVERing innovative therapies for rare tumors: combining genetically accurate disease models with in silico analysis to identify novel therapeutic targets. Clin Cancer Res 22:3903

Hanzlik E et al (2015) A systematic review of neuropsychological outcomes following posterior fossa tumor surgery in children. Childs Nerv Syst 31(10):1869–1875

Hill RM et al (2015) Combined MYC and P53 defects emerge at medulloblastoma relapse and define rapidly progressive, therapeutically targetable disease. Cancer Cell 27(1):72–84

von Hoff K et al (2009) Long-term outcome and clinical prognostic factors in children with medulloblastoma treated in the prospective randomised multicentre trial HIT'91. Eur J Cancer 45(7):1209–1217

Huber JF et al (2006) Long-term effects of transient cerebellar mutism after cerebellar astrocytoma or medulloblastoma tumor resection in childhood. Childs Nerv Syst 22(2):132–138

Hughes EN et al (1988) Medulloblastoma at the joint center for radiation therapy between 1968 and 1984. The influence of radiation dose on the patterns of failure and survival. Cancer 61(10):1992–1998

Jakacki RI et al (2012) Outcome of children with metastatic medulloblastoma treated with carboplatin during craniospinal radiotherapy: a Children's Oncology Group Phase I/II study. J Clin Oncol 30(21):2648–2653

Jones DT et al (2012) Dissecting the genomic complexity underlying medulloblastoma. Nature 488(7409): 100–105

Jones DT et al (2013) The role of chromatin remodeling in medulloblastoma. Brain Pathol 23(2):193–199

Kalifa C, Grill J (2005) The therapy of infantile malignant brain tumors: current status? J Neuro-Oncol 75(3):279–285

Kawauchi D et al (2012) A mouse model of the most aggressive subgroup of human medulloblastoma. Cancer Cell 21(2):168–180

Kieran MW et al (2017) Phase I study of oral sonidegib (LDE225) in pediatric brain and solid tumors and a phase II study in children and adults with relapsed medulloblastoma. Neuro-Oncology 19:1542

Kiltie A, Lashford L, Gattameni H (1997) Survival and late effects in medulloblastoma patients treated with craniospinal irradiation under three years old. Med Pediatr Oncol 28:348–354

Kimura H, Ng JM, Curran T (2008) Transient inhibition of the Hedgehog pathway in young mice causes permanent defects in bone structure. Cancer Cell 13(3):249–260

Kool M et al (2008) Integrated genomics identifies five medulloblastoma subtypes with distinct genetic profiles, pathway signatures and clinicopathological features. PLoS One 3(8):e3088

Kool M et al (2012) Molecular subgroups of medulloblastoma: an international meta-analysis of transcriptome, genetic aberrations, and clinical data of WNT, SHH, Group 3, and Group 4 medulloblastomas. Acta Neuropathol 123(4):473–484

Kool M et al (2014) Genome sequencing of SHH medulloblastoma predicts genotype-related response to smoothened inhibition. Cancer Cell 25(3):393–405

Kortmann RD et al (2000) Postoperative neoadjuvant chemotherapy before radiotherapy as compared to immediate radiotherapy followed by maintenance chemotherapy in the treatment of medulloblastoma in childhood: results of the German prospective randomized trial HIT'91. Int J Radiat Oncol Biol Phys 46(2):269–279

Kotecha RS et al (2015) Rare childhood cancers-an increasing entity requiring the need for global consensus and collaboration. Cancer Med 4(6):819–824

Lam CH et al (2001) Intra-operative MRI-guided approaches to the pediatric posterior fossa tumors. Pediatr Neurosurg 34(6):295–300

Lannering B et al (2012) Hyperfractionated versus conventional radiotherapy followed by chemotherapy in standard-risk medulloblastoma: results from the randomized multicenter HIT-SIOP PNET 4 trial. J Clin Oncol 30(26):3187–3193

Lashford LS et al (1996) An intensive multiagent chemotherapy regimen for brain tumours occurring in very young children. Arch Dis Child 74(3):219–223

Laughton SJ et al (2008) Endocrine outcomes for children with embryonal brain tumors after risk-adapted craniospinal and conformal primary-site irradiation and high-dose chemotherapy with stem-cell rescue on the SJMB-96 trial. J Clin Oncol 26(7):1112–1118

Leary SE et al (2011) Histology predicts a favorable outcome in young children with desmoplastic medulloblastoma: a report from the children's oncology group. Cancer 117(14):3262–3267

Li FP, Fraumeni JF Jr (1969) Soft-tissue sarcomas, breast cancer, and other neoplasms. A familial syndrome? Ann Intern Med 71(4):747–752

Lin CY et al (2016) Active medulloblastoma enhancers reveal subgroup-specific cellular origins. Nature 530(7588):57–62

Lindsey JC et al (2011) TP53 mutations in favorable-risk Wnt/Wingless-subtype medulloblastomas. J Clin Oncol 29(12):e344–e346. author reply e347–8

Louis D et al (2007) The 2007 WHO classification of tumours of the central nervous system. Acta Neuropathol 114(2):97–109

Louis DN et al (2016) The 2016 World Health Organization classification of tumors of the central nervous system: a summary. Acta Neuropathol 131(6):803–820

Marien P et al (2013) Posterior fossa syndrome in adults: a new case and comprehensive survey of the literature. Cortex 49(1):284–300

McManamy CS et al (2003) Morphophenotypic variation predicts clinical behavior in childhood non-desmoplastic medulloblastomas. J Neuropathol Exp Neurol 62(6):627–632

McManamy CS et al (2007) Nodule formation and desmoplasia in medulloblastomas-defining the nodular/desmoplastic variant and its biological behavior. Brain Pathol 17(2):151–164

Meacham LR, Mason PW, Sullivan KM (2004) Auxologic and biochemical characterization of the three phases of growth failure in pediatric patients with brain tumors. J Pediatr Endocrinol Metab 17(5):711–717

Merchant TE et al (2008) Multi-institution prospective trial of reduced-dose craniospinal irradiation (23.4 Gy) followed by conformal posterior fossa (36 Gy) and primary site irradiation (55.8 Gy) and dose-intensive chemotherapy for average-risk medulloblastoma. Int J Radiat Oncol Biol Phys 70(3):782–787

Michalski A, in ISPNO 2016. 2016: Liverpool, UK

Miller RW, Rubinstein JH (1995) Tumors in Rubinstein-Taybi syndrome. Am J Med Genet 56(1):112–115

Miller JH et al (2010) Improved delineation of ventricular shunt catheters using fast steady-state gradient recalled-echo sequences in a rapid brain MR imaging protocol in nonsedated pediatric patients. AJNR Am J Neuroradiol 31(3):430–435

Min HS et al (2013) Genetic grouping of medulloblastomas by representative markers in pathologic diagnosis. Transl Oncol 6(3):265–272

Morfouace M et al (2014) Pemetrexed and gemcitabine as combination therapy for the treatment of Group3 medulloblastoma. Cancer Cell 25(4):516–529

Morrissy AS et al (2016) Divergent clonal selection dominates medulloblastoma at recurrence. Nature 529(7586):351–357

Mostoufi-Moab S, Grimberg A (2010) Pediatric brain tumor treatment: growth consequences and their management. Pediatr Endocrinol Rev 8(1):6–17

Mulhern RK et al (1998) Neuropsychologic functioning of survivors of childhood medulloblastoma randomized to receive conventional or reduced-dose craniospinal irradiation: a Pediatric Oncology Group Study. J Clin Oncol 16(5):1723–1728

Mulhern RK et al (2001) Risks of young age for selected neurocognitive deficits in medulloblastoma are associated with white matter loss. J Clin Oncol 19(2):472–479

Mulhern RK et al (2005) Neurocognitive consequences of risk-adapted therapy for childhood medulloblastoma. J Clin Oncol 23(24):5511–5519

Nazemi KJ et al (2016) High incidence of veno-occlusive disease with myeloablative chemotherapy following craniospinal irradiation in children with newly diagnosed high-risk CNS embryonal tumors: a report from the Children's Oncology Group (CCG-99702). Pediatr Blood Cancer 63:1563

NCT01878617, St. Jude Children's Research Hospital (2013) A clinical and molecular risk-directed therapy for newly diagnosed medulloblastoma. In: ClinicalTrials.gov. National Library of Medicine (US), Bethesda, MD

Nejat F, El Khashab M, Rutka JT (2008) Initial management of childhood brain tumors: neurosurgical considerations. J Child Neurol 23(10):1136–1148

Netson KL et al (2012) A 5-year investigation of children's adaptive functioning following conformal radiation therapy for localized ependymoma. Int J Radiat Oncol Biol Phys 84(1):217–223.e1

Northcott PA et al (2011a) Medulloblastoma comprises four distinct molecular variants. J Clin Oncol 29(11):1408–1414

Northcott PA et al (2011b) Pediatric and adult sonic hedgehog medulloblastomas are clinically and molecularly distinct. Acta Neuropathol 122(2):231–240

Northcott PA et al (2012a) Medulloblastomics: the end of the beginning. Nat Rev Cancer 12(12):818–834

Northcott PA et al (2012b) Subgroup-specific structural variation across 1,000 medulloblastoma genomes. Nature 488(7409):49–56

Northcott PA et al (2014) Enhancer hijacking activates GFI1 family oncogenes in medulloblastoma. Nature 511(7510):428–434

Online Mendelian Inheritance in Man (2012) #605724 ICD+ FANCONI ANEMIA, COMPLEMENTATION GROUP D1; FANCD1 2012

Online Mendelian Inheritance in Man (2013) #109400 BASAL CELL NEVUS SYNDROME; BCNS 2013 4 March 2015 [cited 2015 13 September 2015]. http://www.omim.org/entry/109400?search=gorlin&highlight=gorlin

Online Mendelian Inheritance in Man (2015a) #276300 MISMATCH REPAIR CANCER SYNDROME; MMRCS 10 June 2015 [cited 2015 13 September 2015]. http://www.omim.org/entry/276300

Online Mendelian Inheritance in Man (2015b) #180849 ICD+ RUBINSTEIN-TAYBI SYNDROME 1; RSTS1 2015

Ostrom QT et al (2015a) Alex's lemonade stand foundation infant and childhood primary brain and central nervous system tumors diagnosed in the United States in 2007–2011. Neuro-Oncology 16(Suppl 10):x1–x36

Ostrom QT et al (2015b) CBTRUS Statistical Report: primary brain and central nervous system tumors diagnosed in the United States in 2008–2012. Neuro Oncol 17(Suppl 4):iv1–iv62

Packer RJ et al (1994) Outcome for children with medulloblastoma treated with radiation and cisplatin, CCNU, and vincristine chemotherapy. J Neurosurg 81(5):690–698

Packer RJ et al (1999) Treatment of children with medulloblastomas with reduced-dose craniospinal radiation therapy and adjuvant chemotherapy: a Children's Cancer Group Study. J Clin Oncol 17(7):2127–2136

Packer RJ et al (2006) Phase III study of craniospinal radiation therapy followed by adjuvant chemotherapy for newly diagnosed average-risk medulloblastoma. J Clin Oncol 24(25):4202–4208

Packer RJ et al (2013) Survival and secondary tumors in children with medulloblastoma receiving radiotherapy and adjuvant chemotherapy: results of Children's Oncology Group trial A9961. Neuro-Oncology 15(1):97–103

Palmer SL, Reddick WE, Gajjar A (2007) Understanding the cognitive impact on children who are treated for medulloblastoma. J Pediatr Psychol 32(9):1040–1049

Palmer SL et al (2013) Processing speed, attention, and working memory after treatment for medulloblastoma: an international, prospective, and longitudinal study. J Clin Oncol 31(28):3494–3500

Parsons DW et al (2011) The genetic landscape of the childhood cancer medulloblastoma. Science 331(6016):435–439

Paulino AC et al (2003) Protracted radiotherapy treatment duration in medulloblastoma. Am J Clin Oncol 26(1):55–59

Pei Y et al (2012) An animal model of MYC-driven medulloblastoma. Cancer Cell 21(2):155–167

Pfaff E et al (2010) TP53 mutation is frequently associated with CTNNB1 mutation or MYCN amplification and is compatible with long-term survival in medulloblastoma. J Clin Oncol 28(35):5188–5196

Pfister S, Hartmann C, Korshunov A (2009) Histology and molecular pathology of pediatric brain tumors. J Child Neurol 24(11):1375–1386

Phi JH et al (2011) Cerebrospinal fluid M staging for medulloblastoma: reappraisal of Chang's M staging based on the CSF flow. Neuro-Oncology 13(3):334–344

Phoenix TN et al (2016) Medulloblastoma genotype dictates blood brain barrier phenotype. Cancer Cell 29(4):508–522

Pietsch T et al (2014) Prognostic significance of clinical, histopathological, and molecular characteristics of medulloblastomas in the prospective HIT2000 multicenter clinical trial cohort. Acta Neuropathol 128(1):137–149

Pillai S et al (2012) Intracranial tumors in infants: long-term functional outcome, survival, and its predictors. Childs Nerv Syst 28(4):547–555

Pizer B, Clifford S (2008) Medulloblastoma: new insights into biology and treatment. Arch Dis Child Educ Pract Ed 93(5):137–144

Pizer BL, Clifford SC (2009) The potential impact of tumour biology on improved clinical practice for medulloblastoma: progress towards biologically driven clinical trials. Br J Neurosurg 23(4):364–375

Pizer B et al (2011) Treatment of recurrent central nervous system primitive neuroectodermal tumours in children and adolescents: results of a Children's Cancer and Leukaemia Group study. Eur J Cancer 47(9):1389–1397

Pollack IF et al (1995) Mutism and pseudobulbar symptoms after resection of posterior fossa tumors in children: incidence and pathophysiology. Neurosurgery 37(5):885–893

Pomeroy SL, Sturla LM (2003) Molecular biology of medulloblastoma therapy. Pediatr Neurosurg 39(6):299–304

Pomeroy SL et al (2002) Prediction of central nervous system embryonal tumour outcome based on gene expression. Nature 415(6870):436–442

Poschl J et al (2014) Genomic and transcriptomic analyses match medulloblastoma mouse models to their human counterparts. Acta Neuropathol 128(1):123–136

Puget S et al (2009) Injuries to inferior vermis and dentate nuclei predict poor neurological and neuropsychological outcome in children with malignant posterior fossa tumors. Cancer 115(6):1338–1347

Pugh TJ et al (2012) Medulloblastoma exome sequencing uncovers subtype-specific somatic mutations. Nature 488(7409):106–110

Ramaswamy V et al (2014) Duration of the pre-diagnostic interval in medulloblastoma is subgroup dependent. Pediatr Blood Cancer 61(7):1190–1194

Ramaswamy V et al (2016) Risk stratification of childhood medulloblastoma in the molecular era: the current consensus. Acta Neuropathol 131:821

Rasalkar DD et al (2013) Paediatric intra-axial posterior fossa tumours: pictorial review. Postgrad Med J 89(1047):39–46

Ris MD et al (2001) Intellectual outcome after reduced-dose radiation therapy plus adjuvant chemotherapy for medulloblastoma: a Children's Cancer Group study. J Clin Oncol 19(15):3470–3476

Riva D et al (2002) Intrathecal methotrexate affects cognitive function in children with medulloblastoma. Neurology 59(1):48–53

Robertson PL et al (2006) Incidence and severity of postoperative cerebellar mutism syndrome in children with medulloblastoma: a prospective study by the Children's Oncology Group. J Neurosurg 105(6 Suppl):444–451

Robinson G et al (2012) Novel mutations target distinct subgroups of medulloblastoma. Nature 488(7409):43–48

Robinson GW et al (2015) Vismodegib exerts targeted efficacy against recurrent sonic hedgehog-subgroup medulloblastoma: results from phase II pediatric brain tumor consortium studies PBTC-025B and PBTC-032. J Clin Oncol 33(24):2646–2654

Rohrer TR et al (2010) Growth hormone therapy and the risk of tumor recurrence after brain tumor treatment in children. J Pediatr Endocrinol Metab 23(9):935–942

Rorke LB (1983) The cerebellar medulloblastoma and its relationship to primitive neuroectodermal tumors. J Neuropathol Exp Neurol 42(1):1–15

Roussel MF, Robinson GW (2013) Role of MYC in medulloblastoma. Cold Spring Harb Perspect Med 3(11):a014308

Rudin CM et al (2009) Treatment of medulloblastoma with hedgehog pathway inhibitor GDC-0449. N Engl J Med 361(12):1173–1178

Rutkowski S et al (2005) Treatment of early childhood medulloblastoma by postoperative chemotherapy alone. N Engl J Med 352(10):978–986

Rutkowski S et al (2009) Treatment of early childhood medulloblastoma by postoperative chemotherapy and deferred radiotherapy. Neuro-Oncology 11(2):201–210

Rutkowski S et al (2010) Survival and prognostic factors of early childhood medulloblastoma: an international meta-analysis. J Clin Oncol 28(33):4961–4968

Ryan SL et al (2012) MYC family amplification and clinical risk-factors interact to predict an extremely poor prognosis in childhood medulloblastoma. Acta Neuropathol 123(4):501–513

Saury JM, Emanuelson I (2011) Cognitive consequences of the treatment of medulloblastoma among children. Pediatr Neurol 44(1):21–30

Schneider JF et al (2007) Multiparametric differentiation of posterior fossa tumors in children using diffusion-weighted imaging and short echo-time 1H-MR spectroscopy. J Magn Reson Imaging 26(6):1390–1398

Schwalbe EC et al (2017) Novel molecular subgroups for clinical classification and outcome prediction in childhood medulloblastoma: a cohort study. Lancet Oncol 18(7):958–971

Sexauer CL et al (1985) Cisplatin in recurrent pediatric brain tumors. A POG phase II study. A Pediatric Oncology Group Study. Cancer 56(7):1497–1501

Shih DJ et al (2014) Cytogenetic prognostication within medulloblastoma subgroups. J Clin Oncol 32(9):886–896

SIOPE Medulloblastoma/PNET Working Group (2015) 16/2/2015 [cited 2016 23/11/2016]. https://www.siope.eu/european-research-and-standards/clinical-research-council/siopecrc/european-clinical-study-groups/siope-brain-tumour-group/structure/medulloblastomapnet-wg/

Sklar CA, Constine LS (1995) Chronic neuroendocrinological sequelae of radiation therapy. Int J Radiat Oncol Biol Phys 31(5):1113–1121

Smith MJ et al (2014) Germline mutations in SUFU cause Gorlin syndrome-associated childhood medulloblastoma and redefine the risk associated with PTCH1 mutations. J Clin Oncol 32(36):4155–4161

Spiller SE et al (2008) Response of preclinical medulloblastoma models to combination therapy with 13-cis retinoic acid and suberoylanilide hydroxamic acid (SAHA). J Neuro-Oncol 87(2):133–141

St Jude's Children's Research Hospital (2013) A clinical and molecular risk-directed therapy for newly diagnosed medulloblastoma. 30 March 2017 [cited 2015 22 August 2017]. https://clinicaltrials.gov/ct2/show/study/NCT01878617?view=record

Stiller CA, Bunch KJ (1992) Brain and spinal tumours in children aged under two years: incidence and survival in Britain, 1971–85. Br J Cancer Suppl 18:S50–S53

Swartling FJ et al (2012) Distinct neural stem cell populations give rise to disparate brain tumors in response to N-MYC. Cancer Cell 21(5):601–613

Tabori U et al (2010) Universal poor survival in children with medulloblastoma harboring somatic TP53 mutations. J Clin Oncol 28(8):1345–1350

Tait DM et al (1990) Adjuvant chemotherapy for medulloblastoma: the first multi-centre control trial of the International Society of Paediatric Oncology (SIOP I). Eur J Cancer 26(4):464–469

Tang Y et al (2014) Epigenetic targeting of Hedgehog pathway transcriptional output through BET bromodomain inhibition. Nat Med 20(7):732–740

Tarbell NJ et al (2013) High-risk medulloblastoma: a pediatric oncology group randomized trial of chemotherapy before or after radiation therapy (POG 9031). J Clin Oncol 31(23):2936–2941

Taylor RE et al (2003) Results of a randomized study of preradiation chemotherapy versus radiotherapy alone for nonmetastatic medulloblastoma: the International Society of Paediatric Oncology/United Kingdom Children's Cancer Study Group PNET-3 Study. J Clin Oncol 21(8):1581–1591

Taylor RE et al (2005) Outcome for patients with metastatic (M2-3) medulloblastoma treated with SIOP/UKCCSG PNET-3 chemotherapy. Eur J Cancer 41(5):727–734

Taylor MD et al (2012) Molecular subgroups of medulloblastoma: the current consensus. Acta Neuropathol 123(4):465–472

Thames HD Jr et al (1982) Changes in early and late radiation responses with altered dose fractionation: implications for dose-survival relationships. Int J Radiat Oncol Biol Phys 8(2):219–226

Thomas PR et al (2000) Low-stage medulloblastoma: final analysis of trial comparing standard-dose with reduced-dose neuraxis irradiation. J Clin Oncol 18(16):3004–3011

Thompson MC et al (2006) Genomics identifies medulloblastoma subgroups that are enriched for specific genetic alterations. J Clin Oncol 24(12):1924–1931

Turcot J, Despres JP, Pierre FS (1959) Malignant tumors of the central nervous system associated with familial polyposis of the colon: report of two cases. Dis Colon Rectum 2:465–468

Uday S et al (2015) Endocrine sequelae beyond 10 years in survivors of medulloblastoma. Clin Endocrinol 83:663

Valteau-Couanet D et al (2005) High-dose busulfan and thiotepa followed by autologous stem cell transplantation (ASCT) in previously irradiated medulloblastoma patients: high toxicity and lack of efficacy. Bone Marrow Transplant 36(11):939–945

Wilne SH et al (2006) The presenting features of brain tumours: a review of 200 cases. Arch Dis Child 91(6):502–506

Wilne S et al (2010) The diagnosis of brain tumours in children: a guideline to assist healthcare professionals in the assessment of children who may have a brain tumour. Arch Dis Child 95(7):534–539

Xu W et al (2004) Endocrine outcome in children with medulloblastoma treated with 18 Gy of craniospinal radiation therapy. Neuro-Oncology 6(2):113–118

Yang ZJ et al (2008) Medulloblastoma can be initiated by deletion of patched in lineage-restricted progenitors or stem cells. Cancer Cell 14(2):135–145

Zeltzer PM et al (1999) Metastasis stage, adjuvant treatment, and residual tumor are prognostic factors for medulloblastoma in children: conclusions from the Children's Cancer Group 921 randomized phase III study. J Clin Oncol 17(3):832–845

Zhao X et al (2012) Global gene expression profiling confirms the molecular fidelity of primary tumor-based orthotopic xenograft mouse models of medulloblastoma. Neuro-Oncology 14(5):574–583

Zhukova N et al (2013) Subgroup-specific prognostic implications of TP53 mutation in medulloblastoma. J Clin Oncol 31(23):2927–2935

Ependymoma

8

Hendrik Witt and Kristian W. Pajtler

8.1 Epidemiology

Ependymomas account for approximately 12% of all childhood brain tumors (Louis et al. 2007). In the United States, about 170 new ependymomas per year were diagnosed in children and young adult patients below the age of 25 years (Allen et al. 1998). In a cohort of ependymal tumors of central nervous system (CNS) of the Central Brain Tumor Registry of the United States (CBTRUS), the annual age-adjusted incidence rate was 0.41/100,000 in adult and pediatric patients (Villano et al. 2013). In a study by the Canadian Pediatric Brain Tumor Consortium (CPBTC) of the incidence, management, and outcomes of Canadian infant brain tumor patients, a mean annual age-adjusted incidence rate for infant ependymomas of 4.6 per 100,000 children years was described (Purdy et al. 2014). The mean age at diagnosis ranges from 4 to 6 years, and 12 to 30% are diagnosed in children below 36 months of age (Purdy et al. 2014; Reni et al. 2007). There is a male predominance for developing an intracranial ependymoma, with a male/female ratio of 1.8 (Pajtler et al. 2015; Purdy et al. 2014).

About 70% of childhood ependymomas arise within the posterior fossa (PF), 25% within the supratentorial (ST) compartment, and about 5% within the spinal (SP) canal (Kilday et al. 2012; Modena et al. 2012). The majority of spinal cord ependymomas arise in adolescents; ependymoma of the spine or cauda equina is a rarity in children under 10 years. In contrast, the primary location of ependymal tumors in adult patients is the spinal cord or cauda equina in approximately 50–60% of cases (Pajtler et al. 2015; Villano et al. 2013).

Overall, the outcome of intracranial ependymoma in children still remains unsatisfactory. The clinical outcome varies across several pediatric ependymoma studies; however, approximately 40% of childhood patients cannot be cured with current treatment regimens, the majority of whom are young children under 4 years of age (Gajjar et al. 2014; Korshunov et al. 2010; Merchant et al. 2009). Within the entire childhood ependymoma population up to the age of 18 years, 5-year progression-free survival (PFS) rates range from 23% to 74%, and overall survival (OS) varies between 40 and 75% (Cage et al. 2013; Pajtler et al. 2015; Pejavar et al. 2012; Witt et al. 2011). Spinal ependymomas, including myxopapillary (SP-MPE) and classic ependymomas (SP-EPN), are rare in children. Spinal ependymomas have excellent long-term survival

H. Witt (✉) · K. W. Pajtler
Hopp-Children's Cancer Center at the NCT Heidelberg (KiTZ), Heidelberg, Germany

Division of Pediatric Neurooncology, German Cancer Research Center (DKFZ), Heidelberg, Germany

Department of Pediatric Oncology, Hematology and Immunology, University Hospital Heidelberg, Heidelberg, Germany
e-mail: h.witt@dkfz.de; h.witt@Dkfz-Heidelberg.de

© Springer International Publishing AG, part of Springer Nature 2018
A. Gajjar et al. (eds.), *Brain Tumors in Children*, https://doi.org/10.1007/978-3-319-43205-2_8

rates, although relapses are seen regularly; myxopapillary and classic spinal ependymoma have 10-year OS rates of nearly 100% (Bandopadhayay et al. 2015; Mack et al. 2014; Pajtler et al. 2015).

Recurrences and metastases are serious consequences of intracranial ependymomas; about 50% of children with intracranial ependymomas develop a relapse (Antony et al. 2014). The majority of relapses develop within the first 3 years, typically at the site of the primary tumor (Witt et al. 2011; Zacharoulis et al. 2008). About 20% of failures have isolated distant recurrence (Merchant et al. 2004). Even late recurrences are not uncommon (Witt et al. 2011); in particular, patients with ST-RELA-EPN have a significant relapse rate 5 years following diagnosis (Pajtler et al. 2015). The OS drops from 75% at 5 years to only 49% at 10 years in patients with a *RELA* fusion positive ependymoma. Meningeal dissemination occurs with an incidence of 9–20% in pediatric ependymomas (Zacharoulis et al. 2008). Twenty-nine percentage of patients with metastatic disease at diagnosis are infants (Purdy et al. 2014). In the vast majority of patients (90%) with primary metastatic dissemination, the primary tumor is a Group A tumor of the posterior fossa, while only 10% have supratentorial localization and harbor the *RELA* fusion (Zacharoulis et al. 2008).

8.2　Pathogenesis and Molecular Subgroups

Ependymal tumors comprise a heterogeneous group of neuroepithelial malignancies of the CNS with variable prognosis that can occur in children and adults along the entire neuraxis, including the spine, posterior fossa, and supratentorial brain regions. Accurate histopathological diagnosis according to the World Health Organization (WHO) classification for CNS tumors (Louis et al. 2007) is challenging for ependymal tumors. In particular, distinction between grade II ependymomas and grade III anaplastic ependymomas is often difficult, with poor interobserver reproducibility even if performed by experienced neuropathologists (Ellison et al. 2011; Tihan et al. 2008).

In addition, many tumors contain isolated areas and each represents a distinct grade, resulting in the challenge of predicting which component of the tumor will influence the overall biologic behavior. Although histopathological similarities can be recognized among variants of ependymoma at different anatomical sites, the underlying molecular biology is heterogeneous, with distinct genetic and epigenetic alterations as well as diverse transcriptional programs (Cashman et al. 2002; Dyer et al. 2002; Korshunov et al. 2010; Mack et al. 2014; Mendrzyk et al. 2006; Parker et al. 2014; Wani et al. 2012; Witt et al. 2011).

Ependymomas, as many cancers, are characterized by chromosome copy number aberrations (CNAs), which illustrates a hallmark of the development of malignant tumors. Many different CNAs, representing chromosomal instability, affect all subtypes of pediatric ependymomas: ST-EPN-RELA, ST-EPN-YAP1, Group A ependymomas, and especially Group B tumors (Pajtler et al. 2015; Witt et al. 2011). The only chromosomal aberration that is associated with Group A ependymomas is gain of chromosome 1q; more often these high-risk tumors represent a balanced chromosomal profile (Witt et al. 2011).

The single molecular marker that has repeatedly shown an association with unfavorable outcome is gain of chromosome arm 1q (Godfraind et al. 2012; Kilday et al. 2012; Korshunov et al. 2010; Mendrzyk et al. 2006; Modena et al. 2012; Witt et al. 2011), particularly in PF ependymomas of childhood. Accordingly, a multivariable analysis within a large molecular classification study of ependymal tumors identified gain of chromosome arm 1q to be of independent prognostic value for both OS and PFS in PF-EPN-A patients (Pajtler et al. 2015). Hence, chromosome 1q may host candidate genes involved in ependymoma tumorigenesis or tumor progression. This particular region is quite large, which makes it difficult to pinpoint specific genes that represent drivers or passengers of ependymoma development. Potential transforming oncogenes located on chromosome 1q, especially within the hotspot region 1q21–32, include *DUSP12* (1q23.3), *S100A10* (1q21), *CHI3L1* (1q32.1), *TPR, SHC1, JTB*, and *HSPA6* (1q32) (Kilday et al. 2009).

One other frequently described genomic aberration in high-risk ependymomas is homozygous deletion of *CDKN2A/p16^{INK4a}*, which has repeatedly been detected in supratentorial ST-EPN-RELA ependymomas (Korshunov et al. 2010; Milde et al. 2011; Poppleton and Gilbertson 2007; Taylor et al. 2005; Witt et al. 2011). *CDKN2A/p16^{INK4a}*, a tumor suppressor gene located at 9p21.3, regulates neural stem cell proliferation, and its deletion has been shown to rapidly expand progenitor cell numbers in developing neural tissue (Johnson et al. 2010; Poppleton and Gilbertson 2007). The first evidence that homozygous deletion of *CDKN2A/p16^{INK4a}* is a key factor of ependymoma pathogenesis was delivered by Johnson and colleagues (Johnson et al. 2010). They developed a genetic engineered mouse model based on neural stem cells from an *Ink4a/Arf-null* background and including amplification of *EPHB2*. Interestingly, this model delivered supratentorial ependymomas in vivo, representing a *RELA* fusion negative subtype (Atkinson et al. 2011; Johnson et al. 2010; Wright et al. 2015).

In spinal ependymoma, the neurofibromatosis type 2 gene (NF2) has long been known to be a hallmark genetic aberration occurring either as hereditary germline or as sporadic mutation (Ebert et al. 1999; Rubio et al. 1994). Since CNAs most likely do not occur randomly and might therefore contain drivers of cancer, Mohankumar et al. performed a cross-species in vivo screen of 84 candidate oncogenes and 39 candidate tumor suppressor genes (TSG), located within 28 recurrent CNAs in ependymoma (Mohankumar et al. 2015). In this study, the authors identified eight new ependymoma oncogenes and ten new ependymoma TSGs, which converged on dysregulation of specific cell functions, including trafficking of the growth factor receptors FGFR and EGFR, and epigenetic modifiers known to be oncogenic in ependymoma. The next step is to analyze whether any of these newly identified ependymoma oncogenes or TSGs may generate ependymomas that faithfully model distinct molecular subgroups.

The first evidence of localization-specific molecular subgroups was presented by Korshunov and colleagues based on gene expression analysis (Korshunov et al. 2003). This study delivered novel findings of biochemical pathways that are particularly intriguing in the pathogenesis of ependymomas and suggested that ependymomas comprise molecularly distinct and localization-specific diseases. In a complex cross-species study, Johnson et al. provided evidence that these molecular differences are based on different cells of origin (Johnson et al. 2010). Additional studies were published afterwards, which identified distinct molecular subtypes within each anatomical compartment (Johnson et al. 2010; Pajtler et al. 2015; Wani et al. 2012; Witt et al. 2011). The study by Johnson and colleagues performed a gene expression analysis of 83 ependymomas, including tumors from supratentorial, infratentorial, and spinal locations (Johnson et al. 2010). They were able to identify nine molecular subgroups in total, although their clinical relevance was uncertain, as detailed patient information and outcome data was not available.

For the first time, two molecular subtypes of posterior fossa ependymomas were described as two distinct diseases. Group A (PF-EPN-A) and Group B (PF-EPN-B) tumors are demographically, transcriptionally, genetically, and clinically distinct entities (Witt et al. 2011). Group A patients are most often young children and the tumors are located laterally within the posterior fossa and harbor a balanced genome, and are much more likely to exhibit recurrence, metastasis at recurrence, and death compared with Group B patients. These two distinct molecular subgroups were consistently described in other independent studies using different methodologies and non-overlapping patient cohorts (Mack et al. 2014; Pajtler et al. 2015; Wani et al. 2012; Witt et al. 2011). Group A ependymomas show overexpression and activation of classic cancer-related signaling pathways, such as EGFR, PDGF, RAS, ECM, VEGF, MAPK, and integrins. Interestingly, Group B ependymomas comprise very instable chromosomes, featuring large chromosomal aberrations, partially affecting whole p- or q-arms of a chromosome or the entire chromosome. Gene expression analyses of Group B ependymomas revealed activation of genes involved in ciliogenesis and microtubule assembly, as well as mitochondrial metabolism (Witt et al. 2011). A following study confirmed the identification of two molecular subtypes. Group 1 (Group A) tumors demonstrated overexpression of genes associated with mesenchyme, and were associated with younger age and poor event-free survival (EFS), similar to the findings by Witt and colleagues in Group A ependymomas (Wani et al. 2012). Group 2 (Group B) tumors were associated with favorable clinical outcome, tended to occur in adolescent children and young adults, and did not express genes associated with altered gene ontology terms in their transcriptomes (Wani et al. 2012).

A recent study by Mack and colleagues detected no recurrent mutations and an overall very low mutation rate, with an average of five somatic mutations per tumor, in both molecular subgroups Group A and Group B (Mack et al. 2014). In contrast, DNA methylation patterns were dissimilar between the subgroups. Since Group A displayed a higher proportion of methylated CpG-islands within promoter regions as compared to Group B, Group A was identified as CpG-island methylator phenotype (CIMP). Remarkably, transcriptional silencing in Group A tumors driven by CpG methylation converged on targets of the polycomb repressive 2 complex (PRC2), which represses differential gene expression through trimethylation of the H3K27 histone mark. This prompted speculation that PRC2 complex hyperactivity might cause tumor suppressor gene silencing with subsequent gene silencing by DNA CpG hypermethylation contributing to PF-EPN-A tumor pathogenesis (Mack et al. 2014). In this study, epigenetic agents were investigated as a potential novel treatment option for Group A tumors both in vitro and in vivo in patient-derived xenograft models. The preclinical treatment approaches using either 5-aza-2′-deoxycytidine, 3-deazaneplanocin A, or GSK343 (a selective inhibitor of the H3K27 methyltransferase, EZH2) demonstrated good response in cells and mice bearing Group A tumors, accompanied by marked de-repression of gene sets enriched for *EZH2* targets upon treatment with epigenetic modifying agents. These results are promising for treatment strategies targeting DNA CpG-methylation, PRC2/EZH2, and histone deacetylases of this chemotherapy-resistant disease. Since Group A and B subgroups harbor distinct transcriptomic, genetic, epigenetic, and clinical features, these features are substantially more informative than the WHO grading alone (Archer and Pomeroy 2011).

Notably, in a recent large-scale genomic study of supratentorial ependymomas, Parker and colleagues discovered a fusion between *RELA*, which encodes an NF-κB component, and the poorly characterized gene *C11orf95* caused by chromothripsis on chromosome 11 as the first driver event in ST ependymomas. Chromothripsis is a recently discovered phenomenon of genomic rearrangement arising during a single genome-shattering event. This fusion was found to drive tumorigenesis in the absence of any other genetic alteration when aberrantly expressed in neural stem cells (NSCs) and could be identified in more than 70% of ST ependymomas. The *RELA* gene encodes for p65, which is a downstream target of the NF-κB signaling pathway, acting as a transcription factor and regulating several biological actions of cell maintenance. Importantly, a genetically engineered mouse model was successfully developed based on the *C11orf95-RELA* gene fusion. NSCs from an Ink4a/Arf-null background were transduced with the retroviruses carrying the C11orf95-RELA fusion. These transgenic NSCs were then implanted into the cerebrum and developed supratentorial ependymomas within a few days. Hence, this supratentorial ependymoma subtype model delivers excellent opportunities for preclinical drug testing in vivo. In line with findings of the study by Mack and colleagues, no recurrent somatic mutations were detected in posterior fossa ependymomas, including Group A and Group B. Drivers of PF ependymomas have not yet been identified.

A powerful clinical stratification system comprising all ependymal tumors is still lacking. A recent comprehensive study addressed this challenge by developing an unbiased, robust, and uniform molecular classification of ependymal tumors that adequately reflects the full biological, clinical, and histopathological heterogeneity across all age groups, grades, and major anatomical CNS compartments (Pajtler et al. 2015). DNA methylation patterns of tumor cells were found to represent a very stable molecular memory of the respective cell of origin throughout the disease course (Hoadley et al. 2014; Hovestadt et al. 2014), thus making this assessment particularly suitable for tumor classification. By applying an integrated analysis including genome-wide DNA methylation profiles for 500 ependymal tumors, Pajtler et al. identified nine distinct molecular subgroups, three within each CNS compartment (Fig. 8.1). One of the subgroups within each compartment was enriched with grade I subependymomas (SE), designated SP-SE, PF-SE, and ST-SE, comprising only adult patients. Other molecular

subgroups within the spine showed a relatively good concordance with the histopathological subtypes myxopapillary ependymoma (SP-MPE) and classic ependymoma (SP-EPN). The two remaining molecular subgroups within the hindbrain were identified as the above-described PF-EPN-A and B subgroups (Fig. 8.2). Consistent with findings by Parker et al., the largest supratentorial subgroup was characterized by *RELA-C11orf95* gene fusions and therefore termed ST-EPN-RELA. The third ST subgroup was characterized by highly recurrent fusions to the oncogene *YAP1*, thus designated ST-EPN-YAP1 (Fig. 8.2). Importantly, it was also shown that subgroup classification remains stable at the time of recurrence (Pajtler et al. 2015). Genome-wide DNA copy number

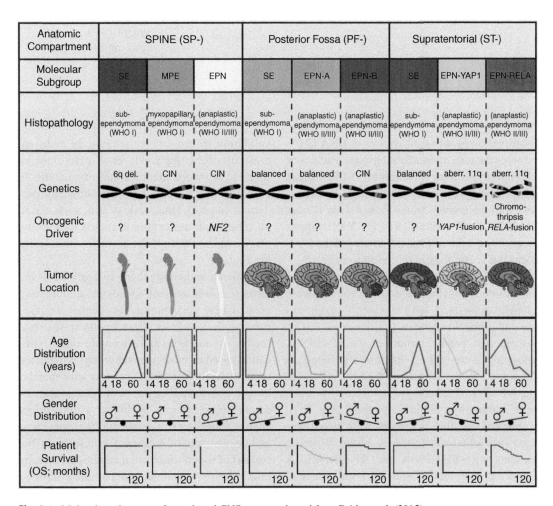

Fig. 8.1 Molecular subgroups of ependymal CNS tumors adapted from Pajtler et al. (2015)

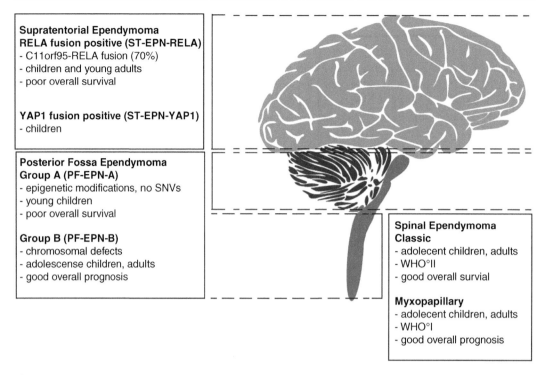

Supratentorial Ependymoma
RELA fusion positive (ST-EPN-RELA)
- C11orf95-RELA fusion (70%)
- children and young adults
- poor overall survival

YAP1 fusion positive (ST-EPN-YAP1)
- children

Posterior Fossa Ependymoma
Group A (PF-EPN-A)
- epigenetic modifications, no SNVs
- young children
- poor overall survival

Group B (PF-EPN-B)
- chromosomal defects
- adolescense children, adults
- good overall prognosis

Spinal Ependymoma
Classic
- adolecent children, adults
- WHO°II
- good overall survial

Myxopapillary
- adolecent children, adults
- WHO°I
- good overall prognosis

Fig. 8.2 An overview of molecular subgroups of pediatric ependymomas

profiles showed strong differences of DNA CNAs between the nine molecular subgroups. Patterns of chromothripsis were only seen in ST-EPN-RELA tumors, mainly involving chromosome 11, consistent with the findings of the Parker study (Parker et al. 2014). In contrast, ST-EPN-YAP1 tumors frequently displayed focal CNAs around the *YAP1* locus that is also located on chromosome 11.

The nine molecular subgroups identified in the study by Pajtler and colleagues were closely associated with distinct demographics and clinical outcomes (Pajtler et al. 2015). As reported before, tumors of the PF-EPN-A subgroup were almost exclusively found in young children, but the ST-EPN-YAP1 and the ST-EPN-RELA subgroups were also much more common in pediatric patients (Fig. 8.2). Tumors of the other subgroups were more common or exclusively found in adults. Whereas patients with PF-EPN-A and ST-EPN-RELA tumors predominantly showed poor outcome, patients in the other subgroups mostly had an excellent prognosis. These data require further

validation in prospective studies. In addition, molecular subgroup and level of resection were found to be independent markers of outcome. In contrast, WHO grading did not show any predictive impact. Thus, risk stratification based on robust and uniform molecular subgrouping was found to be superior to histopathological grading.

In-depth and comprehensive analyses of the molecular landscape of ependymal tumors have created new opportunities to identify relevant therapeutic targets in these treatment-resistant tumors. In addition, more accurate risk stratification based on molecular subgroups is expected to improve clinical care of patients with ependymoma. Future application of molecular classification approaches in a clinical setting might enable adjustment of treatment aggressiveness and assessment of treatment efficacies in the context of specific molecular subgroups, thereby refining current treatments and ultimately allowing for direct implementation of targeted therapies.

8.3 Preclinical Models

Apart from oncogenic aberrations in the three molecular subtypes of ependymal tumors, including recurrent fusions to *RELA* and *YAP1* (in ST-EPN-RELA and ST-EPN-YAP1, respectively) as well as frequent mutations of the *NF2* gene (in SP-EPN), little is known about the aberrant cellular and molecular processes that drive ependymal brain tumors. Limited availability of in vitro and in vivo model systems has especially hampered efforts to understand tumor biology and to test novel therapies for ependymoma. Efforts to establish permanent ependymoma cell lines have largely been unsuccessful, as many of the cultured ependymoma cells can only survive for a short period of time (Jennings et al. 1994).

Brisson and colleagues were able to maintain two of their 11 cultures, one from a grade III hindbrain ependymoma in a 3-year-old child and one from a grade II ependymoma in a 63-year-old patient, long-term in vitro. However, these cells proliferated unusually slowly, requiring 2 years to reach passage 18 (Brisson et al. 2002). In addition, relatively complex culture conditions were needed for successful propagation of tumoral ependymocytes since they had to be cocultured in a 3D culture with endothelial cells. Only very few groups have reported successful establishment of permanent ependymal cell lines growing as monolayers. Interestingly, most of these in vitro models were derived from xenograft models of ependymal tumors. The cell line BXD-1425EPN, which was generated from a passage II xenograft tumor, expressed similar differentiation markers to the ependymal xenograft tumor, maintained identical chromosomal abnormalities, and was capable of forming tumors in the brains of immunodeficient mice (Yu et al. 2010). Guan et al. successfully established two in vitro models, BT-44 and BT-57, using human xenografts. Both models stained positive for GFAP and vimentin in the cytoplasm, harbored ultrastructural characteristics of ependymal cells, including numerous microvilli and microfilaments, and displayed aberrant activation of typical signaling pathways, such as EGFR (Guan et al. 2011). Whereas BXD-1425EPN was pas-

saged in vitro more than 70 times, BT-44 and BT-57 cells could only be passaged serially for 15–20 passages before the cells underwent senescence (Guan et al. 2011; Yu et al. 2010). Bobola et al. (2005) examined the contribution of the DNA repair protein O6-methylguanine-DNA methyltransferase (MGMT) to BCNU and temozolomide resistance in newly characterized ependymoma cell lines Res196, 253, and 254. These cell were grown as monolayers and could be maintained in continuous culture for >50–100 passages. The cells were reported to form spheroids if maintained under suspension culture conditions. Immunohistochemistry revealed strong to moderate expression of glial fibrillary acidic protein and neuron-specific nuclear protein as well as moderate expression of synaptophysin, except for Res254.

It has been reported that multipotent CD133 positive cells, which show features of radial glia (the progenitors that are known to give rise to ependymal cells), are cancer-initiating cells (CSC) and can be cultured from human ependymomas using the neurosphere assay (Taylor et al. 2005). Since the defining characteristics of stemness, that is self-renewal and tumor propagation, are often lost in serum-cultured cell lines of brain tumors (Lee et al. 2006), other groups tried to more closely mirror the phenotype of primary ependymal tumors by culturing cells as neurospheres rather than as monolayers. In order to elucidate the role of CSCs in pediatric brain tumor drug resistance, ependymoma cell lines nEPN1 and nEPN2 were established from a recurrent supratentorial and a primary posterior fossa ependymoma, respectively (Hussein et al. 2011). Both cell lines rapidly formed neurospheres when cultured under appropriate conditions and retained CNAs of the original corresponding tumor. A comparison of neurosphere culture with monolayer culture revealed a higher capacity for multilineage differentiation of neurosphere-derived cells (Hussein et al. 2011). Notably, the neurospheroids also demonstrated an increased resistance to etoposide compared with monolayer-derived cells. The spherogenic and proliferative properties of brain tumor stem cells are known to be dependent on epidermal growth factor (EGF) that binds to the EGF receptor (EGFR) (Vescovi et al. 2006). In addition, ERBB receptor signaling promotes ependymoma cell proliferation (Gilbertson et al. 2002). Based on this knowledge, Servidei et al. analyzed the effects of EGFR blockade on ependymoma CSCs (Servidei et al. 2012). In this study, two ependymoma CSC lines were established from recurrent infratentorial pediatric ependymoma, designated EPP and EPV. Both cell lines expressed markers of radial glia and showed renewal ability as well as multipotency. Interestingly, inhibition of EGFR led to marked reduction of clonogenicity and proliferation accompanied by a strong decrease of CD133 positive cell content. However, although CD133 expression markedly differed between EPP and EPV cell lines (94% vs. 6%, respectively), both lines generated tumors with 100% penetrance when orthotopically transplanted without prior sorting procedures (Servidei et al. 2012). These findings finally prompted the authors to speculate that CD133 might not unambiguously identify tumorigenic cells in ependymoma.

Another stem cell model, DKFZ-EP1NS, was derived from metastasis (malignant ascites) of a patient with highly aggressive supratentorial anaplastic ependymoma WHO III (Milde et al. 2011). DKFZ-EP1NS cells were kept in culture for up to 9 months, corresponding to over 30 passages. Although these cells clearly displayed long-term self-renewal capacity, in contrast to the model described by Servidei and colleagues, they were completely negative for CD133. Cells deriving from this model were intrinsically resistant to temozolomide, vincristine, and cisplatin, thus mimicking the broad chemoresistance of primary ependymal tumors. In clear contrast, DKFZ-EP1NS cells were susceptible to a panel of histone deacetylase inhibitors (HDACi) (Milde et al. 2011). Recent further in-depth molecular analyses could assign this model to one of the supratentorial molecular subgroups of ependymoma, ST-EPN-RELA (Pajtler et al. 2015).

Another approach that allows for a limited number of in vitro experiments, e.g., preclinical drug testing, is short-term cultures of ependymoma. Cells within short-term cultures are destined to undergo senescence after a certain number of passages but have the advantage of being less different from the original tumor than cells from long-term cultures, which often harbor additionally acquired DNA alterations. In order to test the effect of epigenetic modifiers on ependymal tumors, Mack et al. established four short-term, patient-derived primary ependymoma cultures from two PF-EPN-A tumors (E517/E520) and two childhood supratentorial ependymomas (E478/E479) (Mack et al. 2014). Notably, they were unable to grow ependymomas of the less aggressive subtype, PF-EPN-B, in vitro.

To date, approaches to model ependymoma in vivo have been mainly based on patient-derived xenografts. Genetically engineered mouse models that spontaneously develop ependymal tumors are not available. In order to facilitate transplantation and monitoring processes, tumors are often injected subcutaneously. Examples of these subcutaneous xenograft mouse models are D528EP, D612EP, and HxBr5 (Horowitz et al. 1987; McLendon et al. 1996). Other subcutaneous xenograft models, BT-46, -41, -44, -54, are part of the National Cancer Institute supported Pediatric Preclinical Testing Program, which systematically evaluates new agents against childhood solid tumors (Houghton et al. 2007). However, since subcutaneous xenograft models often fail to replicate the complex interactions between tumors and their native microenvironment (Gilbertson and Gutmann 2007; Gutmann et al. 2006, b; Morton and Houghton 2007), attempts have been made to transplant human tumor cells directly into the brains of immunodeficient mice to create orthotopic xenograft mouse models. This direct injection of human primary tumors, ideally into anatomically matched locations of the rodent brain, is expected to better replicate the biology of the original lesion. In addition, this approach does not circumvent the blood brain barrier and might therefore have better predictability of future clinical treatment success when used for preclinical drug testing purposes. Guan et al. developed an intracranial disease model of ependymoma by engrafting xenograft tissue specimens, BT-44 and BT-57 (both from anaplastic posterior fossa ependymomas in children), that were minced into single-cell suspensions and were injected into the caudate nucleus of athymic mice (Guan et al. 2011). All of the mice injected with tumor cells developed signs of neurological deficit or became moribund within a period of 100–150 days after injection. Histopathological examination of the resulting tumors revealed pseudorosette formation, a typical phenotype of ependymoma. Comparing Ki-67 expression of intracranial tumors to its expression in subcutaneous xenografts, the investigators found a higher index in intracranial tumors, suggesting that the microenvironment indeed influences tumor growth. Interestingly, serial transplantation of xenograft tumors led to repeated tumor formation without changes of growth patterns (Guan et al. 2011).

In an attempt to develop clinically relevant animal models of ependymoma, Yu et al. directly injected a fresh surgical specimen (100,000 primary tumor cells) from a recurrent anaplastic ependymoma in a 9-year-old patient into the right cerebrum of RAG2/severe complex immune deficiency (SCID) mice. All five mice receiving the initial transplantation of the patient tumor developed signs of neurological deficit or became moribund within 97–144 days after injection. The orthotopic xenograft tumors, termed IC-1425EPN, shared nearly identical histopathological features with the original tumor and also maintained gene expression profiles resembling that of the original patient tumor. Notably, the model also preserved a small cancer stem cell pool (0.25–2.2%) during repeated in vivo subtransplantations. Similar to the typical growth patterns of primary ependymomas, the xenografts appeared to be well demarcated. However, subtle analyses of the neighboring brain parenchyma could identify infiltrating tumor cells. In another study by Hussein et al., two xenograft models of ependymoma, nEPN1 and 2, were established (Hussein et al. 2011). Although the spindle-cell component of the tumor of origin was retained in nEPN1, ultrastructural examination of the xenograft did not show typical cilia that were present in the primary. In a similar line, nEPN2 xenograft was negative for glial and neu-

ronal markers, was less well differentiated, and lost classical morphological features of ependymoma compared to the primary tumor. This points to the importance of constantly monitoring xenograft tumors used for preclinical testing as their biology might change due to different microenvironmental settings or evolution of certain subclones. Orthotopic xenotransplantation of the CSC models, EPP, EPV, and DKFZ-EP1NS, described above, gave rise to tumors after 67, 95, and 297 days, respectively (Milde et al. 2011; Servidei et al. 2012). All tumors were well demarcated and closely resembled the histopathologic features of the primary tumors.

Milde and colleagues performed a serial transplantation of DKFZ-EP1NS cells from orthotopic xenografts and yielded secondary tumors in half the time compared to the initial transplantation (Milde et al. 2011). The observed acceleration of tumor formation suggests a selection for more aggressive cellular subclones and might therefore represent a model to study progressive disease. In addition, DKFZ-EP1NS cells were found to harbor a certain transcriptome plasticity, since they express a neural stem cell-like program when growing as neuropsheres but recapitulate a profile of primary ependymomas upon in vivo transplantation (Milde et al. 2011). On the basis of previous work showing that intracranial and spinal ependymomas are propagated by radial glia-like cancer stem cells (Taylor et al. 2005), Johnson et al. reasoned that regionally and developmentally distinct radial glia cells, functioning as NSCs in the embryo and being a precursor of adult NSCs, might give rise to individual subgroups of ependymoma (Johnson et al. 2010). Embryonic cerebral NSCs with a deleted Ink4a/Arf locus, which encodes Cdkn2a and b that are frequently lost from human supratentorial ependymomas, were isolated from mice. The NSCs were challenged with overexpression of Ephb2, which is selectively amplified and/or overexpressed in cerebral ependymomas. Fifty percent of mice orthotopically implanted with these cells developed brain tumors within 200 days. The resulting mouse tumors were histologically indistinguishable from human ependymoma and displayed characteristic pseudorosettes, thus representing the first transgenic mouse model of supratentorial ependymoma. A cross-species genomics approach matched the transcriptome of these tumors to the human supratentorial ependymoma subgroup D defined by Johnson et al.; this subgroup showed some overlap with the DNA methylation based molecular subgroups ST-EPN-RELA and ST-SE (Johnson et al. 2010; Pajtler et al. 2015). An integrated in vitro and in vivo high-throughput drug screen using this model identified the generic chemotherapeutic agent 5-fluorouracil as possessing selective toxicity against this specific subtype and therefore clinical trials have begun (Atkinson et al. 2011; Wright et al. 2015).

After having identified that around 70% of supratentorial ependymomas harbor a *RELA-C11orf95* fusion, Parker et al. also used NSCs from Ink4a/Arf-null transgenic mice to test the transforming capacity of RELA fusion proteins (Parker et al. 2014). All mice implanted with NSCs transduced with the *RELA* fusion type 1 developed brain tumors within 20 days that recapitulated the histopathology and molecular patterns of *RELA* fusion positive human supratentorial ependymoma, proving this as an accurate model for the aggressive subtype of ST-EPN-RELA tumors (Parker et al. 2014). Aside from the advantage for biological and preclinical studies that these mouse models closely recapitulate characteristics of primary human ependymoma, large-scale testing of potential new drug-leads might rapidly lead to expensive and labor-intensive endeavors. In this context, Eden et al. recently reported on an intermediary platform between high-throughput drug screens and mice by adapting mouse models of pediatric brain tumors to grow as orthotopic xenografts in the brains of zebrafish (Eden et al. 2015). Red fluorescence protein (RFP)-expressing tumor cells were isolated from ependymal tumors that were generated from Ink4a/Arf deleted NSCs retrovirally transduced either with *EPHB2*, as described by Johnson et al. (Johnson et al. 2010), or with RTBDN, a novel potential ependymoma oncogene (Mohankumar et al. 2015). Cells that were injected via the intranasal route into the cerebrum of anesthetized, 30-day-old, dexamethasone immunosuppressed zebrafish formed tumors that recapitulated the histology of the parent ependymal tumor with pseudorosettes and immunoreactivity for GFAP. In the future, the described model might therefore serve as an inexpensive and rapid method to study drug efficacy in large cohorts of brain tumor-bearing zebrafish prior to further formal efficacy testing in mice.

Accurate in vitro and in vivo models of ependymoma subtypes are crucial to gain further insights into the biological mechanisms that are underlying this disease, as well as to adequately reflect ependymoma heterogeneity during preclinical drug testing. However, diagnoses of most primary tumors from which the above-described models were generated are based on histopathological findings only and lack further molecular characterization. In most cases, the resulting preclinical models were not further molecularly analyzed either. This involves the danger that promising novel therapeutic approaches against ependymoma are tested in unselected and potentially even inadequate tumor models, resulting in the rejection of drugs that otherwise might have been taken further. Comprehensive molecular profiling studies conducted in recent years have identified distinct molecular subgroups that are defined by different genetic alterations and largely differ in patient age and outcome (Mack et al. 2014; Pajtler et al. 2015; Wani et al. 2012; Witt et al. 2011). Existing and upcoming model systems of ependymoma should be analyzed for subgroup affiliation to allow for molecularly informed preclinical studies, which is expected to ultimately increase the likelihood for successful clinical studies.

8.4 Clinical Studies

Currently, the therapeutic strategy for pediatric ependymomas is maximal neurosurgical resection, followed by irradiation and in some cases chemotherapy. The clinical presentation is often nonspecific, especially in young children. The most common presentation (56%) is vomiting, which is related to increased intracranial pressure from obstructive hydrocephalus (Purdy et al.

2014). Patients may also present with headache or with cerebellar or lower cranial nerve dysfunction; in young children, lethargy and irritability may be the only presenting symptoms.

Complete neurosurgical resection is still the most important prognostic factor of overall outcome of ependymoma (Korshunov et al. 2010; Merchant et al. 2009; Pajtler et al. 2015; Witt et al. 2011). Considerable advances have been made in the past decades to cure a substantial proportion of children with these tumors. However, many children still succumb to their disease, and many survivors suffer from severe long-term cognitive, neurological, endocrine, and psychosocial sequelae of the intensive multimodal treatment that includes surgery and radiochemotherapy. Although the standard of care for intracranial ependymomas often includes chemotherapy, the results of chemotherapy efficacy studies vary and therefore its use as an adjuvant part of treatment is still controversial (Bouffet and Foreman 1999; Grundy et al. 2007; Massimino et al. 2004; Venkatramani et al. 2013). Prolonged dose-intensive chemotherapy, including the drugs cyclophosphamide, vincristine, cisplatin, and etoposide, applied to patients with malignant brain tumors resulted in increased EFS only for patients with ependymoma (Strother et al. 2014).

The role of chemotherapy in the treatment of ependymoma is not well established, and response rates to single agent or combination chemotherapy in recurrent ependymoma are disappointing (Bouffet et al. 2009). It has been shown, however, that chemotherapy can be effectively used to delay the beginning of radiotherapy in very young children, without compromising their prognosis (Grundy et al. 2007). Recent and ongoing clinical trials are examining the role of neoadjuvant chemotherapy in unresectable or disseminated disease, as well as in the adjuvant setting post-radiation therapy for high-risk patients (Gajjar et al. 2013).

In North America and across Europe, pediatric patients with a diagnosis of an ependymoma are commonly enrolled in one of two clinical studies: in North America the Children's Oncology Group trial ACNS0831 (NCT01096368) and in Europe SIOP Ependymoma II trial (EudraCT No. 2013-002766-39). The ACNS0831 study is a phase III randomized trial of post-radiation chemotherapy in patients with newly diagnosed ependymomas between the ages of 1 and 21 years. This study aims to answer whether the application of maintenance chemotherapy after radiation will increase PFS and OS rates or will generate additional toxicity. Endocrine, neuropsychological, and neurological long-term side effects of treatment are evaluated in detail. Prospectively, molecular classification and genetic alterations of distinct molecular subtypes of ependymomas are studied.

The ACNS0831 comprises three major treatment arms; for each arm, the level of neurosurgical resection is an essential part of stratification. The first arm includes patients with subtotal resected tumor, independent of age, histological WHO grade or localization. Their treatment begins with induction chemotherapy consisting of: Cycle A—vincristine, carboplatin, and cyclophosphamide, and Cycle B—vincristine, carboplatin, and etoposide. After 7 weeks of the induction regimen, a response assessment is scheduled and, in selected cases, a second look surgery is performed. Depending on the response to chemotherapy and level of resection, patients may receive conformal radiation therapy and then be randomized to receive maintenance chemotherapy or observation. Patients with stable or progressive disease or with residual disease after second look surgery are treated with conformal radiation therapy and maintenance chemotherapy. Maintenance chemotherapy consists of four cycles of vincristine, carboplatin, and cyclophosphamide, and etoposide. The second arm includes children with gross or near total resected ependymomas, of any histological grade for infratentorial tumors and only anaplastic supratentorial tumors. This treatment cohort will receive conformal radiotherapy, followed by randomization to maintenance chemotherapy versus observation. Only microscopically completely resected supratentorial ependymoma patients with classic histology are stratified into the third arm. These children will be observed without any further treatment approaches. The major goal of the

ACNS0831 trial is the determination of EFS and OS of children with completely resected tumors after treatment with postoperative conformal radiation therapy. Additionally, to address the question of whether chemotherapy improves clinical outcome, patients will be randomized to treatment arms with or without maintenance chemotherapy.

The SIOP Ependymoma Program II is a European clinical study that includes patients diagnosed with ependymoma until 22 years of age. This trial aims to improve the precision of the primary diagnosis of ependymoma and to evaluate distinct therapeutic regimens in children and young adults. An important advantage of this study is the precise analyses of molecular patterns as an integral biological study. This high priority initiative is an essential element of the overall program to improve the future treatment of ependymoma. Patients will be enrolled in one of three different strata according to the result of the neurosurgical resection, and their age or eligibility and suitability to receive radiotherapy. Each therapeutic strata will be evaluated in a specific randomized fashion to verify the proposed therapeutic strategies. Before the final strata assignment, another evaluation to determine whether second look surgery is indicated will be performed. This step underlines the importance of gross total resection of these tumors. Stratum 1 is designed as a randomized phase III study. Children and young adults between the age of 1 year and 22 years with no measurable tumor residue will be included in this treatment cohort. These patients will be randomized to receive conformal radiotherapy followed by either 16 weeks of maintenance chemotherapy, including the drugs vincristine, etoposide, cyclophosphamide, and cisplatin, or observation. The aim of this stratum is to determine the clinical impact of maintenance chemotherapy after surgical complete resection followed by conformal radiotherapy in terms of PFS of intracranial ependymomas. Stratum 2 is designed as a randomized phase II trial for patients between 1 year and 22 years of age who have inoperable measurable residual disease. The initial randomization includes induction chemotherapy with vincristine, etoposide, and cyclophosphamide with or without

high-dose methotrexate. A subsequent response assessment will evaluate the possibility of second look surgery. If no residual disease is detected, conformal radiotherapy will be performed followed by maintenance chemotherapy. If there is residual inoperable tumor, a boost of radiotherapy to the residual tumor will be delivered after conformal radiotherapy and maintenance chemotherapy. The application of high-dose methotrexate will generate results that will guide decisions regarding whether methotrexate should be investigated in future phase III trials. Stratum 3 is designed as a randomized phase II chemotherapy study in children <12 months of age or those not eligible to receive radiotherapy. Within this treatment cohort, all patients will receive intensified chemotherapy including vincristine, carboplatin, cyclophosphamide, and cisplatin, and will then be randomized to receive the HDACi, valproate. The goal of this stratum is the evaluation of the benefit of postoperative dose intense chemotherapy administered alone or in combination with valproate. In very young children, the chemotherapeutic treatment is maximized while aiming to minimize the risk of drug resistance. The information collected about the outcome of infants enrolled in this study will be of considerable benefit toward informing future international studies for the ependymoma population. In stratum 3, children under 12 month of age comprise definitively high-risk tumors including the Group A subtype. These tumors potentially could profit from HDACi therapy, based on evidence from preclinical models in which epigenetic therapies of Group-A tumors in vivo showed good response rates (Mack et al. 2014). Both of the above mentioned studies will document the molecular subtype classification up-front, and will try to implement risk stratification based on molecular subgroup information in the near future.

An exemplary translational approach was demonstrated by the preclinical development of a supratentorial subtype model (Johnson et al. 2010), followed by a comprehensive drug screen discovery (Atkinson et al. 2011), and finally the generation of a phase I 5-fluorouracil study for recurrent ependymoma (Wright et al. 2015), which demonstrated antitumor activity of 5-fluorouracil in human intracranial ependymoma. The preclinical rationale to translate this approach into a clinical trial was based on a genetic model, which recapitulated a subtype of fusion-negative supratentorial ependymomas, but not tumors with a *C11orf95-RELA* fusion. In preclinical analyses it was discussed that 5-FU treatment of a *C11orf95-RELA* human xenograft was not successful (Wright et al. 2015). Hence, it has to be clarified which molecular subtype of supratentorial ependymomas possibly can profit from 5-FU therapy. Additionally, a selection approach has to be developed that allows the identification of those patients who will profit from this particular experimental treatment approach.

Clinical outcome in children with recurrent disease from intracranial ependymoma remains extremely poor, regardless of age and initial treatment (Messahel et al. 2009; Zacharoulis et al. 2010). In relapsing children, phase II studies overall report a low response rate with standard (Bouffet and Foreman 1999) or high-dose chemotherapy (Grill and Kalifa 1998). Metronomic therapies have produced long-term stabilizations (Robison et al. 2014). The use of targeted treatment strategies has shown disappointing results so far. Most recently, the Collaborative Ependymoma Research Network (CERN) developed an open-label trial using the drugs bevacizumab and lapatinib in the framework of a phase II study in children with recurrent or refractory ependymomas (DeWire et al. 2015). The dual therapy was well tolerated by the patients, but was ineffective in children with recurrent ependymomas. The improved understanding of ependymoma molecular biology by comprehensive genetic and epigenetic studies has provided a large source of preclinical testing modalities. Several new targets and pathways have been identified during recent years, such as *RELA-C11orf95* fusion and NF-kappaB activation in supratentorial ependymomas (Parker et al. 2014), and the response of epigenetic modifiers, e.g., HDACi and inhibitors of the polycomb repressive complex 2 (PRC2) in vitro and in vivo (Mack et al. 2014; Milde et al. 2011). Other preclinical studies have proposed that response to poly ADP ribose polymerase (PARP) inhibitors, e.g., olaparib which has been shown to be a radiosensitizer in childhood ependymoma (van Vuurden et al. 2011), or Hippo signaling pathway inhibitors in *YAP1* fusion positive ependymomas (Pajtler et al. 2015) could be future areas for targeted therapy approaches. However, the translation process from preclinical studies into clinical phase I or II trials is a time consuming challenge.

Based on experience with the comprehensive spectrum of newly discovered genetic and epigenetic alterations in pediatric ependymomas, combination targeted treatment approaches are promising. In terms of the low numbers of this rare disease, multi-center studies should be more effectively employed to increase the enrollment numbers of ependymoma patients. Future treatment approaches for ependymomas should include up-front stratification of subtypes. Further novel targeted treatment decisions should be made based on preclinical experiences with in vitro and in vivo treatment of subtype-specific ependymoma models. Eventually, novel treatment approaches will broaden and replace current chemotherapy trials in the foreseeable future.

References

Allen JC, Siffert J, Hukin J (1998) Clinical manifestations of childhood ependymoma: a multitude of syndromes. Pediatr Neurosurg 28:49–55

Antony R, Wong KE, Patel M, Olch AJ, McComb G, Krieger M, Gilles F, Sposto R, Erdreich-Epstein A, Dhall G et al (2014) A retrospective analysis of recurrent intracranial ependymoma. Pediatr Blood Cancer 61:1195–1201

Archer TC, Pomeroy SL (2011) Posterior fossa ependymomas: a tale of two subtypes. Cancer Cell 20: 133–134

Atkinson JM, Shelat AA, Carcaboso AM, Kranenburg TA, Arnold LA, Boulos N, Wright K, Johnson RA, Poppleton H, Mohankumar KM et al (2011) An integrated in vitro and in vivo high-throughput screen identifies treatment leads for ependymoma. Cancer Cell 20:384–399

Bandopadhayay P, Silvera VM, Ciarlini PD, Malkin H, Bi WL, Bergthold G, Faisal AM, Ullrich NJ, Marcus K, Scott RM et al (2016) Myxopapillary ependymomas in children: imaging, treatment and outcomes. J Neuro-Oncol 126(1):165–174

Bobola MS, Silber JR, Ellenbogen RG, Geyer JR, Blank A, Goff RD (2005) O6-methylguanine-DNA methyltransferase, O6-benzylguanine, and resistance to clinical alkylators in pediatric primary brain tumor cell lines. Clin Cancer Res 11:2747–2755

Bouffet E, Foreman N (1999) Chemotherapy for intracranial ependymomas. Childs Nerv Syst 15:563–570

Bouffet E, Tabori U, Huang A, Bartels U (2009) Ependymoma: lessons from the past, prospects for the future. Childs Nerv Syst 25:1383–1384. author reply 1385

Brisson C, Lelong-Rebel I, Mottolese C, Jouvet A, Fevre-Montange M, Saint Pierre G, Rebel G, Belin MF (2002) Establishment of human tumoral ependymal cell lines and coculture with tubular-like human endothelial cells. Int J Oncol 21:775–785

Cage TA, Clark AJ, Aranda D, Gupta N, Sun PP, Parsa AT, Auguste KI (2013) A systematic review of treatment outcomes in pediatric patients with intracranial ependymomas. J Neurosurg Pediatr 11:673–681

Cashman PM, Kitney RI, Gariba MA, Carter ME (2002) Automated techniques for visualization and mapping of articular cartilage in MR images of the osteoarthritic knee: a base technique for the assessment of microdamage and submicro damage. IEEE Trans Nanobioscience 1:42–51

DeWire M, Fouladi M, Turner DC, Wetmore C, Hawkins C, Jacobs C, Yuan Y, Liu D, Goldman S, Fisher P et al (2015) An open-label, two-stage, phase II study of bevacizumab and lapatinib in children with recurrent or refractory ependymoma: a collaborative ependymoma research network study (CERN). J Neuro-Oncol 123:85–91

Dyer S, Prebble E, Davison V, Davies P, Ramani P, Ellison D, Grundy R (2002) Genomic imbalances in pediatric intracranial ependymomas define clinically relevant groups. Am J Pathol 161:2133–2141

Ebert C, von Haken M, Meyer-Puttlitz B, Wiestler OD, Reifenberger G, Pietsch T, von Deimling A (1999) Molecular genetic analysis of ependymal tumors. NF2 mutations and chromosome 22q loss occur preferentially in intramedullary spinal ependymomas. Am J Pathol 155:627–632

Eden CJ, Ju B, Murugesan M, Phoenix TN, Nimmervoll B, Tong Y, Ellison DW, Finkelstein D, Wright K, Boulos N et al (2015) Orthotopic models of pediatric brain tumors in zebrafish. Oncogene 34:1736–1742

Ellison DW, Kocak M, Figarella-Branger D, Felice G, Catherine G, Pietsch T, Frappaz D, Massimino M, Grill J, Boyett JM, Grundy RG (2011) Histopathological grading of pediatric ependymoma: reproducibility and clinical relevance in European trial cohorts. J Negat Results Biomed 10:7

Gajjar A, Packer RJ, Foreman NK, Cohen K, Haas-Kogan D, Merchant TE (2013) Children's Oncology Group's 2013 blueprint for research: central nervous system tumors. Pediatr Blood Cancer 60:1022–1026

Gajjar A, Pfister SM, Taylor MD, Gilbertson RJ (2014) Molecular insights into pediatric brain tumors have the potential to transform therapy. Clin Cancer Res 20:5630–5640

Gilbertson RJ, Bentley L, Hernan R, Junttila TT, Frank AJ, Haapasalo H, Connelly M, Wetmore C, Curran T, Elenius K, Ellison DW (2002) ERBB receptor signaling promotes ependymoma cell proliferation and represents a potential novel therapeutic target for this disease. Clin Cancer Res 8:3054–3064

Gilbertson RJ, Gutmann DH (2007) Tumorigenesis in the brain: location, location, location. Cancer Res 67:5579–5582

Godfraind C, Kaczmarska JM, Kocak M, Dalton J, Wright KD, Sanford RA, Boop FA, Gajjar A, Merchant TE, Ellison DW (2012) Distinct disease-risk groups in pediatric supratentorial and posterior fossa ependymomas. Acta Neuropathol 124:247–257

Grill J, Kalifa C (1998) High dose chemotherapy for childhood ependymona. J Neuro-Oncol 40:97

Grundy RG, Wilne SA, Weston CL, Robinson K, Lashford LS, Ironside J, Cox T, Chong WK, Campbell RH, Bailey CC et al (2007) Primary postoperative chemotherapy without radiotherapy for intracranial ependymoma in children: the UKCCSG/SIOP prospective study. Lancet Oncol 8:696–705

Guan S, Shen R, Lafortune T, Tiao N, Houghton P, Yung WK, Koul D (2011) Establishment and characterization of clinically relevant models of ependymoma: a true challenge for targeted therapy. Neuro-Oncology 13:748–758

Gutmann DH, Hunter-Schaedle K, Shannon KM (2006) Harnessing preclinical mouse models to inform human clinical cancer trials. J Clin Invest 116:847–852

Gutmann DH, Maher EA, Van Dyke T (2006) Mouse models of human cancers consortium workshop on nervous system tumors. Cancer Res 66:10–13

Hoadley KA, Yau C, Wolf DM, Cherniack AD, Tamborero D, Ng S, Leiserson MD, Niu B, McLellan MD, Uzunangelov V et al (2014) Multiplatform analysis of 12 cancer types reveals molecular classification within and across tissues of origin. Cell 158:929–944

Horowitz ME, Parham DM, Douglass EC, Kun LE, Houghton JA, Houghton PJ (1987) Development and characterization of human ependymoma xenograft HxBr5. Cancer Res 47:499–504

Houghton PJ, Morton CL, Tucker C, Payne D, Favours E, Cole C, Gorlick R, Kolb EA, Zhang W, Lock R et al (2007) The pediatric preclinical testing program: description of models and early testing results. Pediatr Blood Cancer 49:928–940

Hovestadt V, Jones DT, Picelli S, Wang W, Kool M, Northcott PA, Sultan M, Stachurski K, Ryzhova M, Warnatz HJ et al (2014) Decoding the regulatory landscape of medulloblastoma using DNA methylation sequencing. Nature 510:537–541

Hussein D, Punjaruk W, Storer LC, Shaw L, Othman R, Peet A, Miller S, Bandopadhyay G, Heath R, Kumari R et al (2011) Pediatric brain tumor cancer stem cells: cell cycle dynamics, DNA repair, and etoposide extrusion. Neuro-Oncology 13:70–83

Jennings MT, Kaariainen IT, Gold L, Maciunas RJ, Commers PA (1994) TGF beta 1 and TGF beta 2 are potential growth regulators for medulloblastomas, primitive neuroectodermal tumors, and ependymomas: evidence in support of an autocrine hypothesis. Hum Pathol 25:464–475

Johnson RA, Wright KD, Poppleton H, Mohankumar KM, Finkelstein D, Pounds SB, Rand V, Leary SE, White E, Eden C et al (2010) Cross-species genomics matches driver mutations and cell compartments to model ependymoma. Nature 466:632–636

Kilday JP, Mitra B, Domerg C, Ward J, Andreiuolo F, Osteso-Ibanez T, Mauguen A, Varlet P, Le Deley MC, Lowe J et al (2012) Copy number gain of 1q25 predicts poor progression-free survival for pediatric intracranial ependymomas and enables patient risk stratification: a prospective European clinical trial cohort analysis on behalf of the Children's Cancer Leukaemia Group (CCLG), Societe Francaise d'Oncologie Pediatrique (SFOP), and International Society for Pediatric Oncology (SIOP). Clin Cancer Res 18:2001–2011

Kilday JP, Rahman R, Dyer S, Ridley L, Lowe J, Coyle B, Grundy R (2009) Pediatric ependymoma: biological perspectives. Mol Cancer Res 7:765–786

Korshunov A, Neben K, Wrobel G, Tews B, Benner A, Hahn M, Golanov A, Lichter P (2003) Gene expression patterns in ependymomas correlate with tumor location, grade, and patient age. Am J Pathol 163:1721–1727

Korshunov A, Witt H, Hielscher T, Benner A, Remke M, Ryzhova M, Milde T, Bender S, Wittmann A, Schottler A et al (2010) Molecular staging of intracranial ependymoma in children and adults. J Clin Oncol 28:3182–3190

Lee J, Kotliarova S, Kotliarov Y, Li A, Su Q, Donin NM, Pastorino S, Purow BW, Christopher N, Zhang W et al (2006) Tumor stem cells derived from glioblastomas cultured in bFGF and EGF more closely mirror the phenotype and genotype of primary tumors than do serum-cultured cell lines. Cancer Cell 9:391–403

Louis DN, Ohgaki H, Wiestler OD, Cavenee WK, Burger PC, Jouvet A, Scheithauer BW, Kleihues P (2007) The 2007 WHO classification of tumours of the central nervous system. Acta Neuropathol 114:97–109

Mack SC, Witt H, Piro RM, Gu L, Zuyderduyn S, Stutz AM, Wang X, Gallo M, Garzia L, Zayne K et al (2014) Epigenomic alterations define lethal CIMP-positive ependymomas of infancy. Nature 506:445–450

Massimino M, Gandola L, Giangaspero F, Sandri A, Valagussa P, Perilongo G, Garre ML, Ricardi U, Forni M, Genitori L et al (2004) Hyperfractionated radiotherapy and chemotherapy for childhood ependymoma: final results of the first prospective AIEOP (Associazione Italiana di Ematologia-Oncologia Pediatrica) study. Int J Radiat Oncol Biol Phys 58: 1336–1345

McLendon RE, Fung KM, Bentley RC, Ahmed Rasheed BK, Trojanowski JQ, Bigner SH, Bigner DD, Friedman HS (1996) Production and characterization of two ependymoma xenografts. J Neuropathol Exp Neurol 55:540–548

Mendrzyk F, Korshunov A, Benner A, Toedt G, Pfister S, Radlwimmer B, Lichter P (2006) Identification of gains on 1q and epidermal growth factor receptor overexpression as independent prognostic markers in intracranial ependymoma. Clin Cancer Res 12:2070–2079

Merchant TE, Li C, Xiong X, Kun LE, Boop FA, Sanford RA (2009) Conformal radiotherapy after surgery for paediatric ependymoma: a prospective study. Lancet Oncol 10:258–266

Merchant TE, Mulhern RK, Krasin MJ, Kun LE, Williams T, Li C, Xiong X, Khan RB, Lustig RH, Boop FA, Sanford RA (2004) Preliminary results from a phase II trial of conformal radiation therapy and evaluation of radiation-related CNS effects for pediatric patients with localized ependymoma. J Clin Oncol 22:3156–3162

Messahel B, Ashley S, Saran F, Ellison D, Ironside J, Phipps K, Cox T, Chong WK, Robinson K, Picton S et al (2009) Relapsed intracranial ependymoma in children in the UK: patterns of relapse, survival and therapeutic outcome. Eur J Cancer 45:1815–1823

Milde T, Kleber S, Korshunov A, Witt H, Hielscher T, Koch P, Kopp HG, Jugold M, Deubzer HE, Oehme I et al (2011) A novel human high-risk ependymoma stem cell model reveals the differentiation-inducing potential of the histone deacetylase inhibitor Vorinostat. Acta Neuropathol 122:637–650

Modena P, Buttarelli FR, Miceli R, Piccinin E, Baldi C, Antonelli M, Morra I, Lauriola L, Di Rocco C, Garre ML et al (2012) Predictors of outcome in an AIEOP series of childhood ependymomas: a multifactorial analysis. Neuro-Oncology 14:1346–1356

Mohankumar KM, Currle DS, White E, Boulos N, Dapper J, Eden C, Nimmervoll B, Thiruvenkatam R, Connelly M, Kranenburg TA et al (2015) An in vivo screen identifies ependymoma oncogenes and tumor-suppressor genes. Nat Genet 47:878–887

Morton CL, Houghton PJ (2007) Establishment of human tumor xenografts in immunodeficient mice. Nat Protoc 2:247–250

Pajtler KW, Witt H, Sill M, Jones DT, Hovestadt V, Kratochwil F, Wani K, Tatevossian R, Punchihewa C, Johann P et al (2015) Molecular classification of ependymal tumors across all CNS compartments, histopathological grades, and age groups. Cancer Cell 27:728–743

Parker M, Mohankumar KM, Punchihewa C, Weinlich R, Dalton JD, Li Y, Lee R, Tatevossian RG, Phoenix TN, Thiruvenkatam R et al (2014) C11orf95-RELA fusions drive oncogenic NF-kappaB signalling in ependymoma. Nature 506:451–455

Pejavar S, Polley MY, Rosenberg-Wohl S, Chennupati S, Prados MD, Berger MS, Banerjee A, Gupta N, Haas-Kogan D (2012) Pediatric intracranial ependymoma: the roles of surgery, radiation and chemotherapy. J Neuro-Oncol 106:367–375

Poppleton H, Gilbertson RJ (2007) Stem cells of ependymoma. Br J Cancer 96:6–10

Purdy E, Johnston DL, Bartels U, Fryer C, Carret AS, Crooks B, Eisenstat DD, Lafay-Cousin L, Larouche V, Wilson B et al (2014) Ependymoma in children under the age of 3 years: a report from the Canadian Pediatric Brain Tumour Consortium. J Neuro-Oncol 117:359–364

Reni M, Gatta G, Mazza E, Vecht C (2007) Ependymoma. Crit Rev Oncol Hematol 63:81–89

Robison NJ, Campigotto F, Chi SN, Manley PE, Turner CD, Zimmerman MA, Chordas CA, Werger AM, Allen JC, Goldman S et al (2014) A phase II trial of a multi-agent oral antiangiogenic (metronomic) regimen in children with recurrent or progressive cancer. Pediatr Blood Cancer 61:636–642

Rubio MP, Correa KM, Ramesh V, MacCollin MM, Jacoby LB, von Deimling A, Gusella JF, Louis DN (1994) Analysis of the neurofibromatosis 2 gene in human ependymomas and astrocytomas. Cancer Res 54:45–47

Servidei T, Meco D, Trivieri N, Patriarca V, Vellone VG, Zannoni GF, Lamorte G, Pallini R, Riccardi R (2012) Effects of epidermal growth factor receptor blockade on ependymoma stem cells in vitro and in orthotopic mouse models. Int J Cancer 131:E791–E803

Strother DR, Lafay-Cousin L, Boyett JM, Burger P, Aronin P, Constine L, Duffner P, Kocak M, Kun LE, Horowitz ME, Gajjar A (2014) Benefit from prolonged dose-intensive chemotherapy for infants with malignant brain tumors is restricted to patients with ependymoma: a report of the Pediatric Oncology Group randomized controlled trial 9233/34. Neuro-Oncology 16:457–465

Taylor MD, Poppleton H, Fuller C, Su X, Liu Y, Jensen P, Magdaleno S, Dalton J, Calabrese C, Board J et al (2005) Radial glia cells are candidate stem cells of ependymoma. Cancer Cell 8:323–335

Tihan T, Zhou T, Holmes E, Burger PC, Ozuysal S, Rushing EJ (2008) The prognostic value of histological grading of posterior fossa ependymomas in children: a Children's Oncology Group study and a review of prognostic factors. Mod Pathol 21:165–177

van Vuurden DG, Hulleman E, Meijer OL, Wedekind LE, Kool M, Witt H, Vandertop PW, Wurdinger T, Noske DP, Kaspers GJ, Cloos J (2011) PARP inhibition sensitizes childhood high grade glioma, medulloblastoma and ependymoma to radiation. Oncotarget 2:984–996

Venkatramani R, Ji L, Lasky J, Haley K, Judkins A, Zhou S, Sposto R, Olshefski R, Garvin J, Tekautz T et al (2013) Outcome of infants and young children with newly diagnosed ependymoma treated on the "Head Start" III prospective clinical trial. J Neuro-Oncol 113:285–291

Vescovi AL, Galli R, Reynolds BA (2006) Brain tumour stem cells. Nat Rev Cancer 6:425–436

Villano JL, Parker CK, Dolecek TA (2013) Descriptive epidemiology of ependymal tumours in the United States. Br J Cancer 108:2367–2371

Wani K, Armstrong TS, Vera-Bolanos E, Raghunathan A, Ellison D, Gilbertson R, Vaillant B, Goldman S, Packer RJ, Fouladi M et al (2012) A prognostic gene expression signature in infratentorial ependymoma. Acta Neuropathol 123:727–738

Witt H, Mack SC, Ryzhova M, Bender S, Sill M, Isserlin R, Benner A, Hielscher T, Milde T, Remke M et al (2011) Delineation of two clinically and molecularly distinct subgroups of posterior fossa ependymoma. Cancer Cell 20:143–157

Wright KD, Daryani VM, Turner DC, Onar-Thomas A, Boulos N, Orr BA, Gilbertson RJ, Stewart CF, Gajjar A (2015) Phase I study of 5-fluorouracil in children and young adults with recurrent ependymoma. Neuro-Oncology 17:1620–1627

Yu L, Baxter PA, Voicu H, Gurusiddappa S, Zhao Y, Adesina A, Man TK, Shu Q, Zhang YJ, Zhao XM et al (2010) A clinically relevant orthotopic xenograft model of ependymoma that maintains the genomic signature of the primary tumor and preserves cancer stem cells in vivo. Neuro-Oncology 12:580–594

Zacharoulis S, Ashley S, Moreno L, Gentet JC, Massimino M, Frappaz D (2010) Treatment and outcome of children with relapsed ependymoma: a multi-institutional retrospective analysis. Childs Nerv Syst 26:905–911

Zacharoulis S, Ji L, Pollack IF, Duffner P, Geyer R, Grill J, Schild S, Jaing TH, Massimino M, Finlay J, Sposto R (2008) Metastatic ependymoma: a multi-institutional retrospective analysis of prognostic factors. Pediatr Blood Cancer 50:231–235

High-Grade Glioma, Including Diffuse Intrinsic Pontine Glioma

9

Matthias A. Karajannis, Matija Snuderl,
Brian K. Yeh, Michael F. Walsh, Rajan Jain,
Nikhil A. Sahasrabudhe, and Jeffrey H. Wisoff

9.1 Introduction

High-grade (malignant) gliomas are relatively rare, and comprise approximately 10% of all brain tumors diagnosed in children, with no gender predilection. Following the World Health Organization (WHO) Classification of Tumors of the Central Nervous System, the vast majority of pediatric high-grade gliomas can be classified

M. A. Karajannis (✉) · M. F. Walsh
Department of Pediatrics, Memorial Sloan Kettering Cancer Center, New York, NY, USA
e-mail: karajanm@mskcc.org; walshm2@mskcc.org

M. Snuderl
Department of Pathology, NYU Langone Health, New York, NY, USA
e-mail: matija.snuderl@nyumc.org

B. K. Yeh
Department of Radiation Oncology, NYU Langone Health, New York, NY, USA

Department of Radiation Oncology, Mount Sinai Health System, New York, NY, USA
e-mail: brian.yeh@mountsinai.org

R. Jain
Department of Radiology, NYU Langone Health, New York, NY, USA

Department of Neurosurgery, NYU Langone Health, New York, NY, USA
e-mail: rajan.jain@nyumc.org

N. A. Sahasrabudhe · J. H. Wisoff
Department of Neurosurgery, NYU Langone Health, New York, NY, USA
e-mail: nikhil.sahasrabudhe@nyumc.org; jeffrey.wisoff@nyumc.org

histologically as either anaplastic astrocytoma (WHO grade III) or glioblastoma (WHO grade IV). Refining the traditional histology-based classification and grading schema, the recently updated WHO classification has introduced several molecularly defined HGG entities based on key discoveries in molecular genetics of HGG over the past decade (Louis et al. 2016).

The vast majority of pediatric HGG are considered "primary" HGG, whereas HGG in adults often arise from low-grade gliomas that underwent stepwise malignant transformation ("secondary" HGG) (Lai et al. 2011). Radiation-induced HGG may occur in both children and adults, with a median latency period of approximately 9 years (Elsamadicy et al. 2015), and ionizing radiation remains the only proven exposure risk factor for HGG. Interestingly, atopy has been linked to a risk reduction of up to 40% in developing glioma (Linos et al. 2007).

A unifying biological feature of HGG is the diffuse infiltration of tumor cells into the central nervous system (CNS), representing a major therapeutic challenge (Kelly et al. 1987). This means that even in patients in whom a radical tumor resection can be achieved at diagnosis, disseminated tumor cells remain well beyond the areas of signal abnormalities seen on MRI.

The molecular features and dismal clinical outcome of diffuse intrinsic pontine glioma (DIPG) are highly similar to pediatric HGG arising in other anatomical midline structures of the CNS, such as thalamic or spinal cord HGG. As a result, these "midline pediatric HGGs" can be viewed as a spectrum along a single molecular and clinicopathological entity (Sturm et al. 2012; Fontebasso et al. 2014).

HGG are relatively resistant to standard therapies, including radiation therapy (RT) and chemotherapy. As a result, the prognosis remains dismal and little progress in terms of outcome has been achieved over the past decades. However, recent major advances in our understanding of the molecular genetics and biology of pediatric HGG provide hope for the future by opening multiple avenues for the development of novel therapeutic approaches.

9.2   Clinical Presentation and Diagnosis

HGG can develop at any age, and while the most common locations include the cerebral white matter and deep midline structures, HGG may arise anywhere in the CNS. The clinical presentation is dependent on the anatomical location of the tumor, as well as on the age of the patient. The signs and symptoms prior to diagnosis are usually rapidly evolving, and may include raised intracranial pressure, focal neurological deficits, and/or seizures.

Depending on the suspected tumor location, an MRI (with and without contrast) of the brain and/or spine is typically performed initially. CNS dissemination at diagnosis, including distant sites, is present in approximately 3% of HGG patients (Benesch et al. 2005), and secondary dissemination can be observed in over 20% (Wagner et al. 2006). In DIPG patients, leptomeningeal dissemination is present in up to 20% of patients at diagnosis (Sethi et al. 2011). Therefore, complete neuroimaging of the entire neuraxis (brain and total spine) in all pediatric patients with HGG, including DIPG, is recommended. Although tumor cells can occasionally be found in the CSF (Benesch et al. 2005), a diagnostic lumbar puncture is not considered a standard part of initial staging. With very rare exceptions, HGG do not disseminate outside the CNS.

In patients with a compatible clinical history and imaging findings, the diagnosis of DIPG can be established without tissue confirmation. Onset of clinical symptoms is generally rapid, within weeks to a few months. A history of long-standing or slowly progressive symptoms should prompt investigations to rule out other diagnoses, including nonneoplastic conditions such as Alexander disease (Tavasoli et al. 2017). A classic triad of symptoms on DIPG patients includes *cerebellar signs* (e.g., ataxia, dysmetria, dysarthria), *long-tract signs* (e.g., increased tone, hyperreflexia, clonus, Babinski sign, hemiparesis), and unilateral or bilateral *cranial nerve palsies* (e.g., abducens and facial palsy). In addition, hemiparesis and ataxia are frequently present. Obstructive hydrocephalus is present in approximately 10% of patients with DIPG at the time of diagnosis. Although there are no formally established standard diagnostic criteria for DIPG, commonly suggested imaging characteristics include an intrinsic, central location involving more than 50% of the axial diameter of the pons, indistinct tumor margins, T1 hypointensity, T2 hyperintensity; partial or enhancement following gadolinium administration; encasement of the basilar artery and the absence of cystic or exophytic components (Hankinson et al. 2011). These imaging characteristics help differentiate DIPGs from other brain stem tumors, such as low-grade gliomas including dorsally exophytic brain stem gliomas, cervicomedullary junction tumors, and focal low-grade gliomas of the midbrain or brain stem, which require tissue confirmation.

The recognition of unique molecular genetic drivers of DIPG and paucity of tissue samples for research, especially pretreatment, has prompted a resurgence of diagnostic biopsies for DIPG, predominantly in the setting of clinical trials (Hamisch et al. 2017). As novel therapies are being developed to target unique molecular drivers present in subsets of DIPGs, the role for biopsy at diagnosis as part of "precision medicine" efforts will likely increase in the future.

In non-DIPG patients, initial treatment is generally surgical, with maximal safe resection of the tumor. In patients for whom this is not possible, a tumor biopsy should be performed to obtain diagnostic tissue. The clinical prognostic factors that are linked to outcome include extent of resection and histological grade, with gross total resection and anaplastic astrocytoma histology (WHO grade III) being associated with a more favorable prognosis (Pollack et al. 2003; Cohen et al. 2011).

Several heritable tumor predisposition syndromes (see Chap. 5) have been found to be associated with HGG in children. Patients with Li-Fraumeni syndrome (LFS), an autosomal-dominant condition caused by mutations in the tumor suppressor p53, have an increased risk of developing HGG (Li et al. 1988), and somatic mutations in p53 (*TP53*) are also commonly found in pediatric HGG in non-LFS patients (Pollack et al. 1997, 2002; Schwartzentruber et al. 2012), which can usually be differentiated through integrated tumor normal sequencing (Zhang et al. 2015). While patients with neurofibromatosis type 1 (NF1) most commonly develop low-grade (i.e., optic pathway) gliomas, they are also at increased risk for HGG (Byrne et al. 2017), especially secondary HGG if treated with prior RT. Patients with the autosomal recessive constitutional mismatch repair deficiency syndrome (CMMR-D) are also predisposed to developing HGG and frequently have café-au-lait macules similar to NF1, which can result in misdiagnosis (Bakry et al. 2014; Wimmer and Kratz 2010; Wimmer et al. 2017; Suerink et al. 2017). CMMR-D is caused by germline *biallelic* (homozygous or compound heterozygous) mutations in one of the DNA mismatch repair (MMR) genes: *MLH1, MSH2, MSH6,* and *PMS2.* Germline *monoallelic* mutations in MMR genes are found in hereditary nonpolyposis colon cancer, Lynch syndrome, and brain tumor polyposis syndrome type 1 (BTPS1 or Turcot type 1). Patients with CMMR-D are at increased risk for developing malignant brain tumors including HGG, as well as gastrointestinal and hematological cancers, typically within the first two decades of life. This information is highly relevant to therapy, as children with CMMR-D are excellent candidates for immunotherapy with immune checkpoint inhibitors (Bouffet et al. 2016).

Given the considerable prevalence of undiagnosed or underdiagnosed heritable tumor predisposition syndromes, referral to a clinical geneticist should be offered to all families affected by childhood HGG.

9.3 Neuroimaging

Magnetic resonance imaging (MRI) of the brain, and preferably the entire neuraxis should be performed at diagnosis and to monitor response to treatment. At the very minimum, it should include T1-weighted sequences (both before and after contrast), T2-weighted and fluid attenuated inversion recovery (FLAIR) sequences, and diffusion-weighted imaging (DWI). Pediatric HGG generally enhance after contrast injection, and appear hypointense on T1-weighted images and hyperintense on T2-weighted sequences. Areas of necrosis, seen as low-density regions on T1-weighted images, may be present. Most HGG demonstrate peritumoral edema, which appears as a surrounding, hyperintense region of signal abnormality on T2-weighted images, but may be minimal to absent, as shown in Figs. 9.1 and 9.2. Depending on location, the differential diagnosis based on imaging alone can be very broad, and may include low-grade gliomas, ependymomas, and germ cell tumors, among others.

9.3.1 MR Perfusion Imaging

MR perfusion imaging is a technology that provides hemodynamic parameters such as relative cerebral blood volume (rCBV) and cerebral blood flow (CBF), and can be applied to specific regions of interest. MR perfusion studies are typically obtained using gadolinium contrast agents, and perfusion imaging with dynamic susceptibility contrast (DSC)-MRI applies kinetic modeling to generate perfusion maps of various hemodynamic parameters and assess the cerebral microvasculature (Cha et al. 2002; Griffith and Jain 2015). Malignant brain tumors, including HGG, typically have elevated rCVB values compared to normal brain, as shown in Fig. 9.3. The utility of DSC-MRI in differentiating low-grade gliomas from HGG in the pediatric population is limited, however, mainly due to the frequently elevated perfusion values seen in pilocytic astrocytomas.

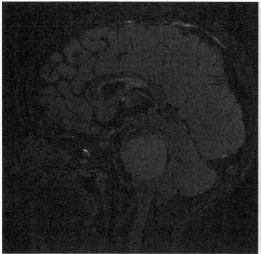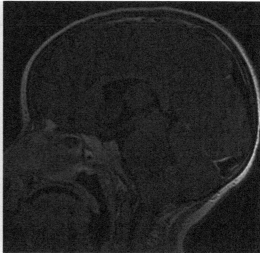

Fig. 9.1 DIPG—conventional MRI. Upper Panels: 4-year-old male presenting with 3-week history of left-sided facial droop, head tilt, and ataxia. MRI brain shows an expansile, T2/FLAIR hyperintense, infiltrating, expansile mass located in the pons (left panel), with no contrast enhancement on T1-weighted post-contrast imaging (right panel). The history and imaging characteristics were consistent with DIPG, establishing the diagnosis. The patient was subsequently treated with involved-field external beam radiation therapy

9.3.2 MR Spectroscopy

MR Spectroscopy (MRS) allows for the measurement of the relative composition of metabolites, including N-acetylaspartate (NAA), choline, creatinine, lipid, and lactate. In select cases, MRS can be a useful adjunct to standard MRI to help differentiate tumor from normal tissue and recurrent disease from treatment-related changes (Guzman-De-Villoria et al. 2014). HGG is often associated with lower levels of NAA and creatine and higher levels of choline and lactate (Guzman-De-Villoria et al. 2014), as shown in Fig. 9.4.

9.3.3 18F-Fluorodeoxyglucose Positron Emission Tomography (FDG-PET)

Metabolic imaging using FDG-PET has been explored in pediatric brain tumors (Zukotynski et al. 2014), but generally is of limited utility in the management of children with HGG and therefore rarely performed.

9.4 Surgical Considerations

HGG have historically been considered to be a nonsurgical disease since surgical resection alone is rarely, if ever, curative. However, multiple studies over the past two decades have shown that the extent of surgical resection is an independent determinant of survival, and when combined with chemotherapy and radiation, offers the best chance of durable disease control.

Although the data on surgical resection is less robust in the pediatric population, it is the current standard of practice that gross total or radical resection should be attempted when possible based on tumor location and the acceptability of postoperative deficits. In experienced centers, it is feasible to obtain a radical resection in deep tumors. In those midline tumors for which open resection is not considered to be feasible, tissue diagnosis should be obtained with a stereotactic or endoscopic biopsy.

When determining the appropriate surgical management plan, the most important factor in determining the feasibility of radical resection

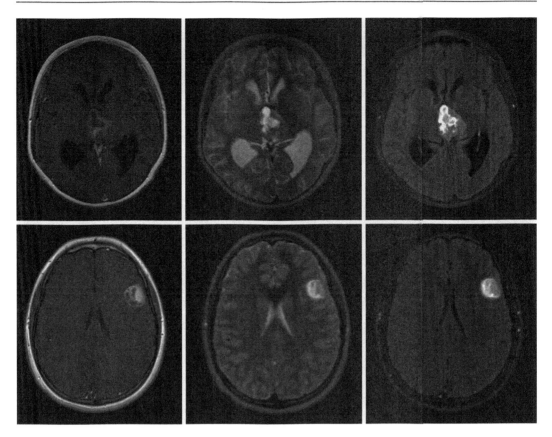

Fig. 9.2 HGG—conventional MRI. *Upper Panels*: 10-year-old female presenting with obstructive hydrocephalus due to a midbrain mass. The tumor is heterogeneously enhancing on T1-weighted post-contrast imaging with areas of cystic/necrotic change (left), and further signal abnormality is seen extending into the left thalamus on pre-contrast T2 (middle panel) and post-contrast FLAIR (right panel). Dynamic perfusion imaging demonstrated rCBV values of the enhancing component up to 12 times of normal-appearing white matter of the right frontal lobe. The nonenhancing FLAIR abnormality showed rCBV values 4 times of normal white matter. Histology was anaplastic astrocytoma (WHO grade III) and molecular testing revealed a K27 subgroup glioblastoma with driver mutations in *H3F3A* (K28M), *FGFR1* (N546K), and NF1 (E1436fs*4, W2317*). *Lower Panels*: 13-year-old male presenting with a seizure and a left frontal lobe mass. The tumor is partially cystic/necrotic and heterogeneously enhancing on T1-weighted post-contrast imaging (left), and no appreciable peritumoral edema seen on pre-contrast T2 (middle panel) or post-contrast FLAIR (right panel). Histology was glioblastoma (WHO grade IV) and molecular testing revealed an RTK-I subgroup glioblastoma with loss of *CDKN2A/B* and *RB1*, as well as amplification of *MDM2* and *CDK4*

is tumor location and relationship to eloquent cortex and white matter pathways. Supratentorial tumors within the cerebral hemispheres not involving eloquent cortex have been amenable to radical or gross total resections. Extensive resections have not previously been attempted with deeper lesions near midline structures, such as thalamic tumors, due to potential for significant postoperative neurologic deficit. This likely contributes to the historically poorer survival outcomes associated with midline tumors (Eisenstat et al. 2015; McCrea et al. 2015). In one study, age < 3 years was shown to predict greater likelihood of survival in patients with high-grade gliomas (Qaddoumi et al. 2009). Gross total resection has also been shown to have improved survival in females versus males (McCrea et al. 2015).

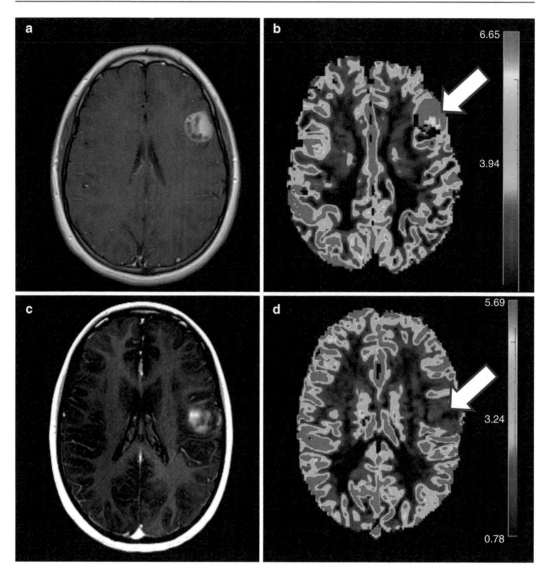

Fig. 9.3 Utility of MR perfusion imaging in differentiating high-grade from low-grade gliomas. (**a**) 10-year-old male with glioblastoma, same patient shown as in Fig. 9.1, lower panel. (**b**) Perfusion analysis (DSC T2* CBV parametric map) demonstrating marked hyper-perfusion of the enhancing lesion with rCBV measuring in the range of 6.0–8.5 relative to the normal-appearing white matter, suggesting a high-grade tumor. (**c**) 9-year-old male presenting with headaches and a left frontal lobe mass, heterogeneously enhancing on post-contrast T1-weighted image, similar in appearance to the glioblastoma shown in the upper row (**a**). (**d**) Perfusion analysis demonstrated low rCBV in the range of 1.5 relative to the normal-appearing white matter, suggesting a low-grade glioma which was subsequently confirmed by histopathology

9.4.1 Extent of Resection

The positive impact of surgical resection on survival has been well documented in the adult HGG literature due to the larger patient population. Sanai et al. showed that even a 78% reduction in tumor volume has survival benefit, with survival increasing as percent of resection increases (Sanai et al. 2011). A review of 21,783 adult GBM patients also showed improved survival with gross total resection compared to subtotal resection (Zinn et al. 2013).

Given the lower incidence of HGG in the pediatric population, there are only limited studies

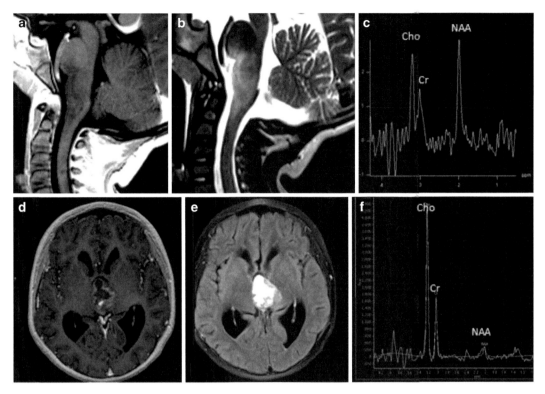

Fig. 9.4 Utility of MR spectroscopy in differentiating high-grade from low-grade gliomas. Upper panel: 9-year-old male presenting with headache and a nonenhancing, diffuse brain stem low-grade glioma noted on sagittal (**a**) post-contrast T1-weighted and (**b**) T2-weighted images. (**c**) Single-voxel MR spectroscopy demonstrated mildly increased choline/creatine ratio and relatively normal-appearing NAA, consistent with a low-grade glioma. Lower panel: 10-year-old female presenting with obstructive hydrocephalus due to a necrotic enhancing midbrain mass as seen on axial (**d**) post-contrast T1-weighted and (**e**) T2-weighted images. (**f**) Single-voxel MR spectroscopy demonstrated markedly increased Cho/Cr ratio and markedly decreased NAA consistent with HGG. Histology was anaplastic astrocytoma (WHO grade III) and molecular testing revealed a K27 subgroup glioblastoma

with small sample sizes that assess the effect of extent of resection on survival. However, these studies confirm that there is survival benefit with greater extent of resection (Walston et al. 2015). Radical tumor resection (>90%) correlated with improved disease-free and overall survival (OS) in a prospective Children's Cancer Study Group (CCSG) study (Wisoff et al. 1998). 5-year progression-free survival (PFS) rates were 35 ± 7% in radical resection versus 17 ± 4% in less extensive resections. In a retrospective review of 37 patients with glioblastoma, gross total resection was associated with a median OS of 45.1 months compared to 8.7 months for subtotal resection (Yang et al. 2013). An analysis of 6212 pediatric glioma patients from the Surveillance, Epidemiology, and End Results (SEER) database also showed extent of resection to be positively correlated with survival outcomes (Qaddoumi et al. 2009). A more recent retrospective review of 97 patients also showed improved median OS at 3.4 years for radical resection versus 1.6 years for subtotal resection (McCrea et al. 2015).

9.4.2 Surgical Adjuncts

Recent advances in surgical adjuncts are now being utilized to increase extent of resection while reducing morbidity. Stereotactic navigation, real-time neurophysiologic monitoring, cortical mapping, identification of critical white matter pathways with diffusion tensor tractography, and intraoperative MRI have allowed increasingly radical removal of glial tumors with preservation of neurological function. Tumor resection can be brought to the edge of functional cortex and deep lesions can be resected through neurophysiologic and neuro-anatomic corridors that were previously not appreciated.

Diffusion tensor tractography (DTT) is increasingly part of the preoperative planning. This imaging modality allows for visualization of specific white matter tracts, such as the corticospinal tract, in order to spare these areas during surgery (Kupper et al. 2015). In a prospective study of 11 pediatric patients with optic pathway gliomas, DTT was used to differentiate the optic pathways from surrounding tumor (Ge et al. 2015). Moshel et al. showed that DTT combined with stereotactic navigation could be used to identify the posterior limb of the internal capsule in order to avoid it during the resection of thalamic tumors (Moshel et al. 2009).

Choudhri et al. performed a retrospective review of 194 patients who had intraoperative MRI during resection of various primary CNS tumors (Choudhri et al. 2014). In this series, 21% of patients underwent more extensive resection after intraoperative MRI. Increased operative time was offset by eliminating the need for a postoperative MRI.

Another intraoperative adjunct is the use of 5-aminolevulinic acid (5-ALA). 5-ALA is currently not part of the standard of care in the US, but internationally has been shown to increase extent of resection in adult HGG by causing fluorescence of the tumor tissue. Small series have shown the same fluorescence in pediatric HGG with no negative side effects (Beez et al. 2014; Barbagallo et al. 2014).

9.5 Histopathology and Molecular Pathology

Historically, the World Health Organization (WHO) classification of tumors of the nervous system did not distinguish "pediatric" from "adult" HGG. Recent major discoveries, however, have led to significant changes in our understanding of the molecular genetics and biology of pediatric gliomas, and it has become evident that adult and pediatric HGG can be subdivided into molecular entities with distinct biology and clini-

cal behavior (Sturm et al. 2014; Mackay et al. 2017). While all of these entities have specific age predilections, the notion of two distinct and separate entities of "adult" and "pediatric" HGG has become outdated. Furthermore, the molecular classification of gliomas has revealed major limitations of the historical histology-based WHO grading system for diffuse gliomas (Reuss et al. 2015). As a result, the recently updated 2016 WHO classification of tumors of the nervous system has introduced several important changes relevant to the diagnostic classification of pediatric HGG (Louis et al. 2016).

9.5.1 Molecular Genetics and Molecular Subgroups

Pediatric HGG can be divided into molecular subgroups characterized by distinct oncogenic driver mutations, DNA methylation profiles, and gene expression. These subgroups, which are summarized in Fig. 9.5, differ substantially in regard to clinical behavior, including age predilection, anatomical locations, and survival (Sturm et al. 2012; Korshunov et al. 2015; Mackay et al. 2017). Each subgroup is linked to recurrent oncogenic driver mutations, including histone H3 K27M and G34R/V mutations, isocitrate dehydrogenase (IDH1/2) mutations, and BRAF[V600E] mutations. Recent further refinements in the molecular subclassification pediatric HGG have revealed additional epigenetically distinct subgroups within H3-/IDH-wild-type tumors that are associated with recurrent amplifications of the MYCN, EGFR, and PDGFRA oncogenes (Korshunov et al. 2017; Mackay et al. 2017).

Overall mutation frequency in pediatric HGG is relatively low compared to adult GBM (61 mutations per sample) (Wu et al. 2014). Interestingly, pediatric HGG show an overall higher mutation rate than other pediatric cancers, with a median of 15 non-synonymous coding mutations per tumor. This number is highly variable, with infant HGG showing an extremely low number of mutations, with a median of 2, while children with mismatch repair abnormalities show the highest mutational burden of all tumors, with a median of >6000 non-synonymous coding mutations per tumor.

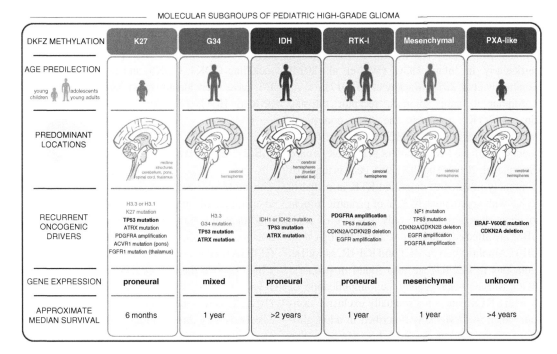

Fig. 9.5 Molecular subgroups of pediatric high-grade glioma, including diffuse intrinsic pontine glioma. Pediatric grade gliomas grouped by genome-wide methylation cluster and associated hotspot mutations, and annotated with key clinical and genomic features. Modified from Gajjar et al. (2015)

Pediatric HGG harbor genetic alterations in the same canonical cancer pathways as adult diffuse gliomas, including the TP53 pathway, the PI3K pathway, and the RB pathway, although the frequency of specific alterations differs between pediatric and adult tumors (Sturm et al. 2014; Mackay et al. 2017). For example, loss of PTEN function via deletion and/or mutation is rare in pediatric HGG, while it is one of the most common alterations in adult GBM. The BRAF^{V600E} mutation is occasionally found in pediatric supratentorial HGG, most commonly in the context of secondary pediatric HGG arising from tumors that were originally low-grade, such as gangliogliomas (Lassaletta et al. 2017; Mistry et al. 2015). Secondary high-grade gliomas in children may also arise from pleomorphic xanthoastrocytoma (PXA), which is a usually slow-growing tumor of the cerebral hemispheres with marked nuclear pleomorphism and assigned WHO grade II. The majority of PXA harbor the BRAF^{V600E} mutations (Schindler et al. 2011), and lack MGMT promoter methylation (Marucci and Morandi 2011). As an alternative mechanism of constitutive activation of BRAF, some PXAs occurring in children harbor oncogenic fusions involving BRAF (Hsiao et al. 2017; Kline et al. 2017). The prognosis for patients with radically resectable PXA is generally excellent, but residual and/or recurrent tumors have a strong propensity for aggressive behavior with malignant transformation towards glioblastoma (Ida et al. 2015; Kahramancetin and Tihan 2013; Rao et al. 2010). A subset of tumors with histopathological features of glioblastoma occurring in infants and young children with a methylation profile resembling PXA and frequent BRAF^{V600E} mutations as well as CDKN2A/B deletions have recently been described and termed "PXA-like" (Korshunov et al. 2015; Mackay et al. 2017), and similar genetic features have also been reported in secondary pediatric HGG arising from low-grade astrocytomas (Mistry et al. 2015).

Chromosomal structural abnormalities are common in pediatric HGG. The copy number alterations (CNA) landscape in pediatric HGG is highly variable, and can range from balanced genomes to simple rearrangements and complex abnormalities caused by chromothripsis phenomena (Wu et al. 2014). For example, NTRK fusions are typically involved and can be the sole molecular aberration, particularly in infant HGG (Wu et al. 2014; Korshunov et al. 2015; Mackay et al. 2017).

Similar to adult gliomas, receptor tyrosine kinases (RTKs) represent the most commonly amplified genes in pediatric HGG; however, the frequency of affected genes differs across age groups (Sturm et al. 2014). The PDGFRA gene is the most commonly mutated or amplified RTK in pediatric HGG, with approximately 30% of pediatric tumors showing alterations, while only 10–15% of adult GBM are affected (Paugh et al. 2010; Phillips et al. 2013). Amplification of MET and IGF1R, as well as mutations in FGFR1, are also found in pediatric HGG. Mosaic heterogeneity, i.e., amplification of different RTK genes in a mutually exclusive fashion, which was originally described in adult glioblastoma (Snuderl et al. 2011), has also been also observed in pediatric gliomas, with coexisting tumor cell subclones harboring either PDGFRA or MET amplification. Recent genomics-based "evolutionary reconstruction" studies in DIPG have revealed high-fidelity obligate partners with histone H3 mutations from diagnosis to end-stage disease involving alterations in TP53 cell-cycle (TP53/ PPM1D) or specific growth factor pathways (ACVR1/PIK3R1), whereas later oncogenic alterations arise in subclones and often affect the PI3K pathway (Nikbakht et al. 2016). Alterations of EGFR, including amplification and mutations commonly seen in adult glioblastomas, are relatively rare in pediatric HGG (Pollack et al. 2006; Bax et al. 2009; Paugh et al. 2010). The TP53 gene is affected in almost 55% of pediatric HGGs. Up to 20% of DIPGs and midline HGGs carry mutations in PPM1D, which is downstream in the pathway, and mutations of TP53 and PPM1D are mutually exclusive in HGG (Zhang et al. 2014). The RB pathway is commonly affected in adult glioblastoma and although homozygous loss of RB is extremely rare in pediatric HGG, loss of chromosome 13q is found in approximately one-third of pediatric HGGs regardless of location (Paugh et al. 2011; Wu et al. 2014). In children, homozygous deletions of CDKN2A/B are found in approximately 25% of supratentorial HGG, but are rare in midline tumors

(Paugh et al. 2010; Wu et al. 2014; Korshunov et al. 2015). Amplification of the components of the cyclin–CDK complex that phosphorylates RB, including CDK4, CDK6, and cyclins D1, D2, or D3, have been identified across all subgroups of pediatric HGGs (Nikbakht et al. 2016).

9.5.2 Epigenetics

The molecular hallmarks of pediatric HGG are aberrations of the genes regulating epigenetic modifications of the genome, including recurrent hotspot mutations in H3 histone, family 3A (H3F3A) and histone cluster 1, H3b (HIST1H3B), which encode the histone H3 variants H3.3 and H3.1, respectively (Schwartzentruber et al. 2012). This was the first example of a human disease driven by direct mutation of histones. Point mutations of H3F3A and HIST1H3B genes occur at hotspots either at amino acid residue 27 resulting in lysine to methionine (K27M) amino acid change or 34 resulting in either glycine to arginine (G34R) or glycine to valine (G34V) amino acid change. The H3 mutations are mutually exclusive with IDH1/2 mutations. Interestingly, both IDH1/2 and H3 mutations appear to drive oncogenesis via genome-wide epigenomic changes. Clinically, different H3 histone mutations are associated with strikingly different age of onset and survival. Younger children (median age 6–7) are predominantly affected by K27M mutated tumors, while older children (median age 13–14) are predominantly affected by G34R/V mutants (Schwartzentruber et al. 2012; Sturm et al. 2012; Wu et al. 2014). Median survival of patients with K27M mutated tumors is 12 months while the median survival of patients with G34R/V mutation is 24 months (Sturm et al. 2012; Korshunov et al. 2015). These mutations can also be present in rare gliomas of young adults, and are mutually exclusive with IDH1/2 mutations. The current WHO Classification recognizes K27M mutant infiltrating glioma as a separate entity, "diffuse midline glioma, H3 K27M mutant" (Louis et al. 2016), and assigns a grade IV irrespective of histological features. Although the vast majority of children with

K27M mutant glioma do poorly with standard therapies, a small subset of patients with K27M mutant glioma who lack other typical genomic features of HGG, i.e., oncogene amplifications and chromosomal gains and losses, may have a more favorable outcome (Orillac et al. 2016).

Other chromatin regulators can also be mutated in pediatric HGG. The ATRX or DAXX genes, which are strongly associated with a telomerase-independent alternative lengthening of telomeres, are mutated in approximately 20% of pediatric HGG, often with concurrent G34 mutations (Schwartzentruber et al. 2012; Wu et al. 2014). Mutations of the telomerase reverse transcriptase (TERT) promoter, which represent different mechanisms to lengthen telomeres and are highly prevalent in adult glioblastoma, can be found in subsets of pediatric HGG as well (Koelsche et al. 2013; Korshunov et al. 2017; Mackay et al. 2017).

There is a striking anatomic predilection for particular driver mutations in pediatric HGG, which points to neurodevelopmental origins of pediatric HGG. Histone H3.3 G34R or G34V mutations are predominantly found in supratentorial hemispheric tumors that can vary considerably in histological appearance; the histologic variation does not appear to impact outcome (Korshunov et al. 2016). Histone H3 K27M mutations are found in midline tumors, including the thalamus and brain stem, with the highest frequency in DIPG (Sturm et al. 2012; Wu et al. 2014; Buczkowicz et al. 2014; Taylor et al. 2014; Fontebasso et al. 2014). In midline tumors, FGFR1 mutations are found in thalamic HGGs while ACVR1 mutations are restricted to DIPG. DIPGs are also characterized by PIK3CA and PIK3R1 mutations and FGF1R and MET amplifications, while loss of CDKN2A and NF1 aberrations are more prevalent in supratentorial HGG.

9.5.3 MGMT Promoter Methylation

Promoter methylation of the O^6-methylguanine-DNA methyltransferase (MGMT) gene, which encodes a DNA repair protein implicated in resistance to alkylating chemotherapy and is considered of prognostic and predictive value in gliomas, can be detected by a variety of assays (Wick et al. 2014), with methylation-specific PCR (MSP) being one of the most widely used. It has recently been shown that MGMT promoter status may also be reliably determined from data generated by genome-wide methylation arrays (Bady et al. 2012).

While in adult glioblastoma, MGMT promoter methylation status has been well established as a strong independent prognostic factor regardless of therapy, as well as a predictive biomarker for significant survival benefit from TMZ (Wick et al. 2014), the role of MGMT promoter methylation status as independent prognostic or therapeutic biomarker in pediatric HGG is unclear. No randomized controlled HGG trials comparing XRT + TMZ to XRT alone have been performed in children; hence, the value of MGMT promoter methylation as a predictive biomarker for benefit from TMZ is unknown. While the Children's Oncology Group (COG) ACNS0126 trial showed improved survival in patients with strong MGMT expression (Cohen et al. 2011), no such difference was observed on ACNS0423 (Jakacki et al. 2016). Of note, MGMT status on both trials was determined using immunohistochemistry, which is unreliable and no longer considered an acceptable test to determine MGMT status in glioma (Wick et al. 2014). Remarkably, data from a retrospective pediatric HGG study (Korshunov et al. 2015) showed that while MGMT promoter methylation was tightly associated with K27M and IDH1 mutational status, it was not an independent prognostic factor in multivariate analysis. This finding is in striking contrast to adult glioblastoma patients, where MGMT promoter methylation status has been validated as a highly reproducible prognostic and predictive biomarker across prospective, randomized clinical trials using XRT and XRT + TMZ (Wick et al. 2014). Therefore, the utility of MGMT promoter methylation status as an independent prognostic biomarker in pediatric HGG is not supported by the current data, and its role as a predictive biomarker for benefit from TMZ in this population is unproven as well. Taken together, there currently is insufficient data to support the use of *MGMT* status for clinical decision-making in children with HGG.

9.5.4 Clinical Implications

Considering major molecular, biological, and clinical differences between HGG subgroups, the limitations of traditional histological grading, the discovery that molecular classification may significantly outperform histopathological grading in terms of prognosis (Reuss et al. 2015; Eckel-Passow et al. 2015; Sturm et al. 2012; Korshunov et al. 2015, 2017; Mackay et al. 2017), and the availability of novel therapeutic options for subsets of patients, the diagnosis of a pediatric HGG based on histology and WHO grade alone can no longer be regarded as sufficient.

The recent development and validation of reliable, mutation-specific antibodies has greatly facilitated the diagnosis of IDH, K27, and BRAF mutant gliomas (Bechet et al. 2014; Capper et al. 2010, 2011). Fluorescence in situ hybridization (FISH) is useful in detecting focal genomic

changes, including oncogene amplifications, such as PDGFRA, and loss of tumor suppressor genes, such as CDKN2A/B. Although several molecular subgroups of HGG can be distinguished using RNA-based gene expression arrays, genome-wide DNA methylation profiling using the Illumina Infinium Human Methylation 450 Bead Chip ("Illumina 450k") has been shown to be of value to recognize clinically relevant molecular subgroups of pediatric HGG (Sturm et al. 2012; Korshunov et al. 2015), as well as to provide valuable additional diagnostic information. The methylation data can be processed to reveal focal copy number changes, such as amplifications of oncogene and loss of tumor suppressors, similar to array comparative genomic hybridization (array CGH), as illustrated in Fig. 9.6. In addition, MGMT promoter methylation status can be readily derived from the data (Bady et al. 2012).

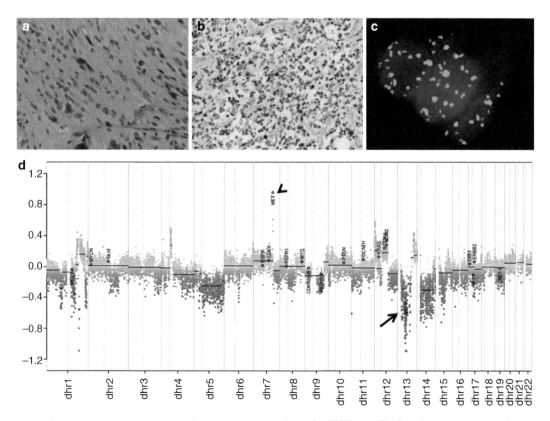

Fig. 9.6 Molecular diagnostics in pediatric high-grade glioma. (DIPG, **a–c**): H&E (**a**), detection of K27M by IHC using a mutant-specific antibody yielding intense brown nuclear staining (**b**), and PDGFRA amplification shown by FISH (**c**). (**d**): Complex chromosomal aberrations in a supratentorial HGG using genome-wide methylation profiling. Arrow head points to MET amplification and arrow to RB loss

9.6　Radiation Therapy

Radiation therapy is an important component of the adjuvant treatment of pediatric high-grade gliomas. Adult randomized controlled studies from the 1970s to the 1990s demonstrated a survival benefit for postoperative radiotherapy with doses from 60 to 64 Gy (Andersen 1978; Kristiansen et al. 1981; Walker et al. 1978). Radiotherapy with or without chemotherapy was found to be more effective than chemotherapy alone in adults (Sandberg-Wollheim et al. 1991; Walker et al. 1978, 1980). However, attempts to augment adjuvant radiation therapy with either brachytherapy or stereotactic radiosurgery in adult patients have not demonstrated a survival benefit (Laperriere et al. 1998; Selker et al. 2002; Souhami et al. 2004).

A Brain Tumor Cooperative Group (BTCG) meta-analysis revealed a statistically significant improvement in median survival for adult patients who received doses of 50–60 Gy as compared to patients who received 45 Gy or less (Walker et al. 1979). A Medical Research Council study of adult patients also demonstrated a statistically significant survival advantage with 60 Gy as compared to 45 Gy (Bleehen and Stenning 1991). These results have been extrapolated to the pediatric population, and standard RT for pediatric high-grade gliomas consists of a total dose of 60 Gy in 30–33 fractions. An initial clinical target volume (CTV1) is treated to 45–54 Gy, followed by a "boost" to a smaller CTV (CTV2) to a total dose of 60 Gy (Fig. 9.7).

Due to the possibility that high-grade gliomas may disseminate widely (Matsukado et al. 1961), whole brain irradiation was initially used in early studies of adult high-grade gliomas. However, concerns about radiation-induced brain necrosis and cognitive impairment have led to increasingly localized treatment volumes. A BTCG randomized study demonstrated that whole brain irradia-

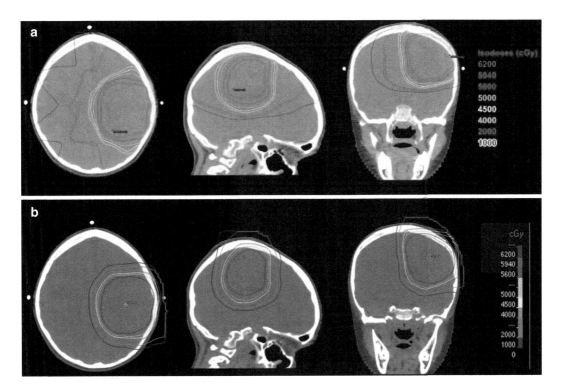

Fig. 9.7 Radiation therapy treatment planning and dosimetry. Dose distribution of an intensity-modulated radiation therapy plan (**a**) and a proton therapy plan (**b**) for an 11-year-old male with anaplastic astrocytoma status post gross total resection

tion with 43 Gy followed by a coned-down boost of 17.2 Gy was as effective as whole brain irradiation with 60.2 Gy (Shapiro et al. 1989). Other adult studies demonstrated that limited volume RT was as effective as whole brain irradiation (A study of the effect of misonidazole in conjunction with radiotherapy for the treatment of grades 3 and 4 astrocytomas. A report from the MRC Working Party on misonidazole in gliomas 1983; Bleehen et al. 1981; Payne et al. 1982; Ramsey and Brand 1973; Sheline 1975; Urtasun et al. 1982). Autopsy series have shown that the volume at highest risk of local failure is within 2–3 cm of the primary tumor bed (Halperin et al. 1989; Hochberg and Pruitt 1980; Wallner et al. 1989). Therefore, CTV1 is usually defined by a 2 cm expansion beyond the tumor, tumor bed, and associated T2 (or FLAIR) signal. CTV2 is usually defined by a 0.5- to 1-cm margin beyond the residual enhancing tumor and tumor bed. 3D conformal RT has been the standard modality for pediatric high-grade gliomas; however, intensity-modulated radiation therapy (IMRT) and proton therapy may provide better sparing of critical normal structures, such as normal brain, optic apparatus, cochlea, and brain stem (Hermanto et al. 2007; Narayana et al. 2006). Modeling studies have demonstrated improved neurocognitive functioning at 5 years for proton therapy compared to 3D conformal RT (Merchant et al. 2008). Therefore, proton therapy may be most appropriate for patients with an expected survival of 5 years or greater, such as patients with IDH mutant glioma.

9.6.1   Dose Escalation and Fractionation

Retrospective patterns-of-failure studies have demonstrated that 89–93% of local failures after RT occur within the high-dose region (Chang et al. 2007; Lee et al. 1999; McDonald et al. 2011). This finding has led some investigators to explore the use of higher RT doses in the treatment of high-grade gliomas. RTOG 9803 was a phase I dose-escalation study that examined four dose levels—66, 72, 78, and 84 Gy—with concurrent BCNU (Tsien et al. 2009). No dose-limited

toxicities were observed at any dose level. However, this study was conducted with concurrent BCNU, which is not currently considered the standard concurrent chemotherapy agent. Dose escalation beyond 84 Gy has been examined using proton therapy. A phase II study at Massachusetts General Hospital treated 23 patients with twice-daily fractions of 1.8–1.92 CGE (Cobalt-60 Gy Equivalent) to a median total dose of 93.5 CGE (range, 81.6–94.2) using a combination of X-ray and proton therapy (Fitzek et al. 1999). The median OS was 20 months, and all the patients were considered to have developed radiation necrosis. Another study at the Proton Medical Research Center in Tsukuba, Japan, treated 23 patients with twice-daily fractions of 1.65–1.8 CGE to a total dose of 96.6 CGE using a combination of X-ray and proton therapy (Mizumoto et al. 2015). Twenty-one patients received concurrent nimustine, and two patients received concurrent temozolomide. The median OS was 21 months; six patients developed radiation necrosis, and two patients developed leukoencephalopathy.

Late-responding normal tissues, such as normal brain, are generally considered to be more sensitive to dose per fraction than tumors. Hyperfractionation attempts to improve the therapeutic ratio by increasing the total dose while reducing the fractional dose. Typically, hyperfractionated RT regimens use twice-daily fractional doses of 1.6 Gy or less. A randomized study at University of California, San Francisco compared standard fractionation (1.8 Gy per fraction, once a day, to 59.4 Gy) with a hyperfractionated regimen (1.6 Gy per fraction, twice a day, to 70.4 Gy) (Prados et al. 2001). No difference in OS or PFS was seen between the two arms. Furthermore, a meta-analysis of altered fractionation for high-grade gliomas revealed no significant improvement in OS for altered fractionation (Nieder et al. 2004).

9.6.2   Pseudoprogression and Radiation Necrosis

Radiographic progression, consisting of increasing edema or contrast-enhancement, on the first posttreatment MRI within 2 months after RT occurs in about 40% of patients after concurrent chemotherapy and RT (Taal et al. 2008). Approximately half of these lesions represent true tumor progression, while the other half represent pseudoprogression. Pseudoprogressive lesions are usually visible on the first posttreatment MRI within 2 months after RT. Radiation necrosis, which can also appear radiographically as increasing edema or contrast-enhancement, can occur in up to 24% of patients; it typically occurs within 3–12 months after RT, but can also occur many years afterwards (Giglio and Gilbert 2003; Kumar et al. 2000; Ruben et al. 2006; Sheline et al. 1980). Steroids are usually recommended in the initial management of asymptomatic pseudoprogression or radiation necrosis. Surgery should be considered in clinically symptomatic patients. Bevacizumab and hyperbaric oxygen therapy have also been shown to be effective in reducing edema associated with radiation necrosis (Gonzalez et al. 2007; Furuse et al. 2016; Chuba et al. 1997; Drezner et al. 2016).

9.6.3 Radiation Therapy for Recurrence

Several therapeutic options, including repeat RT, exist for recurrent high-grade gliomas. Repeat external beam radiotherapy, radiosurgery, and brachytherapy may be considered in carefully selected patients. In a retrospective study of 147 patients treated with hypofractionated stereotactic radiation therapy (HFSRT) with a median dose of 35 Gy in 3.5 Gy fractions, repeat RT was well tolerated with a median OS of 11 months (Fogh et al. 2010). HFSRT consisting of 30 Gy in 5 fractions with bevacizumab has also been shown to be well tolerated with a median OS of 12.5 months (Gutin et al. 2009). In a retrospective review of 11 patients treated with Gamma Knife radiosurgery (median dose, 16 Gy) and bevacizumab, the authors report a median PFS of 15 months and a median OS of 18 months (Park et al. 2012). Studies of interstitial I-125 brachy-

therapy for recurrent high-grade gliomas have reported median OS from 10 to 20 months (Gutin et al. 1987; Lucas et al. 1991; Scharfen et al. 1992; Shrieve et al. 1995).

9.7 Chemotherapy

9.7.1 Chemotherapy for HGG (Excluding DIPG and Infant HGG) at Initial Diagnosis

The first prospective, randomized clinical trial including chemotherapy for children with newly diagnosed HGG was conducted by the Children's Cancer Study Group (CCSG) during the 1980's and showed a significant improvement in outcome using adjuvant RT followed by pCV chemotherapy (prednisone, chloroethyl-cyclohexyl nitrosourea (CCNU), and vincristine), as compared to RT alone (Sposto et al. 1989). In this study, the addition of chemotherapy led to a dramatic increase in 5-year PFS from 16 to 46%. As a result, adjuvant chemotherapy in addition to RT became the standard of care and no subsequent pediatric cooperative group study included an "RT-only" standard arm. Of note, the survival rates reported from the CCSG trial, especially in the chemotherapy arm, far exceeded what has been observed in all subsequent studies. This discrepancy can be explained by the misclassification and inclusion of a large number of low-grade gliomas on older HGG studies (Pollack et al. 2003). As a result, contemporary trials with more stringent neuropathology criteria, including central review, have shown 3-year event-free survival (EFS) and OS rates of approximately 20% and 10%, respectively (Cohen et al. 2011), with long-term survivors beyond 5 years from diagnosis being exceedingly rare.

In a landmark phase 3 trial, single-agent temozolomide (TMZ), when administered during and after RT (the "Stupp regimen"), was shown to significantly prolong EFS and OS in adults with glioblastoma compared to RT alone, with a median survival of 14.6 months with RT + TMZ and 12.1 months with RT alone (Stupp et al.

2005). The subset of patients with MGMT promoter methylation benefitted the most from the addition of TMZ, with an increase of median survival from 15.3 to 21.7 months (Hegi et al. 2005). In contrast, there was only a statistically nonsignificant trend towards improved OS in those patients with MGMT promoter unmethylated tumors, and a subsequent study showed similar results (Weller et al. 2009). Perhaps not surprisingly, the use of adjuvant chemoradiotherapy similar to the "Stupp regimen" in the Children's Oncology Group (COG) single-arm study ACNS0126 did not lead to an improved outcome when compared to historical controls treated with different adjuvant chemotherapy regimens that included alkylators (Cohen et al. 2011). While MGMT expression was confirmed as a prognostic marker in children in this study, the predictive value for benefit from TMZ remains unproven since no recent pediatric studies included an RT-only control arm.

In the subsequent COG HGG trial, ACNS0423, CCNU was added to temozolomide during maintenance. The study did not meet the predefined endpoint, with a 1-year EFS of 49% similar to the original CCG-945-based design model (Jakacki et al. 2016). Although EFS and OS were noted to be significantly improved in ACNS0423 compared to ACNS0126, molecular data on both studies is very limited, with IDH mutational status available on a subset of patients on ACNS0423 only, but not on ACNS0126. Of note, IDH mutations were observed in 16.3% tumors analyzed on ACNS0423 (Pollack et al. 2011), which represents a relatively high percentage compared to other pediatric HGG series. In ACNS0423 patients with IDH mutant tumors, 1-year OS was reported as 100%, underscoring the strong prognostic value of IDH mutations in pediatric HGG patients, in keeping with adult data. Given the paucity of molecular data available on both the ACNS0126 and ANCS0423 cohorts, the relatively small numbers of patients, the sequential study design and lack of randomization, comparisons in outcome between the two studies should be interpreted with caution.

The most recent COG HGG trial, ACNS0822, compared two different experimental arms with vorinostat or bevacizumab during RT to a "control arm" with TMZ during RT. Of note, patients on all three arms received bevacizumab post RT during maintenance therapy. The trial was initially planned as a phase 2 "pick-the-winner" design followed by phase 3 testing, but the study was permanently closed in 2014 during phase 2 after an interim analysis showed that the predefined endpoint (i.e., improved 1-year EFS compared to standard therapy) could not be met (Hoffman et al. 2015). Given these findings, along with the disappointing results of up-front therapy with bevacizumab in adults with glioblastoma (Chinot et al. 2014; Gilbert et al. 2014), bevacizumab is unlikely to play a role in future clinical trials for newly diagnosed pediatric HGG patients.

In pediatric patients with HGG treated on the German "HIT-GBM-C" cooperative group study with intensive chemotherapy during and after RT, survival appeared superior compared to prior HIT-GBM studies in the subgroup of patients with HGG who had undergone gross total resection (Wolff et al. 2010). Although the results were provocative, the data is difficult to interpret given that molecular data on this cohort is unavailable.

9.7.2 Chemotherapy for DIPG at Initial Diagnosis

Disappointingly, numerous strategies using adjuvant chemotherapy to treat patients with DIPG over the past decade, including high-dose chemotherapy followed by stem cell rescue, neoadjuvant chemotherapy (single or multi-agent), concurrent chemotherapy with RT, and adjuvant chemotherapy given post RT, have not demonstrated any survival benefit when compared to conventional RT alone [reviewed in (Jansen et al. 2012)]. Novel preclinical models of DIPG have allowed for in vitro and in vivo drug screening (Grasso et al. 2015; Funato et al. 2014), and are hoped to lead to identification of more effective treatment strategies that can be translated into clinical trials.

To summarize, the historical data suggests a modest benefit of the addition of alkylator-based chemotherapy to adjuvant RT in unselected cohorts of pediatric patients with HGG, but not in patients with DIPG. Given the more favorable toxicity profile of TMZ compared to CCNU, adjuvant RT and TMZ have become the "de facto" standard treatment of pediatric patients with non-brain stem HGG. For DIPG patients, adjuvant RT without chemotherapy remains the standard of care.

9.7.3 Chemotherapy for Infant HGG at Initial Diagnosis

It has been long recognized that HGG arising in infants and very young children (<3 years of age, also termed "infant HGG") have a much better survival compared to HGG seen in older children, hinting at a different biology. As a result of this observation, and the fact that RT is generally avoided in very young children, HGG patients <3 years of age are generally excluded from pediatric HGG studies and typically treated with intensive chemotherapy regimens, such as the "Baby POG" protocol and others (Duffner et al. 1993, 1996, 1999; Dufour et al. 2006; Geyer et al. 1995; Sanders et al. 2007). As discussed in the "Histopathology and Molecular Pathology" section of this chapter, recent data has shed light on the molecular genetics and biology of "infant HGG." Excluding K27M mutant tumors, which can also be seen in very young children and have a dismal prognosis, the majority of "infant HGG" lack the molecular features seen in other HGG and resemble low-grade gliomas genomically (Korshunov et al. 2015; Wu et al. 2014), which likely explains their more favorable response to chemotherapy and improved outcome.

The optimal type and timing of adjuvant therapy for patients with IDH mutant gliomas is unclear. IDH mutant gliomas in children correspond to IDH mutant astrocytomas seen in young adults, which are distinct from adult IDH mutant oligodendrogliomas that harbor the pathognomonic co-deletion of chromosomes 11p and 19q (Cancer Genome Atlas Research et al. 2015). IDH mutant astrocytomas are not seen in young children, but do occur in adolescents (Pollack et al. 2011; Korshunov et al. 2015; Sturm et al. 2012; Mackay et al. 2017), and their molecular and clinical features are indistinguishable from IDH mutant astrocytomas occurring in adults, which have a relatively favorable prognosis with median OS of approximately 10 years reported across large datasets (Reuss et al. 2015; Cancer Genome Atlas Research et al. 2015). The MGMT promoter is methylated in the vast majority of IDH mutant astrocytomas, but data from adult studies indicate that the favorable outcome may be more strongly linked to an intrinsically more favorable biology and natural history of IDH mutant tumors rather than a superior response to therapy (Beiko et al. 2014).

A simplified overview of initial key diagnostic and management considerations for children with newly diagnosed HGG is shown in Fig. 9.8.

9.7.4 Chemotherapy at Recurrence/ Progression

A large number of single-agent and combination chemotherapy salvage regimens, including bevacizumab-containing protocols, have been studied in pediatric HGG patients, with generally disappointing results (Narayana et al. 2010; Gururangan et al. 2014). Oral etoposide, either alone or in combination with TMZ (Korones et al. 2006) and carboplatin (Yung et al. 1991; Prados et al. 1996), appear to have modest activity in a subset of children with recurrent HGG. Re-treatment with dose-intensified TMZ may represent a reasonable treatment option for patients with MGMT promoter methylated glioblastoma (Weller et al. 2015). If available, enrollment on an open clinical trial should be strongly considered for children with HGG at first disease progression or recurrence.

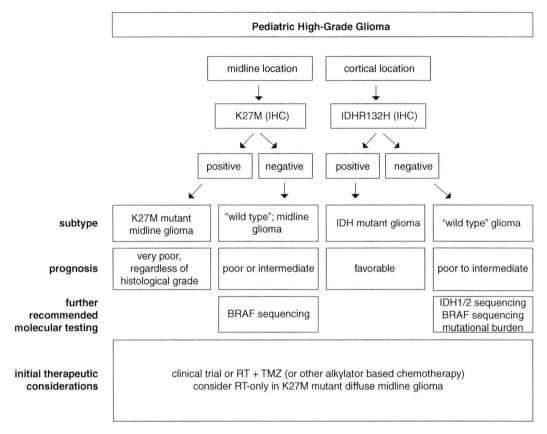

Fig. 9.8 Simplified algorithm for recommended molecular testing and initial therapeutic considerations. A limited molecular diagnostic workup is shown, with consideration given to the most relevant biomarkers to inform clinical management. Of note, IDH mutant gliomas are not seen in patients younger than 10 years of age. Additional molecular testing, based on availability, is recommended and may include FISH, targeted sequencing, array CGH and/or methylation profiling

9.8 Molecular Targeted Therapies

Although a number of "actionable" mutations can be found in both adult and pediatric HGG, treatment of unselected patients with single-agent, molecular targeted therapies has been unsuccessful (Vanan and Eisenstat 2014; Olson et al. 2014). While the selection of "target-enriched" populations is a rational next step being incorporated into recent trials (Lassman et al. 2015), the formidable challenges that remain include intra-tumor heterogeneity with molecular pathway redundancy (Snuderl et al. 2011; Patel et al. 2014) and clonal evolution during therapy (Johnson et al. 2014), as well as issues with drug delivery such as poor blood–brain barrier penetration of many molecular targeted agents (Woodworth et al. 2014). Currently, BRAF[V600E] represents the single most "actionable" oncogenic driver in pediatric HGG and PXA (Chamberlain 2013; Robinson et al. 2014; Lee et al. 2014; Hyman et al. 2015), and clinical trials with BRAF and/or MEK inhibitors are currently ongoing. Unfortunately, the BRAF[V600E] mutation is present in a small subset of pediatric HGG only (Wu et al. 2014; Korshunov et al. 2015), leaving the majority of patients without promising targets for currently available molecular targeted therapies.

9.9 Immunotherapy

There is considerable and growing interest in developing immunotherapy approaches to treat brain tumors including HGG, but until recently, only a very limited number of studies including pediatric patients with HGG have been published (Ardon et al. 2010; Pollack et al. 2014). In the small subset of pediatric HGG patients with hypermutant glioblastoma in the context of constitutional biallelic mismatch repair deficiency (CMMR-D) syndrome, exceptional treatment responses to immune checkpoint blockade using the anti-programmed death-1 (PD-1) inhibitor nivolumab have recently been reported (Bouffet et al. 2016). Several institutional and commercial tumor sequencing platforms are currently available to assess mutational burden and help the clinician in identifying these patients.

An international multicenter trial exploring the use of single and dual immune checkpoint inhibitors in pediatric patients with brain tumors, including HGG, is currently ongoing (ClinicalTrials.gov Identifier: NCT03130959).

A large number of immunotherapy trials for adult patients with glioblastoma, including immune checkpoint blockade and adoptive cellular therapy, are currently being conducted, representing a rapidly emerging field that is beyond the scope of this chapter (Maxwell et al. 2017; Sampson et al. 2017; Weller et al. 2017; Srinivasan et al. 2017).

9.10 Future Directions

The recently generated wealth of data and knowledge regarding the molecular genetics and biology of pediatric HGG, including important prognostic and predictive biomarkers, have greatly enhanced the diagnostic accuracy and opened multiple avenues for novel therapeutic approaches. However, several key challenges for future pediatric HGG clinical trial development remain: (1) lack of currently pharmacologically actionable targets (i.e., recurrent genomic alterations) in the majority of pediatric GBM; (2) inter-tumor heterogeneity, with molecularly and biologically distinct subgroups; (3) intra-tumor heterogeneity, including clonal evolution and molecular pathway redundancy; and (4) issues with drug delivery, including poor blood–brain barrier penetration of many molecular targeted agents. Future clinical trials will have to successfully tackle these challenges to improve the dismal outcome for children with HGG. The rapidly evolving field of immunotherapy, including for solid tumors and brain tumors, also holds significant promise for the future.

References

Andersen AP (1978) Postoperative irradiation of glioblastomas. Results in a randomized series. Acta Radiol Oncol Radiat Phys Biol 17(6):475–484

Ardon H, De Vleeschouwer S, Van Calenbergh F, Claes L, Kramm CM, Rutkowski S, Wolff JE, Van Gool SW (2010) Adjuvant dendritic cell-based tumour vaccination for children with malignant brain tumours. Pediatr Blood Cancer 54(4):519–525. https://doi.org/10.1002/pbc.22319

Bady P, Sciuscio D, Diserens AC, Bloch J, van den Bent MJ, Marosi C, Dietrich PY, Weller M, Mariani L, Heppner FL, McDonald DR, Lacombe D, Stupp R, Delorenzi M, Hegi ME (2012) MGMT methylation analysis of glioblastoma on the Infinium methylation BeadChip identifies two distinct CpG regions associated with gene silencing and outcome, yielding a prediction model for comparisons across datasets, tumor grades, and CIMP-status. Acta Neuropathol 124(4):547–560. https://doi.org/10.1007/s00401-012-1016-2

Bakry D, Aronson M, Durno C, Rimawi H, Farah R, Alharbi QK, Alharbi M, Shamvil A, Ben-Shachar S, Mistry M, Constantini S, Dvir R, Qaddoumi I, Gallinger S, Lerner-Ellis J, Pollett A, Stephens D, Kelies S, Chao E, Malkin D, Bouffet E, Hawkins C, Tabori U (2014) Genetic and clinical determinants of constitutional mismatch repair deficiency syndrome: report from the constitutional mismatch repair deficiency consortium. Eur J Cancer 50(5):987–996. https://doi.org/10.1016/j.ejca.2013.12.005

Barbagallo GM, Certo F, Heiss K, Albanese V (2014) 5-ALA fluorescence-assisted surgery in pediatric brain tumors: report of three cases and review of the literature. Br J Neurosurg 28(6):750–754. https://doi.org/10.3109/02688697.2014.913779

Bax DA, Gaspar N, Little SE, Marshall L, Perryman L, Regairaz M, Viana-Pereira M, Vuononvirta R, Sharp SY, Reis-Filho JS, Stavale JN, Al-Sarraj S, Reis RM, Vassal G, Pearson AD, Hargrave D, Ellison DW, Workman P, Jones C (2009) EGFRvIII deletion mutations in pediatric high-grade glioma and response to targeted therapy in pediatric glioma cell lines. Clin Cancer Res 15(18):5753–5761. https://doi.org/10.1158/1078-0432.CCR-08-3210

Bechet D, Gielen GG, Korshunov A, Pfister SM, Rousso C, Faury D, Fiset PO, Benlimane N, Lewis PW, Lu C, David Allis C, Kieran MW, Ligon KL, Pietsch T, Ellezam B, Albrecht S, Jabado N (2014) Specific detection of methionine 27 mutation in histone 3 variants (H3K27M) in fixed tissue from high-grade astrocytomas. Acta Neuropathol 128(5):733–741. https://doi.org/10.1007/s00401-014-1337-4

Beez T, Sarikaya-Seiwert S, Steiger HJ, Hanggi D (2014) Fluorescence-guided surgery with 5-aminolevulinic acid for resection of brain tumors in children--a technical report. Acta Neurochir 156(3):597–604. https://doi.org/10.1007/s00701-014-1997-9

Beiko J, Suki D, Hess KR, Fox BD, Cheung V, Cabral M, Shonka N, Gilbert MR, Sawaya R, Prabhu SS, Weinberg J, Lang FF, Aldape KD, Sulman EP, Rao G, McCutcheon IE, Cahill DP (2014) IDH1 mutant malignant astrocytomas are more amenable to surgical resection and have a survival benefit associated with maximal surgical resection. Neuro-Oncology 16(1):81–91. https://doi.org/10.1093/neuonc/not159

Benesch M, Wagner S, Berthold F, Wolff JE (2005) Primary dissemination of high-grade gliomas in children: experiences from four studies of the Pediatric Oncology and Hematology Society of the German Language Group (GPOH). J Neuro-Oncol 72(2):179–183. https://doi.org/10.1007/s11060-004-3546-5

Bleehen NM, Stenning SP (1991) A Medical Research Council trial of two radiotherapy doses in the treatment of grades 3 and 4 astrocytoma. The Medical Research Council Brain Tumour Working Party. Br J Cancer 64(4):769–774

Bleehen NM, Wiltshire CR, Plowman PN, Watson JV, Gleave JR, Holmes AE, Lewin WS, Treip CS, Hawkins TD (1981) A randomized study of misonidazole and radiotherapy for grade 3 and 4 cerebral astrocytoma. Br J Cancer 43(4):436–442

Bouffet E, Larouche V, Campbell BB, Merico D, de Borja R, Aronson M, Durno C, Krueger J, Cabric V, Ramaswamy V, Zhukova N, Mason G, Farah R, Afzal S, Yalon M, Rechavi G, Magimairajan V, Walsh MF, Constantini S, Dvir R, Elhasid R, Reddy A, Osborn M, Sullivan M, Hansford J, Dodgshun A, Klauber-Demore N, Peterson L, Patel S, Lindhorst S, Atkinson J, Cohen Z, Laframboise R, Dirks P, Taylor M, Malkin D, Albrecht S, Dudley RW, Jabado N, Hawkins CE, Shlien A, Tabori U (2016) Immune checkpoint inhibition for hypermutant glioblastoma multiforme resulting from germline biallelic mismatch repair deficiency. J Clin Oncol 34(19):2206–2211. https://doi.org/10.1200/JCO.2016.66.6552

Buczkowicz P, Hoeman C, Rakopoulos P, Pajovic S, Letourneau L, Dzamba M, Morrison A, Lewis P, Bouffet E, Bartels U, Zuccaro J, Agnihotri S, Ryall S, Barszczyk M, Chornenkyy Y, Bourgey M, Bourque G, Montpetit A, Cordero F, Castelo-Branco P, Mangerel J, Tabori U, Ho KC, Huang A, Taylor KR, Mackay A, Bendel AE, Nazarian J, Fangusaro JR, Karajannis MA, Zagzag D, Foreman NK, Donson A, Hegert JV, Smith A, Chan J, Lafay-Cousin L, Dunn S, Hukin J, Dunham C, Scheinemann K, Michaud J, Zelcer S, Ramsay D, Cain J, Brennan C, Souweidane MM, Jones C, Allis CD, Brudno M, Becher O, Hawkins C (2014) Genomic analysis of diffuse intrinsic pontine gliomas identifies three molecular subgroups and recurrent activating ACVR1 mutations. Nat Genet 46(5):451–456. https://doi.org/10.1038/ng.2936

Byrne S, Connor S, Lascelles K, Siddiqui A, Hargrave D, Ferner RE (2017) Clinical presentation and prognostic indicators in 100 adults and children with neurofibromatosis 1 associated non-optic pathway brain gliomas. J Neuro-Oncol 133(3):609–614. https://doi.org/10.1007/s11060-017-2475-z

Cancer Genome Atlas Research N, Brat DJ, Verhaak RG, Aldape KD, Yung WK, Salama SR, Cooper LA, Rheinbay E, Miller CR, Vitucci M, Morozova O, Robertson AG, Noushmehr H, Laird PW, Cherniack AD, Akbani R, Huse JT, Ciriello G, Poisson LM, Barnholtz-Sloan JS, Berger MS, Brennan C, Colen RR, Colman H, Flanders AE, Giannini C, Grifford M, Iavarone A, Jain R, Joseph I, Kim J, Kasaian K, Mikkelsen T, Murray BA, O'Neill BP, Pachter L, Parsons DW, Sougnez C, Sulman EP, Vandenberg SR, Van Meir EG, von Deimling A, Zhang H, Crain D, Lau K, Mallery D, Morris S, Paulauskis J, Penny R, Shelton T, Sherman M, Yena P, Black A, Bowen J, Dicostanzo K, Gastier-Foster J, Leraas KM, Lichtenberg TM, Pierson CR, Ramirez NC, Taylor C, Weaver S, Wise L, Zmuda E, Davidsen T, Demchok JA, Eley G, Ferguson ML, Hutter CM, Mills Shaw KR, Ozenberger BA, Sheth M, Sofia HJ, Tarnuzzer R, Wang Z, Yang L, Zenklusen JC, Ayala B, Baboud J, Chudamani S, Jensen MA, Liu J, Pihl T, Raman R, Wan Y, Wu Y, Ally A, Auman JT, Balasundaram M, Balu S, Baylin SB, Beroukhim R, Bootwalla MS, Bowlby R, Bristow CA, Brooks D, Butterfield Y, Carlsen R, Carter S, Chin L, Chu A, Chuah E, Cibulskis K, Clarke A, Coetzee SG, Dhalla N, Fennell T, Fisher S, Gabriel S, Getz G, Gibbs R, Guin R, Hadjipanayis A, Hayes DN, Hinoue T, Hoadley K, Holt RA, Hoyle AP, Jefferys SR, Jones S, Jones CD, Kucherlapati R, Lai PH, Lander E, Lee S, Lichtenstein L, Ma Y, Maglinte DT, Mahadeshwar HS, Marra MA, Mayo M, Meng S, Meyerson ML, Mieczkowski PA, Moore RA, Mose LE, Mungall AJ, Pantazi A, Parfenov M, Park PJ, Parker JS, Perou CM, Protopopov A, Ren X, Roach J, Sabedot TS, Schein J, Schumacher SE, Seidman JG, Seth S, Shen H, Simons JV, Sipahimalani P, Soloway MG, Song X, Sun H, Tabak B, Tam A, Tan D, Tang J, Thiessen N, Triche T Jr, Van Den Berg DJ, Veluvolu U, Waring S, Weisenberger DJ, Wilkerson MD, Wong T, Wu J, Xi L, Xu AW, Yang L, Zack TI, Zhang J, Aksoy BA, Arachchi H, Benz C, Bernard B, Carlin D, Cho J, DiCara D, Frazer S, Fuller GN, Gao J, Gehlenborg N, Haussler D, Heiman DI, Iype L, Jacobsen A, Ju Z, Katzman S, Kim H, Knijnenburg T, Kreisberg RB, Lawrence MS, Lee W, Leinonen K, Lin P, Ling S, Liu

W, Liu Y, Liu Y, Lu Y, Mills G, Ng S, Noble MS, Paull E, Rao A, Reynolds S, Saksena G, Sanborn Z, Sander C, Schultz N, Senbabaoglu Y, Shen R, Shmulevich I, Sinha R, Stuart J, Sumer SO, Sun Y, Tasman N, Taylor BS, Voet D, Weinhold N, Weinstein JN, Yang D, Yoshihara K, Zheng S, Zhang W, Zou L, Abel T, Sadeghi S, Cohen ML, Eschbacher J, Hattab EM, Raghunathan A, Schniederjan MJ, Aziz D, Barnett G, Barrett W, Bigner DD, Boice L, Brewer C, Calatozzolo C, Campos B, Carlotti CG Jr, Chan TA, Cuppini L, Curley E, Cuzzubbo S, Devine K, DiMeco F, Duell R, Elder JB, Fehrenbach A, Finocchiaro G, Friedman W, Fulop J, Gardner J, Hermes B, Herold-Mende C, Jungk C, Kendler A, Lehman NL, Lipp E, Liu O, Mandt R, McGraw M, McLendon R, McPherson C, Neder L, Nguyen P, Noss A, Nunziata R, Ostrom QT, Palmer C, Perin A, Pollo B, Potapov A, Potapova O, Rathmell WK, Rotin D, Scarpace L, Schilero C, Senecal K, Shimmel K, Shurkhay V, Sifri S, Singh R, Sloan AE, Smolenski K, Staugaitis SM, Steele R, Thorne L, Tirapelli DP, Unterberg A, Vallurupalli M, Wang Y, Warnick R, Williams F, Wolinsky Y, Bell S, Rosenberg M, Stewart C, Huang F, Grimsby JL, Radenbaugh AJ, Zhang J (2015) Comprehensive, integrative genomic analysis of diffuse lower-grade gliomas. N Engl J Med 372(26):2481–2498. https://doi.org/10.1056/NEJMoa1402121

Capper D, Weissert S, Balss J, Habel A, Meyer J, Jager D, Ackermann U, Tessmer C, Korshunov A, Zentgraf H, Hartmann C, von Deimling A (2010) Characterization of R132H mutation-specific IDH1 antibody binding in brain tumors. Brain Pathol 20(1):245–254. https://doi.org/10.1111/j.1750-3639.2009.00352.x

Capper D, Preusser M, Habel A, Sahm F, Ackermann U, Schindler G, Pusch S, Mechtersheimer G, Zentgraf H, von Deimling A (2011) Assessment of BRAF V600E mutation status by immunohistochemistry with a mutation-specific monoclonal antibody. Acta Neuropathol 122(1):11–19. https://doi.org/10.1007/s00401-011-0841-z

Cha S, Knopp EA, Johnson G, Wetzel SG, Litt AW, Zagzag D (2002) Intracranial mass lesions: dynamic contrast-enhanced susceptibility-weighted echo-planar perfusion MR imaging. Radiology 223(1):11–29

Chamberlain MC (2013) Salvage therapy with BRAF inhibitors for recurrent pleomorphic xanthoastrocytoma: a retrospective case series. J Neuro-Oncol 114(2):237–240. https://doi.org/10.1007/s11060-013-1176-5

Chang EL, Akyurek S, Avalos T, Rebueno N, Spicer C, Garcia J, Famiglietti R, Allen PK, Chao KS, Mahajan A, Woo SY, Maor MH (2007) Evaluation of peritumoral edema in the delineation of radiotherapy clinical target volumes for glioblastoma. Int J Radiat Oncol Biol Phys 68(1):144–150. https://doi.org/10.1016/j.ijrobp.2006.12.009

Chinot OL, Wick W, Mason W, Henriksson R, Saran F, Nishikawa R, Carpentier AF, Hoang-Xuan K, Kavan P, Cernea D, Brandes AA, Hilton M, Abrey L, Cloughesy T (2014) Bevacizumab plus radiotherapy-temozolomide for newly diagnosed glioblastoma. N Engl J Med 370(8):709–722. https://doi.org/10.1056/NEJMoa1308345

Choudhri AF, Klimo P Jr, Auschwitz TS, Whitehead MT, Boop FA (2014) 3T intraoperative MRI for management of pediatric CNS neoplasms. AJNR Am J Neuroradiol 35(12):2382–2387. https://doi.org/10.3174/ajnr.A4040

Chuba PJ, Aronin P, Bhambhani K, Eichenhorn M, Zamarano L, Cianci P, Muhlbauer M, Porter AT, Fontanesi J (1997) Hyperbaric oxygen therapy for radiation-induced brain injury in children. Cancer 80(10):2005–2012

Cohen KJ, Pollack IF, Zhou T, Buxton A, Holmes EJ, Burger PC, Brat DJ, Rosenblum MK, Hamilton RL, Lavey RS, Heideman RL (2011) Temozolomide in the treatment of high-grade gliomas in children: a report from the Children's Oncology Group. Neuro-Oncology 13(3):317–323. https://doi.org/10.1093/neuonc/noq191

Drezner N, Hardy KK, Wells E, Vezina G, Ho CY, Packer RJ, Hwang EI (2016) Treatment of pediatric cerebral radiation necrosis: a systematic review. J Neuro-Oncol 130(1):141–148. https://doi.org/10.1007/s11060-016-2219-5

Duffner PK, Horowitz ME, Krischer JP, Friedman HS, Burger PC, Cohen ME, Sanford RA, Mulhern RK, James HE, Freeman CR et al (1993) Postoperative chemotherapy and delayed radiation in children less than three years of age with malignant brain tumors. N Engl J Med 328(24):1725–1731

Duffner PK, Krischer JP, Burger PC, Cohen ME, Backstrom JW, Horowitz ME, Sanford RA, Friedman HS, Kun LE (1996) Treatment of infants with malignant gliomas: the Pediatric Oncology Group experience. J Neuro-Oncol 28(2–3):245–256

Duffner PK, Horowitz ME, Krischer JP, Burger PC, Cohen ME, Sanford RA, Friedman HS, Kun LE (1999) The treatment of malignant brain tumors in infants and very young children: an update of the Pediatric Oncology Group experience. Neuro-Oncology 1(2):152–161

Dufour C, Grill J, Lellouch-Tubiana A, Puget S, Chastagner P, Frappaz D, Doz F, Pichon F, Plantaz D, Gentet JC, Raquin MA, Kalifa C (2006) High-grade glioma in children under 5 years of age: a chemotherapy only approach with the BBSFOP protocol. Eur J Cancer 42(17):2939–2945. https://doi.org/10.1016/j.ejca.2006.06.021

Eckel-Passow JE, Lachance DH, Molinaro AM, Walsh KM, Decker PA, Sicotte H, Pekmezci M, Rice T, Kosel ML, Smirnov IV, Sarkar G, Caron AA, Kollmeyer TM, Praska CE, Chada AR, Halder C, Hansen HM, McCoy LS, Bracci PM, Marshall R, Zheng S, Reis GF, Pico AR, O'Neill BP, Buckner JC, Giannini C, Huse JT, Perry A, Tihan T, Berger MS, Chang SM, Prados MD, Wiemels J, Wiencke JK, Wrensch MR, Jenkins RB (2015) Glioma Groups based on 1p/19q, IDH, and TERT promoter mutations in Tumors. N Engl J Med 372(26):2499–2508. https://doi.org/10.1056/NEJMoa1407279

Eisenstat DD, Pollack IF, Demers A, Sapp MV, Lambert P, Weisfeld-Adams JD, Burger PC, Gilles F, Davis RL, Packer R, Boyett JM, Finlay JL (2015) Impact of tumor location and pathological discordance on survival of children with midline high-grade gliomas treated on Children's Cancer Group high-grade glioma study CCG-945. J Neuro-Oncol 121(3):573–581. https://doi.org/10.1007/s11060-014-1669-x

Elsamadicy AA, Babu R, Kirkpatrick JP, Adamson DC (2015) Radiation-induced malignant gliomas: a current review. World Neurosurg 83(4):530–542. https://doi.org/10.1016/j.wneu.2014.12.009

Fitzek MM, Thornton AF, Rabinov JD, Lev MH, Pardo FS, Munzenrider JE, Okunieff P, Bussiere M, Braun I, Hochberg FH, Hedley-Whyte ET, Liebsch NJ, Harsh GR 4th (1999) Accelerated fractionated proton/photon irradiation to 90 cobalt gray equivalent for glioblastoma multiforme: results of a phase II prospective trial. J Neurosurg 91(2):251–260. https://doi.org/10.3171/jns.1999.91.2.0251

Fogh SE, Andrews DW, Glass J, Curran W, Glass C, Champ C, Evans JJ, Hyslop T, Pequignot E, Downes B, Comber E, Maltenfort M, Dicker AP, Werner-Wasik M (2010) Hypofractionated stereotactic radiation therapy: an effective therapy for recurrent high-grade gliomas. J Clin Oncol 28(18):3048–3053. https://doi.org/10.1200/JCO.2009.25.6941

Fontebasso AM, Papillon-Cavanagh S, Schwartzentruber J, Nikbakht H, Gerges N, Fiset PO, Bechet D, Faury D, De Jay N, Ramkissoon LA, Corcoran A, Jones DT, Sturm D, Johann P, Tomita T, Goldman S, Nagib M, Bendel A, Goumnerova L, Bowers DC, Leonard JR, Rubin JB, Alden T, Browd S, Geyer JR, Leary S, Jallo G, Cohen K, Gupta N, Prados MD, Carret AS, Ellezam B, Crevier L, Klekner A, Bognar L, Hauser P, Garami M, Myseros J, Dong Z, Siegel PM, Malkin H, Ligon AH, Albrecht S, Pfister SM, Ligon KL, Majewski J, Jabado N, Kieran MW (2014) Recurrent somatic mutations in ACVR1 in pediatric midline high-grade astrocytoma. Nat Genet 46(5):462–466. https://doi.org/10.1038/ng.2950

Funato K, Major T, Lewis PW, Allis CD, Tabar V (2014) Use of human embryonic stem cells to model pediatric gliomas with H3.3K27M histone mutation. Science 346(6216):1529–1533. https://doi.org/10.1126/science.1253799

Furuse M, Nonoguchi N, Kuroiwa T, Miyamoto S, Arakawa Y, Shinoda J, Miwa K, Iuchi T, Tsuboi K, Houkin K, Terasaka S, Tabei Y, Nakamura H, Nagane M, Sugiyama K, Terasaki M, Abe T, Narita Y, Saito N, Mukasa A, Ogasawara K, Beppu T, Kumabe T, Nariai T, Tsuyuguchi N, Nakatani E, Kurisu S, Nakagawa Y, Miyatake SI (2016) A prospective, multicentre, single-arm clinical trial of bevacizumab for patients with surgically untreatable, symptomatic brain radiation necrosisdagger. Neurooncol Pract 3(4):272–280. https://doi.org/10.1093/nop/npv064

Gajjar A, Bowers DC, Karajannis MA, Leary S, Witt H, Gottardo NG (2015) Pediatric brain tumors: innovative genomic information is transforming the diagnostic and clinical landscape. J Clin Oncol 33(27):2986–2998. https://doi.org/10.1200/JCO.2014.59.9217

Ge M, Li S, Wang L, Li C, Zhang J (2015) The role of diffusion tensor tractography in the surgical treatment of pediatric optic chiasmatic gliomas. J Neuro-Oncol 122(2):357–366. https://doi.org/10.1007/s11060-015-1722-4

Geyer JR, Finlay JL, Boyett JM, Wisoff J, Yates A, Mao L, Packer RJ (1995) Survival of infants with malignant astrocytomas. A report from the Children's Cancer Group. Cancer 75(4):1045–1050

Giglio P, Gilbert MR (2003) Cerebral radiation necrosis. Neurologist 9(4):180–188. https://doi.org/10.1097/01.nrl.0000080951.78533.c4

Gilbert MR, Dignam JJ, Armstrong TS, Wefel JS, Blumenthal DT, Vogelbaum MA, Colman H, Chakravarti A, Pugh S, Won M, Jeraj R, Brown PD, Jaeckle KA, Schiff D, Stieber VW, Brachman DG, Werner-Wasik M, Tremont-Lukats IW, Sulman EP, Aldape KD, Curran WJ Jr, Mehta MP (2014) A randomized trial of bevacizumab for newly diagnosed glioblastoma. N Engl J Med 370(8):699–708. https://doi.org/10.1056/NEJMoa1308573

Gonzalez J, Kumar AJ, Conrad CA, Levin VA (2007) Effect of bevacizumab on radiation necrosis of the brain. Int J Radiat Oncol Biol Phys 67(2):323–326. https://doi.org/10.1016/j.ijrobp.2006.10.010

Grasso CS, Tang Y, Truffaux N, Berlow NE, Liu L, Debily MA, Quist MJ, Davis LE, Huang EC, Woo PJ, Ponnuswami A, Chen S, Johung TB, Sun W, Kogiso M, Du Y, Qi L, Huang Y, Hutt-Cabezas M, Warren KE, Le Dret L, Meltzer PS, Mao H, Quezado M, van Vuurden DG, Abraham J, Fouladi M, Svalina MN, Wang N, Hawkins C, Nazarian J, Alonso MM, Raabe EH, Hulleman E, Spellman PT, Li XN, Keller C, Pal R, Grill J, Monje M (2015) Functionally defined therapeutic targets in diffuse intrinsic pontine glioma. Nat Med 21(7):827. https://doi.org/10.1038/nm0715-827a

Griffith B, Jain R (2015) Perfusion imaging in neurooncology: basic techniques and clinical applications. Radiol Clin N Am 53(3):497–511. https://doi.org/10.1016/j.rcl.2015.01.004

Gururangan S, Fangusaro J, Poussaint TY, McLendon RE, Onar-Thomas A, Wu S, Packer RJ, Banerjee A, Gilbertson RJ, Fahey F, Vajapeyam S, Jakacki R, Gajjar A, Goldman S, Pollack IF, Friedman HS, Boyett JM, Fouladi M, Kun LE (2014) Efficacy of bevacizumab plus irinotecan in children with recurrent low-grade gliomas--a pediatric brain tumor consortium study. Neuro-Oncology 16(2):310–317. https://doi.org/10.1093/neuonc/not154

Gutin PH, Leibel SA, Wara WM, Choucair A, Levin VA, Philips TL, Silver P, Da Silva V, Edwards MS, Davis RL et al (1987) Recurrent malignant gliomas: survival following interstitial brachytherapy with high-activity iodine-125 sources. J Neurosurg 67(6):864–873. https://doi.org/10.3171/jns.1987.67.6.0864

Gutin PH, Iwamoto FM, Beal K, Mohile NA, Karimi S, Hou BL, Lymberis S, Yamada Y, Chang J, Abrey

LE (2009) Safety and efficacy of bevacizumab with hypofractionated stereotactic irradiation for recurrent malignant gliomas. Int J Radiat Oncol Biol Phys 75(1):156–163. https://doi.org/10.1016/j.ijrobp.2008.10.043

Guzman-De-Villoria JA, Mateos-Perez JM, Fernandez-Garcia P, Castro E, Desco M (2014) Added value of advanced over conventional magnetic resonance imaging in grading gliomas and other primary brain tumors. Cancer Imaging 14(1):35. https://doi.org/10.1186/s40644-014-0035-8

Halperin EC, Bentel G, Heinz ER, Burger PC (1989) Radiation therapy treatment planning in supratentorial glioblastoma multiforme: an analysis based on post mortem topographic anatomy with CT correlations. Int J Radiat Oncol Biol Phys 17(6):1347–1350

Hamisch C, Kickingereder P, Fischer M, Simon T, Ruge MI (2017) Update on the diagnostic value and safety of stereotactic biopsy for pediatric brainstem tumors: a systematic review and meta-analysis of 735 cases. J Neurosurg Pediatr 20(3):261–268. https://doi.org/10.3171/2017.2.PEDS1665

Hankinson TC, Campagna EJ, Foreman NK, Handler MH (2011) Interpretation of magnetic resonance images in diffuse intrinsic pontine glioma: a survey of pediatric neurosurgeons. J Neurosurg Pediatr 8(1):97–102. https://doi.org/10.3171/2011.4.PEDS1180

Hegi ME, Diserens AC, Gorlia T, Hamou MF, de Tribolet N, Weller M, Kros JM, Hainfellner JA, Mason W, Mariani L, Bromberg JE, Hau P, Mirimanoff RO, Cairncross JG, Janzer RC, Stupp R (2005) MGMT gene silencing and benefit from temozolomide in glioblastoma. N Engl J Med 352(10):997–1003. https://doi.org/10.1056/NEJMoa043331

Hermanto U, Frija EK, Lii MJ, Chang EL, Mahajan A, Woo SY (2007) Intensity-modulated radiotherapy (IMRT) and conventional three-dimensional conformal radiotherapy for high-grade gliomas: does IMRT increase the integral dose to normal brain? Int J Radiat Oncol Biol Phys 67(4):1135–1144. https://doi.org/10.1016/j.ijrobp.2006.10.032

Hochberg FH, Pruitt A (1980) Assumptions in the radiotherapy of glioblastoma. Neurology 30(9):907–911

Hoffman LM, Geller J, Leach J, Boue D, Drissi R, Chen L, Krailo M, Panandiker AP, Chow L, Haas-Kogan D, Jogal S, Nelson M, Jakacki R, Kieran M, Cohen K, Pollack I, Gajjar A, Fouladi M (2015) A feasibility and randomized phase II study of Vorinostat, Bevacizumab, or Temozolomide during radiation followed by maintenance chemotherapy in newly-diagnosed pediatric high-grade glioma: Children's Oncology Group Study Acns0822. Neuro-Oncology 17:39–40

Hsiao SJ, Karajannis MA, Diolaiti D, Mansukhani MM, Bender JG, Kung AL, Garvin JH Jr (2017) A novel, potentially targetable TMEM106B-BRAF fusion in pleomorphic xanthoastrocytoma. Cold Spring Harb Mol Case Stud 3(2):a001396. https://doi.org/10.1101/mcs.a001396

Hyman DM, Puzanov I, Subbiah V, Faris JE, Chau I, Blay JY, Wolf J, Raje NS, Diamond EL, Hollebecque A,

Gervais R, Elez-Fernandez ME, Italiano A, Hofheinz RD, Hidalgo M, Chan E, Schuler M, Lasserre SF, Makrutzki M, Sirzen F, Veronese ML, Tabernero J, Baselga J (2015) Vemurafenib in multiple nonmelanoma cancers with BRAF V600 mutations. N Engl J Med 373(8):726–736. https://doi.org/10.1056/NEJMoa1502309

Ida CM, Rodriguez FJ, Burger PC, Caron AA, Jenkins SM, Spears GM, Aranguren DL, Lachance DH, Giannini C (2015) Pleomorphic Xanthoastrocytoma: natural history and long-term follow-up. Brain Pathol 25(5):575–586. https://doi.org/10.1111/bpa.12217

Jakacki RI, Cohen KJ, Buxton A, Krailo MD, Burger PC, Rosenblum MK, Brat DJ, Hamilton RL, Eckel SP, Zhou T, Lavey RS, Pollack IF (2016) Phase 2 study of concurrent radiotherapy and temozolomide followed by temozolomide and lomustine in the treatment of children with high-grade glioma: a report of the Children's Oncology Group ACNS0423 study. Neuro-Oncology 18(10):1442–1450. https://doi.org/10.1093/neuonc/now038

Jansen MH, van Vuurden DG, Vandertop WP, Kaspers GJ (2012) Diffuse intrinsic pontine gliomas: a systematic update on clinical trials and biology. Cancer Treat Rev 38(1):27–35. https://doi.org/10.1016/j.ctrv.2011.06.007

Johnson BE, Mazor T, Hong C, Barnes M, Aihara K, McLean CY, Fouse SD, Yamamoto S, Ueda H, Tatsuno K, Asthana S, Jalbert LE, Nelson SJ, Bollen AW, Gustafson WC, Charron E, Weiss WA, Smirnov IV, Song JS, Olshen AB, Cha S, Zhao Y, Moore RA, Mungall AJ, Jones SJ, Hirst M, Marra MA, Saito N, Aburatani H, Mukasa A, Berger MS, Chang SM, Taylor BS, Costello JF (2014) Mutational analysis reveals the origin and therapy-driven evolution of recurrent glioma. Science 343(6167):189–193. https://doi.org/10.1126/science.1239947

Kahramancetin N, Tihan T (2013) Aggressive behavior and anaplasia in pleomorphic xanthoastrocytoma: a plea for a revision of the current WHO classification. CNS Oncol 2(6):523–530. https://doi.org/10.2217/cns.13.56

Kelly PJ, Daumas-Duport C, Kispert DB, Kall BA, Scheithauer BW, Illig JJ (1987) Imaging-based stereotaxic serial biopsies in untreated intracranial glial neoplasms. J Neurosurg 66(6):865–874. https://doi.org/10.3171/jns.1987.66.6.0865

Kline CN, Joseph NM, Grenert JP, van Ziffle J, Talevich E, Onodera C, Aboian M, Cha S, Raleigh DR, Braunstein S, Torkildson J, Samuel D, Bloomer M, Campomanes AGA, Banerjee A, Butowski N, Raffel C, Tihan T, Bollen AW, Phillips JJ, Korn WM, Yeh I, Bastian BC, Gupta N, Mueller S, Perry A, Nicolaides T, Solomon DA (2017) Targeted next-generation sequencing of pediatric neuro-oncology patients improves diagnosis, identifies pathogenic germline mutations, and directs targeted therapy. Neuro-Oncology 19(5):699–709. https://doi.org/10.1093/neuonc/now254

Koelsche C, Sahm F, Capper D, Reuss D, Sturm D, Jones DT, Kool M, Northcott PA, Wiestler B, Bohmer K,

Meyer J, Mawrin C, Hartmann C, Mittelbronn M, Platten M, Brokinkel B, Seiz M, Herold-Mende C, Unterberg A, Schittenhelm J, Weller M, Pfister S, Wick W, Korshunov A, von Deimling A (2013) Distribution of TERT promoter mutations in pediatric and adult tumors of the nervous system. Acta Neuropathol 126(6):907–915. https://doi.org/10.1007/s00401-013-1195-5

Korones DN, Smith A, Foreman N, Bouffet E (2006) Temozolomide and oral VP-16 for children and young adults with recurrent or treatment-induced malignant gliomas. Pediatr Blood Cancer 47(1):37–41. https://doi.org/10.1002/pbc.20510

Korshunov A, Ryzhova M, Hovestadt V, Bender S, Sturm D, Capper D, Meyer J, Schrimpf D, Kool M, Northcott PA, Zheludkova O, Milde T, Witt O, Kulozik AE, Reifenberger G, Jabado N, Perry A, Lichter P, von Deimling A, Pfister SM, Jones DT (2015) Integrated analysis of pediatric glioblastoma reveals a subset of biologically favorable tumors with associated molecular prognostic markers. Acta Neuropathol 129(5):669–678. https://doi.org/10.1007/s00401-015-1405-4

Korshunov A, Capper D, Reuss D, Schrimpf D, Ryzhova M, Hovestadt V, Sturm D, Meyer J, Jones C, Zheludkova O, Kumirova E, Golanov A, Kool M, Schuller U, Mittelbronn M, Hasselblatt M, Schittenhelm J, Reifenberger G, Herold-Mende C, Lichter P, von Deimling A, Pfister SM, Jones DT (2016) Histologically distinct neuroepithelial tumors with histone 3 G34 mutation are molecularly similar and comprise a single nosologic entity. Acta Neuropathol 131(1):137–146. https://doi.org/10.1007/s00401-015-1493-1

Korshunov A, Schrimpf D, Ryzhova M, Sturm D, Chavez L, Hovestadt V, Sharma T, Habel A, Burford A, Jones C, Zheludkova O, Kumirova E, Kramm CM, Golanov A, Capper D, von Deimling A, Pfister SM, Jones DT (2017) H3-/IDH-wild type pediatric glioblastoma is comprised of molecularly and prognostically distinct subtypes with associated oncogenic drivers. Acta Neuropathol 134(3):507–516. https://doi.org/10.1007/s00401-017-1710-1

Kristiansen K, Hagen S, Kollevold T, Torvik A, Holme I, Nesbakken R, Hatlevoll R, Lindgren M, Brun A, Lindgren S, Notter G, Andersen AP, Elgen K (1981) Combined modality therapy of operated astrocytomas grade III and IV. Confirmation of the value of postoperative irradiation and lack of potentiation of bleomycin on survival time: a prospective multicenter trial of the Scandinavian Glioblastoma Study Group. Cancer 47(4):649–652

Kumar AJ, Leeds NE, Fuller GN, Van Tassel P, Maor MH, Sawaya RE, Levin VA (2000) Malignant gliomas: MR imaging spectrum of radiation therapy- and chemotherapy-induced necrosis of the brain after treatment. Radiology 217(2):377–384. https://doi.org/10.1148/radiology.217.2.r00nv36377

Kupper H, Groeschel S, Alber M, Klose U, Schuhmann MU, Wilke M (2015) Comparison of different tractography algorithms and validation by intraoperative stimulation in a child with a brain tumor. Neuropediatrics 46(1):72–75. https://doi.org/10.1055/s-0034-1395346

Lai A, Kharbanda S, Pope WB, Tran A, Solis OE, Peale F, Forrest WF, Pujara K, Carrillo JA, Pandita A, Ellingson BM, Bowers CW, Soriano RH, Schmidt NO, Mohan S, Yong WH, Seshagiri S, Modrusan Z, Jiang Z, Aldape KD, Mischel PS, Liau LM, Escovedo CJ, Chen W, Nghiemphu PL, James CD, Prados MD, Westphal M, Lamszus K, Cloughesy T, Phillips HS (2011) Evidence for sequenced molecular evolution of IDH1 mutant glioblastoma from a distinct cell of origin. J Clin Oncol 29(34):4482–4490. https://doi.org/10.1200/JCO.2010.33.8715

Laperriere NJ, Leung PM, McKenzie S, Milosevic M, Wong S, Glen J, Pintilie M, Bernstein M (1998) Randomized study of brachytherapy in the initial management of patients with malignant astrocytoma. Int J Radiat Oncol Biol Phys 41(5):1005–1011

Lassaletta A, Zapotocky M, Mistry M, Ramaswamy V, Honnorat M, Krishnatry R, Guerreiro Stucklin A, Zhukova N, Arnoldo A, Ryall S, Ling C, McKeown T, Loukides J, Cruz O, de Torres C, Ho CY, Packer RJ, Tatevossian R, Qaddoumi I, Harreld JH, Dalton JD, Mulcahy-Levy J, Foreman N, Karajannis MA, Wang S, Snuderl M, Nageswara Rao A, Giannini C, Kieran M, Ligon KL, Garre ML, Nozza P, Mascelli S, Raso A, Mueller S, Nicolaides T, Silva K, Perbet R, Vasiljevic A, Faure Conter C, Frappaz D, Leary S, Crane C, Chan A, Ng HK, Shi ZF, Mao Y, Finch E, Eisenstat D, Wilson B, Carret AS, Hauser P, Sumerauer D, Krskova L, Larouche V, Fleming A, Zelcer S, Jabado N, Rutka JT, Dirks P, Taylor MD, Chen S, Bartels U, Huang A, Ellison DW, Bouffet E, Hawkins C, Tabori U (2017) Therapeutic and prognostic implications of BRAF V600E in pediatric low-grade gliomas. J Clin Oncol 35(25):2934–2941. https://doi.org/10.1200/JCO.2016.71.8726

Lassman AB, Pugh SL, Gilbert MR, Aldape KD, Geinoz S, Beumer JH, Christner SM, Komaki R, DeAngelis LM, Gaur R, Youssef E, Wagner H, Won M, Mehta MP (2015) Phase 2 trial of dasatinib in target-selected patients with recurrent glioblastoma (RTOG 0627). Neuro-Oncology 17(7):992–998. https://doi.org/10.1093/neuonc/nov011

Lee SW, Fraass BA, Marsh LH, Herbort K, Gebarski SS, Martel MK, Radany EH, Lichter AS, Sandler HM (1999) Patterns of failure following high-dose 3-D conformal radiotherapy for high-grade astrocytomas: a quantitative dosimetric study. Int J Radiat Oncol Biol Phys 43(1):79–88

Lee EQ, Ruland S, LeBoeuf NR, Wen PY, Santagata S (2014) Successful treatment of a progressive BRAF V600E-mutated anaplastic pleomorphic xanthoastrocytoma with vemurafenib monotherapy. J Clin Oncol 34(10):e87–e89. https://doi.org/10.1200/JCO.2013.51.1766

Li FP, Fraumeni JF Jr, Mulvihill JJ, Blattner WA, Dreyfus MG, Tucker MA, Miller RW (1988) A cancer family syndrome in twenty-four kindreds. Cancer Res 48(18):5358–5362

Linos E, Raine T, Alonso A, Michaud D (2007) Atopy and risk of brain tumors: a meta-analysis. J Natl Cancer Inst 99(20):1544–1550. https://doi.org/10.1093/jnci/djm170

Louis DN, Perry A, Reifenberger G, von Deimling A, Figarella-Branger D, Cavenee WK, Ohgaki H, Wiestler OD, Kleihues P, Ellison DW (2016) The 2016 World Health Organization classification of tumors of the central nervous system: a summary. Acta Neuropathol 131(6):803–820. https://doi.org/10.1007/s00401-016-1545-1

Lucas GL, Luxton G, Cohen D, Petrovich Z, Langholz B, Apuzzo ML, Sapozink MD (1991) Treatment results of stereotactic interstitial brachytherapy for primary and metastatic brain tumors. Int J Radiat Oncol Biol Phys 21(3):715–721

Mackay A, Burford A, Carvalho D, Izquierdo E, Fazal-Salom J, Taylor KR, Bjerke L, Clarke M, Vinci M, Nandhabalan M, Temelso S, Popov S, Molinari V, Raman P, Waanders AJ, Han HJ, Gupta S, Marshall L, Zacharoulis S, Vaidya S, Mandeville HC, Bridges LR, Martin AJ, Al-Sarraj S, Chandler C, Ng HK, Li X, Mu K, Trabelsi S, Brahim DH, Kisljakov AN, Konovalov DM, Moore AS, Carcaboso AM, Sunol M, de Torres C, Cruz O, Mora J, Shats LI, Stavale JN, Bidinotto LT, Reis RM, Entz-Werle N, Farrell M, Cryan J, Crimmins D, Caird J, Pears J, Monje M, Debily MA, Castel D, Grill J, Hawkins C, Nikbakht H, Jabado N, Baker SJ, Pfister SM, Jones DTW, Fouladi M, von Bueren AO, Baudis M, Resnick A, Jones C (2017) Integrated molecular meta-analysis of 1,000 pediatric high-grade and diffuse intrinsic pontine glioma. Cancer Cell 32(4):520–537. https://doi.org/10.1016/j.ccell.2017.08.017

Marucci G, Morandi L (2011) Assessment of MGMT promoter methylation status in pleomorphic xanthoastrocytoma. J Neuro-Oncol 105(2):397–400. https://doi.org/10.1007/s11060-011-0605-6

Matsukado Y, Maccarty CS, Kernohan JW (1961) The growth of glioblastoma multiforme (astrocytomas, grades 3 and 4) in neurosurgical practice. J Neurosurg 18:636–644. https://doi.org/10.3171/jns.1961.18.5.0636

Maxwell R, Jackson CM, Lim M (2017) Clinical trials investigating immune checkpoint blockade in glioblastoma. Curr Treat Options in Oncol 18(8):51. https://doi.org/10.1007/s11864-017-0492-y

McCrea HJ, Bander ED, Venn RA, Reiner AS, Iorgulescu JB, Puchi LA, Schaefer PM, Cederquist G, Greenfield JP (2015) Sex, age, anatomic location, and extent of resection influence outcomes in children with high-grade glioma. Neurosurgery 77(3):443–452.; discussion 452–443. https://doi.org/10.1227/NEU.0000000000000845

McDonald MW, Shu HK, Curran WJ Jr, Crocker IR (2011) Pattern of failure after limited margin radiotherapy and temozolomide for glioblastoma. Int J Radiat Oncol Biol Phys 79(1):130–136. https://doi.org/10.1016/j.ijrobp.2009.10.048

Merchant TE, Hua CH, Shukla H, Ying X, Nill S, Oelfke U (2008) Proton versus photon radiotherapy for common pediatric brain tumors: comparison of models of dose characteristics and their relationship to cognitive function. Pediatr Blood Cancer 51(1):110–117. https://doi.org/10.1002/pbc.21530

Mistry M, Zhukova N, Merico D, Rakopoulos P, Krishnatry R, Shago M, Stavropoulos J, Alon N, Pole JD, Ray PN, Navickiene V, Mangerel J, Remke M, Buczkowicz P, Ramaswamy V, Guerreiro Stucklin A, Li M, Young EJ, Zhang C, Castelo-Branco P, Bakry D, Laughlin S, Shlien A, Chan J, Ligon KL, Rutka JT, Dirks PB, Taylor MD, Greenberg M, Malkin D, Huang A, Bouffet E, Hawkins CE, Tabori U (2015) BRAF mutation and CDKN2A deletion define a clinically distinct subgroup of childhood secondary high-grade glioma. J Clin Oncol 33(9):1015–1022. https://doi.org/10.1200/JCO.2014.58.3922

Mizumoto M, Yamamoto T, Takano S, Ishikawa E, Matsumura A, Ishikawa H, Okumura T, Sakurai H, Miyatake S, Tsuboi K (2015) Long-term survival after treatment of glioblastoma multiforme with hyperfractionated concomitant boost proton beam therapy. Pract Radiat Oncol 5(1):e9–e16. https://doi.org/10.1016/j.prro.2014.03.012

Moshel YA, Elliott RE, Monoky DJ, Wisoff JH (2009) Role of diffusion tensor imaging in resection of thalamic juvenile pilocytic astrocytoma. J Neurosurg Pediatr 4(6):495–505. https://doi.org/10.3171/2009.7.PEDS09128

MRC Working Party (1983) A study of the effect of misonidazole in conjunction with radiotherapy for the treatment of grades 3 and 4 astrocytomas. A report from the MRC Working Party on misonidazole in gliomas. Br J Radiol 56(669):673–682. https://doi.org/10.1259/0007-1285-56-669-673

Narayana A, Yamada J, Berry S, Shah P, Hunt M, Gutin PH, Leibel SA (2006) Intensity-modulated radiotherapy in high-grade gliomas: clinical and dosimetric results. Int J Radiat Oncol Biol Phys 64(3):892–897. https://doi.org/10.1016/j.ijrobp.2005.05.067

Narayana A, Kunnakkat S, Chacko-Mathew J, Gardner S, Karajannis M, Raza S, Wisoff J, Weiner H, Harter D, Allen J (2010) Bevacizumab in recurrent high-grade pediatric gliomas. Neuro-Oncology 12(9):985–990. https://doi.org/10.1093/neuonc/noq033

Nieder C, Andratschke N, Wiedenmann N, Busch R, Grosu AL, Molls M (2004) Radiotherapy for high-grade gliomas. Does altered fractionation improve the outcome? Strahlenther Onkol 180(7):401–407. https://doi.org/10.1007/s00066-004-1220-7

Nikbakht H, Panditharatna E, Mikael LG, Li R, Gayden T, Osmond M, Ho CY, Kambhampati M, Hwang EI, Faury D, Siu A, Papillon-Cavanagh S, Bechet D, Ligon KL, Ellezam B, Ingram WJ, Stinson C, Moore AS, Warren KE, Karamchandani J, Packer RJ, Jabado N, Majewski J, Nazarian J (2016) Spatial and temporal homogeneity of driver mutations in diffuse intrinsic pontine glioma. Nat Commun 7:11185. https://doi.org/10.1038/ncomms11185

Olson JJ, Nayak L, Ormond DR, Wen PY, Kalkanis SN, Ryken TC, Committee ACJG (2014) The role of targeted therapies in the management of progressive glioblastoma : a systematic review and evidence-based clinical practice guideline. J Neuro-Oncol 118(3):557–599. https://doi.org/10.1007/s11060-013-1339-4

Orillac C, Thomas C, Dastagirzada Y, Hidalgo ET, Golfinos JG, Zagzag D, Wisoff JH, Karajannis MA, Snuderl M (2016) Pilocytic astrocytoma and glioneuronal tumor with histone H3 K27M mutation. Acta Neuropathol Commun 4(1):84. https://doi.org/10.1186/s40478-016-0361-0

Park KJ, Kano H, Iyer A, Liu X, Niranjan A, Flickinger JC, Lieberman FS, Lunsford LD, Kondziolka D (2012) Salvage gamma knife stereotactic radiosurgery followed by bevacizumab for recurrent glioblastoma multiforme: a case-control study. J Neuro-Oncol 107(2):323–333. https://doi.org/10.1007/s11060-011-0744-9

Patel AP, Tirosh I, Trombetta JJ, Shalek AK, Gillespie SM, Wakimoto H, Cahill DP, Nahed BV, Curry WT, Martuza RL, Louis DN, Rozenblatt-Rosen O, Suva ML, Regev A, Bernstein BE (2014) Single-cell RNA-seq highlights intratumoral heterogeneity in primary glioblastoma. Science 344(6190):1396–1401. https://doi.org/10.1126/science.1254257

Paugh BS, Qu C, Jones C, Liu Z, Adamowicz-Brice M, Zhang J, Bax DA, Coyle B, Barrow J, Hargrave D, Lowe J, Gajjar A, Zhao W, Broniscer A, Ellison DW, Grundy RG, Baker SJ (2010) Integrated molecular genetic profiling of pediatric high-grade gliomas reveals key differences with the adult disease. J Clin Oncol 28(18):3061–3068. https://doi.org/10.1200/JCO.2009.26.7252

Paugh BS, Broniscer A, Qu C, Miller CP, Zhang J, Tatevossian RG, Olson JM, Geyer JR, Chi SN, da Silva NS, Onar-Thomas A, Baker JN, Gajjar A, Ellison DW, Baker SJ (2011) Genome-wide analyses identify recurrent amplifications of receptor tyrosine kinases and cell-cycle regulatory genes in diffuse intrinsic pontine glioma. J Clin Oncol 29(30):3999–4006. https://doi.org/10.1200/JCO.2011.35.5677

Payne DG, Simpson WJ, Keen C, Platts ME (1982) Malignant astrocytoma: hyperfractionated and standard radiotherapy with chemotherapy in a randomized prospective clinical trial. Cancer 50(11):2301–2306

Phillips JJ, Aranda D, Ellison DW, Judkins AR, Croul SE, Brat DJ, Ligon KL, Horbinski C, Venneti S, Zadeh G, Santi M, Zhou S, Appin CL, Sioletic S, Sullivan LM, Martinez-Lage M, Robinson AE, Yong WH, Cloughesy T, Lai A, Phillips HS, Marshall R, Mueller S, Haas-Kogan DA, Molinaro AM, Perry A (2013) PDGFRA amplification is common in pediatric and adult high-grade astrocytomas and identifies a poor prognostic group in IDH1 mutant glioblastoma. Brain Pathol 23(5):565–573. https://doi.org/10.1111/bpa.12043

Pollack IF, Hamilton RL, Finkelstein SD, Campbell JW, Martinez AJ, Sherwin RN, Bozik ME, Gollin SM (1997) The relationship between TP53 mutations and overexpression of p53 and prognosis in malignant gliomas of childhood. Cancer Res 57(2):304–309

Pollack IF, Finkelstein SD, Woods J, Burnham J, Holmes EJ, Hamilton RL, Yates AJ, Boyett JM, Finlay JL, Sposto R, Children's Cancer G (2002) Expression of p53 and prognosis in children with malignant gliomas. N Engl J Med 346(6):420–427. https://doi.org/10.1056/NEJMoa012224

Pollack IF, Boyett JM, Yates AJ, Burger PC, Gilles FH, Davis RL, Finlay JL, Children's Cancer G (2003) The influence of central review on outcome associations in childhood malignant gliomas: results from the CCG-945 experience. Neuro-Oncology 5(3):197–207. https://doi.org/10.1215/S1152-8517-03-00009-7

Pollack IF, Hamilton RL, James CD, Finkelstein SD, Burnham J, Yates AJ, Holmes EJ, Zhou T, Finlay JL, Children's Oncology G (2006) Rarity of PTEN deletions and EGFR amplification in malignant gliomas of childhood: results from the Children's Cancer Group 945 cohort. J Neurosurg 105(5 Suppl):418–424. https://doi.org/10.3171/ped.2006.105.5.418

Pollack IF, Hamilton RL, Sobol RW, Nikiforova MN, Lyons-Weiler MA, LaFramboise WA, Burger PC, Brat DJ, Rosenblum MK, Holmes EJ, Zhou T, Jakacki RI, Children's Oncology G (2011) IDH1 mutations are common in malignant gliomas arising in adolescents: a report from the Children's Oncology Group. Childs Nerv Syst 27(1):87–94. https://doi.org/10.1007/s00381-010-1264-1

Pollack IF, Jakacki RI, Butterfield LH, Hamilton RL, Panigrahy A, Potter DM, Connelly AK, Dibridge SA, Whiteside TL, Okada H (2014) Antigen-specific immune responses and clinical outcome after vaccination with glioma-associated antigen peptides and polyinosinic-polycytidylic acid stabilized by lysine and carboxymethylcellulose in children with newly diagnosed malignant brainstem and nonbrainstem gliomas. J Clin Oncol 32(19):2050–2058. https://doi.org/10.1200/JCO.2013.54.0526

Prados MD, Warnick RE, Mack EE, Chandler KL, Rabbitt J, Page M, Malec M (1996) Intravenous carboplatin for recurrent gliomas. A dose-escalating phase II trial. Am J Clin Oncol 19(6):609–612

Prados MD, Wara WM, Sneed PK, McDermott M, Chang SM, Rabbitt J, Page M, Malec M, Davis RL, Gutin PH, Lamborn K, Wilson CB, Phillips TL, Larson DA (2001) Phase III trial of accelerated hyperfractionation with or without difluromethylornithine (DFMO) versus standard fractionated radiotherapy with or without DFMO for newly diagnosed patients with glioblastoma multiforme. Int J Radiat Oncol Biol Phys 49(1):71–77

Qaddoumi I, Sultan I, Gajjar A (2009) Outcome and prognostic features in pediatric gliomas: a review of 6212 cases from the surveillance, epidemiology, and end results database. Cancer 115(24):5761–5770. https://doi.org/10.1002/cncr.24663

Ramsey RG, Brand WN (1973) Radiotherapy of glioblastoma multiforme. J Neurosurg 39(2):197–202. https://doi.org/10.3171/jns.1973.39.2.0197

Rao AA, Laack NN, Giannini C, Wetmore C (2010) Pleomorphic xanthoastrocytoma in children and adolescents. Pediatr Blood Cancer 55(2):290–294. https://doi.org/10.1002/pbc.22490

Reuss DE, Mamatjan Y, Schrimpf D, Capper D, Hovestadt V, Kratz A, Sahm F, Koelsche C, Korshunov A, Olar A, Hartmann C, Reijneveld JC, Wesseling P, Unterberg A, Platten M, Wick W, Herold-Mende C, Aldape K, von Deimling A (2015) IDH mutant diffuse and anaplastic astrocytomas have similar age at presentation and little difference in survival: a grading problem for WHO. Acta Neuropathol 129(6):867–873. https://doi.org/10.1007/s00401-015-1438-8

Robinson GW, Orr BA, Gajjar A (2014) Complete clinical regression of a BRAF V600E-mutant pediatric glioblastoma multiforme after BRAF inhibitor therapy. BMC Cancer 14:258. https://doi.org/10.1186/1471-2407-14-258

Ruben JD, Dally M, Bailey M, Smith R, McLean CA, Fedele P (2006) Cerebral radiation necrosis: incidence, outcomes, and risk factors with emphasis on radiation parameters and chemotherapy. Int J Radiat Oncol Biol Phys 65(2):499–508. https://doi.org/10.1016/j.ijrobp.2005.12.002

Sampson JH, Maus MV, June CH (2017) Immunotherapy for brain tumors. J Clin Oncol 35(21):2450–2456. https://doi.org/10.1200/JCO.2017.72.8089

Sanai N, Polley MY, McDermott MW, Parsa AT, Berger MS (2011) An extent of resection threshold for newly diagnosed glioblastomas. J Neurosurg 115(1):3–8. https://doi.org/10.3171/2011.2.JNS10998

Sandberg-Wollheim M, Malmstrom P, Stromblad LG, Anderson H, Borgstrom S, Brun A, Cronqvist S, Hougaard K, Salford LG (1991) A randomized study of chemotherapy with procarbazine, vincristine, and lomustine with and without radiation therapy for astrocytoma grades 3 and/or 4. Cancer 68(1):22–29

Sanders RP, Kocak M, Burger PC, Merchant TE, Gajjar A, Broniscer A (2007) High-grade astrocytoma in very young children. Pediatr Blood Cancer 49(7):888–893. https://doi.org/10.1002/pbc.21272

Scharfen CO, Sneed PK, Wara WM, Larson DA, Phillips TL, Prados MD, Weaver KA, Malec M, Acord P, Lamborn KR et al (1992) High activity iodine-125 interstitial implant for gliomas. Int J Radiat Oncol Biol Phys 24(4):583–591

Schindler G, Capper D, Meyer J, Janzarik W, Omran H, Herold-Mende C, Schmieder K, Wesseling P, Mawrin C, Hasselblatt M, Louis DN, Korshunov A, Pfister S, Hartmann C, Paulus W, Reifenberger G, von Deimling A (2011) Analysis of BRAF V600E mutation in 1,320 nervous system tumors reveals high mutation frequencies in pleomorphic xanthoastrocytoma, ganglioglioma and extra-cerebellar pilocytic astrocytoma. Acta Neuropathol 121(3):397–405. https://doi.org/10.1007/s00401-011-0802-6

Schwartzentruber J, Korshunov A, Liu XY, Jones DT, Pfaff E, Jacob K, Sturm D, Fontebasso AM, Quang DA, Tonjes M, Hovestadt V, Albrecht S, Kool M, Nantel A, Konermann C, Lindroth A, Jager N, Rausch T, Ryzhova M, Korbel JO, Hielscher T, Hauser P, Garami M, Klekner A, Bognar L, Ebinger M,

Schuhmann MU, Scheurlen W, Pekrun A, Fruhwald MC, Roggendorf W, Kramm C, Durken M, Atkinson J, Lepage P, Montpetit A, Zakrzewska M, Zakrzewski K, Liberski PP, Dong Z, Siegel P, Kulozik AE, Zapatka M, Guha A, Malkin D, Felsberg J, Reifenberger G, von Deimling A, Ichimura K, Collins VP, Witt H, Milde T, Witt O, Zhang C, Castelo-Branco P, Lichter P, Faury D, Tabori U, Plass C, Majewski J, Pfister SM, Jabado N (2012) Driver mutations in histone H3.3 and chromatin remodelling genes in paediatric glioblastoma. Nature 482(7384):226–231. https://doi.org/10.1038/nature10833

Selker RG, Shapiro WR, Burger P, Blackwood MS, Arena VC, Gilder JC, Malkin MG, Mealey JJ Jr, Neal JH, Olson J, Robertson JT, Barnett GH, Bloomfield S, Albright R, Hochberg FH, Hiesiger E, Green S, Brain Tumor Cooperative G (2002) The brain tumor cooperative group NIH trial 87-01: a randomized comparison of surgery, external radiotherapy, and carmustine versus surgery, interstitial radiotherapy boost, external radiation therapy, and carmustine. Neurosurgery 51(2):343–355. discussion 355–347

Sethi R, Allen J, Donahue B, Karajannis M, Gardner S, Wisoff J, Kunnakkat S, Mathew J, Zagzag D, Newman K, Narayana A (2011) Prospective neuraxis MRI surveillance reveals a high risk of leptomeningeal dissemination in diffuse intrinsic pontine glioma. J Neuro-Oncol 102(1):121–127. https://doi.org/10.1007/s11060-010-0301-y

Shapiro WR, Green SB, Burger PC, Mahaley MS Jr, Selker RG, VanGilder JC, Robertson JT, Ransohoff J, Mealey J Jr, Strike TA et al (1989) Randomized trial of three chemotherapy regimens and two radiotherapy regimens in postoperative treatment of malignant glioma. Brain tumor cooperative group trial 8001. J Neurosurg 71(1):1–9. https://doi.org/10.3171/jns.1989.71.1.0001

Sheline GE (1975) Radiation therapy of primary tumors. Semin Oncol 2(1):29–42

Sheline GE, Wara WM, Smith V (1980) Therapeutic irradiation and brain injury. Int J Radiat Oncol Biol Phys 6(9):1215–1228

Shrieve DC, Alexander E 3rd, Wen PY, Fine HA, Kooy HM, Black PM, Loeffler JS (1995) Comparison of stereotactic radiosurgery and brachytherapy in the treatment of recurrent glioblastoma multiforme. Neurosurgery 36(2):275–282. discussion 282–274

Snuderl M, Fazlollahi L, Le LP, Nitta M, Zhelyazkova BH, Davidson CJ, Akhavanfard S, Cahill DP, Aldape KD, Betensky RA, Louis DN, Iafrate AJ (2011) Mosaic amplification of multiple receptor tyrosine kinase genes in glioblastoma. Cancer Cell 20(6):810–817. https://doi.org/10.1016/j.ccr.2011.11.005

Souhami L, Seiferheld W, Brachman D, Podgorsak EB, Werner-Wasik M, Lustig R, Schultz CJ, Sause W, Okunieff P, Buckner J, Zamorano L, Mehta MP, Curran WJ Jr (2004) Randomized comparison of stereotactic radiosurgery followed by conventional radiotherapy with carmustine to conventional radiotherapy with carmustine for patients with glioblastoma multiforme:

report of Radiation Therapy Oncology Group 93-05 protocol. Int J Radiat Oncol Biol Phys 60(3):853–860. https://doi.org/10.1016/j.ijrobp.2004.04.011

Sposto R, Ertel IJ, Jenkin RD, Boesel CP, Venes JL, Ortega JA, Evans AE, Wara W, Hammond D (1989) The effectiveness of chemotherapy for treatment of high grade astrocytoma in children: results of a randomized trial. A report from the Children's Cancer Study Group. J Neuro-Oncol 7(2):165–177

Srinivasan VM, Ferguson SD, Lee S, Weathers SP, Kerrigan BCP, Heimberger AB (2017) Tumor vaccines for malignant gliomas. Neurotherapeutics 14(2):345–357. https://doi.org/10.1007/s13311-017-0522-2

Stupp R, Mason WP, van den Bent MJ, Weller M, Fisher B, Taphoorn MJ, Belanger K, Brandes AA, Marosi C, Bogdahn U, Curschmann J, Janzer RC, Ludwin SK, Gorlia T, Allgeier A, Lacombe D, Cairncross JG, Eisenhauer E, Mirimanoff RO, European Organisation for R, Treatment of Cancer Brain T, Radiotherapy G, National Cancer Institute of Canada Clinical Trials G (2005) Radiotherapy plus concomitant and adjuvant temozolomide for glioblastoma. N Engl J Med 352(10):987–996. https://doi.org/10.1056/NEJMoa043330

Sturm D, Witt H, Hovestadt V, Khuong-Quang DA, Jones DT, Konermann C, Pfaff E, Tonjes M, Sill M, Bender S, Kool M, Zapatka M, Becker N, Zucknick M, Hielscher T, Liu XY, Fontebasso AM, Ryzhova M, Albrecht S, Jacob K, Wolter M, Ebinger M, Schuhmann MU, van Meter T, Fruhwald MC, Hauch H, Pekrun A, Radlwimmer B, Niehues T, von Komorowski G, Durken M, Kulozik AE, Madden J, Donson A, Foreman NK, Drissi R, Fouladi M, Scheurlen W, von Deimling A, Monoranu C, Roggendorf W, Herold-Mende C, Unterberg A, Kramm CM, Felsberg J, Hartmann C, Wiestler B, Wick W, Milde T, Witt O, Lindroth AM, Schwartzentruber J, Faury D, Fleming A, Zakrzewska M, Liberski PP, Zakrzewski K, Hauser P, Garami M, Klekner A, Bognar L, Morrissy S, Cavalli F, Taylor MD, van Sluis P, Koster J, Versteeg R, Volckmann R, Mikkelsen T, Aldape K, Reifenberger G, Collins VP, Majewski J, Korshunov A, Lichter P, Plass C, Jabado N, Pfister SM (2012) Hotspot mutations in H3F3A and IDH1 define distinct epigenetic and biological subgroups of glioblastoma. Cancer Cell 22(4):425–437. https://doi.org/10.1016/j.ccr.2012.08.024

Sturm D, Bender S, Jones DT, Lichter P, Grill J, Becher O, Hawkins C, Majewski J, Jones C, Costello JF, Iavarone A, Aldape K, Brennan CW, Jabado N, Pfister SM (2014) Paediatric and adult glioblastoma: multiform (epi)genomic culprits emerge. Nat Rev Cancer 14(2):92–107. https://doi.org/10.1038/nrc3655

Suerink M, Potjer TP, Versluijs AB, Ten Broeke SW, Tops CM, Wimmer K, Nielsen M (2017) Constitutional mismatch repair deficiency in a healthy child: on the spot diagnosis? Clin Genet 93(1):134–137. https://doi.org/10.1111/cge.13053

Taal W, Brandsma D, de Bruin HG, Bromberg JE, Swaak-Kragten AT, Smitt PA, van Es CA, van den Bent MJ (2008) Incidence of early pseudo-progression in a cohort of malignant glioma patients treated with chemoirradiation with temozolomide. Cancer 113(2):405–410. https://doi.org/10.1002/cncr.23562

Tavasoli A, Armangue T, Ho CY, Whitehead M, Bornhorst M, Rhee J, Hwang EI, Wells EM, Packer R, van der Knaap MS, Bugiani M, Vanderver A (2017) Alexander disease. J Child Neurol 32(2):184–187. https://doi.org/10.1177/0883073816673263

Taylor KR, Mackay A, Truffaux N, Butterfield YS, Morozova O, Philippe C, Castel D, Grasso CS, Vinci M, Carvalho D, Carcaboso AM, de Torres C, Cruz O, Mora J, Entz-Werle N, Ingram WJ, Monje M, Hargrave D, Bullock AN, Puget S, Yip S, Jones C, Grill J (2014) Recurrent activating ACVR1 mutations in diffuse intrinsic pontine glioma. Nat Genet 46(5):457–461. https://doi.org/10.1038/ng.2925

Tsien C, Moughan J, Michalski JM, Gilbert MR, Purdy J, Simpson J, Kresel JJ, Curran WJ, Diaz A, Mehta MP, Radiation Therapy Oncology Group T (2009) Phase I three-dimensional conformal radiation dose escalation study in newly diagnosed glioblastoma: radiation therapy oncology group trial 98-03. Int J Radiat Oncol Biol Phys 73(3):699–708. https://doi.org/10.1016/j.ijrobp.2008.05.034

Urtasun R, Feldstein ML, Partington J, Tanasichuk H, Miller JD, Russell DB, Agboola O, Mielke B (1982) Radiation and nitroimidazoles in supratentorial high grade gliomas: a second clinical trial. Br J Cancer 46(1):101–108

Vanan MI, Eisenstat DD (2014) Management of high-grade gliomas in the pediatric patient: past, present, and future. Neurooncol Pract 1(4):145–157. https://doi.org/10.1093/nop/npu022

Wagner S, Benesch M, Berthold F, Gnekow AK, Rutkowski S, Strater R, Warmuth-Metz M, Kortmann RD, Pietsch T, Wolff JE (2006) Secondary dissemination in children with high-grade malignant gliomas and diffuse intrinsic pontine gliomas. Br J Cancer 95(8):991–997. https://doi.org/10.1038/sj.bjc.6603402

Walker MD, Alexander E Jr, Hunt WE, MacCarty CS, Mahaley MS Jr, Mealey J Jr, Norrell HA, Owens G, Ransohoff J, Wilson CB, Gehan EA, Strike TA (1978) Evaluation of BCNU and/or radiotherapy in the treatment of anaplastic gliomas. A cooperative clinical trial. J Neurosurg 49(3):333–343. https://doi.org/10.3171/jns.1978.49.3.0333

Walker MD, Strike TA, Sheline GE (1979) An analysis of dose-effect relationship in the radiotherapy of malignant gliomas. Int J Radiat Oncol Biol Phys 5(10):1725–1731

Walker MD, Green SB, Byar DP, Alexander E Jr, Batzdorf U, Brooks WH, Hunt WE, MacCarty CS, Mahaley MS Jr, Mealey J Jr, Owens G, Ransohoff J 2nd, Robertson JT, Shapiro WR, Smith KR Jr, Wilson CB, Strike TA (1980) Randomized comparisons of radiotherapy and nitrosoureas for the treatment of malignant glioma after surgery. N Engl J Med 303(23):1323–1329. https://doi.org/10.1056/NEJM198012043032303

Wallner KE, Galicich JH, Krol G, Arbit E, Malkin MG (1989) Patterns of failure following treatment for glioblastoma multiforme and anaplastic astrocytoma. Int J Radiat Oncol Biol Phys 16(6):1405–1409

Walston S, Hamstra DA, Oh K, Woods G, Guiou M, Olshefski RS, Chakravarti A, Williams TM (2015) A multi-institutional experience in pediatric high-grade glioma. Front Oncol 5:28. https://doi.org/10.3389/fonc.2015.00028

Weller M, Felsberg J, Hartmann C, Berger H, Steinbach JP, Schramm J, Westphal M, Schackert G, Simon M, Tonn JC, Heese O, Krex D, Nikkhah G, Pietsch T, Wiestler O, Reifenberger G, von Deimling A, Loeffler M (2009) Molecular predictors of progression-free and overall survival in patients with newly diagnosed glioblastoma: a prospective translational study of the German Glioma Network. J Clin Oncol 27(34):5743–5750. https://doi.org/10.1200/JCO.2009.23.0805

Weller M, Tabatabai G, Kastner B, Felsberg J, Steinbach JP, Wick A, Schnell O, Hau P, Herrlinger U, Sabel MC, Wirsching HG, Ketter R, Bahr O, Platten M, Tonn JC, Schlegel U, Marosi C, Goldbrunner R, Stupp R, Homicsko K, Pichler J, Nikkhah G, Meixensberger J, Vajkoczy P, Kollias S, Husing J, Reifenberger G, Wick W, Group DS (2015) MGMT promoter methylation is a strong prognostic biomarker for benefit from dose-intensified temozolomide rechallenge in progressive Glioblastoma: the DIRECTOR trial. Clin Cancer Res 21(9):2057–2064. https://doi.org/10.1158/1078-0432.CCR-14-2737

Weller M, Roth P, Preusser M, Wick W, Reardon DA, Platten M, Sampson JH (2017) Vaccine-based immunotherapeutic approaches to gliomas and beyond. Nat Rev Neurol 13(6):363–374. https://doi.org/10.1038/nrneurol.2017.64

Wick W, Weller M, van den Bent M, Sanson M, Weiler M, von Deimling A, Plass C, Hegi M, Platten M, Reifenberger G (2014) MGMT testing--the challenges for biomarker-based glioma treatment. Nat Rev Neurol 10(7):372–385. https://doi.org/10.1038/nrneurol.2014.100

Wimmer K, Kratz CP (2010) Constitutional mismatch repair-deficiency syndrome. Haematologica 95(5):699–701. https://doi.org/10.3324/haematol.2009.021626

Wimmer K, Rosenbaum T, Messiaen L (2017) Connections between constitutional mismatch repair deficiency syndrome and neurofibromatosis type 1. Clin Genet 91(4):507–519. https://doi.org/10.1111/cge.12904

Wisoff JH, Boyett JM, Berger MS, Brant C, Li H, Yates AJ, McGuire-Cullen P, Turski PA, Sutton LN, Allen JC, Packer RJ, Finlay JL (1998) Current neurosurgical management and the impact of the extent of resection in the treatment of malignant gliomas of childhood: a report of the Children's Cancer Group trial no. CCG-945. J Neurosurg 89(1):52–59. https://doi.org/10.3171/jns.1998.89.1.0052

Wolff JE, Driever PH, Erdlenbruch B, Kortmann RD, Rutkowski S, Pietsch T, Parker C, Metz MW, Gnekow A, Kramm CM (2010) Intensive chemotherapy improves survival in pediatric high-grade glioma after gross total resection: results of the HIT-GBM-C proto-col. Cancer 116(3):705–712. https://doi.org/10.1002/cncr.24730

Woodworth GF, Dunn GP, Nance EA, Hanes J, Brem H (2014) Emerging insights into barriers to effective brain tumor therapeutics. Front Oncol 4:126. https://doi.org/10.3389/fonc.2014.00126

Wu G, Diaz AK, Paugh BS, Rankin SL, Ju B, Li Y, Zhu X, Qu C, Chen X, Zhang J, Easton J, Edmonson M, Ma X, Lu C, Nagahawatte P, Hedlund E, Rusch M, Pounds S, Lin T, Onar-Thomas A, Huether R, Kriwacki R, Parker M, Gupta P, Becksfort J, Wei L, Mulder HL, Boggs K, Vadodaria B, Yergeau D, Russell JC, Ochoa K, Fulton RS, Fulton LL, Jones C, Boop FA, Broniscer A, Wetmore C, Gajjar A, Ding L, Mardis ER, Wilson RK, Taylor MR, Downing JR, Ellison DW, Baker SJ (2014) The genomic landscape of diffuse intrinsic pontine glioma and pediatric non-brainstem high-grade glioma. Nat Genet 46(5):444–450. https://doi.org/10.1038/ng.2938

Yang T, Temkin N, Barber J, Geyer JR, Leary S, Browd S, Ojemann JG, Ellenbogen RG (2013) Gross total resection correlates with long-term survival in pediatric patients with glioblastoma. World Neurosurg 79(3–4):537–544. https://doi.org/10.1016/j.wneu.2012.09.015

Yung WK, Mechtler L, Gleason MJ (1991) Intravenous carboplatin for recurrent malignant glioma: a phase II study. J Clin Oncol 9(5):860–864

Zhang L, Chen LH, Wan H, Yang R, Wang Z, Feng J, Yang S, Jones S, Wang S, Zhou W, Zhu H, Killela PJ, Zhang J, Wu Z, Li G, Hao S, Wang Y, Webb JB, Friedman HS, Friedman AH, McLendon RE, He Y, Reitman ZJ, Bigner DD, Yan H (2014) Exome sequencing identifies somatic gain-of-function PPM1D mutations in brainstem gliomas. Nat Genet 46(7):726–730. https://doi.org/10.1038/ng.2995

Zhang J, Walsh MF, Wu G, Edmonson MN, Gruber TA, Easton J, Hedges D, Ma X, Zhou X, Yergeau DA, Wilkinson MR, Vadodaria B, Chen X, McGee RB, Hines-Dowell S, Nuccio R, Quinn E, Shurtleff SA, Rusch M, Patel A, Becksfort JB, Wang S, Weaver MS, Ding L, Mardis ER, Wilson RK, Gajjar A, Ellison DW, Pappo AS, Pui CH, Nichols KE, Downing JR (2015) Germline mutations in predisposition genes in pediatric cancer. N Engl J Med 373(24):2336–2346. https://doi.org/10.1056/NEJMoa1508054

Zinn PO, Colen RR, Kasper EM, Burkhardt JK (2013) Extent of resection and radiotherapy in GBM: a 1973 to 2007 surveillance, epidemiology and end results analysis of 21,783 patients. Int J Oncol 42(3):929–934. https://doi.org/10.3892/ijo.2013.1770

Zukotynski K, Fahey F, Kocak M, Kun L, Boyett J, Fouladi M, Vajapeyam S, Treves T, Poussaint TY (2014) 18F-FDG PET and MR imaging associations across a spectrum of pediatric brain tumors: a report from the pediatric brain tumor consortium. J Nucl Med 55(9):1473–1480. https://doi.org/10.2967/jnumed.114.139626

Low-Grade Gliomas

10

Anna K. Paulsson, Michael A. Garcia,
David A. Solomon, and Daphne A. Haas-Kogan

10.1 Introduction

Tumors of the central nervous system (CNS) are the most common solid tumors in childhood and the second most common overall malignancy in children. The majority of pediatric CNS tumors are gliomas and they are most frequently low-grade. Of the pediatric low-grade gliomas (PLGG), astrocytomas are the predominating histopathologic diagnosis, and include the more prevalent pilocytic astrocytoma and diffuse astrocytoma as well as less common tumors, such as pleomorphic xanthoastrocytoma (PXA), subependymal giant cell astrocytoma (SEGA), and pilomyxoid astrocytoma. Other PLGGs include oligodendroglioma, angiocentric glioma, astroblastoma, and mixed glioneuronal tumors, such as ganglioglioma and dysembryoplastic neuroepithelial tumor (DNT).

A. K. Paulsson · M. A. Garcia
Department of Radiation Oncology, University of California, San Francisco, CA, USA

D. A. Solomon
Division of Neuropathology, Department of Pathology, University of California, San Francisco, CA, USA

D. A. Haas-Kogan (✉)
Department of Radiation Oncology, Dana-Farber Cancer Institute, Brigham and Women's Hospital, Boston Children's Hospital, Harvard Medical School, Boston, MA, USA
e-mail: Dhaas-kogan@lroc.harvard.edu

Evaluation and treatment of PLGG is complex due to the wide variety of tumor types and tumor locations. Surgical removal is often complicated and chemotherapy and radiation treatment have long-term significant side effects and sequelae. Overall prognosis, however, is very good and recent advances in molecular profiling of the tumors have presented an increasing armamentarium of targeted agents with the potential to improve outcomes for young patients.

10.2 Epidemiology

Overall, CNS malignancies account for 20–25% of childhood malignancies, with the highest incidence in children 1–4 years of age and the lowest among children 10–14 years of age. In the United States the annual incidence of PLGG is 2.1 per 100,000, accounting for 1600 new diagnoses every year (Bergthold et al. 2014).

The etiology of PLGG is unknown for the majority of patients. However, 2–5% of CNS tumors are attributed to genetic syndromes (Halperin et al. 2013) (discussed further in Sect. 11.3). Ionizing radiation is a known and established environmental risk and is associated with a 2.6-fold increase in risk of developing a glioma (Ron et al. 1988). Other potential risk factors that have been studied, but that are less clear-cut, include parental exposure to pesticides, dietary exposure to nitrosamines, parental exposure to excessive heat in the 3 months prior to conception, increased birth weight, mother having a prior abortion, and exposure to antiretroviral medication during pregnancy. However, these risk factors have not been reproducible, and the relative risk is rarely greater than 2 (Dulac et al. 2013).

Low-grade astrocytomas (LGAs) can occur anywhere within the cerebral hemispheres, cerebellum, brainstem, or spinal cord. Most commonly, they are found in the posterior fossa (15–20%), followed by the cerebral hemispheres, midline structures such as the ventricles, hypothalamus, thalamus, and brainstem (10–15% for each sub-site), and finally 3–6% are found in the spinal cord (Gupta et al. 2004).

Pilocytic astrocytomas (WHO grade I) are the most common type of PLGG. They account for approximately 35% of pediatric posterior fossa and optic pathway lesions, though they can be found in the deep midline structures and cerebral hemispheres as well (Gupta et al. 2004). Pilomyxoid astrocytoma is a histologic variant of pilocytic astrocytoma with a more aggressive clinical course that has been described in infants and young children. This tumor is often centered within the optic chiasm or hypothalamus. Another PLGG histological subtype is subependymal giant cell astrocytoma (SEGA, WHO grade I), which arises almost exclusively in patients with tuberous sclerosis (TS) and invariably is centered within the lateral ventricles (Gupta et al. 2004).

Among the infiltrative PLGG, diffuse astrocytomas (WHO grade II) most often arise in the cerebral hemispheres and make up a relatively higher proportion of lesions seen in infants and adolescents (Gupta et al. 2004). Oligodendrogliomas are a rare subtype of PLGG. The relative incidence ranges from 4 to 33% depending on the study series; however, they represent only 2% of brain tumors in patients under the age of 14 (Sievert and Fisher 2009).

Approximately 20–30% of PLGG arise within the optic pathway; these are most frequently pilocytic astrocytomas, or less commonly diffuse astrocytomas (Dulac et al. 2013). The peak incidence for gliomas involving the optic pathway is during the first decade of life, and there is no gender predilection. Neurofibromatosis type 1 (NF-1, also referred to as peripheral neurofibromatosis

or von Recklinghausen's disease) is present in about one-third to one-half of patients with optic pathway gliomas. Ten percent of gliomas arising within the optic pathway are confined to a single optic nerve, and 30% have bilateral nerve involvement, which is pathognomonic of NF-1 (Gupta et al. 2004; Ris and Beebe 2008). However, the majority involve the posterior optic chiasm or the hypothalamus.

Glioneuronal tumors are uncommon tumors composed of a mixture of both neoplastic ganglion cells and glial cells. Subtypes include ganglioglioma, desmoplastic infantile ganglioglioma (DIG), and dysembryoplastic neuroepithelial tumor (DNT). They most commonly arise within the cerebral hemispheres, most often within the temporal lobes, and are WHO grade I tumors, although rare glioneuronal tumors with anaplastic features (WHO grade III) have been described (Dulac et al. 2013).

Additional information on Epidemiology can be found in Chap. 1.

10.3 Molecular Biology and Genetics of Pediatric Low-Grade Gliomas (PLGG)

Although morphological classification of PLGG has been the mainstay of determining diagnosis and management, morphology alone has limitations in characterizing this heterogeneous tumor group, as there is considerable overlap in histology and clinical behavior. A better approach for guiding management and predicting prognosis may be to integrate histopathology with emerging molecular biology and genomic data (Bergthold et al. 2014). Early insights into the molecular underpinnings of PLGG came from genetic syndromes, namely NF-1 and TS. Recent advances in high-throughput genetic sequencing and gene expression profiling have furthered our understanding of the specific signaling pathway disturbances involved in the pathogenesis of PLGG (Bergthold et al. 2014; Meyerson et al. 2010; Nakamura et al. 2007). Notably, PLGG are genetically distinct from low-grade gliomas in adult patients, particularly the infiltrative gliomas. Some of the most important genetic alterations and signaling pathway alterations in PLGG are discussed here.

10.3.1 Neurofibromatosis Type 1

Up to 15% of patients with NF-1 develop a cerebral neoplasm before adulthood, with the most common tumors being pilocytic astrocytomas and diffuse astrocytomas (Hernaiz Driever et al. 2010). NF-1-associated PLGG appear to have clinical patterns that are distinct from their sporadic counterparts. NF-1-associated pilocytic astrocytomas more commonly occur in the optic pathway, present at a later age, and tend to have better clinical outcomes (Arun and Gutmann 2004; Rodriguez et al. 2008; Parsa et al. 2001; Perilongo et al. 1999; Piccirilli et al. 2006), with some reports of spontaneous regression.

NF-1 is due to a constitutional mutation in the tumor suppressor gene *neurofibromin 1* (*NF1*) located on chromosome 17q. The functional domain of NF1, RasGAP-related domain (Ras-GRD), accelerates the conversion of the active GTP-bound Ras into its inactive GDP form, thus downregulating the Raf and PI3K transduction pathways (Le and Parada 2007) (Fig. 10.1). The majority of *NF1* mutations cause premature truncation of the protein. Disturbances in the Ras-

GRD hinder the ability of NF1 to deactivate Ras-GTP and result in the dysregulation of the Raf and PI3K transduction pathways, thereby promoting cellular proliferation (Le and Parada 2007; Costa et al. 2002).

NF-1 is inherited as an autosomal-dominant trait, and the development of neurofibromas and pilocytic astrocytomas results from loss of heterozygosity (Cichowski et al. 1999), consistent with the Knudson "two-hit" model of tumorigenesis (Le and Parada 2007). However, the development of malignant gliomas in NF-1 patients, either from anaplastic transformation of a pre-existing pilocytic astrocytoma or de novo high-grade infiltrative astrocytomas, requires additional genetic aberrations, such as inactivation of PTEN, ATRX, TP53, CDKN2A, or amplification of EGFR or PDGFRA (Rodriguez et al. 2016) (Le and Parada 2007). This suggests that multiple alterations in cellular proliferation signaling pathways must be disturbed for tumorigenesis.

10.3.2 Tuberous Sclerosis (TS)

Up to 15% of patients with TS develop a SEGA (Hargrave 2009). TS results from germline mutations in one of the two tumor suppressor genes, *TSC1* (*hamartin* on chromosome 9q34) and *TSC2* (*tuberin* on 16p13.3) (Hargrave 2009; van Slegtenhorst et al. 1997; Reuss and von

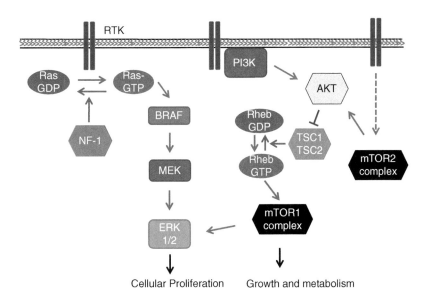

Fig. 10.1 BRAF and mTOR signaling pathways

Deimling 2009). *TSC1* and *TSC2* function together as part of a tumor suppressor complex within the mTOR signaling pathway (Hargrave 2009) (Fig. 10.1). The tuberin–hamartin complex inactivates the GTP-bound Ras-homolog-enhanced-in-the-brain (Rheb) into an inactive GDP-bound state (Hargrave 2009; Rosner et al. 2008). Specific mutations in either tuberin or hamartin can hinder deactivation of Rheb-GTP. Unopposed Rheb-GTP activates mTOR in an unregulated fashion, thus promoting the development of hamartomatous lesions (i.e., tubers) as well tumorigenesis of SEGA (Hargrave 2009; Reuss and von Deimling 2009).

10.3.3 Ras-Raf-MAP Kinase Pathway

As initially implicated by early studies of the NF-1 syndrome, dysregulation of the Ras-Raf-MAP kinase pathway has a pivotal role in the pathobiology of PLGG (Dasgupta and Haas-Kogan 2013). Within this pathway, Raf regulates the MEK/MAP kinase cascade, a regulator of cellular differentiation and proliferation (Dasgupta and Haas-Kogan 2013; Gilheeney and Kieran 2012) (Fig. 10.1). There has been considerable attention over the last decade focused on a specific member of the Raf family, BRAF, one of the most commonly mutated genes in human cancer (Bergthold et al. 2014; Dasgupta and Haas-Kogan 2013; Lawrence et al. 2014). Two major genomic alterations of BRAF have been observed in PLGG: V600E mutation and kinase domain duplication/fusion.

A mutation at codon 600 of the BRAF gene occurs in up to 40% of sporadic PLGG tumors (Dougherty et al. 2010), most commonly in pleomorphic xanthoastrocytoma, ganglioglioma, pilocytic astrocytoma, and pilomyxoid astrocytoma (Bergthold et al. 2014; Schindler et al. 2011). The BRAF V600E mutation involves the replacement of valine by glutamic acid within the activation loop of the enzyme, which mimics phosphorylation of the activation site (Dasgupta and Haas-Kogan 2013) and results in constitutive activation of BRAF serine/threonine kinase domain (Bergthold et al.

2014), leading to disinhibition of the MEK/MAP kinase cascade (Fig. 10.1). The V600E mutation is sufficient to transform NIH3T3 fibroblasts in vitro and also results in proliferative transformation of human neural stem cells followed by senescence (Raabe et al. 2011). Intriguingly, it has been hypothesized that this "oncogene-induced senescence" may partly account for the low-grade pathobiology of pilocytic astrocytomas (Raabe et al. 2011; Jacob et al. 2011).

In addition to the V600E missense mutation, genetic rearrangements and duplications of the kinase domain of BRAF are common in PLGG, including pilocytic astrocytoma, pilomyxoid astrocytoma, and ganglioglioma, and lead to dysregulated kinase activity. Comparative genomic hybridization studies have shown that the gain of chromosomal region 7q34, which contains the *BRAF* locus, is the most common copy number alteration in sporadic PLGG, with frequent tandem insertion into the *KIAA1549* gene (Bergthold et al. 2014; Hemmati et al. 2003; Jacob et al. 2009). Greater than 90% of pilocytic astrocytomas arising in the cerebellum in patients without NF-1 have KIAA1549-BRAF gene fusions, while pilocytic astrocytomas outside the cerebellum (e.g., hypothalamus) have a lower frequency of KIAA1549-BRAF gene fusions, reportedly around 50% (Zhang et al. 2013; Jones et al. 2013). Pilomyxoid astrocytomas also have been reported to harbor KIAA1549-BRAF gene fusions (Lin et al. 2012; Gierke et al. 2016), demonstrating that this entity has similar genetics to pilocytic astrocytoma and providing support that pilomyxoid astrocytoma represents a more aggressive histologic variant of pilocytic astrocytoma rather than a distinct entity. Other *BRAF* fusion transcripts have been found to involve *GNA11*, *MKRN1, CLCN6, SRGAP3, FAM131B, MACF1*, and *RNF130*, and all known *BRAF* fusion transcripts are characterized by the loss of the N-terminal inhibitory domain of BRAF, resulting in constitutive activation of the kinase domain and dysregulation of the downstream MAP kinase signaling pathway (Bergthold et al. 2014).

10.3.4 PI3-Kinase-AKT-mTOR Pathway

As suggested by early studies of TS, genetic aberrations in the PI3K-Akt-mTOR signaling pathway predispose to PLGG. This pathway normally integrates intracellular and extracellular signals to regulate cellular metabolism, proliferation, and survival (Hassan et al. 2013). mTOR is a multi-protein serine-threonine kinase, composed of two protein complexes (mTORC1 and mTORC2), that is a master regulator of protein translation (Laplante and Sabatini 2012). In high nutritional states, conformational changes allow mTORC1 to interact with Rheb, stimulating mTORC1, which itself activates p70S6 kinase. This results in formation of phospho-S6 and phospho-4EBP1, leading to protein translation and cellular proliferation (Dasgupta and Haas-Kogan 2013) (Fig. 10.1).

The importance of the mTORC1 pathway in PLGG pathogenesis is highlighted by the fact that approximately half of these tumors show enhanced expression of phospho-S6 and phospho-4EBP1 (Dasgupta and Haas-Kogan 2013). Furthermore, overexpression of these two proteins is associated with significantly worse progression-free survival (Populo et al. 2012), with a trend toward shorter overall survival as well (McBride et al. 2010).

The mTORC2 component is also an important regulator of cellular proliferation in response to cell nutritional status and redox states. A critical function of mTORC2 is phosphorylative activation of Akt. Akt has a role in multiple cellular processes, including metabolism, cell cycle regulation, and apoptosis. Abnormal activation of Akt is implicated in many human cancers (Schindler et al. 2011) and may be important in both management and prognosis. In a series of 92 pilocytic astrocytomas, Akt phosphorylation was associated with more aggressive histology and worse clinical outcomes (Rodriguez et al. 2011). Like Akt, other members of the PI3K-AKT-mTOR and Ras-Raf-MAPK pathways are being targeted by novel agents that are currently being developed and used in the treatment of PLGG. These and other new agents will be discussed in Sect. 11.6.4.

10.3.5 Genetic Alterations in Pediatric Infiltrative Gliomas

The genetic alterations that drive infiltrative gliomas are highly specific, depending on patient age and site of origin within the CNS. Infiltrative gliomas arising sporadically within the cerebral hemispheres in older pediatric patients in their late teenage years (i.e., 15–20 years of age) often have genetic alterations similar to those found in adult patients. In diffuse astrocytomas, these include mutations in TP53, ATRX, and either IDH1 or IDH2 in the majority of tumors (Cancer Genome Atlas Research Network 2015; Eckel-Passow et al. 2015; Suzuki et al. 2015). In oligodendrogliomas, these include co-deletion of chromosomes 1p and 19q, TERT promoter mutation, and mutation of either IDH1 or IDH2 in the majority of tumors (Suzuki et al. 2015; Eckel-Passow et al. 2015; Cancer Genome Atlas Research Network 2015). Further discussion of the genetic alterations that drive these adult-type infiltrative gliomas is beyond the scope of this review, and interested readers should refer to the three references above and other references therein for more information on the molecular mechanisms by which IDH, TP53, ATRX, and TERT promoter mutations drive gliomagenesis.

In contrast, diffuse astrocytomas arising in the cerebral hemispheres in younger pediatric patients lack these adult-type molecular alterations and instead harbor rearrangements involving MYB or MYBL1 genes or, less commonly, BRAF-V600E mutation (Ramkissoon et al. 2013; Zhang et al. 2013). MYB and MYBL1 are proto-oncogenes that encode transcriptional activator proteins, and the rearrangements in pediatric gliomas involving these genes typically lead to truncation of their C-terminal negative regulatory domains causing constitutive activation and altered gene transcription (Zhang et al. 2013; Ramkissoon et al. 2013). The rearrangements present in MYB and MYBL1 genes have only been found in PLGGs within the cerebral hemispheres and have not been found in pediatric high-grade gliomas (Zhang et al. 2013). Recent studies have shown that angiocentric glioma, an epilepsy-associated cortical neoplasm of childhood, also is genetically characterized by MYB rearrangement, most commonly as MYB-QKI gene fusion (Bandopadhayay et al. 2016).

As opposed to those infiltrative gliomas arising in the cerebral hemispheres, infiltrative astrocytomas arising within midline structures, including the thalamus, pons, and spinal cord, from both pediatric patients and young adults often harbor a missense mutation at codon 27 in either of the H3F3A or HIST1H3B genes, which encode the histone H3 variants, H3.3 and H3.1, respectively (Schwartzentruber et al. 2012; Khuong-Quang et al. 2012; Sturm et al. 2012; Gielen et al. 2013; Wu et al. 2014; Aihara et al. 2014). These missense mutations cause a lysine to methionine substitution (K27M) that alters an important site of posttranslational modification in these histone H3 variants and leads to altered gene expression profiles thought to drive gliomagenesis (Bender et al. 2013; Chan et al. 2013). These diffuse midline gliomas with histone H3 K27M mutations are associated with a poor prognosis irrespective of the histologic grade seen at the time of biopsy or resection (Aihara et al. 2014; Khuong-Quang et al. 2012; Schwartzentruber et al. 2012; Sturm et al. 2012; Wu et al. 2014; Gielen et al. 2013). As such, "Diffuse midline glioma, H3 K27M-mutant" was included as a grade IV entity in the 2016 WHO Classification of Tumors of the Central Nervous System, which is the recommended designation for all diffuse midline gliomas with H3 K27M mutation regardless of the presence or absence of high grade histologic features (e.g. increased mitotic activity, necrosis, and microvascular proliferation). A mutant-specific antibody for the detection of histone H3-K27M mutant protein has now been developed and is routinely being using in the practice of surgical neuropathology and has been highly effective in the identification of diffuse midline

gliomas with this important molecular alteration (Bechet et al. 2014; Venneti et al. 2014).

Pediatric oligodendrogliomas are a rare entity, and the largest case series reported to date has found that they do not harbor IDH mutations and deletion of chromosomes 1p and 19q typical of oligodendrogliomas in adult patients (Rodriguez et al. 2014). Genome-wide analysis of pediatric oligodendrogliomas has revealed alterations in the FGFR1 oncogene in the majority of cases, either through tandem duplication of the kinase domain, gene fusions such as FGFR1-TACC1, or hotspot missense mutations that localize within the kinase domain, typically either N546K or K656E (Zhang et al. 2013). Dysembryoplastic neuroepithelial tumors also frequently harbor FGFR1 alterations through either kinase domain mutation or tandem duplication (Rivera et al. 2016). A recent study integrating histologic features with underlying genetic alterations in PLGG demonstrated that tumors with astrocytic morphology most commonly harbor alterations in BRAF or MYB/MYBL1, whereas those tumors with oligodendroglial morphology most commonly harbor FGFR1 alterations (Qaddoumi et al. 2016).

Additional information regarding predisposition syndromes and molecular classification can be found in Chaps. 5 and 6, respectively.

10.4 Clinical Features

Presenting symptoms of low-grade gliomas in the pediatric population are highly variable and are dependent on location of the lesion, age at presentation, and tumor biology. Symptoms can be divided into generalized and localized symptoms.

Seizures are the most common general symptom and occur in more than 50% of children at any age who have hemispheric tumors (Gupta et al. 2004). Generalized seizures are more common with slowly progressive disease, whereas rapidly growing tumors are more likely to produce complex partial motor or sensory seizures. Gangliogliomas, due to their location, often present with seizures, which are often refractory until the lesion is surgically removed (Dulac et al. 2013). Other general signs and symptoms include increased intracranial pressure that can manifest as headache, hydrocephalus, or nausea and vomiting in a more acute setting. This constellation of symptoms is common in posterior fossa tumors where an enlarging lesion can cause blockage of the fourth ventricle (Dulac et al. 2013).

In infants with open cranial sutures, enlarging head circumference can be a sign of a CNS lesion. As children age, failure to meet developmental milestones can warrant further neurologic evaluation (Gupta et al. 2004). Finally, in school-age children, gradual changes such as developmental delay, personality changes, irritability, altered psychomotor function, apathy, and declining school performance can be seen as well (Gupta et al. 2004).

Focal neurologic deficits, including hemiparesis, monoparesis, aphasia, dysphasia, and other cranial nerve or long tract signs, can represent localizing signs of an intracranial tumor. Optic pathway lesions in the nerves or chiasm can lead to decreased visual acuity, strabismus, proptosis, hemianopsia, and quadrantanopsia (Sievert and Fisher 2009). Cortical blindness can be noted when the lesion involves bilateral occipital lobes. Ataxia or dysmetria can present as difficulty with balance and is associated with patients who have cerebellar tumors (Sievert and Fisher 2009). Hypothalamic lesions or pituitary lesions can result in endocrine disturbances leading to precocious puberty, growth retardation, diabetes insipidus, or visual field deficits due to compression of the optic chiasm.

Since many of these symptoms are nonspecific for pediatric gliomas, thorough neurologic evaluation is paramount in children who present with deficits to aid in early diagnosis and treatment.

10.5 Imaging and Workup

At the time of presentation with concerning neurologic symptoms, MRI should be obtained in all cases. Important sequences to obtain include T1 axial and coronal images, both pre- and post-gadolinium contrast (Fig. 10.2), and T2 axial and coronal fluid-attenuated inversion recovery (FLAIR) sequences (Fig. 10.3a, b). Sagittal sequences are often helpful to define the anatomy of supra-sellar and midline tumors (Fig. 10.2a, b). Newer sequences, such as diffusion weighted imaging (DWI), MR spectroscopy, and functional MRI, are noninvasive modalities used to glean biochemical and functional information that may contribute to obtaining a pathologic diagnosis in the future and could be of prognostic importance. Of note, many children may need conscious sedation or anesthesia to obtain an MRI.

PLGGs tend to be T1 iso- to hypointense, T2 hyperintense and non-enhancing post-gadolinium administration. The lack of contrast enhancement makes FLAIR sequences ideal for delineating tumor extent (Gupta et al. 2004; Alkonyi et al. 2015).

Gliomas involving the optic pathway have a fusiform appearance and are typified by enlargement of the optic nerve(s) and chiasm (Avery et al. 2011). FLAIR sequences demonstrate an infiltrative component extending along the optic tracts. For all gliomas involving the optic pathways, detailed fine cuts of the sella should be obtained (Gupta et al. 2004). In patients with NF-1, there is often extensive streaking along the optic pathway and/or involvement of the optic nerve at the time of diagnosis, in addition to nonspecific T2 white matter abnormalities. Tumor can spread into the perivascular space along the circle of Willis, as well as posteriorly toward the brainstem with rostral invasion into the third ventricle. Chiasmatic and hypothalamic lesions have an increased risk for neuraxis dissemination (Gupta et al. 2004). In children without NF-1, tumors tend to be more globular and restricted to a single anatomic location without significant

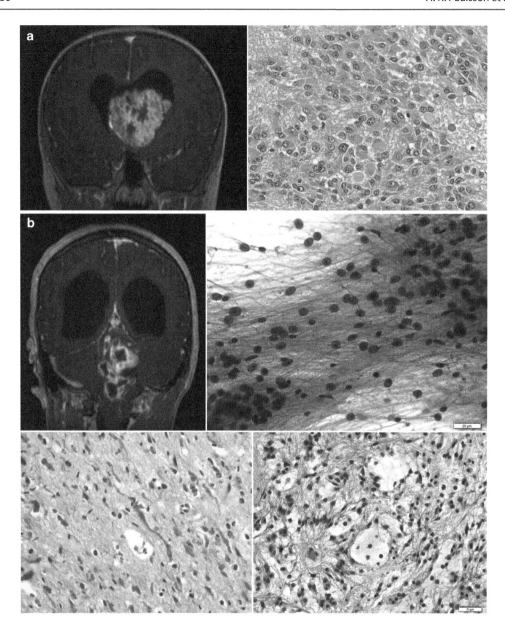

Fig. 10.2 Representative examples of circumscribed gliomas. (**a**) Subependymal giant cell astrocytoma (SEGA), WHO grade I. Coronal T1-weighted MR image post-gadolinium administration (left) demonstrating a solidly enhancing intraventricular mass lesion without invasion of the adjacent brain parenchyma. H&E stained section (right) demonstrating a solid neoplasm composed of large epithelioid astrocytes with abundant eosinophilic cytoplasm within a densely fibrillar background. (**b**) Pilocytic astrocytoma, WHO grade I. Coronal T1-weighted MR image post-gadolinium administration (top left) demonstrating a complex solid and cystic lesion with peripheral enhancement centered in the midline of the posterior fossa. Intraoperative cytologic preparation (top right) demonstrating a proliferation of bipolar astrocytes with elongate ("piloid") cytoplasmic processes. H&E stained section (bottom left) demonstrating a compact area of the neoplasm of piloid astrocytes containing numerous Rosenthal fibers. H&E stained section (bottom right) demonstrating a loose area of the neoplasm with microcysts and oligodendroglioma-like cells with round nuclei. (**c**) Pleomorphic xanthoastrocytoma (PXA), WHO grade II. Sagittal T1-weighted MR image post-gadolinium administration (top left) demonstrating a solid and cystic lesion in the parieto-occipital lobes. H&E stained section (top right) demonstrating a solid neoplasm of markedly pleomorphic astrocytes including occasional cells with lipidized cytoplasm and scattered eosinophilic granular bodies in the background. Laidlaw reticulin stain (bottom left) demonstrating abundant pericellular reticulin deposition among the tumor cells. Immunohistochemical stain using a mutant-specific antibody against BRAF-V600E mutant protein (bottom right) demonstrating cytoplasmic staining within the neoplastic astrocytes, indicative of *BRAF* gene mutation

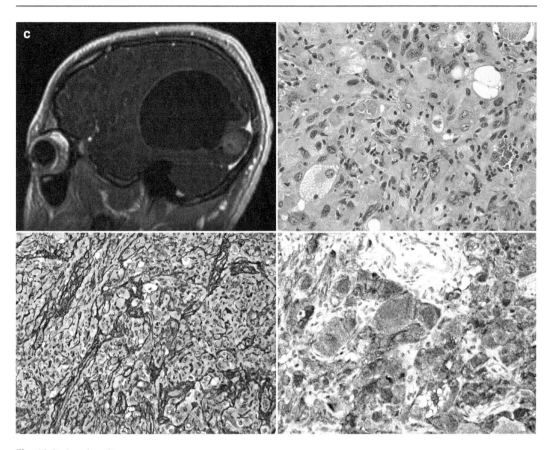

Fig. 10.2 (continued)

involvement of the meninges. Gadolinium enhancement and cyst formation is also more common in sporadic gliomas involving the optic pathway (Avery et al. 2011).

Oligodendrogliomas are lesions with involvement of the superficial cortex and are typically non-enhancing on MR-based imaging. 60–90% of these lesions have characteristic intrinsic calcification (Gupta et al. 2004). Pilocytic astrocytomas are well-circumscribed lesions (Fig. 10.2b) that have characteristic cystic changes and an enhancing mural nodule (Alkonyi et al. 2015). Diffuse astrocytomas (Fig. 10.4a) by definition are infiltrative lesions that appear less circumscribed and typically do not enhance unless a higher-grade component of the tumor is present (Sievert and Fisher 2009).

If unable to obtain an MRI, CT imaging of the brain with and without contrast can detect an intracranial abnormality. Low-grade gliomas typically appear as non-enhancing iso- or hypodense masses on CT. Mild to moderate nonhomogeneous contrast enhancement may be seen in up to 40% of cases. Calcifications are seen in 15–20% of cases and CT imaging represents the best modality with which to visualize calcified lesions (Gupta et al. 2004).

Obtaining serial imaging over time is paramount since many lesions can progress or recur. It is important to obtain a postoperative baseline MRI 24–48 h after surgery to distinguish residual tumor from postoperative changes. Quality imaging scans should subsequently be obtained every 3–6 months or as neurologic symptoms dictate (Gupta et al. 2004). Differentiating between treatment changes, radiation necrosis, and tumor recurrence can present a radiologic challenge. Notable findings concerning for progression or recurrence include increase in volume of T2-weighted abnormality on MRI or new enhancement on the post-contrast images (Gupta et al. 2004).

Example MRI sequences with corresponding histopathologic images from select pediatric low-grade gliomas are demonstrated in Figs. 10.2, 10.3, and 10.4.

10.6 Treatment and Outcomes

Overall survival is generally excellent for the majority of PLGG (Wisoff et al. 2011), with 20-year overall survival rates up to 87% (Bandopadhayay et al. 2014). Therefore, the treatment goals should not only include long-term tumor control, but also minimization of treatment-related morbidity. Management options include surgery, radiation, and chemotherapy. In addition, our growing understanding of the pathobiology of PLGG is leading to the establishment of novel targeted molecular agents (Dasgupta and Haas-Kogan 2013; Nageswara Rao and Packer 2014).

10.6.1 Surgery

Historically, surgery has been the cornerstone of PLGG management (Bergthold et al. 2014). The goal of surgery is maximal safe removal of tumor and decompression of adjacent normal tissue structures (Sutton et al. 1995). Deep lesions in the brain, such as those located in the hypothalamus, optic pathways, or brainstem, are many times not amenable to surgical resection; therefore, alternate therapeutic options such as radiation and chemotherapy come into play as primary treatment.

In a prospective natural history trial of patients treated with primary surgery and subsequent observation by Wisoff and colleagues, the 5-year overall survival (OS) rate was 97%, and progression-free survival (PFS) rate was 80%. Gross total resection (GTR) without residual disease was a strong and independent predictor of PFS. The ability to obtain a GTR varied significantly by location. About 75% of patients with cerebral and cerebellar hemisphere tumors had a GTR, while less than a quarter of children with chiasmic-hypothalamic and midline tumors had a complete resection. For subtotal resections (STR), the volume of residual tumor was predictive of disease progression (Fig. 10.5). However, the degree of surgical resection (including GTR) was not predictive of OS when tumor location, histology, and age were taken into account. This is thought to be due to the indolent nature of PLGG (Wisoff et al. 2011). In this series, only histology and tumor location were independently associated with OS.

Fig. 10.3 Representative examples of glioneuronal tumors. (**a**) Dysembryoplastic neuroepithelial tumor (DNT), WHO grade I. Coronal T2-weighted fluid-attenuated inversion recovery MR image (top left) demonstrating a well-circumscribed, cortically based mass lesion in the temporal lobe with internal nodularity. H&E stained section at low power (top right) demonstrating a sharply demarcated mucin-rich nodule within the cortex. H&E stained section at high power (bottom left) demonstrating a neoplasm of round oligodendrocyte-like cells arranged in linear columns along capillaries and neuronal processes within a mucin-rich stroma containing "floating" neurons. Immunohistochemical stain for neurofilament protein (bottom right) highlighting a background of neuronal processes within the nodules and showing cytoplasmic staining with the neurons floating in the mucin-rich stroma. (**b**) Ganglioglioma, WHO grade I. Sagittal T2-weighted fluid-attenuated inversion recovery MR image (top left) demonstrating a well-circumscribed, cortically based solid and cystic mass lesion in the occipital lobe. H&E stained section (top right) demonstrating a biphasic tumor composed of large dysmorphic ganglion cells admixed with neoplastic astrocytes. Immunohistochemical stain for neurofilament protein (bottom left) highlighting the delicate neuronal processes in the background and showing staining in the cells bodies of the neoplastic ganglion cells. Immunohistochemical stain using a mutant-specific antibody against BRAF-V600E mutant protein (bottom right) demonstrating cytoplasmic staining within the tumor with accentuated staining in the neoplastic ganglion cells, indicative of *BRAF* gene mutation

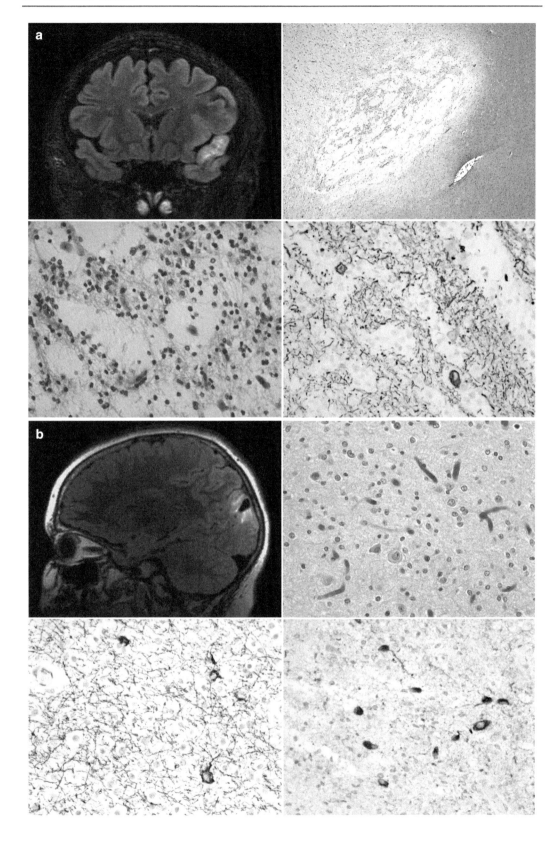

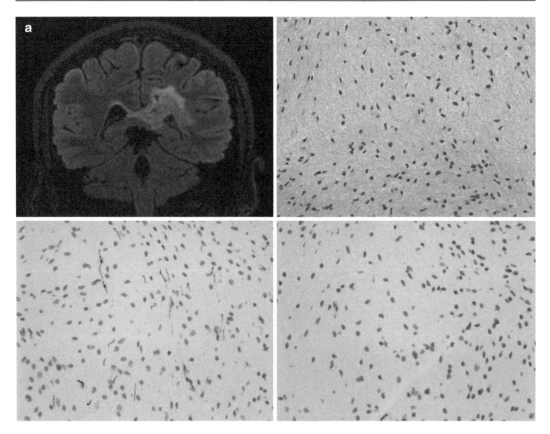

Fig. 10.4 Representative examples of infiltrative gliomas. (**a**), Diffuse astrocytoma with *MYB* gene rearrangement, WHO grade II. Coronal T2-weighted fluid-attenuated inversion recovery MR image (top left) demonstrating an infiltrative hyperintense lesion within the deep white matter of the parietal lobe and crossing over the splenium of the corpus callosum into the contralateral cerebral hemisphere. H&E stained section (top right) demonstrating infiltrating neoplastic astrocytes with elongate nuclei in a background of densely fibrillar glial processes. Immunohistochemical stain for neurofilament protein (bottom left) highlighting the presence of infiltrated axons among the tumor cells. Immunohistochemical stain using a mutant-specific antibody against IDH1-R132H mutant protein (bottom right) demonstrating absence of staining in the neoplastic astrocytes. Fluorescence in situ hybridization (not shown) demonstrated rearrangement of the *MYB* gene in this diffuse astrocytoma. (**b**) Diffuse astrocytoma, IDH-mutant, WHO grade II. Sagittal T2-weighted fluid-attenuated inversion recovery MR image (top left) demonstrating an irregular mass-like area of hyperintensity expanding the gyri of the frontal lobe. H&E stained section (top right) demonstrating neoplastic astrocytes with ovoid nuclei containing coarse chromatin infiltrating through the cortex with satellitosis of preexisting neurons. Immunohistochemical stain using a mutant-specific antibody against IDH1-R132H mutant protein (bottom left) demonstrating cytoplasmic staining within the neoplastic astrocytes, indicative of *IDH1* gene mutation. Immunohistochemical stain for ATRX protein (bottom right) demonstrating loss of staining in the tumor cells with retained expression in the entrapped, preexisting neurons suggestive of *ATRX* gene mutation. (**c**) Diffuse midline glioma, H3 K27M-mutant, WHO grade IV. Coronal (top left) and sagittal (top right) T2-weighted fluid-attenuated inversion recovery MR image demonstrating a hyperintense mass lesion expanding the pons. H&E stained section (bottom left) demonstrating neoplastic astrocytes with elongate nuclei and coarse chromatin infiltrating through the parenchyma of the pons, with a couple of entrapped neurons seen. Immunohistochemical stain using a mutant-specific antibody against histone H3-K27M mutant protein (bottom right) demonstrating nuclear staining in the neoplastic astrocytes, indicative of *H3F3A* gene mutation. Despite lacking significant mitotic activity, necrosis, or microvascular proliferation, this tumor should be classified as grade IV per the 2016 WHO Classification of Tumors of the Central Nervous System

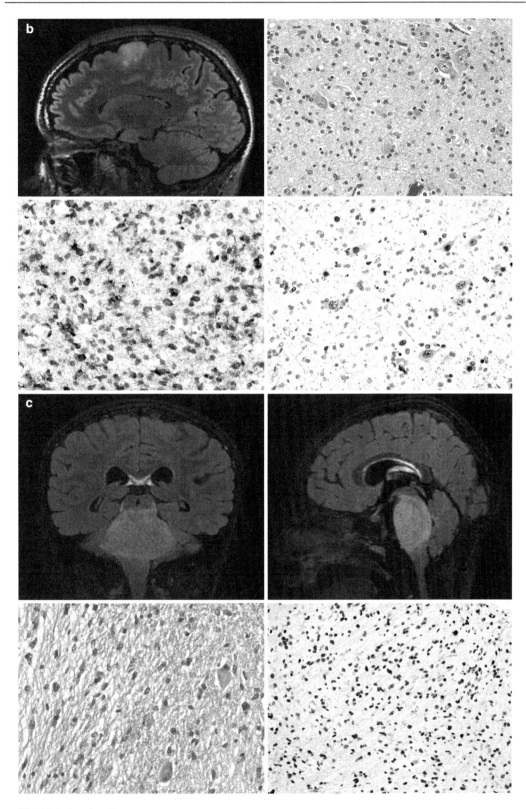

Fig. 10.4 (continued)

Fig. 10.5 Progression-free survival by postsurgical residual disease. In this prospective natural history trial, Wisoff and colleagues followed postsurgical patients with any pediatric low-grade glial neoplasm. Tumors with anaplastic features were excluded. All intracranial sites were included except for intrinsic brainstem tumors and tumors limited to the optic nerves. Wisoff et al. Neurosurgery. 2011;68(6):1548–1555

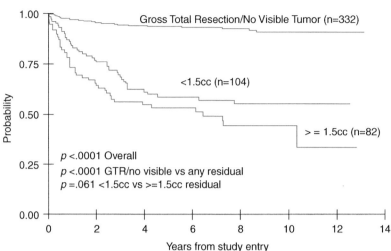

Progression-Free Survival by Post-Surgical Residual

Gross Total Resection/No Visible Tumor (n=332)

<1.5cc (n=104)

> = 1.5cc (n=82)

p <.0001 Overall
p <.0001 GTR/no visible vs any residual
p =.061 <1.5cc vs >=1.5cc residual

Probability — Years from study entry

Notably, over 50% of children with residual tumor volume after resection have no disease progression at 5 years (Wisoff et al. 2011), and these patients have excellent long-term survival. Therefore, even though complete resection should be a goal, the benefit of possibly prolonging PFS should be carefully weighed with the risk of neurologic deficit caused by an aggressive resection. In addition, because not all patients will progress after resection most are observed expectantly (Benesch et al. 2006), reserving chemotherapy, radiation, and re-resection for salvage therapies.

10.6.2 Radiation

Radiation therapy has been used as up-front treatment and as salvage therapy in PLGG. However, the observance of cognitive effects, endocrine deficiencies, secondary malignancies, vascular damage, and growth abnormalities associated with older radiation techniques have largely led to the avoidance of radiation therapy in the up-front management setting of PLGG. In addition, old retrospective studies that evaluated more historic radiation delivery techniques showed poor 5-year PFS (less than 50%) (Fisher et al. 2008).

However, advancements in three-dimensional treatment planning have allowed for highly conformal radiation delivery with the sparing of normal adjacent tissue structures. The role and safety of these radiation therapy techniques for PLGG is being re-evaluated.

A prospective study by Marcus and colleagues at Dana Farber Cancer Institute evaluated the efficacy of highly conformal radiotherapy for small (less than 5 cm) tumors either as up-front treatment or as salvage therapy. The mean radiation dose delivered to the gross tumor volume with a 2 mm planning treatment margin was 52.2 Gy in 1.8 Gy fractions. PFS was 82.5% at 5 years, and OS was 97.8% at 5 years. At a median follow-up of 6.9 years, 7 of 81 patients had local progression. There were no marginal failures observed. Other than rare temporary hair thinning, no acute radiation-related toxicities occurred. One child developed a primitive neuroectodermal tumor 6 years after radiation, and four children developed moyamoya syndrome during follow-up. The authors concluded that stereotactic radiotherapy provides excellent local control for children with small, localized PLGG, and limiting the treatment margins may protect against radiation-related toxicity while not compromising local control (Marcus et al. 2005).

A phase II trial at St. Jude Children's Research Hospital also evaluated the efficacy of conformal radiation therapy. In this study, 54 Gy was delivered to the tumor with a 10 mm margin. This trial demonstrated a 5-year PFS of 87% and OS of 96%. During the 89-month follow-up, the cumulative vasculopathy rate was less than 6% (Merchant et al. 2009). Cognitive function was largely preserved with the use of conformal radiotherapy. However, cognitive decline did appear to be strongly associated with age, with the steepest decline in IQ among the youngest children. At 5 years of follow-up, a 5-year-old child would be predicted to have an IQ drop of 10 points, and each year of increasing age decreased the decline in IQ by 0.03 points per month (Merchant et al. 2009). There is a more detailed discussion of radiation toxicity below.

These two studies highlight the ability to achieve excellent local control using highly conformal radiation techniques that spare normal tissues and decrease the risk of radiation-related toxicities. Figure 10.6 demonstrates an example of the ability of highly conformal radiation therapy to spare the optic chiasm. Of note, the patient population in these two prospective studies was somewhat heterogeneous and included both children who were treated in the up-front and the salvage settings.

Mishra and colleagues at the University of California, San Francisco, retrospectively evaluated the role of radiation therapy in the up-front setting for children with incompletely resected WHO grade II PLGG. After subtotal resection, PFS and OS did not differ between children who received adjuvant radiation therapy (median dose 54 Gy) and those who did not (Mishra et al. 2006). The series reproduced previous observations that extent of resection affects PFS.

Overall, highly conformal radiation therapy appears to be a safe and effective way to achieve local control, likely best reserved for the salvage setting. At this time there does not appear to be clear benefit in the immediate postoperative setting since many children may not go on to have disease progression. When radiation therapy is employed for PLGG, doses of 52–54 Gy appear to be effective, and planning setup margin can safely be limited to 1 cm or less to protect adjacent normal tissues.

10.6.3 Chemotherapy

Given the generally favorable outcomes after surgery, chemotherapy is not routinely employed in the adjuvant setting but rather reserved for unresectable or symptomatic progression (Bergthold et al. 2014), especially in younger patients, to

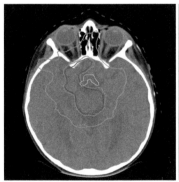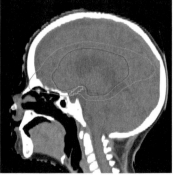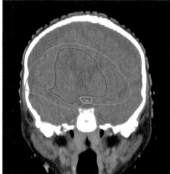

Fig. 10.6 Pediatric patient undergoing radiation treatment for PLGG. The optic chiasm is outlined in light blue. The red line represents the prescription dose, 5220 cGy, the orange line represents the volume receiving 5000 cGy, and the pink line represents the volume receiving 3000 cGy. Using highly conformal radiation treatment (Intensity Modulated Radiation Treatment-IMRT), sparing normal tissue structures such as the optic chiasm can greatly decrease the risk of radiation-related toxicity

Table 10.1 Chemotherapy regimens for PLGG

Study	Chemotherapy regimen	Number of patients	Event-free survival (%)		
			2 years	3 years	5 years
Ater et al. J Clin Oncol. 30:2641–2647, 2012	CV	137			39
	TPCV	137			52 (ns)
Mishra et al. J Neurooncol.100:121–7, 2010	TPD(CCNU)V	33			30
Gnekow et al. Klin Padiatr 216:331–342, 2004	CV	198			61
Massimino et al. J Clin Oncol 20:4209–4216, 2002	CisVP	31		78	
Prados et al. J Neurooncol 32:235–241, 1997	TPCV	42	50		
Packer et al. J Neurosurg 86:747–754, 1997	CV	78		68	

C carboplatin, *V* vincristine, *T* thioguanine, *P* procarbazine, *Cis* cisplatin, *VP* etoposide, *D* dibromodulcitol, *(CCNU)* Lomustine, *ns* not statistically significant. Adapted from: Merchant et al. J Clin Oncol. 2009;27(22):3598–3604

delay or obviate the need for radiation therapy (Merchant et al. 2009). A number of poly-chemotherapy regimens have been used in PLGG, detailed in Table 10.1 (Merchant et al. 2009). With these regimens, 2–3-year PFS rates range from 50 to 78%.

The Children's Oncology Group (COG) published the results of Protocol A9952, which randomized children with progressive or residual PLGG to carboplatin and vincristine (CV) versus thioguanine, procarbazine, lomustine, and vincristine (TPCV) (Table 10.1). The 5-year event-free survival was not significantly different (39% for CV and 52% for TPCV). Toxicity was slightly worse with TPCV (Ater et al. 2012). Because of the potential for long-term morbidity associated with alkylating agents, such as infertility and secondary malignancies, most oncologists favor CV as first line chemotherapy over TPCV (Bergthold et al. 2014).

Monotherapy with temozolomide, vinblastine, or cyclophosphamide has been evaluated in phase II studies, although with mixed results (Bergthold et al. 2014). A COG study of temozolomide for recurrent brain tumors found one partial response in 21 children with PLGG and 41% of these children had stable disease through 12 months of treatment (Nicholson et al. 2007). Another COG phase II trial of cyclophosphamide for progressive low-grade astrocytoma in 14 patients demonstrated a complete response in one patient and disease stability in 8 patients. The excessive number of children (5) with progressive disease prompted the study to close (Kadota et al. 1999). Single agent vinblastine was

evaluated in 51 patients with recurrent or refractory PLGG, among whom 36% had a complete, partial, or minor response and 5-year PFS was 42%. Thirty-eight patients had grade 3 or 4 hematologic toxicity (Bouffet et al. 2012).

Chemotherapy has also been combined with noncytotoxic agents. A recent phase II study evaluating irinotecan with the anti-VEGF monoclonal antibody bevacizumab for progressive PLGG demonstrated a 47.8% PFS at 2 years (Gururangan et al. 2014). Bevacizumab is well tolerated, although children need to be monitored closely for hypertension and proteinuria (Bergthold et al. 2014).

10.6.4 Targeted Systemic Agents

The prevalence of mutations within the Ras-Raf-MAP kinase and PI3-kinase-AKT-mTOR pathways (see Fig. 10.1) has led to the development of antitumor agents that specifically target the oncogenic protein within these pathways (Dasgupta and Haas-Kogan 2013). As described in Sect. 11.3, the BRAF V600E mutation occurs in up to 40% of PLGG. Vemurafenib specifically inhibits BRAF V600E from activating MEK. Vemurafenib has remarkable clinical activity against BRAF V600E mutated melanoma and prolongs OS (Chapman et al. 2011). This has led to great interest in using vemurafenib in other BRAF V600E positive cancers.

A multicenter phase I trial under the auspices of the Pacific Pediatric Neuro-Oncology Consortium (PNOC) is currently enrolling patients with recurrent or refractory gliomas to evaluate the safety and pharmacokinetic characteristics of vemurafenib (http://www.pnoc.us). It is important to note that in addition to the V600E mutation, a significant proportion of BRAF alterations in PLGG involve duplication/gene fusions, and the efficacy of various RAF inhibitors against fusion molecules is unknown, but may be associated with paradoxical activation in some cases (Dasgupta and Haas-Kogan 2013).

BRAF-mutated tumors appear to have sensitivity to MEK inhibition (Flaherty et al. 2012, b). The MEK inhibitor trametinib is now FDA approved for the treatment of melanoma and has demonstrated efficacy against colorectal, hepatocellular, and non-small cell lung cancers in ongoing clinical trials. Another small molecule MEK inhibitor, selumetinib, was shown to have activity against a pilocytic astrocytoma xenograft harboring the BRAF V600E mutation (Kolb et al. 2010). The Pediatric Brain Tumor Consortium (PBTC) protocol PBTC 029 is an open phase I trial evaluating the maximal safe dose of selumetinib in patients with histologically confirmed recurrent or refractory PLGG. In addition, the National Cancer Institute is currently sponsoring a phase II trial of selumetinib for patients with recurrent or refractory PLGGs.

Targeting the mTOR pathway also appears promising. Approximately half of PLGGs have activation of the PI3-kinase-AKT-mTOR pathway. Rapamycin (sirolimus), an allosteric inhibitor of mTORC1, blocks the ability of mTORC1 to activate S6 kinase (a regulator of translation and a critical downstream target) but not 4E-BP1. It has been documented to cause regression of SEGAs in patients with TS harboring TSC1/2 gene mutation (Northrup et al. 1993). Everolimus, a derivative of rapamycin, has been used clinically for cancer therapy (Motzer et al. 2008), and is approved for multiple indications in adults. Among children with TS and progressive SEGA, 75% of tumors exhibited responses to everolimus (Krueger et al. 2010). Indeed, everolimus was recently approved for the treatment of SEGA in patients with TS.

Clinical trials have demonstrated promising results for mTOR inhibition in PLGGs more generally. Yalon et al. examined the activity of siroli-mus and erlotinib in recurrent PLGGs (Yalon et al. 2013). Responses in 19 patients included 1 partial response, 5 stable, and 10 progressive disease (3 discontinued therapy). Six patients had tumor stabilization for ≥12 months, and two experienced tumor control for >1 year after therapy completion. Kieran et al. reported 23 patients with PLGGs who were treated with everolimus after progression following carboplatin-containing chemotherapy regimens. Observed responses included 13 stable, 6 progressive disease, and 4 partial responses (Kieran, M. personal communication). This study met its goal of greater than 25% response rate defined a priori in order to consider everolimus a promising regimen for further study in PLGGs. Copious evidence indicates that molecular markers will define subgroups of PLGGs that are likely to respond to everolimus, but answers to this critical question remain elusive as of yet. A notable manuscript provides a persuasive mechanism for these promising results of mTOR inhibition in sporadic PLGGs. Kaul et al. documented that KIAA1549:BRAF is sufficient to induce glioma-like lesions in vivo in a cell type-specific and mTOR-dependent manner. Rapamycin-mediated mTOR inhibition blocks KIAA1549:BRAF-induced S6 activation and proliferation in neural stem cells. These data provide preclinical evidence for the use of mTOR inhibitors for sporadic PLGGs (Kaul et al. 2012). A PNOC phase II study of everolimus is enrolling children with recurrent or progressive PLGGs with the aim of seeking a molecular signature that will predict responses to mTOR inhibition.

10.7 Late Effects and Follow-Up

Current estimates indicate that approximately one adult in 2500 is a survivor of a childhood brain tumor (Dulac et al. 2013). Due to the combined treatment modalities and the location of the tumors, CNS lesions in children are frequently associated with high morbidity and long-term side effects. Survival, however, ranges from 87 to 99% at 5 years, so while many of these patients are cured of their disease, cure often comes at the price of late sequelae of treatment (Wisoff et al. 2011 and Shaw and Wisoff 2003). The burden of long-term disability is not inconsequential, as reports have shown up to half of patients treated for pediatric brain tumors have mild to severe disabilities, including cognitive and social impairment (Aarsen et al. 2006).

10.7.1 Surgical Toxicity

In children who undergo surgery alone for cerebellar and cerebral lesions, there is an elevated rate of below-average IQ, lower achievement, and difficulties with adaptive behavior. Behavioral and emotional adjustment measures appear to remain intact (Pollack 2011). It is unclear if location of the lesion correlates with the magnitude of poor cognitive performance, though patients with cerebral lesions may perform better than those with posterior fossa lesions (Aarsen et al. 2006; Beebe et al. 2005; Ris et al. 2008; Ris and Noll 1994). This finding implicates the importance of the cerebellum in cognitive and emotional regulatory circuits (Sancak et al. 2016). Patients with left hemispheric lesions tend to have inferior performance, likely due to the impact of a left-sided lesion on language functions (Beebe et al. 2005; Roncadin et al. 2008).

10.7.2 Toxicity Due to Chemotherapy and Other Medical Therapy

Multiple chemotherapeutic options exist for treatment of PLGG, and many have associated long-term morbidity. There is well-known ototoxicity and peripheral neuropathy that result from treatment with platinum analogs and vincristine, respectively. Procarbazine and lomustine have a higher risk of secondary leukemia and are typically avoided in children with NF-1, due to their increased underlying risk of hematologic malignancy (Shannon et al. 1994; Matsui et al. 1993; Leone et al. 1999). Cisplatin and etoposide-based regimens have a risk of secondary leukemia as well (Le Deley et al. 2005).

The risk of neurotoxicity associated with chemotherapy, however, remains an unanswered question. Anti-folates such as methotrexate have been shown to impart delayed neurotoxicity (Cole and Kamen 2006); however, other studies have shown no neuropsychological differences between patients treated with chemotherapy and healthy controls (Anderson et al. 2000; Reddick et al. 1998).

A significant proportion of PLGG patients require anti-epileptic medications that have been implicated in long-term neurocognitive deficits. Patients who were prescribed seizure medication performed worse on delayed list memory tasks (King et al. 2004). However, this finding may be confounded by tumor location as well.

10.7.3 Radiation Associated Toxicity

In a series of studies performed in the last 20 years, chemotherapy has been notable in its ability to delay or obviate the need for radiation therapy in children with subtotal resections or progressive disease (Pollack 2011). When radiation is indicated, though, it is important to note that the late side effects of radiation therapy are pronounced in the pediatric population. In general, children who undergo radiation at a young age are at increased risk for development of infield cranial and spinal meningiomas, gliomas, and sarcomas. Usually these lesions are benign; however, malignant meningiomas can occur as a result as well.

Cranial irradiation also increases the risk of neurovascular disease due to vascular injury, endothelial proliferation, collagen synthesis, and loss of intercellular junctions (Siffert and Allen 2000). These effects in both small and large vessels increase the risk for both hemorrhagic and ischemic strokes, as well as moyamoya disease. Moyamoya disease is radiation-induced vascular injury characterized by progressive bilateral occlusion of the internal carotid arteries and development of anomalous collateral circulation. Highest risk patients are those of Japanese ancestry and those affected by NF-1 treated with radiation to the circle of Willis (Siffert and Allen 2000). In a large 2014 Surveillance, Epidemiology, and End Results (SEER) retrospective study of PLGG, radiation treatment was found to be the greatest predictor of worst survival (Bandopadhayay et al. 2014). However, it is extremely likely this finding is strongly influenced by selection bias since the patients who are treated with radiation have a worse prognosis, regardless of the addition of radiation.

Long-term neurocognitive deficits are notable and are clearly associated with radiation dose and volume (Fuss et al. 2000). Toxicity includes, but is not limited to, a lower average IQ, difficulty with visuospatial skills, and expressive language and verbal memory deficits (Ris and Beebe 2008). Again, tumor location is a confounding factor for interpreting the magnitude with which radiation contributes to long-term disability (Fouladi et al. 2003). Although focal radiation treatment has reduced this risk, over time patients who are treated with radiation remain at an increased risk for social adjustment disorders and withdrawal as well as many other neurocognitive deficits (Aarsen et al. 2006).

A recent phase II study from St. Jude Children's Research Hospital assessed long-term neurocognitive outcomes following focal radiation therapy (Merchant et al. 2009). Cognitive effects, such as internalizing and behavioral problem scores, visual auditory learning, communication and reading and spelling, were followed through 5 years after the completion of radiotherapy using psychological testing. At the 5-year time point, only the decline in ability to spell was clinically significant. Patients with NF-1, on average, had significantly lower baseline performance scores. Those who were treated at a younger age, with higher radiation doses (between 30 and 60 Gy), and those who had larger volumes of brain irradiated experienced more dramatic declines in IQ 5 years after the completion of treatment. Older patients, however, were more likely to have preserved IQ scores over time after the completion of treatment. Extent of surgery impacted psychology scores. Initially, patients who had a biopsy performed better than patients with a subtotal resection, but eventually the patients who had a more complete resection demonstrated superior performance. Overall, conclusions from this study indicate that age at the time of treatment is the most

important factor to consider when weighing the risk of long-term side effects. Delaying adjuvant treatment, such as radiation or chemotherapy, if clinically indicated, can positively impact long-term functional outcome.

10.7.4 Chiasmatic, Hypothalamic, and Diencephalic Toxicity

Endocrine abnormalities and hypothalamic dysfunction are common for tumors that arise in the midline and diencephalic region. In order of decreasing incidence, deficits include growth hormone deficiency, hypothyroidism, glucocorticoid deficiency, and gonadotropin deficiency (Merchant et al. 2010). It is often unclear if the deficit results from the treatment itself or from the structural stress placed on intracranial tissues by the tumor, but the deficits are likely to be multifactorial in nature and are strongly influenced by the extent of surgical resection and dose of radiation (Ris and Beebe 2008; Ris and Noll 1994; Ris et al. 2008; Siffert and Allen 2000; Fouladi et al. 2003).

When the lesion involves the optic nerve or chiasm, visual impairment can occur as a result of tumor infiltration or treatment. These lesions are usually subtotally resected due to their location, and therefore adjuvant chemotherapy or radiation is necessary to stabilize residual disease. Patients with anterior chiasmatic lesions have been noted to have IQ impairment at diagnosis but it is unclear if subsequent chemotherapy or radiation treatment further impair intellectual performance (Lacaze et al. 2003; Fouladi et al. 2003), as these studies include NF-1 patients who many times have baseline neurocognitive deficits.

Diencephalic syndrome (DS) is a rare, but potentially fatal, metabolic syndrome that can be associated with low-grade gliomas that arise from the hypothalamus or chiasm in young children. DS is characterized by profound emaciation and failure to thrive despite adequate caloric intake (Kilday et al. 2014). Long-term care for children with DS frequently includes nutritional support with both nasogastric and subsequent gastrostomy tube to aid in weight gain and recovery and there has been data to suggest that aggressive nutritional support during treatment yields better outcomes. Post-treatment sequelae include significant visual impairment, partial- or panhypopituitarism and learning difficulties, excessive weight gain, motor deficits, psychiatric disturbances, and seizures (Kilday 2014).

10.7.5 Delayed Toxicity

Since PLGGs are associated with very good overall survival, there is a growing population of adult survivors that have been studied. When surveyed, adult patients who were treated with various combinations of treatment (chemotherapy, radiation, and surgery) reported higher incidences of global distress and depression compared to their control siblings (Kilday 2014). Furthermore, some patients were found to have "grown into" a deficit, meaning they experienced normal functioning for a period of time, then developed behavioral and cognitive disabilities years after diagnosis and treatment (Aarsen et al. 2006).

Adult survivors were also less likely to be fully employed, married, to have graduated from college, or to have an annual income over $20,000. Additionally, those affected with pediatric malignancies were also more likely to have reported a major medical condition and to describe their current health as "fair" or "poor" (Zebrack et al. 2004). This effect is likely multifactorial in etiology, related to both tumor and treatment effects.

10.7.6 Approaches to Management of Long-Term Toxicity

Because the pediatric population affected by CNS tumors is at high risk for long-term sequelae from tumor effect and treatment toxicity, it is important to implement a multidisciplinary approach to optimize health and function of survivors. Several studies have documented survivors' knowledge of their diagnosis, prior treatment, and future oncologic screening guidelines (Byrne et al. 1989; Hudson et al. 2002, 2003; Kadan-Lottick et al. 2002; Nathan et al. 2007). At the completion of treatment, providing patients, their families and their primary care providers with a comprehensive treatment summary and recommendations for follow-up is paramount. Oncologists provide an essential role in counseling patients to engage in prevention strategies, risk-stratified medical monitoring, and healthy behavior.

Since many of the survivors of pediatric CNS tumors experience long-term neuropsychological and cognitive difficulties, complete neuropsychological testing prior to treatment and involvement in a follow-up clinic is essential. Communicating the special needs of the child to day-care and school officials helps to ensure adequate resources, aiding the child's ability to adapt and succeed. Involvement of a school psychologist as a liaison between physicians and school administrators can often be helpful.

Multidisciplinary follow-up through adulthood provides these patients with resources and care to optimize their functional outcome. The COG, which consists of over 240 institutions, provides "Long-Term Follow-up Guidelines for Survivors of Childhood, Adolescent and Young-Adult Cancer," available at www.survivorship-guidelines.org.

Conclusion

In conclusion, PLGG are a heterogeneous group of childhood tumors with generally favorable prognosis. Our understanding of the underlying molecular pathobiology of these tumors is allowing us to better define prognosis and guide management. Surgical resection is the hallmark of management, although there is also a role for chemotherapy, radiation, and targeted systemic agents in unresectable or recurrent tumors. Given the young age of PLGG patients, there has been concern regarding long-term side effects of treatment. However, an evolving theory suggests that younger age confers greater resilience to treatment, rather than vulnerability, and that children have a greater potential for recovery due to neuronal plasticity (Kolb and Gibb 2007). Improving outcomes and long-term follow-up of children treated for brain tumors will provide insight into that hypothesis. Furthermore, as therapies are becoming more targeted, both on the anatomic and molecular levels, short- and long-term toxicities may likely be mitigated.

References

Aarsen FK, Paquier PF, Reddingius RE, Streng IC, Arts WF, Evera-Preesman M, Catsman-Berrevoets CE (2006) Functional outcome after low-grade astrocytoma treatment in childhood. Cancer 106(2):396–402. https://doi.org/10.1002/cncr.21612

Aihara K, Mukasa A, Gotoh K, Saito K, Nagae G, Tsuji S, Tatsuno K, Yamamoto S, Takayanagi S, Narita Y, Shibui S, Aburatani H, Saito N (2014) H3F3A K27M mutations in thalamic gliomas from young adult patients. Neuro-Oncology 16(1):140–146. https://doi.org/10.1093/neuonc/not144

Alkonyi B, Nowak J, Gnekow AK, Pietsch T, Warmuth-Metz M (2015) Differential imaging characteristics and dissemination potential of pilomyxoid astrocytomas versus pilocytic astrocytomas. Neuroradiology https://doi.org/10.1007/s00234-015-1498-4

Anderson H, Hopwood P, Stephens RJ, Thatcher N, Cottier B, Nicholson M, Milroy R, Maughan TS, Falk SJ, Bond MG, Burt PA, Connolly CK, McIllmurray MB, Carmichael J (2000) Gemcitabine plus best supportive care (BSC) vs BSC in inoperable non-small cell lung cancer--a randomized trial with quality of life as the primary outcome. UK NSCLC gemcitabine group. Non-small cell lung Cancer. Br J Cancer 83(4):447–453. https://doi.org/10.1054/bjoc.2000.1307

Arun D, Gutmann DH (2004) Recent advances in neurofibromatosis type 1. Curr Opin Neurol 17(2):101–105

Ater JL, Zhou T, Holmes E, Mazewski CM, Booth TN, Freyer DR, Lazarus KH, Packer RJ, Prados M, Sposto R, Vezina G, Wisoff JH, Pollack IF (2012) Randomized study of two chemotherapy regimens for treatment of low-grade glioma in young children: a report from the Children's oncology group. J Clin Oncol 30(21):2641–2647. https://doi.org/10.1200/JCO.2011.36.6054

Avery RA, Fisher MJ, Liu GT (2011) Optic pathway gliomas. J Neuroophthalmol 31(3):269–278. https://doi.org/10.1097/WNO.0b013e31822aef82

Bandopadhayay P, Bergthold G, London WB, Goumnerova LC, Morales La Madrid A, Marcus KJ, Guo D, Ullrich NJ, Robison NJ, Chi SN, Beroukhim R, Kieran MW, Manley PE (2014) Long-term outcome of 4,040 children diagnosed with pediatric low-grade gliomas: an analysis of the surveillance epidemiology and end results (SEER) database. Pediatr Blood Cancer 61(7):1173–1179. https://doi.org/10.1002/pbc.24958

Bandopadhayay P, Ramkissoon LA, Jain P, Bergthold G, Wala J, Zeid R, Schumacher SE, Urbanski L, O'Rourke R, Gibson WJ, Pelton K, Ramkissoon SH, Han HJ, Zhu Y, Choudhari N, Silva A, Boucher K, Henn RE, Kang YJ, Knoff D, Paolella BR, Gladden-Young A, Varlet P, Pages M, Horowitz PM, Federation A, Malkin H, Tracy AA, Seepo S, Ducar M, Van Hummelen P, Santi M, Buccoliero AM, Scagnet M, Bowers DC, Giannini C, Puget S, Hawkins C, Tabori U, Klekner A, Bognar L, Burger PC, Eberhart C, Rodriguez FJ, Ashley Hill D, Mueller S, Haas-Kogan DA, Phillips JJ, Santagata S, Stiles CD, Bradner JE, Jabado N, Goren A, Grill J, Ligon AH, Goumnerova L, Waanders AJ, Storm PB, Kieran MW, Ligon KL, Beroukhim R, Resnick AC (2016) MYB-QKI rearrangements in angiocentric glioma drive tumorigenicity through a tripartite mechanism. Nat Genet 48(3):273–282

Bechet D, Gielen GG, Korshunov A, Pfister SM, Rousso C, Faury D, Fiset PO, Benlimane N, Lewis PW, Lu C, David Allis C, Kieran MW, Ligon KL, Pietsch T, Ellezam B, Albrecht S, Jabado N (2014) Specific detection of methionine 27 mutation in histone 3 variants (H3K27M) in fixed tissue from high-grade astrocytomas. Acta Neuropathol 128(5):733–741. https://doi.org/10.1007/s00401-014-1337-4

Beebe DW, Ris MD, Armstrong FD, Fontanesi J, Mulhern R, Holmes E, Wisoff JH (2005) Cognitive and adaptive outcome in low-grade pediatric cerebellar astrocytomas: evidence of diminished cognitive and adaptive functioning in National Collaborative Research Studies (CCG 9891/POG 9130). J Clin Oncol 23(22):5198–5204. https://doi.org/10.1200/JCO.2005.06.117

Bender S, Tang Y, Lindroth AM, Hovestadt V, Jones DT, Kool M, Zapatka M, Northcott PA, Sturm D, Wang W, Radlwimmer B, Hojfeldt JW, Truffaux N, Castel D, Schubert S, Ryzhova M, Seker-Cin H, Gronych J, Johann PD, Stark S, Meyer J, Milde T, Schuhmann M, Ebinger M, Monoranu CM, Ponnuswami A, Chen S, Jones C, Witt O, Collins VP, von Deimling A, Jabado N, Puget S, Grill J, Helin K, Korshunov A, Lichter P, Monje M, Plass C, Cho YJ, Pfister SM (2013) Reduced H3K27me3 and DNA hypomethylation are major drivers of gene expression in K27M mutant pediatric high-grade gliomas. Cancer Cell 24(5):660–672. https://doi.org/10.1016/j.ccr.2013.10.006

Benesch M, Eder HG, Sovinz P, Raith J, Lackner H, Moser A, Urban C (2006) Residual or recurrent cerebellar low-grade glioma in children after tumor resection: is re-treatment needed? A single center experience from 1983 to 2003. Pediatr Neurosurg 42(3):159–164. https://doi.org/10.1159/000091859

Bergthold G, Bandopadhayay P, Bi WL, Ramkissoon L, Stiles C, Segal RA, Beroukhim R, Ligon KL, Grill J, Kieran MW (2014) Pediatric low-grade gliomas: how modern biology reshapes the clinical field. Biochim Biophys Acta 1845(2):294–307. https://doi.org/10.1016/j.bbcan.2014.02.004

Bouffet E, Jakacki R, Goldman S, Hargrave D, Hawkins C, Shroff M, Hukin J, Bartels U, Foreman N, Kellie

S, Hilden J, Etzl M, Wilson B, Stephens D, Tabori U, Baruchel S (2012) Phase II study of weekly vinblastine in recurrent or refractory pediatric low-grade glioma. J Clin Oncol 30(12):1358–1363. https://doi.org/10.1200/JCO.2011.34.5843

Byrne J, Lewis S, Halamek L, Connelly RR, Mulvihill JJ (1989) Childhood cancer survivors' knowledge of their diagnosis and treatment. Ann Intern Med 110(5):400–403

Cancer Genome Atlas Research N, Brat DJ, Verhaak RG, Aldape KD, Yung WK, Salama SR, Cooper LA, Rheinbay E, Miller CR, Vitucci M, Morozova O, Robertson AG, Noushmehr H, Laird PW, Cherniack AD, Akbani R, Huse JT, Ciriello G, Poisson LM, Barnholtz-Sloan JS, Berger MS, Brennan C, Colen RR, Colman H, Flanders AE, Giannini C, Grifford M, Iavarone A, Jain R, Joseph I, Kim J, Kasaian K, Mikkelsen T, Murray BA, O'Neill BP, Pachter L, Parsons DW, Sougnez C, Sulman EP, Vandenberg SR, Van Meir EG, von Deimling A, Zhang H, Crain D, Lau K, Mallery D, Morris S, Paulauskis J, Penny R, Shelton T, Sherman M, Yena P, Black A, Bowen J, Dicostanzo K, Gastier-Foster J, Leraas KM, Lichtenberg TM, Pierson CR, Ramirez NC, Taylor C, Weaver S, Wise L, Zmuda E, Davidsen T, Demchok JA, Eley G, Ferguson ML, Hutter CM, Mills Shaw KR, Ozenberger BA, Sheth M, Sofia HJ, Tarnuzzer R, Wang Z, Yang L, Zenklusen JC, Ayala B, Baboud J, Chudamani S, Jensen MA, Liu J, Pihl T, Raman R, Wan Y, Wu Y, Ally A, Auman JT, Balasundaram M, Balu S, Baylin SB, Beroukhim R, Bootwalla MS, Bowlby R, Bristow CA, Brooks D, Butterfield Y, Carlsen R, Carter S, Chin L, Chu A, Chuah E, Cibulskis K, Clarke A, Coetzee SG, Dhalla N, Fennell T, Fisher S, Gabriel S, Getz G, Gibbs R, Guin R, Hadjipanayis A, Hayes DN, Hinoue T, Hoadley K, Holt RA, Hoyle AP, Jefferys SR, Jones S, Jones CD, Kucherlapati R, Lai PH, Lander E, Lee S, Lichtenstein L, Ma Y, Maglinte DT, Mahadeshwar HS, Marra MA, Mayo M, Meng S, Meyerson ML, Mieczkowski PA, Moore RA, Mose LE, Mungall AJ, Pantazi A, Parfenov M, Park PJ, Parker JS, Perou CM, Protopopov A, Ren X, Roach J, Sabedot TS, Schein J, Schumacher SE, Seidman JG, Seth S, Shen H, Simons JV, Sipahimalani P, Soloway MG, Song X, Sun H, Tabak B, Tam A, Tan D, Tang J, Thiessen N, Triche T Jr, Van Den Berg DJ, Veluvolu U, Waring S, Weisenberger DJ, Wilkerson MD, Wong T, Wu J, Xi L, Xu AW, Yang L, Zack TI, Zhang J, Aksoy BA, Arachchi H, Benz C, Bernard B, Carlin D, Cho J, DiCara D, Frazer S, Fuller GN, Gao J, Gehlenborg N, Haussler D, Heiman DI, Iype L, Jacobsen A, Ju Z, Katzman S, Kim H, Knijnenburg T, Kreisberg RB, Lawrence MS, Lee W, Leinonen K, Lin P, Ling S, Liu W, Liu Y, Liu Y, Lu Y, Mills G, Ng S, Noble MS, Paull E, Rao A, Reynolds S, Saksena G, Sanborn Z, Sander C, Schultz N, Senbabaoglu Y, Shen R, Shmulevich I, Sinha R, Stuart J, Sumer SO, Sun Y, Tasman N, Taylor BS, Voet D, Weinhold N, Weinstein JN, Yang D, Yoshihara K, Zheng S, Zhang W, Zou L, Abel T, Sadeghi S, Cohen ML, Eschbacher J, Hattab EM, Raghunathan A, Schniederjan MJ, Aziz D, Barnett G,

Barrett W, Bigner DD, Boice L, Brewer C, Calatozzolo C, Campos B, Carlotti CG Jr, Chan TA, Cuppini L, Curley E, Cuzzubbo S, Devine K, DiMeco F, Duell R, Elder JB, Fehrenbach A, Finocchiaro G, Friedman W, Fulop J, Gardner J, Hermes B, Herold-Mende C, Jungk C, Kendler A, Lehman NL, Lipp E, Liu O, Mandt R, McGraw M, McLendon R, McPherson C, Neder L, Nguyen P, Noss A, Nunziata R, Ostrom QT, Palmer C, Perin A, Pollo B, Potapov A, Potapova O, Rathmell WK, Rotin D, Scarpace L, Schilero C, Senecal K, Shimmel K, Shurkhay V, Sifri S, Singh R, Sloan AE, Smolenski K, Staugaitis SM, Steele R, Thorne L, Tirapelli DP, Unterberg A, Vallurupalli M, Wang Y, Warnick R, Williams F, Wolinsky Y, Bell S, Rosenberg M, Stewart C, Huang F, Grimsby JL, Radenbaugh AJ, Zhang J (2015) Comprehensive, integrative genomic analysis of diffuse lower-grade gliomas. N Engl J Med 372(26):2481–2498. https://doi.org/10.1056/NEJMoa1402121

Chan KM, Fang D, Gan H, Hashizume R, Yu C, Schroeder M, Gupta N, Mueller S, James CD, Jenkins R, Sarkaria J, Zhang Z (2013) The histone H3.3K27M mutation in pediatric glioma reprograms H3K27 methylation and gene expression. Genes Dev 27(9):985–990. https://doi.org/10.1101/gad.217778.113

Chapman PB, Hauschild A, Robert C, Haanen JB, Ascierto P, Larkin J, Dummer R, Garbe C, Testori A, Maio M, Hogg D, Lorigan P, Lebbe C, Jouary T, Schadendorf D, Ribas A, O'Day SJ, Sosman JA, Kirkwood JM, Eggermont AM, Dreno B, Nolop K, Li J, Nelson B, Hou J, Lee RJ, Flaherty KT, McArthur GA, Group B-S (2011) Improved survival with vemurafenib in melanoma with BRAF V600E mutation. N Engl J Med 364(26):2507–2516. https://doi.org/10.1056/NEJMoa1103782

Cichowski K, Shih TS, Schmitt E, Santiago S, Reilly K, McLaughlin ME, Bronson RT, Jacks T (1999) Mouse models of tumor development in neurofibromatosis type 1. Science 286(5447):2172–2176

Cole PD, Kamen BA (2006) Delayed neurotoxicity associated with therapy for children with acute lymphoblastic leukemia. Ment Retard Dev Disabil Res Rev 12(3):174–183. https://doi.org/10.1002/mrdd.20113

Costa RM, Federov NB, Kogan JH, Murphy GG, Stern J, Ohno M, Kucherlapati R, Jacks T, Silva AJ (2002) Mechanism for the learning deficits in a mouse model of neurofibromatosis type 1. Nature 415(6871):526–530. https://doi.org/10.1038/nature711

Dasgupta T, Haas-Kogan DA (2013) The combination of novel targeted molecular agents and radiation in the treatment of pediatric gliomas. Front Oncol 3:110. https://doi.org/10.3389/fonc.2013.00110

Dougherty MJ, Santi M, Brose MS, Ma C, Resnick AC, Sievert AJ, Storm PB, Biegel JA (2010) Activating mutations in BRAF characterize a spectrum of pediatric low-grade gliomas. Neuro-Oncology 12(7):621–630. https://doi.org/10.1093/neuonc/noq007

Dulac O, Lassonde M, Sarnat H (2013) Pediatric neurology, part II. In: Handbook of clinical neurology, vol 112. Elsevier, Amsterdam

Eckel-Passow JE, Lachance DH, Molinaro AM, Walsh KM, Decker PA, Sicotte H, Pekmezci M, Rice T, Kosel ML, Smirnov IV, Sarkar G, Caron AA, Kollmeyer TM, Praska CE, Chada AR, Halder C, Hansen HM, McCoy LS, Bracci PM, Marshall R, Zheng S, Reis GF, Pico AR, O'Neill BP, Buckner JC, Giannini C, Huse JT, Perry A, Tihan T, Berger MS, Chang SM, Prados MD, Wiemels J, Wiencke JK, Wrensch MR, Jenkins RB (2015) Glioma groups based on 1p/19q, IDH, and TERT promoter mutations in tumors. N Engl J Med 372(26):2499–2508. https://doi.org/10.1056/NEJMoa1407279

Fisher PG, Tihan T, Goldthwaite PT, Wharam MD, Carson BS, Weingart JD, Repka MX, Cohen KJ, Burger PC (2008) Outcome analysis of childhood low-grade astrocytomas. Pediatr Blood Cancer 51(2):245–250. https://doi.org/10.1002/pbc.21563

Flaherty KT, Infante JR, Daud A, Gonzalez R, Kefford RF, Sosman J, Hamid O, Schuchter L, Cebon J, Ibrahim N, Kudchadkar R, Burris HA 3rd, Falchook G, Algazi A, Lewis K, Long GV, Puzanov I, Lebowitz P, Singh A, Little S, Sun P, Allred A, Ouellet D, Kim KB, Patel K, Weber J (2012) Combined BRAF and MEK inhibition in melanoma with BRAF V600 mutations. N Engl J Med 367(18):1694–1703

Flaherty KT, Robert C, Hersey P, Nathan P, Garbe C, Milhem M, Demidov LV, Hassel JC, Rutkowski P, Mohr P, Dummer R, Trefzer U, Larkin JM, Utikal J, Dreno B, Nyakas M, Middleton MR, Becker JC, Casey M, Sherman LJ, Wu FS, Ouellet D, Martin AM, Patel K, Schadendorf D, METRIC study group (2012) Improved survival with MEK inhibition in BRAF-mutated melanoma. N Engl J Med 367(2):107–114

Fouladi M, Wallace D, Langston JW, Mulhern R, Rose SR, Gajjar A, Sanford RA, Merchant TE, Jenkins JJ, Kun LE, Heideman RL (2003) Survival and functional outcome of children with hypothalamic/chiasmatic tumors. Cancer 97(4):1084–1092

Fuss M, Poljanc K, Hug EB (2000) Full scale IQ (FSIQ) changes in children treated with whole brain and partial brain irradiation. A review and analysis. Strahlenther Onkol 176(12):573–581

Gielen GH, Gessi M, Hammes J, Kramm CM, Waha A, Pietsch T (2013) H3F3A K27M mutation in pediatric CNS tumors: a marker for diffuse high-grade astrocytomas. Am J Clin Pathol 139(3):345–349. https://doi.org/10.1309/AJCPABOHBC33FVMO

Gierke M, Sperveslage J, Schwab D, Beschorner R, Ebinger M, Schuhmann MU, Schittenhelm J (2016) Analysis of IDH1-R132 mutation, BRAF V600 mutation and KIAA1549-BRAF fusion transcript status in central nervous system tumors supports pediatric tumor classification. J Cancer Res Clin Oncol 142(1):89–100. https://doi.org/10.1007/s00432-015-2006-2

Gilheeney SW, Kieran MW (2012) Differences in molecular genetics between pediatric and adult malignant astrocytomas: age matters. Future Oncol 8(5):549–558. https://doi.org/10.2217/fon.12.51

Gnekow AK, Kortmann RD, Pietsch T et al (2004) Low grade chiasmatic-hypothalamic glioma- carboplatin and vincristin chemotherapy effectively defers radio- therapy within a comprehensive treatment strategy: report from the multicenter treatment study for children and adolescents with a low grade glioma, HIT-LGG 1996, of the Society of Pediatric Oncology and Hematology (GPOH). Klin Padiatr 216:331–342

Gupta N, Banerjee A, Haas-Kogen D (eds) (2004) Pediatric CNS tumors. Springer, New York

Gururangan S, Fangusaro J, Poussaint TY, McLendon RE, Onar-Thomas A, Wu S, Packer RJ, Banerjee A, Gilbertson RJ, Fahey F, Vajapeyam S, Jakacki R, Gajjar A, Goldman S, Pollack IF, Friedman HS, Boyett JM, Fouladi M, Kun LE (2014) Efficacy of bevacizumab plus irinotecan in children with recurrent low-grade gliomas--a pediatric brain tumor consortium study. Neuro-Oncology 16(2):310–317. https://doi.org/10.1093/neuonc/not154

Halperin EC, Wazer DE, Perez CA, Brady LW (eds) (2013) Perez and Brady's principles and practice of radiation oncology, 6th edn. Lippincott Williams & Wilkins, Philadelphia

Hargrave D (2009) Paediatric high and low grade glioma: the impact of tumour biology on current and future therapy. Br J Neurosurg 23(4):351–363

Hassan B, Akcakanat A, Holder AM, Meric-Bernstam F (2013) Targeting the PI3-kinase/Akt/mTOR signaling pathway. Surg Oncol Clin N Am 22(4):641–664. https://doi.org/10.1016/j.soc.2013.06.008

Hemmati HD, Nakano I, Lazareff JA, Masterman-Smith M, Geschwind DH, Bronner-Fraser M, Kornblum HI (2003) Cancerous stem cells can arise from pediatric brain tumors. Proc Natl Acad Sci U S A 100(25):15178–15183. https://doi.org/10.1073/pnas.2036535100

Hernaiz Driever P, von Hornstein S, Pietsch T, Kortmann R, Warmuth-Metz M, Emser A, Gnekow AK (2010) Natural history and management of low-grade glioma in NF-1 children. J Neuro-Oncol 100(2):199–207. https://doi.org/10.1007/s11060-010-0159-z

Hudson MM, Mertens AC, Yasui Y, Hobbie W, Chen H, Gurney JG, Yeazel M, Recklitis CJ, Marina N, Robison LR, Oeffinger KC, Childhood Cancer Survivor Study I (2003) Health status of adult long-term survivors of childhood cancer: a report from the childhood cancer survivor study. JAMA 290(12):1583–1592. https://doi.org/10.1001/jama.290.12.1583

Hudson MM, Tyc VL, Srivastava DK, Gattuso J, Quargnenti A, Crom DB, Hinds P (2002) Multicomponent behavioral intervention to promote health protective behaviors in childhood cancer survivors: the protect study. Med Pediatr Oncol 39(1):2–1.; discussion 2. https://doi.org/10.1002/mpo.10071

Jacob K, Albrecht S, Sollier C, Faury D, Sader E, Montpetit A, Serre D, Hauser P, Garami M, Bognar L, Hanzely Z, Montes JL, Atkinson J, Farmer JP, Bouffet E, Hawkins C, Tabori U, Jabado N (2009) Duplication of 7q34 is specific to juvenile pilocytic astrocytomas and a hallmark of cerebellar and optic pathway tumours. Br J Cancer 101(4):722–733. https://doi.org/10.1038/sj.bjc.6605179

Jacob K, Quang-Khuong DA, Jones DT, Witt H, Lambert S, Albrecht S, Witt O, Vezina C, Shirinian M, Faury D, Garami M, Hauser P, Klekner A,

Bognar L, Farmer JP, Montes JL, Atkinson J, Hawkins C, Korshunov A, Collins VP, Pfister SM, Tabori U, Jabado N (2011) Genetic aberrations leading to MAPK pathway activation mediate oncogene-induced senescence in sporadic pilocytic astrocytomas. Clin Cancer Res 17(14):4650–4660. https://doi.org/10.1158/1078-0432.CCR-11-0127

Jones DT, Hutter B, Jager N, Korshunov A, Kool M, Warnatz HJ, Zichner T, Lambert SR, Ryzhova M, Quang DA, Fontebasso AM, Stutz AM, Hutter S, Zuckermann M, Sturm D, Gronych J, Lasitschka B, Schmidt S, Seker-Cin H, Witt H, Sultan M, Ralser M, Northcott PA, Hovestadt V, Bender S, Pfaff E, Stark S, Faury D, Schwartzentruber J, Majewski J, Weber UD, Zapatka M, Raeder B, Schlesner M, Worth CL, Bartholomae CC, von Kalle C, Imbusch CD, Radomski S, Lawerenz C, van Sluis P, Koster J, Volckmann R, Versteeg R, Lehrach H, Monoranu C, Winkler B, Unterberg A, Herold-Mende C, Milde T, Kulozik AE, Ebinger M, Schuhmann MU, Cho YJ, Pomeroy SL, von Deimling A, Witt O, Taylor MD, Wolf S, Karajannis MA, Eberhart CG, Scheurlen W, Hasselblatt M, Ligon KL, Kieran MW, Korbel JO, Yaspo ML, Brors B, Felsberg J, Reifenberger G, Collins VP, Jabado N, Eils R, Lichter P, Pfister SM, International Cancer Genome Consortium PedBrain Tumor P (2013) Recurrent somatic alterations of FGFR1 and NTRK2 in pilocytic astrocytoma. Nat Genet 45(8):927–932. https://doi.org/10.1038/ng.2682

Kadan-Lottick NS, Robison LL, Gurney JG, Neglia JP, Yasui Y, Hayashi R, Hudson M, Greenberg M, Mertens AC (2002) Childhood cancer survivors' knowledge about their past diagnosis and treatment: childhood cancer survivor study. JAMA 287(14):1832–1839

Kadota RP, Kun LE, Langston JW, Burger PC, Cohen ME, Mahoney DH, Walter AW, Rodman JH, Parent A, Buckley E, Kepner JL, Friedman HS (1999) Cyclophosphamide for the treatment of progressive low-grade astrocytoma: a pediatric oncology group phase II study. J Pediatr Hematol Oncol 21(3):198–202

Kaul A, Chen YH, Emnett RJ, Dahiya S, Gutmann DH (2012) Pediatric glioma-associated KIAA1549:BRAF expression regulates neuroglial cell growth in a cell type-specific and mTOR-dependent manner. Genes Dev 26(23):2561–2566. https://doi.org/10.1101/gad.200907.112

Khuong-Quang DA, Buczkowicz P, Rakopoulos P, Liu XY, Fontebasso AM, Bouffet E, Bartels U, Albrecht S, Schwartzentruber J, Letourneau L, Bourgey M, Bourque G, Montpetit A, Bourret G, Lepage P, Fleming A, Lichter P, Kool M, von Deimling A, Sturm D, Korshunov A, Faury D, Jones DT, Majewski J, Pfister SM, Jabado N, Hawkins C (2012) K27M mutation in histone H3.3 defines clinically and biologically distinct subgroups of pediatric diffuse intrinsic pontine gliomas. Acta Neuropathol 124(3):439–447. https://doi.org/10.1007/s00401-012-0998-0

Kilday JP, Bartels U, Huang A, Barron M, Shago M, Mistry M, Zhukova N, Laperriere N, Dirks P, Hawkins C, Bouffet E, Tabori U (2014) Favorable survival and metabolic outcome for children with diencephalic syndrome using a radiation-sparing approach. J Neurooncol 116(1):195–204

Kilday JP, Bouffet E (2014) Curr Pediatr Rep 2:38

King TZ, Fennell EB, Williams L, Algina J, Boggs S, Crosson B, Leonard C (2004) Verbal memory abilities of children with brain tumors. Child Neuropsychol 10(2):76–88. https://doi.org/10.1080/092970404909110

Kolb B, Gibb R (2007) Brain plasticity and recovery from early cortical injury. Dev Psychobiol 49(2):107–118. https://doi.org/10.1002/dev.20199

Kolb EA, Gorlick R, Houghton PJ, Morton CL, Neale G, Keir ST, Carol H, Lock R, Phelps D, Kang MH, Reynolds CP, Maris JM, Billups C, Smith MA (2010) Initial testing (stage 1) of AZD6244 (ARRY-142886) by the pediatric preclinical testing program. Pediatr Blood Cancer 55(4):668–677. https://doi.org/10.1002/pbc.22576

Krueger DA, Care MM, Holland K, Agricola K, Tudor C, Mangeshkar P, Wilson KA, Byars A, Sahmoud T, Franz DN (2010) Everolimus for subependymal giant-cell astrocytomas in tuberous sclerosis. N Engl J Med 363(19):1801–1811. https://doi.org/10.1056/NEJMoa1001671

Lacaze E, Kieffer V, Streri A, Lorenzi C, Gentaz E, Habrand JL, Dellatolas G, Kalifa C, Grill J (2003) Neuropsychological outcome in children with optic pathway tumours when first-line treatment is chemotherapy. Br J Cancer 89(11):2038–2044. https://doi.org/10.1038/sj.bjc.6601410

Laplante M, Sabatini DM (2012) mTOR signaling in growth control and disease. Cell 149(2):274–293. https://doi.org/10.1016/j.cell.2012.03.017

Lawrence MS, Stojanov P, Mermel CH, Robinson JT, Garraway LA, Golub TR, Meyerson M, Gabriel SB, Lander ES, Getz G (2014) Discovery and saturation analysis of cancer genes across 21 tumour types. Nature 505(7484):495–501. https://doi.org/10.1038/nature12912

Le Deley MC, Vassal G, Taibi A, Shamsaldin A, Leblanc T, Hartmann O (2005) High cumulative rate of secondary leukemia after continuous etoposide treatment for solid tumors in children and young adults. Pediatr Blood Cancer 45(1):25–31. https://doi.org/10.1002/pbc.20380

Le LQ, Parada LF (2007) Tumor microenvironment and neurofibromatosis type I: connecting the GAPs. Oncogene 26(32):4609–4616. https://doi.org/10.1038/sj.onc.1210261

Leone G, Mele L, Pulsoni A, Equitani F, Pagano L (1999) The incidence of secondary leukemias. Haematologica 84(10):937–945

Lin A, Rodriguez FJ, Karajannis MA, Williams SC, Legault G, Zagzag D, Burger PC, Allen JC, Eberhart CG, Bar EE (2012) BRAF alterations in primary glial and glioneuronal neoplasms of the central nervous system with identification of 2 novel KIAA1549:BRAF fusion variants. J Neuropathol

Exp Neurol 71(1):66–72. https://doi.org/10.1097/NEN.0b013e31823f2cb0

Marcus KJ, Goumnerova L, Billett AL, Lavally B, Scott RM, Bishop K, Xu R, Young Poussaint T, Kieran M, Kooy H, Pomeroy SL, Tarbell NJ (2005) Stereotactic radiotherapy for localized low-grade gliomas in children: final results of a prospective trial. Int J Radiat Oncol Biol Phys 61(2):374–379. https://doi.org/10.1016/j.ijrobp.2004.06.012

Massimino M, Spreafico F, Cefalo G et al (2002) High response rate to cisplatin/etoposide regimen in childhood lowgrade glioma. J Clin Oncol 20:4209–4216

Matsui I, Tanimura M, Kobayashi N, Sawada T, Nagahara N, Akatsuka J (1993) Neurofibromatosis type 1 and childhood cancer. Cancer 72(9):2746–2754

McBride SM, Perez DA, Polley MY, Vandenberg SR, Smith JS, Zheng S, Lamborn KR, Wiencke JK, Chang SM, Prados MD, Berger MS, Stokoe D, Haas-Kogan DA (2010) Activation of PI3K/mTOR pathway occurs in most adult low-grade gliomas and predicts patient survival. J Neuro-Oncol 97(1):33–40. https://doi.org/10.1007/s11060-009-0004-4

Merchant TE, Conklin HM, Wu S, Lustig RH, Xiong X (2009) Late effects of conformal radiation therapy for pediatric patients with low-grade glioma: prospective evaluation of cognitive, endocrine, and hearing deficits. J Clin Oncol 27(22):3691–3697. https://doi.org/10.1200/JCO.2008.21.2738

Merchant TE, Kun LE, Wu S, Xiong X, Sanford RA, Boop FA (2009) Phase II trial of conformal radiation therapy for pediatric low-grade glioma. J Clin Oncol 27(22):3598–3604. https://doi.org/10.1200/JCO.2008.20.9494

Merchant TE, Pollack IF, Loeffler JS (2010) Brain tumors across the age spectrum: biology, therapy, and late effects. Semin Radiat Oncol 20(1):58–66. https://doi.org/10.1016/j.semradonc.2009.09.005

Meyerson M, Gabriel S, Getz G (2010) Advances in understanding cancer genomes through second-generation sequencing. Nat Rev Genet 11(10):685–696. https://doi.org/10.1038/nrg2841

Mishra KK, Puri DR, Missett BT, Lamborn KR, Prados MD, Berger MS, Banerjee A, Gupta N, Wara WM, Haas-Kogan DA (2006) The role of up-front radiation therapy for incompletely resected pediatric WHO grade II low-grade gliomas. Neuro-Oncology 8(2):166–174. https://doi.org/10.1215/15228517-2005-011

Mishra KK, Squire S, Lamborn K et al (2010) Phase II TPDCV protocol for pediatric low-grade hypothalamic/chiasmatic gliomas: 15-year update. J Neurooncol 100(1):121–127

Motzer RJ, Escudier B, Oudard S, Hutson TE, Porta C, Bracarda S, Grunwald V, Thompson JA, Figlin RA, Hollaender N, Urbanowitz G, Berg WJ, Kay A, Lebwohl D, Ravaud A, Group R-S (2008) Efficacy of everolimus in advanced renal cell carcinoma: a double-blind, randomised, placebo-controlled phase III trial. Lancet 372(9637):449–456. https://doi.org/10.1016/S0140-6736(08)61039-9

Nageswara Rao AA, Packer RJ (2014) Advances in the management of low-grade gliomas. Curr Oncol Rep 16(8):398. https://doi.org/10.1007/s11912-014-0398-9

Nakamura M, Shimada K, Ishida E, Higuchi T, Nakase H, Sakaki T, Konishi N (2007) Molecular pathogenesis of pediatric astrocytic tumors. Neuro-Oncology 9(2):113–123. https://doi.org/10.1215/15228517-2006-036

Nathan PC, Patel SK, Dilley K, Goldsby R, Harvey J, Jacobsen C, Kadan-Lottick N, McKinley K, Millham AK, Moore I, Okcu MF, Woodman CL, Brouwers P, Armstrong FD, Children's Oncology Group Long-term Follow-up Guidelines Task Force on Neurocognitive/Behavioral Complications After Childhood C (2007) Guidelines for identification of, advocacy for, and intervention in neurocognitive problems in survivors of childhood cancer: a report from the Children's oncology group. Arch Pediatr Adolesc Med 161(8):798–806. https://doi.org/10.1001/archpedi.161.8.798

Nicholson HS, Kretschmar CS, Krailo M, Bernstein M, Kadota R, Fort D, Friedman H, Harris MB, Tedeschi-Blok N, Mazewski C, Sato J, Reaman GH (2007) Phase 2 study of temozolomide in children and adolescents with recurrent central nervous system tumors: a report from the Children's oncology group. Cancer 110(7):1542–1550. https://doi.org/10.1002/cncr.22961

Northrup H, Koenig MK, Pearson DA, Au KS (1993) Tuberous Sclerosis Complex. In: Pagon RA, Adam MP, Ardinger HH et al (eds) GeneReviews(R). University of Washington, Seattle, WA

Packer RJ, Ater J, Allen J et al (1997) Carboplatin and vincristine chemotherapy for children with newly diagnosed progressive low-grade gliomas. J Neurosurg 86:747–754

Prados MD, Edwards MS, Rabbitt J et al (1997) Treatment of pediatric low-grade gliomas with a nitrosourea-based multiagent chemotherapy regimen. J Neurooncol 32:235–241

Parsa CF, Hoyt CS, Lesser RL, Weinstein JM, Strother CM, Muci-Mendoza R, Ramella M, Manor RS, Fletcher WA, Repka MX, Garrity JA, Ebner RN, Monteiro ML, McFadzean RM, Rubtsova IV, Hoyt WF (2001) Spontaneous regression of optic gliomas: thirteen cases documented by serial neuroimaging. Arch Ophthalmol 119(4):516–529

Perilongo G, Moras P, Carollo C, Battistella A, Clementi M, Laverda A, Murgia A (1999) Spontaneous partial regression of low-grade glioma in children with neurofibromatosis-1: a real possibility. J Child Neurol 14(6):352–356. https://doi.org/10.1177/088307389901400602

Piccirilli M, Lenzi J, Delfinis C, Trasimeni G, Salvati M, Raco A (2006) Spontaneous regression of optic pathways gliomas in three patients with neurofibromatosis type I and critical review of the literature. Childs Nerv Syst 22(10):1332–1337. https://doi.org/10.1007/s00381-006-0061-3

Pollack IF (2011) Multidisciplinary management of childhood brain tumors: a review of outcomes, recent advances, and challenges. J Neurosurg Pediatr 8(2):135–148. https://doi.org/10.3171/2011.5.PEDS1178

Populo H, Lopes JM, Soares P (2012) The mTOR signalling pathway in human cancer. Int J Mol Sci 13(2):1886–1918. https://doi.org/10.3390/ijms13021886

Qaddoumi I, Orisme W, Ji W, Santiago T, Gupta K, Dalton JD, Bo T, Haupfear K, Punchihewa C, Easton J, Mulder H, Boggs K, Shao Y, Rusch M, Becksfort J, Gupta P, Wang S, Lee RP, Brat D, Peter Collins V, Dahiya S, George D, Konomos W, Kurian KM, McFadden K, Serafini LN, Nickols H, Perry A, Shurtleff S, Gajjar A, Boop FA, Klimo PD, Mardis ER, Wilson RK, Baker SJ, Zhang J, Gang W, Downing JR, Tatevossian RG, Ellison DW (2016) Genetic alterations in uncommon low-grade neuroepithelial tumors: BRAF, FGFR1, and MYB mutations occur at high frequency and align with morphology. Acta Neuropathol 131(6):833–845

Raabe EH, Lim KS, Kim JM, Meeker A, Mao XG, Nikkhah G, Maciaczyk J, Kahlert U, Jain D, Bar E, Cohen KJ, Eberhart CG (2011) BRAF activation induces transformation and then senescence in human neural stem cells: a pilocytic astrocytoma model. Clin Cancer Res 17(11):3590–3599. https://doi.org/10.1158/1078-0432.CCR-10-3349

Ramkissoon LA, Horowitz PM, Craig JM, Ramkissoon SH, Rich BE, Schumacher SE, McKenna A, Lawrence MS, Bergthold G, Brastianos PK, Tabak B, Ducar MD, Van Hummelen P, MacConaill LE, Pouissant-Young T, Cho YJ, Taha H, Mahmoud M, Bowers DC, Margraf L, Tabori U, Hawkins C, Packer RJ, Hill DA, Pomeroy SL, Eberhart CG, Dunn IF, Goumnerova L, Getz G, Chan JA, Santagata S, Hahn WC, Stiles CD, Ligon AH, Kieran MW, Beroukhim R, Ligon KL (2013) Genomic analysis of diffuse pediatric low-grade gliomas identifies recurrent oncogenic truncating rearrangements in the transcription factor MYBL1. Proc Natl Acad Sci U S A 110(20):8188–8193. https://doi.org/10.1073/pnas.1300252110

Reddick WE, Mulhern RK, Elkin TD, Glass JO, Merchant TE, Langston JW (1998) A hybrid neural network analysis of subtle brain volume differences in children surviving brain tumors. Magn Reson Imaging 16(4):413–421

Reuss D, von Deimling A (2009) Hereditary tumor syndromes and gliomas. Recent results in cancer research Fortschritte der Krebsforschung Progres dans les recherches Sur le. Cancer 171:83–102. https://doi.org/10.1007/978-3-540-31206-2_5

Ris MD, Beebe DW (2008) Neurodevelopmental outcomes of children with low-grade gliomas. Dev Disabil Res Rev 14(3):196–202. https://doi.org/10.1002/ddrr.27

Ris MD, Beebe DW, Armstrong FD, Fontanesi J, Holmes E, Sanford RA, Wisoff JH, Children's Oncology G (2008) Cognitive and adaptive outcome in extracerebellar low-grade brain tumors in children: a report from the Children's oncology group. J Clin Oncol 26(29):4765–4770. https://doi.org/10.1200/JCO.2008.17.1371

Ris MD, Noll RB (1994) Long-term neurobehavioral outcome in pediatric brain-tumor patients: review and methodological critique. J Clin

Exp Neuropsychol 16(1):21–42. https://doi.org/10.1080/01688639408402615

Rivera B, Gayden T, Carrot-Zhang J, Nadaf J, Boshari T, Faury D, Zeinieh M, Blanc R, Burk DL, Fahiminiya S, Bareke E, Schüller U, Monoranu CM, Sträter R, Kerl K, Niederstadt T, Kurlemann G, Ellezam B, Michalak Z, Thom M, Lockhart PJ, Leventer RJ, Ohm M, MacGregor D, Jones D, Karamchandani J, Greenwood CMT, Berghuis AM, Bens S, Siebert R, Zakrzewska M, Liberski PP, Zakrzewski K, Sisodiya SM, Paulus W, Albrecht S, Hasselblatt M, Jabado N, Foulkes WD, Majewski J (2016) Germline and somatic FGFR1 abnormalities in dysembryoplastic neuroepithelial tumors. Acta Neuropathol 131(6):847–863

Rodriguez FJ, Perry A, Gutmann DH, O'Neill BP, Leonard J, Bryant S, Giannini C (2008) Gliomas in neurofibromatosis type 1: a clinicopathologic study of 100 patients. J Neuropathol Exp Neurol 67(3):240–249. https://doi.org/10.1097/NEN.0b013e318165eb75

Rodriguez EF, Scheithauer BW, Giannini C, Rynearson A, Cen L, Hoesley B, Gilmer-Flynn H, Sarkaria JN, Jenkins S, Long J, Rodriguez FJ (2011) PI3K/AKT pathway alterations are associated with clinically aggressive and histologically anaplastic subsets of pilocytic astrocytoma. Acta Neuropathol 121(3):407–420. https://doi.org/10.1007/s00401-010-0784-9

Rodriguez FJ, Tihan T, Lin D, McDonald W, Nigro J, Feuerstein B, Jackson S, Cohen K, Burger PC (2014) Clinicopathologic features of pediatric oligodendrogliomas: a series of 50 patients. Am J Surg Pathol 38(8):1058–1070. https://doi.org/10.1097/PAS.0000000000000221

Rodriguez FJ, Adelita Vizcaino M, Blakeley J, Heaphy CM (2016) Frequent alternative lengthening of telomeres and ATRX loss in adult NF1-associated diffuse and high-grade astrocytomas. Acta Neuropathol 132(5):761–763

Ron E, Modan B, Boice JD Jr, Alfandary E, Stovall M, Chetrit A, Katz L (1988) Tumors of the brain and nervous system after radiotherapy in childhood. N Engl J Med 319(16):1033–1039. https://doi.org/10.1056/NEJM198810203191601

Roncadin C, Dennis M, Greenberg ML, Spiegler BJ (2008) Adverse medical events associated with childhood cerebellar astrocytomas and medulloblastomas: natural history and relation to very long-term neurobehavioral outcome. Childs Nerv Syst 24(9):995–1002.; discussion 1003. https://doi.org/10.1007/s00381-008-0658-9

Rosner M, Hanneder M, Siegel N, Valli A, Hengstschläger M (2008) The tuberous sclerosis gene products hamartin and tuberin are multifunctional proteins with a wide spectrum of interacting partners. Mutat Res 658(3):234–246

Sancak S, Gursoy T, Imamoglu EY, Karatekin G, Ovali F (2016) Effect of prematurity on cerebellar growth. J Child Neurol 31(2):138–144. https://doi.org/10.1177/0883073815585350

Schindler G, Capper D, Meyer J, Janzarik W, Omran H, Herold-Mende C, Schmieder K, Wesseling P, Mawrin C, Hasselblatt M, Louis DN, Korshunov A, Pfister S, Hartmann C, Paulus W, Reifenberger G, von Deimling A (2011) Analysis of BRAF V600E mutation in 1,320 nervous system tumors reveals high mutation frequencies in pleomorphic xanthoastrocytoma, ganglioglioma and extra-cerebellar pilocytic astrocytoma. Acta Neuropathol 121(3):397–405. https://doi.org/10.1007/s00401-011-0802-6

Schwartzentruber J, Korshunov A, Liu XY, Jones DT, Pfaff E, Jacob K, Sturm D, Fontebasso AM, Quang DA, Tonjes M, Hovestadt V, Albrecht S, Kool M, Nantel A, Konermann C, Lindroth A, Jager N, Rausch T, Ryzhova M, Korbel JO, Hielscher T, Hauser P, Garami M, Klekner A, Bognar L, Ebinger M, Schuhmann MU, Scheurlen W, Pekrun A, Fruhwald MC, Roggendorf W, Kramm C, Durken M, Atkinson J, Lepage P, Montpetit A, Zakrzewska M, Zakrzewski K, Liberski PP, Dong Z, Siegel P, Kulozik AE, Zapatka M, Guha A, Malkin D, Felsberg J, Reifenberger G, von Deimling A, Ichimura K, Collins VP, Witt H, Milde T, Witt O, Zhang C, Castelo-Branco P, Lichter P, Faury D, Tabori U, Plass C, Majewski J, Pfister SM, Jabado N (2012) Driver mutations in histone H3.3 and chromatin remodelling genes in paediatric glioblastoma. Nature 482(7384):226–231. https://doi.org/10.1038/nature10833

Shannon KM, O'Connell P, Martin GA, Paderanga D, Olson K, Dinndorf P, McCormick F (1994) Loss of the normal NF1 allele from the bone marrow of children with type 1 neurofibromatosis and malignant myeloid disorders. N Engl J Med 330(9):597–601. https://doi.org/10.1056/NEJM199403033300903

Shaw EG, Wisoff JH (2003) Prospective clinical trials of intracranial low-grade glioma in adults and children. Neuro-Oncology 5(3):153–160

Sievert AJ, Fisher MJ (2009) Pediatric low-grade gliomas. J Child Neurol 24(11):1397–1408. https://doi.org/10.1177/0883073809342005

Siffert J, Allen JC (2000) Late effects of therapy of thalamic and hypothalamic tumors in childhood: vascular, neurobehavioral and neoplastic. Pediatr Neurosurg 33(2):105–111. https://doi.org/10.1159/000028985

Sturm D, Witt H, Hovestadt V, Khuong-Quang DA, Jones DT, Konermann C, Pfaff E, Tonjes M, Sill M, Bender S, Kool M, Zapatka M, Becker N, Zucknick M, Hielscher T, Liu XY, Fontebasso AM, Ryzhova M, Albrecht S, Jacob K, Wolter M, Ebinger M, Schuhmann MU, van Meter T, Fruhwald MC, Hauch H, Pekrun A, Radlwimmer B, Niehues T, von Komorowski G, Durken M, Kulozik AE, Madden J, Donson A, Foreman NK, Drissi R, Fouladi M, Scheurlen W, von Deimling A, Monoranu C, Roggendorf W, Herold-Mende C, Unterberg A, Kramm CM, Felsberg J, Hartmann C, Wiestler B, Wick W, Milde T, Witt O, Lindroth AM, Schwartzentruber J, Faury D, Fleming A, Zakrzewska M, Liberski PP, Zakrzewski K, Hauser P, Garami M, Klekner A, Bognar L, Morrissy

S, Cavalli F, Taylor MD, van Sluis P, Koster J, Versteeg R, Volckmann R, Mikkelsen T, Aldape K, Reifenberger G, Collins VP, Majewski J, Korshunov A, Lichter P, Plass C, Jabado N, Pfister SM (2012) Hotspot mutations in H3F3A and IDH1 define distinct epigenetic and biological subgroups of glioblastoma. Cancer Cell 22(4):425–437. https://doi.org/10.1016/j.ccr.2012.08.024

Sutton LN, Molloy PT, Sernyak H, Goldwein J, Phillips PL, Rorke LB, Moshang T Jr, Lange B, Packer RJ (1995) Long-term outcome of hypothalamic/chiasmatic astrocytomas in children treated with conservative surgery. J Neurosurg 83(4):583–589. https://doi.org/10.3171/jns.1995.83.4.0583

Suzuki H, Aoki K, Chiba K, Sato Y, Shiozawa Y, Shiraishi Y, Shimamura T, Niida A, Motomura K, Ohka F, Yamamoto T, Tanahashi K, Ranjit M, Wakabayashi T, Yoshizato T, Kataoka K, Yoshida K, Nagata Y, Sato-Otsubo A, Tanaka H, Sanada M, Kondo Y, Nakamura H, Mizoguchi M, Abe T, Muragaki Y, Watanabe R, Ito I, Miyano S, Natsume A, Ogawa S (2015) Mutational landscape and clonal architecture in grade II and III gliomas. Nat Genet 47(5):458–468. https://doi.org/10.1038/ng.3273

van Slegtenhorst M, de Hoogt R, Hermans C, Nellist M, Janssen B, Verhoef S, Lindhout D, van den Ouweland A, Halley D, Young J, Burley M, Jeremiah S, Woodward K, Nahmias J, Fox M, Ekong R, Osborne J, Wolfe J, Povey S, Snell RG, Cheadle JP, Jones AC, Tachataki M, Ravine D, Sampson JR, Reeve MP, Richardson P, Wilmer F, Munro C, Hawkins TL, Sepp T, Ali JB, Ward S, Green AJ, Yates JR, Kwiatkowska J, Henske EP, Short MP, Haines JH, Jozwiak S, Kwiatkowski DJ (1997) Identification of the tuberous sclerosis gene TSC1 on chromosome 9q34. Science 277(5327):805–808

Venneti S, Santi M, Felicella MM, Yarilin D, Phillips JJ, Sullivan LM, Martinez D, Perry A, Lewis PW, Thompson CB, Judkins AR (2014) A sensitive and specific histopathologic prognostic marker for H3F3A K27M mutant pediatric glioblastomas. Acta Neuropathol 128(5):743–753. https://doi.org/10.1007/s00401-014-1338-3

Wisoff JH, Sanford RA, Heier LA, Sposto R, Burger PC, Yates AJ, Holmes EJ, Kun LE (2011) Primary neurosurgery for pediatric low-grade gliomas: a prospective multi-institutional study from the Children's oncology group. Neurosurgery 68(6):1548–1554.; discussion 1554-1545. https://doi.org/10.1227/NEU.0b013e318214a66e

Wu G, Diaz AK, Paugh BS, Rankin SL, Ju B, Li Y, Zhu X, Qu C, Chen X, Zhang J, Easton J, Edmonson M, Ma X, Lu C, Nagahawatte P, Hedlund E, Rusch M, Pounds S, Lin T, Onar-Thomas A, Huether R, Kriwacki R, Parker M, Gupta P, Becksfort J, Wei L, Mulder HL, Boggs K, Vadodaria B, Yergeau D, Russell JC, Ochoa K, Fulton RS, Fulton LL, Jones C, Boop FA, Broniscer A, Wetmore C, Gajjar A, Ding L, Mardis ER, Wilson RK, Taylor MR, Downing JR, Ellison DW, Zhang J, Baker SJ, St. Jude Children's Research Hospital-

Washington University Pediatric Cancer Genome P (2014) The genomic landscape of diffuse intrinsic pontine glioma and pediatric non-brainstem high-grade glioma. Nat Genet 46(5):444–450. https://doi.org/10.1038/ng.2938

Yalon M, Rood B, MacDonald TJ, McCowage G, Kane R, Constantini S, Packer RJ (2013) A feasibility and efficacy study of rapamycin and erlotinib for recurrent pediatric low-grade glioma (LGG). Pediatr Blood Cancer 60(1):71–76. https://doi.org/10.1002/pbc.24142

Zebrack BJ, Gurney JG, Oeffinger K, Whitton J, Packer RJ, Mertens A, Turk N, Castleberry R, Dreyer Z, Robison LL, Zeltzer LK (2004) Psychological outcomes in long-term survivors of childhood brain cancer: a report from the childhood cancer survivor study. J Clin Oncol 22(6):999–1006. https://doi.org/10.1200/JCO.2004.06.148

Zhang J, Wu G, Miller CP, Tatevossian RG, Dalton JD, Tang B, Orisme W, Punchihewa C, Parker M, Qaddoumi I, Boop FA, Lu C, Kandoth C, Ding L, Lee R, Huether R, Chen X, Hedlund E, Nagahawatte P, Rusch M, Boggs K, Cheng J, Becksfort J, Ma J, Song G, Li Y, Wei L, Wang J, Shurtleff S, Easton J, Zhao D, Fulton RS, Fulton LL, Dooling DJ, Vadodaria B, Mulder HL, Tang C, Ochoa K, Mullighan CG, Gajjar A, Kriwacki R, Sheer D, Gilbertson RJ, Mardis ER, Wilson RK, Downing JR, Baker SJ, Ellison DW, St. Jude Children's Research Hospital-Washington University Pediatric Cancer Genome P (2013) Whole-genome sequencing identifies genetic alterations in pediatric low-grade gliomas. Nat Genet 45(6):602–612. https://doi.org/10.1038/ng.2611

Germ Cell Tumors

11

Kee Kiat Yeo and Girish Dhall

Abbreviations

AFP	Alpha-fetoprotein
AuHCR	Autologous hematopoietic cell rescue
CBTRUS	Central Brain Tumor Registry of the United States
CCKBR	Cholecystokinin B receptor
CGH	Comparative genomic hybridization
CNS	Central nervous system
COG	Children's Oncology Group
CR	Complete response
CSF	Cerebrospinal fluid
CSI	Craniospinal irradiation
CT	Computed tomography
ETV	Endoscopic third ventriculostomy
FISH	Fluorescent in situ hybridization
GCT	Germ cell tumor
Gy	Gray
IFR	Involved field radiation
miRNA	microRNA
MMGCT	Mixed malignant germ cell tumor
MRI	Magnetic resonance imaging

NGGCT	Nongerminomatous germ cell tumor
OS	Overall survival
PFS	Progression-free survival
PLAP	Placental alkaline phosphatase
PR	Partial response
qRT-PCR	Quantitative reverse transcriptase polymerase chain reaction
RT	Radiation therapy
SFOP	Société Française d'Oncologie Pédiatrique
SIOP	Société Internationale d'Oncologie Pédiatrique
SNRPN	Small nuclear ribonucleoprotein polypeptide N
VP	Ventricular peritoneal
WBI	Whole brain irradiation
WES	Whole exome sequencing
WHO	World Health Organization
WVI	Whole ventricular irradiation
YST	Yolk sac tumors
βhCG	β Human chorionic gonadotropin

K. K. Yeo, M.D. · G. Dhall, M.D. (✉)
Children's Hospital Los Angeles,
Los Angeles, CA, USA

Keck School of Medicine of University of Southern
California, Los Angeles, CA, USA

Neuro-Oncology Program, Children's Hospital
Los Angeles, Los Angeles, CA, USA
e-mail: gdhall@chla.usc.edu

11.1 Introduction

Central nervous system (CNS) germ cell tumors (GCT) are a rare and heterogeneous group of malignant tumors that present in children and young adults. According to the Central Brain Tumor Registry of the United States (CBTRUS) 2012 Statistical Report, CNS GCTs accounted for 0.5% of all CNS tumors in adults, 1.3% in young adults (ages 20–34 years), 5.1% in patients ages 15–19 years, and 3.6% in patients 0–14 years of age (Dolecek et al. 2012). The incidence of CNS GCTs is significantly higher in Asian countries where it has been reported to be as high as 9–15% (Kamoshima and Sawamura 2010; Matsutani et al. 1997). CNS GCTs are twice as common in males than in females and 1.5 times more common in Caucasians than in African Americans (Dolecek et al. 2012). Although GCTs typically occur in the gonads, extragonadal sites are more common in children. In older children and adolescents, the brain is the most common site for GCTs. CNS GCTs present predominantly in the pineal and suprasellar regions with basal ganglia being the third most common location. Approximately 5–10% of patients have bifocal tumors involving both pineal and suprasellar regions (Jennings et al. 1985).

The World Health Organization (WHO) classification of CNS GCTs divides these tumors into germinomas and nongerminomatous GCTs (NGGCTs). NGGCTs include teratoma (mature and immature), teratoma with malignant transformation, yolk sac tumor (YST), embryonal carcinoma, choriocarcinoma, and mixed tumors. Whereas germinomas occur as pure tumors in 60–65% of cases, nongerminomatous tumors more frequently occur as mixed tumors, which most commonly include germinoma and teratoma along with other malignant elements (Rosenblum et al. 2007). Hence, the term NGGCTs is a misnomer in this sense and some investigators prefer to use the term "mixed malignant germ cell tumors." NGGCTs account for approximately one-third of CNS GCTs. Germinomas are more prone to occur in the suprasellar region and in older children, adolescents, and young adults, whereas NGGCTs have a predilection for the pineal region and a younger age group (Dolecek et al. 2012). Primary tumors in the basal ganglia as well as bifocal tumors (pineal and suprasellar) are more likely to be germinomas as well. Tumors in infants are more likely to be mature or immature teratomas.

11.2 Diagnosis

11.2.1 Clinical Presentation

In general, clinical presentations of these tumors vary with location and age. Pineal tumors often present with signs and symptoms of increased intracranial pressure secondary to obstructive hydrocephalus. These symptoms include worsening early morning headaches and emesis in older children, with rapidly growing head circumference and sun-setting sign seen in infants. Patients with pineal tumors are also likely to have Parinaud's syndrome at the time of diagnosis— impairment of upward gaze and dilated pupils responsive to accommodation but not to light. Patients with choriocarcinoma may present with sudden intracranial hemorrhage. Suprasellar GCTs often present with hypothalamic/pituitary axis dysfunction, namely diabetes insipidus, delayed sexual development, hypopituitarism, growth hormone deficiency, and precocious puberty. Approximately one-third of patients with isolated endocrinopathy remain asymptomatic for months to years. Patients with isolated pineal tumors can rarely have occult disease within the suprasellar region that is not visible on the MRI at the time of diagnosis. It is therefore very important to perform endocrine function tests in such patients. Patients with a primary tumor within the basal ganglia may present with hemiparesis, seizures, and neurocognitive dysfunction that can go undetected for months to years.

11.2.2 Radiology

A computerized tomography (CT) scan is generally the first imaging study to be performed when the patients present to the emergency room. The utility of CT scans in diagnosing the nature and extent of lesions within the brain is limited with the exception of intracranial hemorrhage or hydrocephalus. Magnetic resonance imaging (MRI) with and without gadolinium administration is the imaging modality of choice for the diagnosis of CNS GCTs. Germinomas tend to enhance diffusely whereas the NGGCTs often have associated hemorrhage and appear more heterogeneous. However, it is typically a challenge to distinguish between the two tumor types (germinomas and NGGCTs) by MRI alone. "Doublet lesions," involving pituitary and suprasellar areas, are most likely to be pure germinomas. Ventricular spread (enhancing nodular disease along the walls of the lateral ventricles) is not uncommon with germinomas. Basal ganglia GCTs typically show minimal to no enhancement on imaging, especially during the early phase of the disease.

11.2.3 Tumor Markers

GCTs secrete proteins into the blood and cerebrospinal fluid (CSF) that can be measured and be used for diagnostic purposes. These include, but are not limited to, beta-human chorionic gonadotropin (βhCG) and alpha-fetoprotein (AFP) in blood and CSF, and placental alkaline phosphatase (PLAP) in CSF (Matsutani 2004). βhCG levels above 50 mIU/mL and/or AFP above 10 ng/mL in the serum or above 2 ng/mL in the CSF are generally considered sufficient for a diagnosis of NGGCT and a biopsy is not considered necessary. However, pure germinomas have been reported to secrete βhCG levels of up to 200 mIU/mL with no adverse impact upon survival (Fujimaki and Matsutani 2005). The current European standard is to consider βhCG levels of <50 mIU/mL as germinomas and >50 mIU/mL as NGGCTs, whereas the Children's Oncology Group (COG) in the United States draws the line at βhCG levels of >100 mIU/mL. Measurement of PLAP in the serum or CSF has been suggested to be a sensitive marker for germinoma; however, its use still remains investigational (Watanabe et al. 2012). Although lumbar CSF is traditionally used for cytology to look for malignant cells, ventricular CSF drawn at the time of endoscopic biopsy or open craniotomy may be used for measurement of tumor markers.

11.2.4 Tissue Diagnosis

For patients with radiographic findings suggestive of a CNS GCT but without tumor marker elevation in the serum and/or CSF, a biopsy to diagnose the exact tumor type is warranted. Conversely, for patients with a midline tumor on the MRI (±basal ganglia), any elevation of AFP above 10 ng/mL (or greater than institutional normal) or with βhCG >100 mIU/mL in serum and/or CSF is consistent with a diagnosis of a NGGCT and no tissue diagnosis is required. AFP levels in the range of 100 s to 1000 s are generally consistent with a diagnosis of yolk sac tumor. Similarly, high βhCG levels are considered to be compatible with a diagnosis of choriocarcinoma. However, the need for histologic diagnosis in patients with tumor markers in the range of 5–100 mIU/mL is still controversial. Some experts believe that low elevation of βhCG is most consistent with a diagnosis of germinoma whereas others argue that low levels of βhCG can be secreted by embryonal carcinoma and immature teratoma elements as well and therefore all tumors with low levels of βhCG should be biopsied.

11.3 Histopathology

11.3.1 Germinoma

The classic germinoma is comprised of large monomorphous tumor cells that have central nuclei and large prominent nucleoli and are separated into lobules by thin fibrous septa. The tumor cells have abundant clear or vacuolated cytoplasm (reflecting high glycogen content) and distinct cell borders. Lymphocytic infiltration is a characteristic finding as well.

11.3.2 Yolk Sac Tumor

These tumors are characterized by large and polygonal cells with faint eosinophilic or clear cytoplasm and well-defined cytoplasmic borders.

Tufts of malignant cuboidal-to-columnar tumor cells surrounding central blood vessels, known as Schiller-Duval bodies, are common though not universal, and not a requirement for the diagnosis. Many different morphologic patterns can be encountered within the same tumor: *reticular* or *microcystic* pattern, *macrocystic* pattern, *polyvesicular vitelline* pattern, *endodermal sinus* pattern, *papillary* pattern, and *hepatoid* pattern.

11.3.3 Embryonal Carcinoma

Tumor cells are highly atypical and are generally larger and more pleomorphic, with oval-to-round nuclei and large single or multiple nucleoli. The malignant cells can be arranged in solid sheets, cords, papillae, or gland-like patterns. Necrosis is common and the mitotic rate is typically high.

11.3.4 Teratoma

Mature teratomas are made up of an admixture of differentiated, adult-type tissues from more than one germ cell layer. Skin and glial tissue are common ectodermal components and enteric, respiratory, or transitional type tissues account for endodermal derivation. Immature teratomas, by definition, contain varying amounts of incompletely differentiated tissues that resemble primitive embryonic tissues. Most commonly, the immature tissue shows neural differentiation with rosette or tubule formation (i.e., primitive or embryonic-type neuroepithelium). Increased mitoses and apoptosis are not features of mature tissue, and can be helpful clues to the identification of immature elements. Any amount of immature component, no matter how small, is sufficient to render the diagnosis of immature teratoma.

11.3.5 Choriocarcinoma

Choriocarcinomas are highly malignant GCTs that are extensively hemorrhagic and highly necrotic and comprised of two cell types: syncy-

tiotrophoblasts and cytotrophoblasts. Syncytiotrophoblasts are easily recognized as large multinucleated cells with smudged vesicular nuclei and dark eosinophilic-to-amphophilic cytoplasm. Cytotrophoblasts are more uniform and have single bland nuclei with vesicular chromatin and pale-to-amphophilic cytoplasm.

11.3.6 Ancillary Immunohistochemical Studies

Due to the limited amount of tumor specimen available for diagnosis, use of immunohistochemical stains is critical for diagnosis of CNS GCTs. βhCG and AFP are the most commonly used stains. βhCG strongly stains the syncytiotrophoblastic cells of choriocarcinoma as well as those intermixed with other germ cell tumors (Ho and Liu 1992; Inoue et al. 1987). OCT4 preferentially highlights germinomas and embryonal carcinomas and has the added advantage of being a nuclear marker allowing for easier interpretation. CD30 shows strong membranous staining in embryonal carcinomas while other GCTs, including germinomas, are negative. C-kit can also be exploited in the differential diagnosis of embryonal carcinoma versus germinoma as it shows strong and diffuse membranous staining in germinoma but focal or weak cytoplasmic staining in embryonal carcinomas (Hattab et al. 2004; Iczkowski et al. 2008; Takeshima et al. 2004). AFP has historically served as the marker of choice for yolk sac tumors. Staining, however, is often focal and patchy and generally varies among the different patterns of tumors. Additionally, abundant background staining is often observed (Mei et al. 2009). Glypican-3 is touted as a superior marker in diagnosing yolk sac tumors of the ovaries and testes. Glypican-3 offers more precise and easy to interpret staining characteristics as well as improved sensitivity (Zynger et al. 2010). Studies evaluating glypican-3 staining in CNS yolk sac tumors, however, are limited (Table 11.1).

Cytotrophoblastic cells often are weakly positive or negative for these markers. Additionally,

Table 11.1 Immunohistochemical markers used in diagnosis of germ cell tumors

	AFP	βhCG	OCT4	PLAP	SALL4	c-kit	CD30
Germinoma	–	±	+	+	+	+	–
Teratoma	+	–	–	–	±	±	–
Choriocarcinoma	–	+	–	±	±	–	–
Yolk sac tumor	+	–	–	±	+	–	–
Embryonal carcinoma	–	–	+	+	+	–	+

AFP alpha-fetoprotein, *βhCG* human chorionic gonadotropin-beta, *PLAP* placental alkaline phosphatase

cytokeratins can also be used to highlight choriocarcinomas.

11.4 Histogenesis

GCTs are thought to arise from progenitor germ cells, mainly due to the following facts: the germinoma component very closely resembles progenitor cells, intracranial GCTs resemble their extracranial counterparts morphologically and immunophenotypically, a single tumor can have multiple components (mixed GCTs) suggestive of differentiation of progenitor cells along various lines (embryonic and extraembryonic), and because none of the progenitor cells in the brain share any morphologic features with CNS GCTs. It is hypothesized that aberrant migration of the germ cell progenitors ventrally along the midline is responsible for the predominant midline location of these tumors throughout the body. Both testicular and CNS GCTs have been shown to have overexpression of wild-type p53 and MDM2 proteins with a low incidence of TP53 gene mutation and a moderate incidence of MDM2 gene amplification, which points towards a common origin of these tumors (Iwato et al. 2000a). Since p14[ARF], a protein coded by the *INK4a/ARF* gene locus, functions as a tumor suppressor and regulates the interaction between the MDM2 and p53 proteins by stimulating degradation of MDM2, Iwato et al. further tested for gene mutations in the *INK4a/ARF* gene in 21 CNS GCTs. They found 71% of tumors (90% of germinomas and 55% of NGGCTs) had either a homozygous deletion (14/15) or a frameshift mutation (1/15) in this gene, pointing towards a more central role for this protein in the development of CNS GCTs

(Iwato et al. 2000b). More evidence linking germ cell progenitors to CNS GCTs is the lack of methylation seen in gonadal and extragonadal GCTs, since the progenitor cells transiently lose methylation of imprinted genes during migration. Small nuclear ribonucleoprotein polypeptide N (*SNRPN*) is an imprinted gene with complete lack of methylation, which is common to GCTs and progenitor cells. However, Lee et al. showed that lack of methylation of *SNRPN* and other imprinted genes is also seen in neural stem cells in the brain, providing an alternate hypothesis about the origin of CNS GCTs (Lee et al. 2011).

11.5 Cytogenetics

The overwhelming majority of intracranial GCTs are sporadic; however, a few conditions, including Klinefelter syndrome and Down syndrome, show higher incidence. Based on the predisposition to GCTs in patients with Klinefelter syndrome, Okada and colleagues studied 25 CNS GCTs with fluorescent in situ hybridization (FISH) for X and Y chromosomes and other chromosomal abnormalities described in systemic GCTs (Okada et al. 2002). They found extra copies of the X chromosome in 23 of 25 cases with extra X chromosomes being hypomethylated in nearly all tumors irrespective of histology. This was suggestive of the potential role of X chromosomes in the etiology of these tumors (Okada et al. 2002). Schneider et al. performed chromosomal comparative genomic hybridization (CGH) analysis on tumor samples from 19 CNS GCT patients (ages newborn to 25 years; median age 11.5 years) and then compared these to the CGH profiles of gonadal and extragonadal GCTs. All 15 malignant CNS GCTs had chromosomal imbalance with the average number of imbalances being higher in NGGCTs than in germinomas and with the CGH profiles of CNS GCTS being identical to gonadal/extragonadal GCTs. Gain of 12p was the most commonly detected abnormality (11 of 19 tumors and 10 of 15 malignant CNS GCTs). Other chromosomal imbalances detected included 1q gain (1q 21–24) and 8q1121 gain (Schneider et al. 2006). In another study, chromosome 12 abnormalities, including 12p gain and isochromosome 12p formation were found at very high frequencies in CNS germinomas (96% and 57%, respectively), but only in 20–40% of cases in two other studies (Okada et al. 2002; Rickert et al. 2000; Hattab et al. 2006).

11.6 Gene Expression Profiling

Palmer et al. performed gene expression analysis on 27 pediatric malignant GCTs, including 3 CNS GCT (2 germinoma and 1 YST), and showed that malignant YSTs had a completely different gene expression signature than testicular seminomas. Self-renewing pluripotency genes (*Nanog*, *OCT3/4*, and *UTF*) were overexpressed in seminomas and genes responsible for tumor growth (cholecystokinin B receptor [*CCKBR*]) and differentiation (*KRT19*, *KRT8*, *GATA3*, and *GATA6*) and genes involved in WNT/β-catenin pathway were upregulated in YSTs. There were no significant differences in gene expression between CNS GCTs of similar histology arising at different sites and different ages within the pediatric age group. In addition, pediatric and adult testicular YSTs exhibited significantly different gene expression signatures, suggesting different biologic behavior (Palmer et al. 2008).

MicroRNAs (miRNAs) are responsible for controlling gene expression and also function as oncogenes as well as tumor suppressor genes within tumor cells. Palmer et al. studied miRNA profiles of 32 pediatric GCTs (gonadal and extragonadal), eight control samples, two adult testicular seminomas, and six GCT cell lines. In unsupervised hierarchical clustering analysis, all

pediatric GCT samples showed clear separation with seminomas, cell lines, YSTs, and embryonal carcinomas, all having clearly different miRNA expression profiles. There was no overlap between malignant and nonmalignant (mature and immature teratoma) GCTs on a heat map based on differentially expressed miRNAs. Nine of the top ten differentially expressed miRNAs belonged to two clusters (miRNA-371 and miRNA-302) and were overexpressed in malignant GCTs compared to nonmalignant GCTs. Similar to the gene expression profile, miRNA expression pattern was comparable in various histologic subtypes irrespective of patient age. Both of these miRNA clusters have been shown to be associated with human embryonic stem cells and their overexpression in turn regulates the expression of various transcription factors involved in oncogenesis and malignant progression. They further showed that YSTs and germinomas had significantly different miRNA expression profiles, with members of the miRNA-2302 cluster overexpressed in YSTs compared to germinomas, resulting in overexpression of transcription factors such as *GATA6*, *GATA3*, *SMARCA1*, and *SOX11*. Additionally, miRNA-451 and miRNA-144 were significantly overexpressed in intracranial compared to extracranial germinomas and miRNA-320, miRNA-487b, and miRNA-491-3p were significantly underexpressed (Palmer et al. 2010).

Murray et al. used TaqMan® quantitative reverse transcriptase polymerase chain reaction (qRT-PCR) to measure miRNA levels in the serum of a 4-year-old boy with a sacrococcygeal mixed GCT with a predominant YST component (serum AFP 82 ng/mL [420 kU/L]) at diagnosis and followed the levels during treatment. miRNA-71~373 and miRNA-302 were significantly overexpressed in the patient's serum when compared to three healthy controls. miRNA-372 and miRNA-373 levels were 703 and 192 times higher, respectively. The level of miRNA-372 dropped to 5.8-fold higher on day 73 (serum AFP 5.8 ng/mL), 2.2-fold higher on day 91 (serum AFP 6 ng/mL), and <1-fold higher on all subsequent follow-up time points (serum AFP <2 ng/mL) (Murray et al. 2011). Terashima and colleagues examined 32

CSF samples from 22 intracranial GCT patients for expression of miRNA-371~373 and miRNA-302~367 clusters. Significantly higher expression levels were found in the CSF of GCT patients compared to controls, as well as pretreatment samples compared to those collected during or after treatment. In addition, miRNA-373 expression was significantly higher in germinomas when compared to NGGCTs (Terashima et al. 2013). These two publications highlighted for the first time the potential for using miRNAs as diagnostic and/or therapeutic biomarkers for CNS GCTs.

11.7 Molecular Signaling Pathways and Targeted Therapies

In recent years, several tumor molecular analysis studies have been reported using next-generation sequencing technology. The Japanese intracranial GCT consortium performed whole exome sequencing (WES) on 33 CNS GCTs and found that *KIT* mutations were the most commonly found abnormality, especially in germinomas (Ichimura et al. 2013). Fukushima et al. screened 52 CNS GCTs for mutations in genes involved in the MAPK pathway and detected mutations only in *KIT* and *RAS* genes (Fukushima et al. 2013). These findings were validated by Wang et al., who performed WES through an international multi-institutional collaboration on 62 cases of CNS GCTs (29 germinomas, 25 NGGCT and 8 mixed GCT). In this study, the *KIT/RAS* signaling pathway was mutated in over 50% of cases, with mutations in *KIT* and *RAS* being mutually exclusive. *KIT* overexpression was seen in the majority of pure germinomas and rarely in NGGCT, consistent with the immunohistochemistry finding of c-kit expression in germinomas (Wang et al. 2014). This has made germinoma an attractive disease for the application of tyrosine kinase inhibitors.

Wang et al. also found somatic alterations in the AKT/mTOR pathway, corresponding with upregulation of AKT1 expression in 19% of patients. In addition, they also found recurrent somatic mutations in BCORL1, TP53, SPTA1, KDM2A, and LAMA4. Interestingly, the authors also identified a novel and rare germline variant in the Jumonji domain-containing (JMJD) gene in ten patients (nine from Japan, one from Hong Kong). JMJD germline variants were significantly enriched in the Japanese population in control cohorts and even more enriched (approximately fivefold) in Japanese CNS GCT patients (Wang et al. 2014). This finding is important given the significant increase in incidence of CNS GCT in Japan (Kamoshima and Sawamura 2010; Matsutani et al. 1997).

Osorio and colleagues reported on six patients with CNS GCTs (five pure germinomas and one mixed CNS GCT with predominant germinoma components) who were treated with dasatinib (KIT inhibitor) in an effort to avoid irradiation and/or to delay recurrence (Osorio et al. 2013). The study could not directly assess the efficacy of dasatinib in this population, since most patients received dasatinib while they were in a minimal residual disease state (i.e., no evaluable target lesions on imaging). However, only 33% of patients received irradiation in conventional dosing, suggesting a possible role for targeted therapy with KIT inhibitors in combination with chemotherapy with or without irradiation (Osorio et al. 2013).

11.8 Treatment

11.8.1 Staging

Since CNS GCTs tend to spread through the subarachnoid space (approximately 15–20% of cases), MRI of the brain and spine with and without contrast and CSF evaluation for malignant cells is used for staging disseminated disease. Lumbar CSF and not ventricular CSF cytology has been traditionally preferred for staging purposes. Similar to the modified Chang staging system for medulloblastoma, M0 stage is assigned to patients with no evidence of tumor dissemination on brain and spine MRI, M1 for patients in whom only CSF cytology is positive with a negative brain and spine MRI, M2 for patients with macroscopic dissemination on the brain MRI and a negative spine MRI, M3 for patients with macroscopic spinal metastases, and M4 for patients with extraneural spread to distant organs, such as bones.

11.8.2 Role of Surgery in CNS Germ Cell Tumors

Pineal GCTs often present with obstructive hydrocephalus requiring an endoscopic third ventriculostomy (ETV) or a ventriculoperitoneal (VP) shunt placement. It is occasionally possible to avoid insertion of a VP shunt after an initial external ventricular drain placement if chemotherapy is initiated expeditiously since germ cell tumors are often sensitive to chemotherapy allowing sufficient shrinkage for normal flow of CSF. Due to the strategic location of pineal GCTs, and no significant differences documented in outcome related to the extent of surgery, biopsy is preferred over aggressive surgical resection as the initial approach; biopsy may be performed at the time of ETV or VP shunt placement (Sawamura et al. 1997). There is definitely a role for second-look surgery in patients with incomplete response to chemotherapy who achieve normalization of tumor markers, since residual masses post-therapy can often be necrosis and fibrosis devoid of tumor or even mature teratoma, a phenomenon known as "the growing teratoma syndrome" (O'Callaghan et al. 1997). It is important to distinguish this entity from residual active or progressive malignancy. Second-look surgery may also help to better assess any residual malignant elements.

11.8.3 Therapeutic Strategies for Intracranial Germinoma

The optimal management of germinomas remains controversial and to date a standard therapeutic strategy has not been established.

11.8.4 Role of Radiation Therapy

Germinomas are exquisitely radiosensitive and treatment with craniospinal irradiation (CSI) plus primary site boost to 50 Gy has been shown to result in 5- and 10-year overall survival (OS) rates ranging from 86% to 100% (Shibamoto et al. 1988; Aoyama et al. 1998). However, undesirable side effects including neurocognitive decline and endocrine and gonadal dysfunction have been consistently documented in these children (Spiegler et al. 2004). In patients with radiographic or cytological evidence of metastasis, CSI continues to be a current recommendation in many centers. Although doses of 30–36 Gy CSI have been used successfully by different investigators (Maity et al. 2000; Kretschmar et al. 2007), the Societé Internationale d'Oncologie Pédiatrique (SIOP) CNS GCT 96 study showed similarly good outcome with a reduced dose of 24 Gy CSI with 16 Gy additional boost to the primary and metastatic sites (Calaminus et al. 2013).

In localized germinoma, recent efforts have been directed towards reducing and redefining the appropriate volume and dose of radiation therapy (RT) to optimize disease control while decreasing the risk of late morbidity. In the aforementioned SIOP CNS GCT 96 study, localized germinoma patients were also treated with 24 Gy CSI with an additional 16 Gy boost to the primary site and had a 5-year progression-free survival (PFS) of 97% (Calaminus et al. 2013). Additionally, there have been several clinical studies showing low risk of spinal relapse after whole brain irradiation (WBI) or whole ventricular irradiation (WVI), supporting the thought that CSI may not necessarily be needed in treatment of localized germinoma (Khatua et al. 2010; Matsutani 2010a). Some data suggest that 45 Gy may be the optimal upper dose limit, although the lowest RT dose that can be delivered without increasing failure rates has not been defined (Rogers et al. 2005). Twenty-one of 51 patients with localized germinoma were treated with WVI to 40 Gy alone in one study. No relapses were noted in these patients over a period of 10 years (Hardenbergh et al. 1997). A recent study evaluating 26 patients with localized germinoma who received a further dose reduction of WVI to 30 Gy showed a 5-year OS of 100%, even without chemotherapy (Yen et al. 2010).

11.8.5 Role of Chemotherapy

The largest chemotherapy only experience stems from the International CNS Germ Cell Tumor Studies. In the first study, 22 of 45 CNS germinoma patients relapsed on this chemotherapy only regimen (Balmaceda et al. 1996). In the second study, 19 germinoma patients were treated with an intensified cisplatin- and cyclophosphamide-based regimen. The 5-year event-free survival (EFS) and OS rates were unsatisfactory at 47 ± 2.3% and 68 ± 2.2%, respectively, with unacceptable morbidity and mortality (four deaths), predominantly in patients with diabetes insipidus (Kellie et al. 2004). Patients with central diabetes insipidus show significant variations in sodium level during hyperhydration with cisplatin/ifosfamide and therefore have an increased risk of neurological complications (Afzal et al. 2008). The third study used carboplatin/etoposide alternating with cyclophosphamide/etoposide for germinoma patients. This chemotherapy regimen was well tolerated with toxicity mainly being hematologic; survival was very similar to the first two studies but was inferior to studies using either RT alone or a combination of chemotherapy and RT (da Silva et al. 2010).

11.8.6 Role of Chemoradiotherapy

Due to the high failure rate of chemotherapy only regimens and the deleterious effects of RT on the developing brain, several investigators have tried to combine chemotherapy with reduced dose and volume RT. The SIOP CNS GCT-96 trial enrolled a total of 235 patients, with 82 patients (65 with localized disease) receiving chemotherapy (carboplatin and etoposide alternating with etoposide and ifosfamide for a total of four cycles) followed by irradiation. Those with localized disease received chemotherapy followed by 40 Gy focal irradiation while patients with metastatic disease received the same chemotherapy followed by CSI to 24 Gy plus a 16 Gy boost to the primary site. 5-year PFS for localized and metastatic patients was 88% and 100%, respectively. Seven

of 65 patients with localized disease experienced a relapse; 6 of 7 patients had ventricular recurrence outside the primary radiotherapy field (Calaminus et al. 2013). In the Japanese cooperative group study, 16 of 23 patients with localized germinoma relapsed within the ventricular system after having been treated with upfront chemotherapy followed by 24 Gy involved field radiation (IFR) (Matsutani 2010a). The French national group (SFOP) published similar results using IFR, with a relapse rate of 16%, mostly in the ventricular system (Alapetite et al. 2008).

This unacceptable rate and pattern of relapse prompted extending the field of RT to include the ventricles. In a publication by Haas-Kogan et al. on 41 patients with localized germinoma, none of the 18 patients who received WVI with a median dose to the ventricles of 32.4 Gy (range 19.8–50.4 Gy) relapsed (Haas-Kogan et al. 2003). At our institution, 19 patients with localized germinoma received WVI to 21.6–25.5 Gy with a boost to 30–30.6 Gy following chemotherapy with carboplatin and etoposide. Our 3-year PFS and OS from that study was 89.5% and 100%, respectively (Khatua et al. 2010).

Treatment of bifocal (pineal and suprasellar) germinomas remains highly controversial with patients subjected to CSI as in the recently closed COG Study, ACNS0232. Data support the contention that bifocal germinomas can be effectively treated with WVI and CSI could be avoided. Six patients with bifocal germinomas and diabetes insipidus were reported as having no recurrences after a median follow-up of 48.1 months after initial chemotherapy followed by WVI (Lafay-Cousin et al. 2006). Another study reported 100% OS at 40 months after initial chemotherapy plus extended focal radiotherapy to the tumor bed plus 1.5 cm margin and WVI of 30 Gy (Huang et al. 2008). Larger prospective trials are required to evaluate these initial outcomes in using chemotherapy along with reduced-dose RT strategies.

Our institutional practice is to treat germinoma patients with four cycles of chemotherapy with carboplatin and etoposide followed by WVI to 21.0–23.4 Gy and a boost to the primary tumor site to a total dose of 30 Gy.

11.8.7 Therapeutic Strategies for Nongerminomatous Germ Cell Tumors (NGGCTs)

The treatment of NGGCTs of the CNS involves a combination of chemotherapy and irradiation; however, the exact regimen including the specific chemotherapeutic drugs and RT dose and volume still remains variable and undefined.

11.8.8 Role of Chemotherapy

Chemotherapy regimens utilizing cisplatin, etoposide, and either ifosfamide or cyclophosphamide have greatly improved the outcomes of patients with GCTs over the last few decades (Williams et al. 1987; Einhorn 1986; Einhorn and Williams 1980). Responses to a variety of chemotherapy agents have been achieved, including vinblastine, etoposide, bleomycin, and carboplatin (Allen et al. 1985, 1987; Chang et al. 1995; Matsukado et al. 1986; Patel et al. 1992). In the Second International CNS GCT Study Group Protocol, 16 of 17 assessable patients achieved a complete or a partial response to two courses of chemotherapy (Kellie et al. 2004). Robertson et al. treated 18 patients with four cycles of platinum-based chemotherapy followed by RT and additional chemotherapy. Nine of 12 patients demonstrated objective responses to neoadjuvant chemotherapy (Robertson et al. 1997). The German cooperative group treated patients with two cycles of cisplatin, etoposide, and bleomycin, followed by RT and two cycles of cisplatin, vinblastine, and ifosfamide. Eighteen of 22 patients who received >400 mg/m^2 of cisplatin were long-term survivors as compared to 5/15 who received <400 mg/m^2 (Calaminus et al. 2004). Carboplatin regimens have shown similar efficacies as compared to cisplatin regimens with the added benefit of easier outpatient administration and less toxicity (Robertson et al. 1997; Baranzelli 1999; Calaminus et al. 1994). The recently completed COG ACNS0121 trial for NGGCT patients used a combination of carboplatin/etoposide alternating with ifosfamide/etoposide. With 104 patients enrolled (and central

imaging review performed in 84 patients), the response rate after three cycles of neoadjuvant chemotherapy was reported to be 90% and no unexpected toxicities were observed (Goldman et al. 2015). Chemotherapy only strategies, despite resulting in high response rates, did not provide a durable PFS in NGGCT patients (Balmaceda et al. 1996; Kellie et al. 2004; da Silva et al. 2010).

11.8.9 Role of Radiation Therapy

Radiation therapy plays an important role in the treatment of NGGCT. However, regimens that use exclusively RT, including CSI to 36 Gy with boost treatment of the primary site to 54 Gy, achieve 5-year survival rates of only 20–40%. Without the added benefit of chemotherapy, most patients relapse within 18 months of diagnosis (Matsutani et al. 1997; Jennings et al. 1985; Dearnaley et al. 1990; Hoffman et al. 1991).

11.8.10 Role of Chemoradiotherapy

Combined modality therapy including chemotherapy and RT is the current standard of care. Since CSI and WBI are associated with neurocognitive and neuroendocrine dysfunction, ototoxicity and secondary malignancies (Constine et al. 1993; Copeland et al. 1985; Mulhern et al. 1998), minimizing exposure to RT by stratifying patients according to risk of disease progression after combined modality therapy has been the hallmark of international clinical trial designs for NGGCT. Risk classification has been based on a variety of factors including histology, degree of tumor marker elevation at diagnosis, and response to chemotherapy (Matsutani et al. 1997; Fuller et al. 1994; Gobel et al. 2000; Matsutani 2010b; Chen et al. 2010).

The SIOP CNS GCT-96 trial enrolled 172 patients. Those with localized disease ($n = 135$) at diagnosis received four courses of chemotherapy with cisplatin, ifosfamide, and etoposide, followed by IFR to 54 Gy. Those with metastatic disease ($n = 37$) received the same chemotherapy regimen followed by CSI to 30 Gy and boost to the primary site. At a median follow-up of 47 months, the reported PFS for the localized and metastatic patients were 69% and 64%, respectively. Of the 34 patients with residual disease after induction chemotherapy, almost half (47%) relapsed and had a much worse PFS (37 ± 12%) than those patients in complete response post-induction (86 ± 4%). Lack of response to induction chemotherapy was a significant adverse prognostic factor in this study (Calaminus et al. 2008, 2010). In addition, patients with AFP of ≥1000 ng/mL in serum and/or CSF (n = 21) had a significantly worse outcome (PFS = 0.35 ± 12%).

Matsutani et al. from the Japanese GCT study group showed that patients with NGGCTs with predominantly germinoma or teratoma elements (Japanese "intermediate group") had 10-year PFS and OS rates of 81.5% and 89.3%, respectively, when treated with five cycles of carboplatin and etoposide followed by WVI to 30 Gy and tumor bed irradiation to 54 Gy. Patients with predominantly malignant germ cell tumor elements (embryonal carcinoma, yolk sac tumor, choriocarcinoma) formed the poor prognosis group and were treated with ICE (ifosfamide, cisplatin, and etoposide) and concurrent CSI. They received additional chemotherapy for five cycles. The 10-year OS and PFS rates were 58.8% and 62.7%, respectively. Patients who achieved a complete response to chemotherapy enjoyed a 10-year PFS of 94.7% compared to 62.2% for patients with less than complete response (Matsutani 2010b).

The recently completed COG trial, ACNS0121, utilized 36 Gy CSI with IFR following six cycles of chemotherapy with carboplatin/etoposide alternating with ifosfamide/etoposide, and resulted in a 5-year EFS and OS of 84% ± 4% and 93% ± 3%, respectively (Goldman et al. 2015). The complete response and partial response rate for this induction regimen was 69%. In this study, increased serum or CSF AFP (≥10 IU/L or within institutional normal rates), but not βhCG, approached statistically significant negative association with EFS (p = 0.063). At a median follow-up of 5 years, 16 patients either recurred or progressed with 10 of 16 being local failures.

Our institutional practice is to treat NGGCT patients with three cycles of carboplatin/etoposide alternating with three cycles of ifosfamide/etoposide followed by response-based irradiation. Patients with localized disease and a complete radiographic and tumor marker response to neoadjuvant chemotherapy receive whole ventricular irradiation to 36 Gy plus an 18 Gy boost to the primary tumor site. Patients with metastatic disease at diagnosis receive full dose CSI (36 Gy) and an 18 Gy additional boost to the primary tumor bed and sites of bulky disease. Patients who fail to achieve a complete response (elevated tumor markers or residual malignant tumor) are treated with myeloablative chemotherapy and autologous hematopoietic progenitor cell rescue (AuHCR) before proceeding to CSI.

11.8.11 Role of Marrow-Ablative Chemotherapy with Autologous Hematopoietic Progenitor Cell Rescue in CNS Germ Cell Tumors

High-dose marrow-ablative chemotherapy with AuHCR has been employed in high risk CNS GCT with recurrent/progressive and refractory disease. Modak et al. reported their data on 21 CNS GCT patients with relapse and progression despite previous chemotherapy and radiotherapy. Most patients were treated with thiotepa-based high-dose chemotherapy regimens followed by AuHCR. OS and EFS for the entire group were 57% and 52%, respectively. Seven of nine patients with germinoma and four of 12 patients with NGGCT remain alive at a median of 35 months (Modak et al. 2004). The SFOP group also reported 14 patients with recurrent germinoma and 10 patients with NGGCT treated with myeloablative chemotherapy; they showed no clear benefit for germinoma patients but a clear survival benefit for NGGCT patients (Bouffet 2000).

Conclusion

Although high survival rates have been achieved in CNS germ cell tumors, the management of these tumors remains controversial. A combined modality approach using lower doses of RT has been shown to provide equivalent survival in germinoma and improved survival in NGGCT patients when compared to RT alone. However, the exact doses and fields of RT still remain undecided and larger prospective, preferably randomized, clinical trials are needed to answer these questions.

References

Afzal S, Wherrett D, Bartels U, Tabori U et al (2008) Challenges and difficulties in management of patients with intracranial germ cell tumor having diabetes insipidus treated with cisplatin and or ifosfamide based chemotherapy. Neuro-Oncology 10:417

Alapetite C, Patte C, Frappaz D, et al (2008) Intracranial germinoma treated with primary chemotherapy followed by focal radiation treatment: the SFOP-90 experience. Final analysis. 40th Congress of the International Society of Paediatric Oncology Berlin, Germany

Allen JC, Bosl G, Walker R (1985) Chemotherapy trials in recurrent primary intracranial germ cell tumors. J Neuro-Oncol 3(2):147–152

Allen JC, Kim JH, Packer RJ (1987) Neoadjuvant chemotherapy for newly diagnosed germ-cell tumors of the central nervous system. J Neurosurg 67(1):65–70

Aoyama H, Shirato H, Kakuto Y, Inakoshi H et al (1998) Pathologically-proven intracranial germinoma treated with radiation therapy. Radiother Oncol 47(2):201–205

Balmaceda C, Heller G, Rosenblum M, Diez B et al (1996) Chemotherapy without irradiation—a novel approach for newly diagnosed CNS germ cell tumors: results of an international cooperative trial. The First International Central Nervous System Germ Cell Tumor Study. J Clin Oncol 14:2908–2915

Baranzelli C (1999) Carboplatin-based chemotherapy (CT) and focal radiation (RT) in primary cerebral germ cell tumor (GCT): A French Society of pediatric Oncology (SFOP) experience. Proc Am Soc Clin Oncol 18:140A

Bouffet E (2000) High dose etoposide and thiotepa for refractory and recurrent malignant intracranial germ cell tumors, No. 38. at 9th International Symposium on Pediatric Neuro-Oncology. San Francisco, CA, USA

Calaminus G, Bamberg M, Barenzelli MC, Benoit Y et al (1994) Intracranial germ cell tumors: a comprehensive update of the European data. Neuropediatrics 25(1):26–32

Calaminus G, Bamberg M, Jurgens H, Kortmann RD et al (2004) Impact of surgery, chemotherapy and irradiation on long-term outcome of intracranial malignant non-germinomatous germ cell tumors: results of the German Cooperative Trial MAKEI 89. Klin Padiatr 216:141–149

Calaminus G, Frappaz D, Kortmann RD et al (2008) Localized and metastatic non-germinoma treated according to SIOP CNS GCT 96 protocol. Update on risk profiles and outcome. [abstract GCT 06]. Neuro-Oncology 10:369–537

Calaminus G, Nicholson J, Frappaz D, Garre M et al (2010) Localized and metastatic non-germinoma (NGGCT) treated according to SIOP CNS GCT 96 protocol. Update on risk profiles and outcome. [abstract GCT 06]. Neuro Oncol 12(6):ii28

Calaminus G, Kortmann R, Worch J, Nicholson JC et al (2013) SIOP CNS GCT 96: final report of outcome of a prospective, multinational nonrandomized trial for children and adults with intracranial germinoma, comparing craniospinal irradiation alone with chemotherapy followed by focal primary site irradiation for patients with localized disease. Neuro-Oncology 15(6):788–796

Chang TK, Wong TT, Hwang B (1995) Combination chemotherapy with vinblastine, bleomycin, cisplatin, and etoposide (VBPE) in children with primary intracranial germ cell tumors. Med Pediatr Oncol 24(6):368–372

Chen MJ, Santos AS, Sakuraba RK, Lopes CP et al (2010) Intensity-modulated and 3D-conformal radiotherapy for whole-ventricular irradiation as compared with conventional whole-brain irradiation in the management of localized central nervous system germ cell tumors. Int J Radiat Oncol Biol Phys 76(2):608–614

Constine LS, Woolf PD, Caan D, Mick G et al (1993) Hypothalamic-pituitary dysfunction after radiation for brain tumors. N Engl J Med 328(2):87–94

Copeland DR, Fletcher JM, Pfeferbaum LB, Jaffe N et al (1985) Neuropsychological sequelae of childhood cancer in long-term survivors. Pediatrics 75(4):745–753

Dearnaley DP, A'Hern RP, Whittaker S, Bloom HJ (1990) Pineal and CNS germ cell tumors: Royal Marsden Hospital experience 1962–1987. Int J Radiat Oncol Biol Phys 18(4):773–781

Dolecek TA, Propp JM, Stroup NE, Kruchko C (2012) CBTRUS statistical report: primary brain and central nervous system tumors diagnosed in the United States in 2005-2009. Neuro-Oncology 14(Suppl 5):v1–v49

Einhorn LH (1986) Cancer of the testis: a new paradigm. Hosp Pract (Off Ed) 21(4):165–172. 175–178

Einhorn LH, Williams SD (1980) Chemotherapy of disseminated testicular cancer. A random prospective study. Cancer 46(6):1339–1344

Fujimaki T, Matsutani M (2005) The Japanese Pediatric Brain Tumor Study Group. HCGβ-producing germinoma: Analysis of Japanese Pediatric Brain Tumor Study Group results. Neurooncology 7:518. abstr G5

Fukushima S, Otsuka A, Suzuki T, et al (eds) (2013) Mutually exclusive mutations of c-kit and RAS are associated with chromosomal instability in primary intracranial germinomas. 3rd International CNS Germ Cell Tumor Symposium, Cambridge, UK

Fuller BG, Kapp DS, Cox R (1994) Radiation therapy of pineal region tumors: 25 new cases and a review of 208 previously reported cases. Int J Radiat Oncol Biol Phys 28(1):229–245

Gobel U, Schneider DT, Calaminus G, Hass RJ et al (2000) Germ-cell tumors in childhood and adolescence. GPOH MAKEI and the MAHO study groups. Ann Oncol 11(3):263–271

Goldman S, Bouffet E, Fisher PG, Allen JC et al (2015) Phase II trial assessing the ability of neoadjuvant chemotherapy with or without second-look surgery to eliminate measurable disease for nongerminomatous germ cell tumors: a children's Oncology Group Study. J Clin Oncol 33(22):2464–2471

Haas-Kogan DA, Missett BT, Wara WM, Donaldson SS et al (2003) Radiation therapy for intracranial germ cell tumors. Int J Radiat Oncol Biol Phys 56:511–518

Hardenbergh PH, Golden J, Billet A, Scott RM et al (1997) Intracranial germinoma: the case for lower dose radiation therapy. Int J Radiat Oncol Biol Phys 39:419–426

Hattab EM, Tu P, Wilson JD, Cheng L (2004) C-kit and HER2/neu expression in primary intracranial germinoma (abstract). J Neuropathol Exp Neurol 63(5):547

Hattab EM, Zhang SB, Wilson JD, Tu PH, Cheng L (2006) Chromosome 12p abnormalities in germinoma of the central nervous system: A FISH analysis of 23 cases (abstract). Brain Pathol 16(Supplement 1):S155

Ho DM, Liu HC (1992) Primary intracranial germ cell tumor. Pathologic study of 51 patients. Cancer 70(6):1577–1584

Hoffman HJ, Otsubo H, Hendrick EB, Humphreys RP et al (1991) Intracranial germ-cell tumors in children. J Neurosurg 74(4):545–551

Huang PI, Chen YW, Wong TT, Lee YY et al (2008) Extended focal radiotherapy of 30Gy alone for intracranial synchronous bifocal germinoma: single institute experience. Childs Nerv Syst 24:315–321

Ichimura K, Fukushima S, Totoki Y, et al (eds) (2013) Exome sequencing of intracranial germ cell tumours. 3rd International CNS Germ Cell Tumor Symposium; Cambridge, UK

Iczkowski KA, Butler SL, Shanks JH, Hossain D et al (2008) Trials of new germ cell immunohistochemical stains in 93 extragonadal and metastatic germ cell tumors. Hum Pathol 39(2):275–281

Inoue HK, Naganuma H, Ono N (1987) Pathobiology of intracranial germ-cell tumors: immunochemical, immunohistochemical, and electron microscopic investigations. J Neuro-Oncol 5(2):105–115

Iwato M, Tachibana O, Tohma Y, Nitta H et al (2000a) Molecular analysis for p53 and mdm2 in intracranial germ cell tumors. Acta Neuropathol 99(1):21–25

Iwato M, Tachibana O, Tohma Y et al (2000b) Alterations of the INK4a/ARF locus in human intracranial germ cell tumors. Cancer Res 60:2113–2115

Jennings MT, Gelman R, Hochberg F (1985) Intracranial germ-cell tumors: natural history and pathogenesis. J Neurosurg 63(2):155–167

Kamoshima Y, Sawamura Y (2010) Update on current standard treatments in central nervous system germ cell tumors. Curr Opin Neurol 23(6):571–575

Kellie SJ, Boyce H, Dunkel IJ, Diez B et al (2004) Intensive cisplatin and cyclophosphamide-based chemotherapy without radiotherapy for intracranial germinomas: failure of a primary chemotherapy approach. Pediatr Blood Cancer 43:126–133

Khatua S, Dhall G, O'Neil S, Jubran R et al (2010) Treatment of primary CNS germinomatous germ cell tumors with chemotherapy prior to reduced dose whole ventricular and local boost irradiation. Pediatr Blood Cancer 55(1):42–46

Kretschmar C, Kleinberg L, Greenberg M, Burger P et al (2007) Pre-radiation chemotherapy with response-based radiation therapy in children with central nervous germ cell tumors: a report from the Children's Oncology group. Pediatr Blood Cancer 48:285–291

Lafay-Cousin L, Millar B-A, Mabbot D, Spiegler B et al (2006) Limited-field radiation for bifocal germinoma. Int J Radiat Oncol Biol Phys 65:486–492

Lee SH, Appleby V, Jeyapalan JN, Palmer RD et al (2011) Variable methylation of the imprinted gene, SNRPN, supports a relationship between intracranial germ cell tumours and neural stem cells. J Neuro-Oncol 101(3):419–428

Maity A, Shu HK, Janss A, Belasco JB et al (2000) Craniospinal radiation in the treatment of biopsy-proven intracranial germinomas: twenty five years experience in a single center. Int J Radiat Oncol Biol Phys 46:1171–1176

Matsukado Y, Abe H, Tanaka R, Kobayashi T et al (1986) Cisplatin, vinblastine and bleomycin (PVB) combination chemotherapy in the treatment of intracranial malignant germ cell tumors—a preliminary report of a phase II study—The Japanese Intracranial Germ Cell Tumor Study Group. Gan No Rinsho 32(11):1387–1393

Matsutani M (2004) Clinical management of primary central nervous system germ cell tumors. Semin Oncol 31:676–683

Matsutani M (2010a) Long-term followup of germinomas treated by ventricular irradiation with 24 Gy and concurrently administered carboplatin and etoposide chemotherapy. [abstract GCT 02]. Neuro Oncol 12(6):ii28

Matsutani M (2010b) Excellent 10-year's OS & PFS of patients with non-germinomatous germ cell tumors treated by surgery, radiation and chemotherapy. Neuro-oncology 112(6):ii28. (abstr GCT 03)

Matsutani M, Sano K, Takakura K, Fujimaki T et al (1997) Primary intracranial germ cell tumors: a clinical analysis of 153 histologically verified cases. J Neurosurg 86(3):446–455

Mei K, Liu A, Allan RW, Wang P et al (2009) Diagnostic utility of SALL4 in primary germ cell tumors of the central nervous system: a study of 77 cases. Mod Pathol 22(12):1628–1636

Modak S, Gardner S, Dunkel IJ, Balmaceda C et al (2004) Thiotepa-based high-dose chemotherapy with autologous stem-cell rescue in patients with recurrent or progressive CNS germ cell tumors. J Clin Oncol 22(10):1934–1943

Mulhern RK, Kepner JL, Thomas PR, Armstrong FD et al (1998) Neuropsychologic functioning of survivors of childhood medulloblastoma randomized to receive conventional or reduced-dose craniospinal irradiation: a Pediatric Oncology Group study. J Clin Oncol 16(5):1723–1728

Murray MJ, Halsall DJ, Hook CE, Williams DM et al (2011) Identification of microRNAs from the miR-371~373 and miR-302 clusters as potential serum biomarkers of malignant germ cell tumors. Am J Clin Pathol 135(1):119–125

O'Callaghan AM, Katapodis O, Ellison DW et al (1997) The growing teratoma syndrome in a nongerminomatous germ cell tumor of the pineal gland: a case report and review. Cancer 80(5):942–947

Okada Y, Nishikawa R, Matsutani M, Louis DN (2002) Hypomethylated X chromosome gain and rare isochromosome 12p in diverse intracranial germ cell tumors. J Neuropathol Exp Neurol 61(6):531–538

Osorio DS, Finlay JL, Dhall G, Goldman S et al (2013) Feasibility of dasatinib in children and adolescents with new or recurrent central nervous system germinoma. Pediatr Blood Cancer 60(9):E100–E102

Palmer RD, Barbosa-Morais NL, Gooding EL, Muralidhar B et al (2008) Pediatric malignant germ cell tumors show characteristic transcriptome profiles. Cancer Res 68(11):4239–4247

Palmer RD, Murray MJ, Saini HK, van Dongen S et al (2010) Malignant germ cell tumors display common microRNA profiles resulting in global changes in expression of messenger RNA targets. Cancer Res 70(7):2911–2923

Patel SR, Buckner JC, Sminthson WA, Scheithauer BW et al (1992) Cisplatin-based chemotherapy in primary central nervous system germ cell tumors. J Neuro-Oncol 12(1):47–52

Rickert CH, Simon R, Bergmann M, Dockhorn-Dworniczak B, Paulus W (2000) Comparative genomic hybridization in pineal germ cell tumors. J Neuropathol Exp Neurol 59(9):815–821

Robertson PL, DaRosso RC, Allen JC (1997) Improved prognosis of intracranial non-germinoma germ cell tumors with multimodality therapy. J Neuro-Oncol 32(1):71–80

Rogers SJ, Mosleh-Shirazi MA, Saran FH (2005) Radiotherapy of localized intracranial germinoma: time to sever historical ties? Lancet Oncol 6:509–519

Rosenblum MK, Nakazato Y, Matsutani M (2007) CNS germ cell tumors. In: Louis DNO, Hiroko O, Wiestler OD, Cavenee WK (eds) WHO classification of tumours of the central nervous system, 4th edn. IARC Press, Lyon, pp 197–204

Sawamura Y, de Tribolet N, Ishi N, Abe H (1997) Management of primary intracranial germinomas: diagnostic surgery or radical resection? J Neurosurg 87:262–266

Schneider DT, Zahn S, Sievers S, Alemazkour K et al (2006) Molecular genetic analysis of central nervous system germ cell tumors with comparative genomic hybridization. Mod Pathol 19(6):864–873

Shibamoto Y, Abe M, Yamashita J, Takahashi M et al (1988) Treatment results of intracranial germinoma as a function of the irradiated volume. Int J Radiat Oncol Biol Phys 15(2):285–290

da Silva NS, Cappellano AM, Diez B, Cavalhiero S et al (2010) Primary chemotherapy for intracranial germ cell tumors : results of the Third International Germ Cell Tumor Study. Pediatr Blood Cancer 54:377–383

Spiegler BJ, Bouffet E, Greenberg ML, Rutka JT et al (2004) Change in neurocognitive functioning after treatment with cranial radiation in childhood. J Clin Oncol 22:706–713

Takeshima H, Kaji M, Uchida H, Hirano H, Kuratsu J (2004) Expression and distribution of c-kit receptor and its ligand in human CNS germ cell tumors: a useful histological marker for the diagnosis of germinoma. Brain Tumor Pathol 21(1):13–16

Terashima KS, Luan J, Yu A, Suzuki T, et al (eds) (2013) microRNA 371–373 and 302A in cerebrospinal fluid are potential tumor-derived biomarkers for intracranial germ cell tumors. 3rd International CNS Germ Cell Tumor Symposium. Cambridge, UK

Wang L, Yamaguchi S, Burstein MD, Terashima K et al (2014) Novel somatic and germline mutations in intracranial germ cell tumours. Nature 511(7508):241–245

Watanabe S, Aihara Y, Kikuno A, Sato T et al (2012) A highly sensitive and specific chemiluminescent enzyme immunoassay for placental alkaline phosphatase in the cerebrospinal fluid of patients with intracranial germinomas. Pediatr Neurosurg 48(3):141–145

Williams SD, Stablein DM, Einhorn LH, Muggia FM et al (1987) Immediate adjuvant chemotherapy versus observation with treatment at relapse in pathological stage II testicular cancer. N Engl J Med 317(23):1433–1438

Yen SH, Chen YW, Huang PI, Wong TT et al (2010) Optimal treatment for intracranial germinoma: can we lower radiation dose without chemotherapy? Int J Radiat Oncol Biol Phys 77(4):980–987

Zynger DL, McCallum JC, Luan C, Chou PM, Yang XJ (2010) Glypican 3 has a higher sensitivity than alpha-fetoprotein for testicular and ovarian yolk sac tumour: immunohistochemical investigation with analysis of histological growth patterns. Histopathology 56(6):750–757

Childhood Craniopharyngioma

12

Thomas E. Merchant

12.1 Introduction

Craniopharyngioma is a unique brain tumor characterized by its consistent midline location and intimate association with the hypothalamic pituitary axis, visual pathways, and central cerebrovasculature. Children diagnosed with craniopharyngioma commonly present with endocrine deficiencies, visual deficits, headaches, and, in more advanced cases, neurological deficits affecting cranial nerves and long-tracts. The more advanced presentations include extensive tumor with mass effect or obstruction of CSF flow. The debilitating effects of this tumor are often noted in young children prior to diagnosis when signs of increased intracranial pressure are overlooked and vision loss occurs. The extent of tumor and its clinical impact affect treatment and prognosis, including both tumor control rates and functional outcomes. The tumor is comprised of solid and cystic components, the latter often responsible for the signs and symptoms observed at presentation.

In North America, the incidence of craniopharyngioma is stable among diverse geographic groups and races with an age adjusted incidence of 0.1 per 100,000 based on the 2000 United States (US) standard population, with a slightly higher incidence of 0.12 for those ages 0–14 or 0–19 years and 0.13 for those ages 55–64 and 65–74 years. The total number of new pediatric cases annually within the US is estimated to be approximately 160 for children ages 0–19 years (Ostrom et al. 2015) (Fig. 12.1). The rarity of this tumor is an important consideration. Few centers have significant experience in the treatment of craniopharyngioma. This fact is made evident by the small numbers in institutional series that describe experiences over many decades (Kiehna and Merchant 2010). By WHO criteria, craniopharyngioma is a grade I tumor and includes both adamantinomatous (ACP) and papillary (PCP) subtypes. The latter is most commonly seen in adults. Despite its designation as a catastrophic disease of childhood with the associated morbidity and mortality, craniopharyngioma is usually not included among cancer center statistics.

12.2 Craniopharyngioma Biology

Craniopharyngioma arises in the sellar region, and is thought to be derived from remnants of the primordium of the anterior pituitary. There are two subtypes of craniopharyngioma: adamantinomatous and papillary. ACP occurs mainly in children under 15 years of age. PCP occurs in adults between the ages of 50 and 74 years. The cell of origin of human ACP remains unknown (Martinez-Barbera 2015).

T. E. Merchant
Department of Radiation Oncology, St. Jude
Children's Research Hospital, Memphis, TN, USA
e-mail: thomas.merchant@stjude.org

© Springer International Publishing AG, part of Springer Nature 2018
A. Gajjar et al. (eds.), *Brain Tumors in Children*, https://doi.org/10.1007/978-3-319-43205-2_12

Fig. 12.1 Annual incidence of craniopharyngioma in the US based on SEER 2008–2012

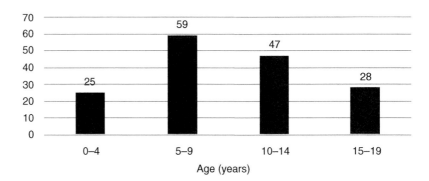

The biology of ACP is understood in the context of the Wnt signal transduction pathway. Wnt signaling is critical in embryonic development, differentiation of pluripotent stem cells, and proliferation of embryonic stem cells, and is known to be involved in carcinogenesis (Anastas and Moon 2013; van Amerongen and Nusse 2009). The pathway begins with the binding of the Wnt ligand to the membrane bound protein Frizzled (Fz). Binding leads to the stabilization of β-catenin. β-Catenin is maintained in the cells at low levels in a complex of proteins. The absence of Wnt causes β-catenin to be degraded though ubiquitination. Stable β-catenin is translocated to the nucleus and induces the expression of target genes, such as *CMYC* and *CCND1* (Serman et al. 2014). The hallmark of ACP is clusters of cells with nuclear-cytoplasmic accumulation of β-catenin. Mutations of Ser/Thr residues in exon 3 of the *CTNNB1* gene prevent ubiquitination. The result is overexpression of the Wnt/β-catenin pathway and uncontrolled cell proliferation.

12.3 Surgery

The treatment of craniopharyngioma has a number of controversies and challenges. Surgical resection is a valid approach and may be characterized as radical or limited. Radical surgery is defined as complete microscopic resection with no evidence of residual disease by surgical or neuroimaging report. Radical surgery may be proposed when the chance of complete resection is high and the morbidity acceptable and limited in its impact on long-term functional outcomes. It may also be proposed for very young children when the alternative, radiation therapy, may have age-related side effects. Surgery is characterized as limited when the goal is to decompress optic structures, reduce mass effect and neurological symptoms, restore CSF flow, and confirm the diagnosis when neuroimaging findings are equivocal. In some cases, the choice of performing radical surgery or limited surgery is made at the time of the operation, since exploration may be required to understand the association of the tumor with critical anatomy and to estimate the potential for surgical morbidity.

Surgery that does not involve tumor resection may play a central and important role in preparing the patient for subsequent radical surgery or limited surgery and radiation therapy. CSF shunting, temporary or permanent, may be considered for selective cases in which outflow is obstructed. Although surgery may be used to open CSF pathways, resection may not be possible under certain conditions or symptomatic hydrocephalus may be observed after surgery and require management when obstruction is not present.

Surgery for craniopharyngioma may also involve cyst drainage through open or closed procedures. Often, a catheter is inserted into the cyst(s) and permanently attached to an extracranial reservoir placed under the skin. Indeed, the use of an Ommaya reservoir is a common practice to manage cyst components of craniopharyngioma in unresectable patients and in preparation for radiation therapy or alternative therapies.

There are many approaches to surgery and techniques available to limit morbidity and mortality. The approaches are driven by tumor extent, size, and shape. Historically, a variety of transcranial approaches have been used; however, more recently transnasal surgery has been considered feasible even in younger patients. Endonasal endoscopic surgery has become increasingly popular and may result in a similar extent of resection as other approaches. It may be preferred under certain circumstances (Dhandapani et al. 2016).

Radical surgery is appropriate for patients with tumors that may be completely removed without damaging the anterior hypothalamus and affecting the quality of life. For other patients, limited surgery followed by conformal, fractionated external beam irradiation should be considered. The side effects of surgery include operative and perioperative morbidity and mortality; patients treated with surgery risk acute complications affecting neurological and endocrine function and late effects involving metabolism, achievement, personality and problem behavior.

Because radical resection and radiation therapy yield similar rates of disease control, more information is required about the morbidity and mortality of the primary surgery approach. Surgical series tend to lack functional outcomes data. Patients treated with radical surgery should be compared to irradiated patients using similar measures to improve patient selection for treatment. It is not considered feasible to randomize patients to these two very different treatment approaches.

12.3.1 Comparing Radical Surgery to Radiation Therapy with or Without Surgery

A comparison of disease control and functional outcomes for patients treated with primary surgery versus those treated with more limited or no surgery and radiation therapy has not been done prospectively because of the small number of patients with this disease and management controversies and concerns that generate selection bias. Despite limited data on morbidity and the factors that influence functional outcomes, radiotherapy avoidance remains a primary goal in the management of these patients at some centers. The literature demonstrates good disease control regardless of treatment approach and modality-specific side effects. Primary surgery patients are more likely to experience acute effects involving neurological function and long-term side effects on personality, depending on the extent of hypothalamic involvement and dissection. Long-term cognitive and vascular effects have been observed in patients treated with limited surgery and radiation therapy. Most patients present with preexisting endocrinopathy, and both treatments have similar rates of anterior pituitary endocrinopathy; however, those who undergo primary surgery are more likely to experience hypothalamic damage, vision loss, or acute stroke (Huang et al. 1997; Lustig et al. 2003; Macdonald and Hoffman 1997). Systematically collecting information about the acute, early, and late effects of both treatment approaches in a prospective protocol would be a rational alternative to randomization.

The rate of gross total resection (GTR) varies widely in the literature, and the rate of tumor recurrence in patients treated primarily with surgery is related to patient selection (Kiehna and Merchant 2010). Even though these patients may be salvaged with a high rate of success using radiation therapy, they tend to suffer the combined effects of both approaches (Merchant et al. 2002b).

It is important to consider the factors that influence patient selection, disease control, and acute, perioperative effects. In one of the largest US series of patients treated with primary surgery, clinical and treatment factors found to negatively affect progression-free (PFS) and overall survival (OS) were subtotal resection (STR), tumor size >5 cm, and the presence of hydrocephalus or CSF shunting (Elliott et al. 2010). It is logical that STR would affect PFS but not OS, since patients who have disease progression after primary surgery may be successfully salvaged with radiation therapy. It may be that patients treated with STR are prone to progression and subsequently undergo a second surgery instead of irradiation and are at increased risk for perioperative morbidity and mortality. The explanation for tumor size, hydrocephalus, and ventriculoperitoneal (VP) shunting impacting PFS suggests more extensive or unresectable disease and a probable association with STR. There is no logical explanation for the relationship between tumor size and OS. This finding may be attributed to the morbidity and mortality of salvage (i.e., second) surgery. It has been noted that recurrent tumors are more likely to lose their tissue planes, making second surgery dangerous (Elliott et al. 2009). There were three deaths in the reported series, two among the 57 primary patients and one among the 29 patients with recurrent tumors. The recurrence rate was 22% among 81 patients who were not among those who died perioperatively ($n = 3$) or were lost to follow-up ($n = 2$). The median time to recurrence was 20 months, and the 2-year PFS rate was 85%. Based on these findings, and because PFS in patients with recurrent tumors was low, it can be concluded that it is not in the best interest of the patient to undergo a second attempt at radical resection unless the patient is young and conditions for resection and complete removal are favorable. The death rate during the interval of this study was 15%. The median follow-up was 8.3 years, ranging from 3 months to 22.8 years. These data support the policy of one attempt at major resection, and postoperative irradiation in patients who undergo STR. Although it may not be detrimental to delay irradiation for an amount of time measured in months, growth will ultimately occur, affecting the target volume and potentially increasing the morbidity arising from irradiation.

There is limited information on cognitive function and quality-of-life outcomes after primary surgery. Quality of life and behavioral follow-up for 29 patients (Sands et al. 2005) were reported from a series that included a primary surgery approach. The authors found that social-emotional and behavioral functions were within the normal range for externalizing problems but borderline for internalizing problems. Tumor recurrence and additional surgery were associated with decreased physical functioning.

Retrochiasmatic tumor location was associated with lower psychosocial quality of life and impaired social-emotional and behavioral function. There was no association between outcome and gender, age, tumor size, or hydrocephalus. These findings differed from the findings of other, much older surgical series and suggest that more patients are needed for such a study. Assessment of quality of life is important in this group, and there needs to be more information about outcomes after the primary surgery approach to better understand the effects of GTR.

Hypothalamic dysfunction may be characterized in patients treated with surgery using acquired variables similar to those used in the grading scale of DeVile (Devile et al. 1996): mild dysfunction—postoperative obesity (BMI > 2SD) and a lack of behavioral or psychological symptoms; moderate dysfunction—obesity with hyperphagia or memory disturbances; and severe dysfunction—extreme obesity and hyperphagia with behavioral disturbances including rage and disturbances of thermoregulation, sleep-wake cycles, or memory. Other classifications include the functional status of patients and acquired variables similar to those of Wen (Wen et al. 1989), whose four-part functional classification index has been used in many surgical series. The classifications are: class I—grossly normal and independent, mild hormone disturbances, seizures well controlled with medication; class II—independent, panhypopituitarism, mild to moderate visual compromise, cranial nerve deficits, mild psychological dysfunction; class III—partially dependent, serious visual compromise, serious neurological deficits including hemiparesis or refractory seizures, learning disabilities, or poorly controlled psychological disorders; and class IV—entirely dependent on others for care. These scales were used by Elliott and Wisoff (2009) in their assessment of 19 very young children with craniopharyngioma. The median age at the time of surgery was 3 years, and very few patients had more than one surgery to achieve GTR, which was successful in 18/19 (94.7%) patients. Hypothalamic morbidity at any level occurred in 4/17 (23.5%) patients for whom data were available. There was no statistical difference between pre- and postoperative functional scores among the group of evaluated patients. Recurrence was noted in 33% of patients after a median time of 16 months. Further assessment of these patients based on presenting signs and symptoms, including presence of headache, vision loss, behavioral changes, diabetes insipidus, endocrine symptoms, or focal neurological deficits, as clinical variables may be helpful. The relationship of the tumor to the optic chiasm (prechiasmatic, retrochiasmatic, complex, lateral, or predominantly third ventricle) should be assessed in planning for surgery.

One important caveat in reviewing surgical data is that radical resection denotes GTR. This is not achievable in all patients, and the rate of progression after GTR at experienced centers approaches 25% (Weiner et al. 1994). GTR is defined as no tumor by visual (GTR-macro) or microscopic (GTR-micro) inspection. No residual disease by imaging and no evidence of enhancement or microscopic calcifications are considered by many to be GTR (Elliott and Wisoff 2009). If blood products obscure the postoperative cavity, imaging, including CT, should be repeated 1 month later as there should be no rush to initiate adjuvant therapy. In the series by Elliot (Elliott et al. 2009), the recurrence rate was 24% among a group of 49 patients with calcification on preoperative CT scan. There was no significant difference in the rate of tumor recurrence based on postoperative calcification, and they found the Hoffman scale was not particularly useful in their study, probably because of small numbers. The Hoffman scale (Hoffman 1985) has five levels: grade 1—a normal CT scan; grade 2—tiny calcific fleck but no residual tumor; grade 3—a small calcific chunk without evidence of enhancement or mass effect; grade 4—a small contrast-enhancing lesion without mass effect; and grade 5—lesion with significant enhancement and mass effect.

The PFS after radical surgery versus limited surgery and radiation therapy should be similar, approximately 75%, when measured between 5 and 10 years after diagnosis and initial treatment. The caveat is that radical surgery means GTR and limited surgery means cyst drainage or decompression with limited dissection and tumor removal or no surgical manipulation of the tumor. It should not be the goal of any study to compare local disease control for these two groups; rather, it is most relevant to compare acute and late effects of treatment. There is another cohort to consider: patients who undergo radical surgery who do not achieve GTR and require postoperative irradiation and those treated primarily with GTR who later have local tumor progression and require radiation therapy. The third cohort can be characterized by surgical extent, which adds value to the analysis of surgical factors by bridging the defined group of limited surgery patients and those treated with radical surgery. There is no difference in outcomes comparing patients treated with immediate postoperative radiation therapy to those treated initially with surgery who experience progression prior to subsequent irradiation (Lo et al. 2014).

12.3.2 Surgery Planning

Neurosurgical input and intervention are integral to the treatment of children with craniopharyngioma before, during, and after radiation therapy. Patients should be evaluated by neurosurgery experts for resection, decompression, biopsy, Ommaya reservoir placement, CSF shunting, or similar procedures. As noted earlier, exploratory surgery may be required. Because craniopharyngioma may undergo spontaneous or radiation-induced cyst enlargement, unplanned neurosurgical intervention may be required after the patient has started treatment. Preoperative evaluation should include, whenever possible, a detailed ophthalmologic examination, including visual field assessment, and endocrinology consultation. Preoperative imaging should include a CT scan and MRI of the brain.

The goal of surgical intervention should be to facilitate tumor control, keeping surgical morbidity to a minimum. Common indications for surgical intervention directed at the tumor include establishing a tissue diagnosis, tumor control by radical resection, relieving tumor mass effect to reduce symptoms, and decreasing the target volume for radiation therapy. Patients should always be selected for radical surgery based on the neurosurgeon's assessment that a GTR may be achieved with acceptable postoperative morbidity. The Wen classification system (I–II) may serve as a guide (Wen et al. 1989). This assessment should include patient and tumor characteristics and consider the treating neurosurgeon's experience. The decision should ultimately be made by the parents with guidance of the multidisciplinary team following a discussion about the risks and benefits of surgery. To avoid operative hypothalamic damage, the degree of preoperative hypothalamic involvement may be assessed clinically or by neuroimaging using systems similar to the grading system proposed by Puget et al. (2007). The Puget Scale: Grade 0—no hypothalamic involvement; Grade 1—tumor abutting or displacing the hypothalamus; Grade 2—hypothalamic involvement with hypothalamus no longer identifiable. Preoperative hypothalamic involvement, clinical or radiographic (Puget Grade 2) (Devile et al. 1996; Puget et al. 2007), should be a contraindication to attempting GTR (Fig. 12.2). In addition, GTR is not recommended for patients who have already had a previous but unsuccessful attempt at a GTR. Patients with poor functional status (Wen Class III–IV) (Wen et al. 1989), previous stroke, or arterial or hypothalamic injury are also not good candidates for GTR. It is recognized that in certain cases, determining the feasibility of radical surgery may initially require exploration (Fig. 12.3).

Patients may be selected for less than radical surgery and subsequent radiation therapy based on the opinion of the neurosurgeon that a GTR cannot be achieved with acceptable morbidity. In some instances, neither radical nor limited surgery may be indicated. These patients, diagnosed based on imaging findings, may proceed directly to radiation therapy in the absence of any attempt to invasively establish a diagnosis; however, the patient and parents need to understand the unique nature of this situation.

Surgical evaluation, including the physical and neurologic examinations and detailed visual examination by ophthalmology, is critical since the surgical method to decompress the visual apparatus is an important part of the decision-

Puget 0

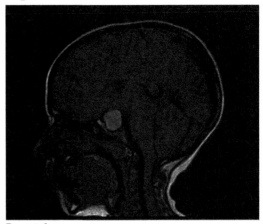

Puget 1

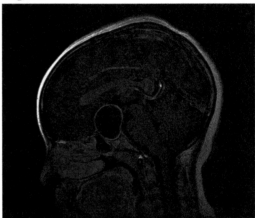

Puget 2

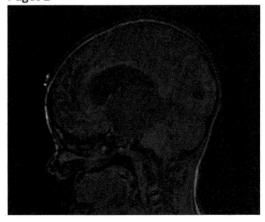

Fig. 12.2 Examples of Puget Scale

making process in choosing the surgical plan. Neuroimaging studies, including CT, which is useful for assessing calcification in the tumor and

T1 MRI pre-operative

T1 MRI after stroke

T2 MRI pre-operative

T2 MRI after stroke

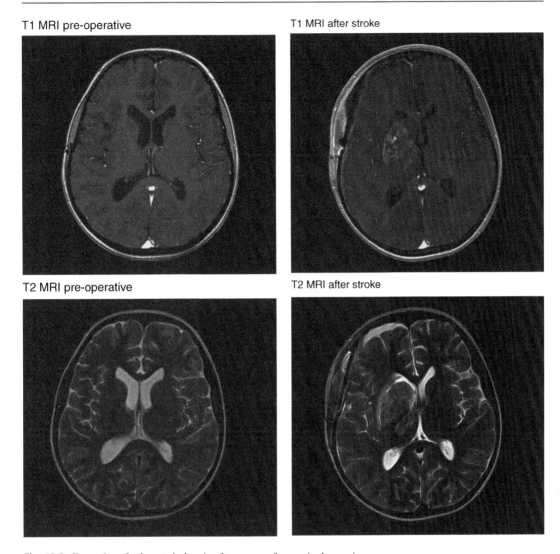

Fig. 12.3 Examples of subacute ischemia after surgery for craniopharyngioma

in the cyst wall, and MRI with and without contrast, should be used. The surgical planning discussion for a patient with presumed craniopharyngioma should include a frank discussion of the risks and benefits of radical surgery versus limited surgery and radiation therapy. Factors supporting radical surgery may include minimal involvement of the hypothalamus with a solid tumor or thick-walled or calcified cyst, or a thin-walled cyst; a favorable chance of total removal; and an experienced neurosurgeon. Factors supporting limited surgery and proton therapy may include involvement of hypothala-

mus with solid tumor, thick-walled cyst, or both, and good vision. Methods for handling poor vision may include correcting hydrocephalus or performing cyst drainage and obtaining tissue to confirm diagnosis. There are a variety of means for performing cyst drainage, including stereotatic or endoscopic placement of an Ommaya reservoir for a thin-walled cyst, or open procedure for a thick-walled cyst or when the cyst wall will not collapse. In any event, a decision must be made regarding the safety of cyst resection, and resection of a cyst on the hypothalamus should be avoided if access is difficult. For thin-walled cysts beneath the optic chiasm, leaving a catheter in place is preferable to resection unless the surgeon can be sure that the cyst is removed, because leaving a catheter with a large amount of cyst wall remaining may allow the cyst to reform with the catheter outside of cyst (Fig. 12.4). Other considerations regarding surgery include: (1) surgical decompression of a solid tumor compressing a nerve is often not necessary, because relief of hydrocephalus and drainage of the cyst will improve vision; (2) if an open procedure is performed, care should be taken to preserve the pituitary stalk to avoid diabetes insipidus; and (3) care must be taken not to disturb the interface of the hypothalamus and solid tumor, or the morbidity will be the same as that of radical surgery.

12.4 Radiation Therapy

Radiation therapy has a long track record of success in the treatment of craniopharyngioma and there are a number of published disease control benchmarks reporting high rates of local tumor control with long-term follow-up. Institutional series highlight the excellent rate of tumor control and the spectrum of side effects that may arise with radiation therapy and long-term follow-up. The rationale for radiation therapy and the potential side effects include long-term disease control with limited morbidity in appropriately selected patient understanding the contribution of tumor and surgery to the latter. When tumors are left intact or minimally disturbed by surgery, their borders are distinct and well-defined which permits the use of highly focused irradiation and limited margins of security around the defined target volume. Prior to the advent of three-dimensional conformal radiation therapy and, later, intensity-modulated radiation therapy—both using photons—and eventually the application of proton therapy, children with craniopharyngioma were irradiated with parallel opposed portals and fairly large margins surrounding the perceived target in an effort to encompass the volume at risk. Not only did the lack of image-guidance risk recurrence because of the possibility that the entire tumor was not

encompassed, the parallel-opposed portals also encompassed a substantial amount of normal tissue, including the temporal lobes, brainstem, entire circle of Willis and substantial vasculature of the middle cerebral arteries and possibly the anterior and posterior cerebral arteries as well.

In an effort to reduce the side effects of radiation therapy, and to take advantage of advances in treatment technology and the often well-defined imaging nature of craniopharyngioma, these tumors were some of the earliest to be subjected to conformal and so-called stereotactic radiation therapy using advanced methods of immobilization in cooperative patients and cone-based circular collimators that apply arc methods of irradiation. In some of the earliest series, craniopharyngioma was treated with margins surrounding the tumor of approximately 2 mm with the caveat that the entire tumor diameter was less than 5–6 cm. With the advent of three-dimensional conformal radiation therapy and later intensity-modulated radiation therapy, investigators were able to treat tumors with conformal therapy regardless of tumor size, initially using customized cerrobend collimation and later multi-leaf collimation.

There is a need to reduce side effects associated with the irradiation of young adults and children with craniopharyngioma because the tumor arises in the suprasellar region and is intimately associated with the diencephalon, optic pathways, and central cerebrovasculature. There is also a need to report on long-term disease control and functional outcomes for patients with craniopharyngioma and develop expanded models of radiation dosimetry that predict functional outcomes. Finally, there is a need to identify factors associated with tumor progression and side effects for patients with craniopharyngioma and to identify new clinical and biological correlates of outcome.

Progression-free and OS rates of 77% and 83% at 10 years and 66% and 79% at 20 years (Rajan et al. 1993) after limited surgery and radiation therapy have been reported from the Royal Marsden Hospital using doses ≥50 Gy. These are considered benchmarks for disease control and the same principals of treatment are now followed more than 50 years after their initial description. Despite the success of photon irra-

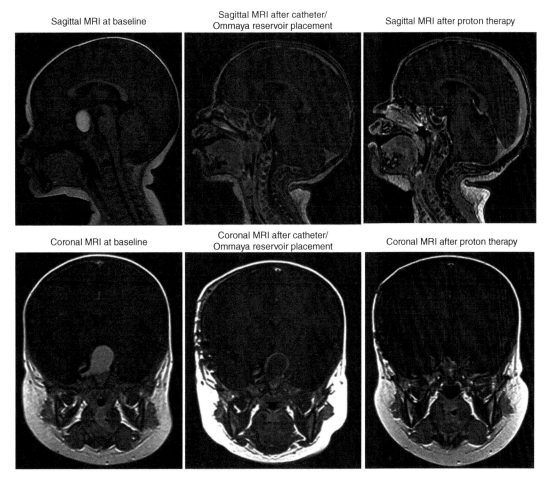

Fig. 12.4   Baseline, after catheter/Ommaya reservoir placement, and after proton therapy

diation, the side effects on neurologic, endocrine, and cognitive function weigh heavily when recommending irradiation because the long-term prospects for survival are excellent. Reducing dose to normal tissue should be a primary goal when radiation therapy is administered. Long-term disease control and toxicity reports from other centers support the use of irradiation and provide evidence of durable disease control. Investigators in Houston reported 5 and 10 year cystic (65.8% and 60.7%) and solid (90.7%) control rates for children treated with a 1 cm clinical target volume (CTV) margin and doses ranging from 49.8 to 54 Gy (Greenfield et al. 2015). Similarly, investigators reported 5, 10, and 20 year disease control (95.3, 92.1, and 88.1%)

and OS (10 year—83.3% and 20 year—67.8%) rates, highlighting excellent local control and the concept that most patients do not die from their tumor but associated complications from treatment (Harrabi et al. 2014). This latter point is also highlighted by recent data from Vancouver that demonstrates that the leading cause of late death is complications arising from tumor and treatment-related morbidity (Lo et al. 2014).

12.4.1   Radiation Dose and Volume

Disease control and functional outcomes have been prospectively defined for patients with craniopharyngioma using advanced methods of photon irradiation, such as intensity-modulated photon therapy, and investigations are now underway using intensity-modulated proton therapy with the goal of limiting side effects. Intensity-modulated proton therapy using discrete spot scanning is the newest form of proton therapy and includes intensity-modulation with iterative planning as well as single-field uniform dose methods. The potential advantages of proton therapy over photon therapy have been highlighted by a number of groups (Bishop et al. 2014; Boehling et al. 2012), despite concern by others about the costs associated with the use of protons (Leroy et al. 2016) and insufficient data, which is likely related to earlier proton therapy methods (Leroy et al. 2016) (Fig. 12.5).

There have been few systematic applications of focused irradiation attempting to define targeting and treatment for craniopharyngioma. A prospective Phase II trial of conformal radiation therapy was conducted at St. Jude Children's Research Hospital between 1998 and 2003. The primary objective was to estimate the local control and patterns of failure for pediatric patients treated with conformal radiation therapy using a 10 mm CTV margin. The trial demonstrated that event-free survival (EFS) with a 10 mm CTV margin and 3–5 mm planning target volume (PTV) margin was similar to treatment with conventional radiation therapy (Merchant et al. 2006). With a median follow-up of 28 months, the 3-year EFS was reported to be $85 \pm 11\%$. This study was the first to prospectively define a minimum target volume for this disease. The secondary objective of the same trial was to estimate the incidence and time to onset of clinically significant CNS effects based on radiation dose distributions in normal tissue, including deficits in neurological, endocrine, and cognitive function. The impact of high-dose irradiation on functional outcomes, specifically cognition, was clearly demonstrated (Merchant et al. 2006) in younger patients. These findings and recent advances in radiation therapy have made further reductions in the irradiated volume warranted and feasible.

A total of 93 patients diagnosed between December 1994 and March 2010 received conformal or intensity-modulated radiation therapy at St. Jude Children's Research Hospital. This number includes patients in the original 1998–2003 prospective series (Merchant 2006). The CTV margin was subsequently reduced to less than 10 mm after 2003 yielding two groups of patients: those treated with a CTV margin greater than (>) 5 mm ($n = 26$) and those treated with a CTV margin less than or equal to ($\leq$) 5 mm ($n = 67$). There was no significant difference in PFS distributions between these groups ($P > 0.70$) with 5-year estimates of $88.1 \pm 6.3\%$ vs. $91.7 \pm 4.9\%$, respectively. There was no significant difference comparing patients on the basis of their PTV or combined CTV + PTV margins. The PTV was systematically reduced during this time period from 5 to 3 mm with the advent of more sophisticated methods of immobilization and verification. All cases of tumor progression were within the target volumes. While not statistically significant, factors that appeared to be associated with improved PFS included Caucasian race ($P = 0.058$) and no permanent CSF shunting requirements ($P = 0.022$). These results suggest that reductions in the targeted volume using photons and smaller margins were feasible and safe as applied (Merchant et al. 2013).

Proton therapy appears to be superior to photon therapy in reducing dose to normal tissue. It has become increasingly available for children with brain tumors and has become a preferred radiation therapy modality (Merchant et al. 2008; Luu et al. 2006; Fitzek et al. 2006; Habrand et al. 2006). Several studies have shown the advantage of proton therapy to reduce dose to normal tissues irrespective of the chosen margin (Alapetite et al. 2010; Baumert et al. 2004; Fitzek et al. 2006; Merchant et al. 2008); however, a minimum CTV margin has not been defined and investigators remain concerned about idiosyncratic tumor cyst expansion during proton therapy that may lead to underdosing of targets (Winkfield et al. 2009). We studied the differences in normal tissue dose distributions comparing protons and photons. Protons spare normal tissues better than photons, especially in patients with small tumors. Small critical structures (chiasm, pituitary, and hypothalamus) adjacent to the

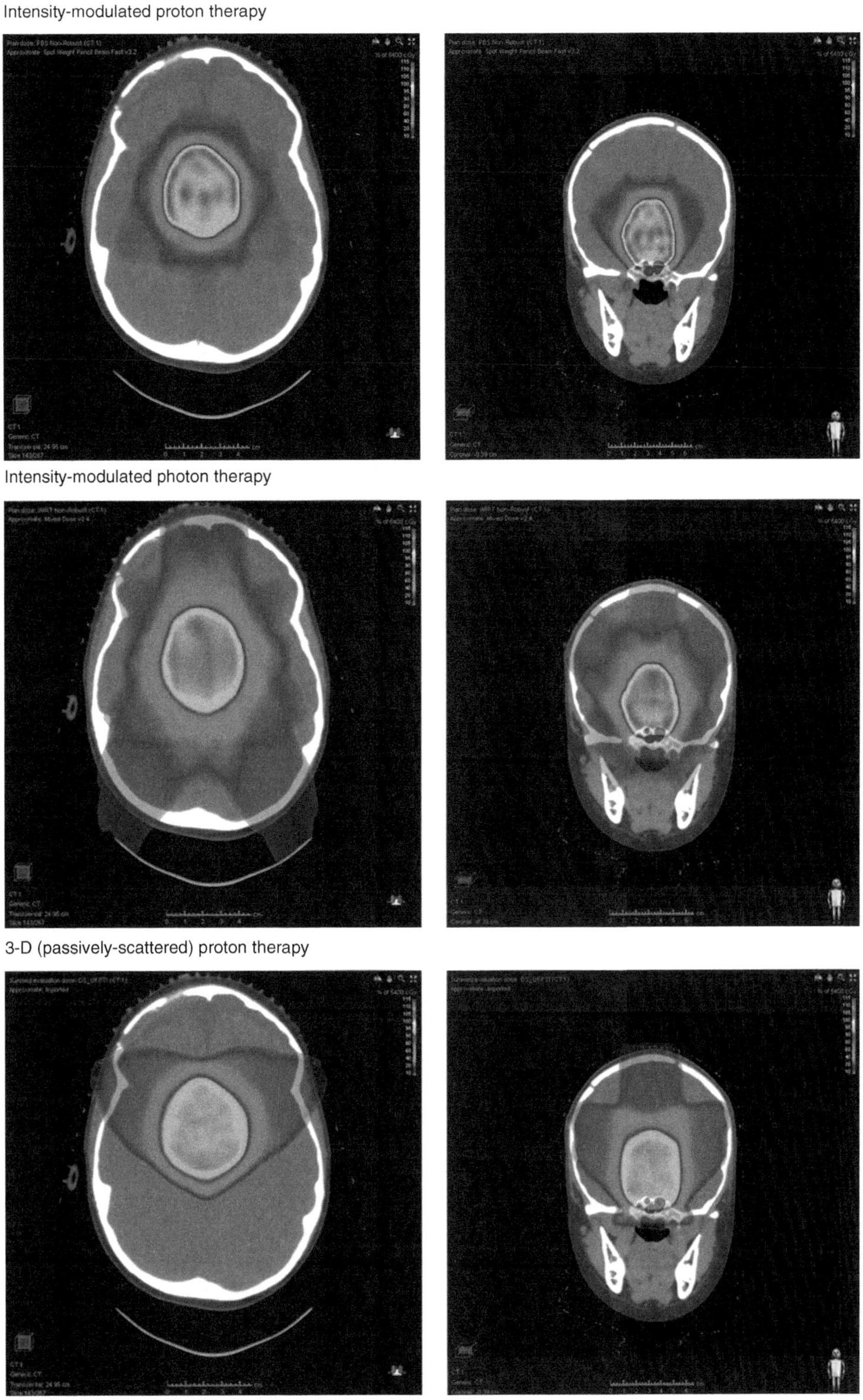

Intensity-modulated proton therapy

Intensity-modulated photon therapy

3-D (passively-scattered) proton therapy

Fig. 12.5 Intensity-modulated photon therapy, 3-D (passively scattered) proton therapy, and intensity-modulated proton therapy

PTV tend to receive the prescription dose; however, those separated from the PTV (cochleae) will receive significantly less or no dose when using proton therapy. Relatively large normal tissue volumes partially (cerebellum and brainstem) or more fully (entire brain or supratentorial volumes) subtended by the PTV are expected to receive minimal reductions in the high-dose volume, moderate reduction in the intermediate dose volume, and significant reductions in the low-dose volume using proton therapy. The differences widen as the volume of the normal tissue structure increases. The magnitude of the difference may be a factor of 3. Models suggest that cognitive function will be preserved using proton therapy in the same setting where a decline in cognitive function is expected using photons. Although the endocrine effects of radiation therapy may not be reduced, it is likely that proton therapy will reduce the risk of secondary neoplasia and vasculopathy because these late effects depend on the volume that receives both high and low doses (Merchant et al. 2008). Vasculopathy and cerebrovascular disease is a concern when considering late effects of irradiation in craniopharyngioma (Lo et al. 2014).

Apart from a number of registries, there is currently only one recently completed study in the US that deployed proton therapy for craniopharyngioma: a Phase II trial of limited surgery and proton therapy for craniopharyngioma and observation for craniopharyngioma after radical resection. This study was known as RT2CR. The proton therapy delivery method for the RT2CR protocol was passive-scattering, otherwise known as double-scattering or three-dimensional proton therapy. A 5 mm CTV margin surrounded the postoperative tumor bed and/or residual tumor. The RT2CR protocol successfully recruited patients from 2011 to 2016. The results have not been published.

It has been shown that with on-treatment monitoring (weekly or periodic MR imaging during radiation therapy), the targeted volume for craniopharyngioma may be safely reduced; however, these data apply only to photons, which are not significantly affected by tissue heterogeneity and which have a wider gradient in therapeutic to nontherapeutic dose coverage. Craniopharyngioma is a heterogeneous cystic and solid (calcified) tumor adjacent to the base of skull. These physical properties may affect proton dose distributions that are susceptible to tissue heterogeneity. The physical characteristics of the proton beam lead to very sharp dose profiles along the lateral aspects of the beam and at the distal edge. The sharp profile may risk marginal miss of craniopharyngioma target volumes that are prone to change in size or position. The importance of monitoring these tumors during treatment has been highlighted in a number of reports (Beltran et al. 2010; Shi et al. 2012).

Proton therapy advantageously reduces dose to normal tissue in children with craniopharyngioma and should reduce or eliminate the side effects of radiation therapy. Considering the vigilance required to reduce the targeted volume using photons, the susceptibility of proton therapy to tissue heterogeneity, and the dynamic nature of the craniopharyngioma target volume, protocol-based systematic monitoring is required with the possibility of adaptive therapy to investigate the feasibility and safety of using intensity-modulated proton therapy (Yang et al. 2014).

12.4.2 Radiation Dose-Effects Models

The objective of using advanced methods of irradiation and monitoring dose to normal tissues is to expand the models of treatment dosimetry and structural and functional outcome. The treatment guidelines in successive trials have included smaller target volume margins than those used in prior studies. Clinical trials that include radiation therapy now seek to prospectively evaluate the use of proton therapy. The goal is to proportionally irradiate less normal tissue and define a new minimum in the irradiated volume. Longitudinal functional assessment on the aforementioned RT1 protocol included a broad range of CNS effects measured before, during, and after irradiation; assessments include audiometry, ophthalmology, neurology, endocrinology, neuropsychology, quantitative neuroimaging, sleep and fatigue assessments and evaluation of physical performance. With a median follow-up of 5 years, the reported incidence of neurologic complications including deficits in hearing and vision was low, endocrine deficits were found to be common before treatment, and imaging changes and cognitive declines were statistically related to treatment dosimetry (Merchant et al. 2002a, 2002c, 2004; Dolson et al. 2009). Because of the paucity of prior prospective data for patients with this type of brain tumor (Merchant et al. 2002b), the benefit of volume reduction could not be proven; however, the acquired data now serve as a benchmark for the specified CTV and PTV margins and the irradiated volume of normal tissue. Data acquired in this study will be used for parametric modeling and future comparison with subsequent volume reductions, dose-escalation or normal tissue protection strategies for these patients.

Despite all attempts to limit dose to normal tissues, side effects will continue to be observed in these patients and it remains an important goal to identify important clinical variables and treatment factors that improve models of radiation dose. It is critical to have large numbers of patients in dose-effect modeling. The number of dose-volume intervals and correlative variables assessed depends on the number of patients. In prior studies we assessed mean dose and intervals of low (0–20 Gy), intermediate (20–40 Gy), and high dose (40–60 Gy). Correlation of radiation dosimetry with IQ has shown a statistically significant relationship with higher doses having the greatest impact. It should be a goal to evaluate more critically the effects of low dose given that this range of dose is the one most likely to differ when comparing proton and photon data. Independent of radiation dose, surgical factors have the greatest impact on cognitive function after radiation therapy. The extent of resection, number of attempts at resection, and the presence of diabetes insipidus, a surrogate marker for surgical morbidity, correlate significantly with decline in IQ (Merchant et al. 2006). These findings demonstrate the importance of considering all variables in dose-effects models. Dose models may be used to compare linear or nonlinear trends in subgroups or historic data; the same models may be used to estimate the proportion of patients falling within deficient ranges on functional measures.

12.4.3 Radiation Therapy Guidelines

The guidelines for radiation therapy have been developed to ensure coverage of the volume at risk and to minimize the side effects of treatment. The guidelines used by most centers are standard in terms of total dose (50.4–54 Gy) and fractionation (1.6–1.8 Gy/day). There is limited data concerning disease control and functional outcomes after treatment with new methods of radiation therapy, including proton therapy, or the impact of target volume reduction. None of the published reports concerning proton therapy describe in detail the method of targeting, immobilization and verification, or treatment assessment of target volume deformity. There has never been a national or international prospective study for the treatment of craniopharyngioma that included radiotherapy. The prescribed dose for craniopharyngioma has evolved to a standard of 54 Gy when using a CTV margin of 5 mm for all children. There are ample data demonstrating that these prescribed doses and target volumes are reasonable and safe. However, the data also suggest that further volume reductions are warranted because of the correlation between radiation dose, treatment volume, and a variety of functional outcomes. With the availability of improved imaging and increased treatment accuracy, the CTV and associated target volumes will be further reduced with the expectation that the dose to normal tissue will be lowered and side effects will be reduced. A single treatment plan is envisioned for most patients early in their course except for those who experience target volume change (most often cystic enlargement) early during treatment. Because of the association of the brainstem, optic chiasm, and optic nerves, prior studies have not specified brainstem dose-volume constraints and few unexpected adverse events have been observed in these patients. Children with craniopharyngioma tend to be young and vulnerable from the events leading to diagnosis and neurosurgery.

Surgery performed prior to proton therapy may reduce the targeted volume depending on the extent of resection and interpretation of the treatment planning guidelines and the definitions of the gross-tumor volume (GTV), CTV, and PTV. The GTV is defined as the edge of the residual disease as determined by pre- and postoperative neuroimaging and does not include the surgical corridor. In some instances, the resection bed may be added to the GTV when the likelihood of microscopic residual is high. The CTV is defined as the margin of security surrounding the GTV and tumor bed, when indicated, which is meant to encompass subclinical microscopic disease. Current institutional preferences include a 3–5 mm margin which is anatomically confined at interfaces where invasion is unlikely, such as the bony base of skull or where a cystic structure may be pushing but not invading a normal tissue structure such as the brainstem, or can be reduced where surgery has not been performed and a clear interface exists between tumor and normal tissue. At the bony interfaces the CTV margin is essentially zero (0 mm); however, for practical purposes it is customary for the CTV contour to appear external to the GTV. At interfaces such as the brainstem, the CTV margin may or may not be altered. A limited survey was conducted regarding target volume margins and treatment parameters at North American proton therapy sites. The survey included recommendations based on non-protocol treatment plans. The consensus is a 3–5 mm CTV margin, 95–100% CTV coverage, 3 mm margin beyond the CTV to define the PTV or equivalent, prescribed dose 54CGE, and dose maximum 100% including point dose to the chiasm (Table 12.1). All investigators would include the postoperative tumor bed in their targeted volume.

12.5 Alternatives to Radical Surgery and Fractionated External Beam Radiation Therapy

Investigators are keen to understand the biology of craniopharyngioma to identify aberrant pathways that might be targeted using existing agents. So far none have been found. Interferon administered systemically is currently being tested through the Pediatric Brain Tumor Consortium for newly diagnosed patients and those recurrent after prior radiation therapy. The Phase II study of peginterferon alfa-2b (PEGIntron) for pediatric patients with unresectable or recurrent craniopharyngioma was activated October 2013 (Goldman 2013. ClinicalTrials.gov Identifier: NCT01964300). Other means to treat craniopharyngioma include intracystic isotopes, bleomycin, and interferon (Bartels et al. 2012; Lafay-Cousin et al. 2007). Phosphorous-32 (^{32}P) brachytherapy can provide local control for growing cysts, but does not supplant the need for surgery or external beam radiation therapy in most cases (Ansari et al. 2016). Radiosurgery may be considered for local residual disease or recurrence. Toxicity of radiosurgery is not insignificant as described (Murphy et al. 2016).

12.5.1 Physical Performance

Children with craniopharyngioma are at risk for physical performance limitations, either related to their tumor or as a result of treatment. Limitations are likely the result of structural or physiological damage to critical normal tissue structures in proximity to the suprasellar region. Hypothalamic obesity, neuroendocrine abnormalities, visual

Table 12.1 Current guidelines for the use of proton therapy

CTV margin[a]	CTV coverage	PTV margin[b]	Prescribed dose	Dose maximum[c]
3–5 mm	95–100%	2–3 mm	50.4–54.0 CGE	100–108%

CTV clinical target volume, *PTV* planning target volume, *CGE* cobalt gray equivalent
[a]Includes margin surrounding postoperative tumor bed and not surgical corridor
[b]Includes margin surrounding CTV for positional and range uncertainty
[c]Chiasm dose maximum ≤100%

deficits, and neuromuscular dysfunction, including muscle weakness and poor flexibility, may contribute to poor physical performance. Poor physical performance may be perpetuated by difficulty with movement. Movement problems encourage inactivity and sedentary behavior, resulting in further deterioration in performance capacity. Reduced physical performance may be compounded by neurocognitive and emotional limitations so that participation in everyday activities is difficult and unrewarding (Fange et al. 2002). Less than optimal participation may result in social isolation and contribute to poor health related quality of life.

12.5.2 Cognitive Effects

Neuropsychological measures have been used to monitor function outcomes regardless of treatment strategy. The typical location of craniopharyngioma in the suprasellar region renders frontal/subcortical pathways vulnerable with respect to tumor infiltration, vascular displacement, surgical disruption (particularly with subfrontal approaches), and radiation effects. Previous studies investigating cognitive outcomes following treatment for craniopharyngioma indicate vulnerabilities in the areas of frontal lobe functioning, including perseveration, inflexibility and disinhibition (Cavazzuti et al. 1983; Riva et al. 1998), attention regulation (Kiehna et al. 2006) and memory (Carpentieri et al. 2003; Niwa et al. 1996; Di Pinto et al. 2012; Dolson et al. 2009; Netson et al. 2013). Findings from the St. Jude RT1 protocol indicate that overall academic achievement may be relatively well preserved with reading achievement more vulnerable than math achievement (Fig. 12.6).

12.5.3 Endocrine Effects

The hypothalamus produces growth hormone releasing hormone (GHRH) and is sensitive to the effects of tumors (hydrocephalus and tumor invasion) and treatment (surgery and irradiation). Thus, growth hormone deficiency is a

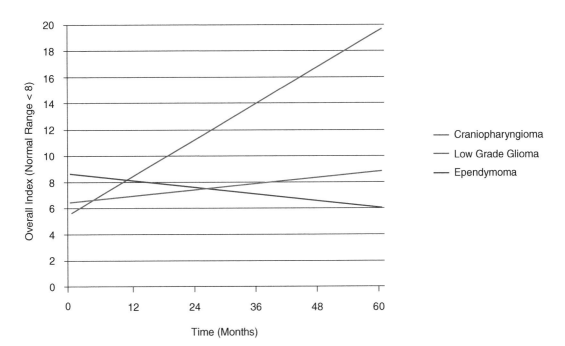

Fig. 12.6 Summary of attentional deficits in children with craniopharyngioma compared to children with other tumor types. Connor's continuous performance test over-

all index after surgery and radiation therapy—normal 0–8, borderline 8–10, abnormal >10

common side effect in patients with craniopharyngioma. The extent and impact of growth hormone deficiency before and after irradiation is largely unknown and is, therefore, an important research focus. Estimating the extent of this underreported problem may prompt research to identify means for intervention and improvement in screening guidelines for those at risk. Growth hormone secretion has shown the greatest sensitivity to the effects of radiation therapy on the hypothalamus. Peak growth hormone levels after radiation therapy decline as an exponential function of time based on the mean dose to the hypothalamus. This conclusion is consistent among patients with craniopharyngioma. However, in contrast to adults, children with craniopharyngioma have a high rate of pre-irradiation growth hormone deficiency. Levels of growth hormone are often undetectable as soon as 12 months after radiation therapy. The assessment of pre- and post-irradiation growth hormone secretion abnormalities in children with brain tumors can be divided according to whether they arise from tumor-related hydrocephalus, tumor invasion, or tumor extension. Among children with craniopharyngioma, pre-irradiation growth hormone deficiency impacts both baseline and longitudinal changes in IQ and reading scores. The treatment of growth hormone deficiency may be a means to improve functional outcomes.

12.5.4 Ophthalmology and Audiology Effects

Vision loss and impairment from tumor and treatment is common in children with craniopharyngioma (Drimtzias et al. 2014). Worsening vision is most often a sign of tumor progression and not treatment effect. Baseline testing and serial follow-up should be considered a standard of care with the findings useful in the assessment of functional outcomes. Visual function does not necessarily impact functional outcomes (Netson et al. 2013). The incidence of hearing loss after radiation therapy for craniopharyngioma is low

based on the assessment of children with this disease (Bass et al. 2016).

12.5.5 Sleep Disorders, Fatigue, and Quality of Life in Craniopharyngioma

Survivors of craniopharyngioma are known to have neuroendocrine deficiencies, visual deficits, and hypothalamic obesity due to tumor location (Rosenfeld et al. 2014). In addition to the tumor location, damage to the hypothalamus by surgery and radiation therapy results in sleep disturbances, daytime hypersomnolence, short-term memory problems, and limited concentration (Palm et al. 1992, van der Klaauw et al. 2008). Sleep disturbances as part of long-term outcomes in survivors have only been reported as case studies or in small cohorts. Poretti et al. (2004) reported on patients with craniopharyngioma who were treated with radical tumor excision and found long-term complications, including sleep disturbances and poor quality of life. Increased daytime sleepiness was noted in 6 of 21 patients with 5 of 6 of these patients having obesity. Other problems beset by this tumor have been documented in the assessment of long-term survivors (Crom et al. 2010).

12.5.6 Neuroimaging

Neuroimaging is critical to the treatment and follow-up of children with craniopharyngioma. The purpose of the diagnostic imaging examination is to ensure the diagnosis of craniopharyngioma, define the extent of disease for surgery and radiation therapy planning, perform surveillance for tumor progression after surgery and during and after radiation therapy, and detect or evaluate treatment-related side effects. Diagnostic imaging should include multi-sequence, multi-planar, multi-dimensionally acquired MR imaging with and without IV gadolinium. The rationale for the chosen sequences is based on their ability to differentiate between the cystic and solid tumor components, the interface between the tumor complex and the base of skull, brain parenchyma and CSF spaces.

Weekly examinations during radiation therapy using a dedicated MR system (1.5 T or 3.0 T) are performed at major institutions during the 6-week proton therapy treatment course to monitor tumor shape and volume. MR imaging during the treatment course is essential to monitor for volumetric changes in the cystic component of the tumor that would reduce target volume coverage and/or increase normal tissue doses. Acquired imaging data during the treatment course may be used to model tumor response to treatment and dosimetry benefits of adaptive therapy. The goal of adaptive planning is to allow the plan to adapt when target volume coverage appears to be compromised by change in the volume or shape of the target during treatment. Some centers will perform imaging frequently during the early phase of therapy and discontinue if no change is observed. Others perform less frequently and as clinically indicated. In some instances CT is used and may be appropriate.

More advanced imaging may be performed in the follow-up of children with craniopharyngioma to monitor for response and changes in normal tissues. Diffusion-weighted imaging (DWI) is the most important MRI technique to investigate tumor cellularity in various brain tumors. Numerous lines of evidence support the use of DWI in studying tumor response. Uh and others used DWI to study radiation-related normal tissue effects in children with craniopharyngioma treated with proton therapy (Uh et al. 2015).

12.5.7 Management of Treatment-Related Effects

When early signs of progressive parenchymal changes representing necrosis are present on imaging, one may consider referral for hyperbaric oxygen therapy (HBOT). HBOT should be considered when progressive parenchymal changes are associated with symptoms regardless of severity. Steroid therapy, most often dexamethasone, may be initiated and tapered according to symptoms. When the dose of dexamethasone has been tapered to approximately 0.5 mg daily, a taper of hydrocortisone is initiated at approximately 25 mg daily administered in divided doses. Dexamethasone is discontinued within 2–3 days of the initiation of the hydrocortisone. Patients are not required to remain on steroid therapy during HBOT. The use of HBOT for non-radiation-induced normal tissue damage resulting from mechanical, ischemic, and other toxic insults is less certain (Fig. 12.7).

Vasculopathy is common among patients with craniopharyngioma and is responsible for some of the devastating effects observed after radiation therapy. The incidence and time to onset and factors predictive of severe and life-threatening vasculopathy have not been studied systematically (Bitzer and Topka 1995; Ishikawa et al. 1997; Lui et al. 2007; Mori et al. 1978; Murakami et al. 2002; Pereira et al. 2002; Rossi et al. 2006; Sutton 1994). Perioperative vasospasm and ischemia have been attributed to effects of surgery, whereas late events are largely attributable to radiation dose and volume. Managing vasculopathy is often difficult because medical or surgical intervention is instituted or considered after the process has become established. Three-dimensional time-of-flight MRA of the brain is the standard MRI technique for evaluation of the arteries of the Circle of Willis and its branches. This technique is used to evaluate for stenosis, dilatations and aneurysms of the principle components of the intracranial arterial circulation. It should be considered that the MRA is a screening tool and represents physiology as well as structure at the time of the examination. An abnormal MRA should be triaged by an experienced interventional team to determine the value of evaluation of the vasculature by digital subtraction angiography or CT angiography. In some cases, additional MR studies evaluating small vessels and tissue perfusion may be indicated and can be used to determine the need for revascularization surgery (Fig. 12.8)

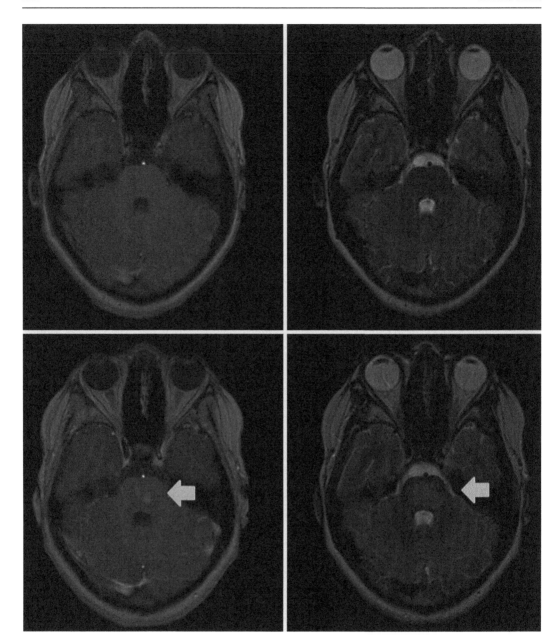

Fig. 12.7 Example of brainstem necrosis and response to hyperbaric oxygen therapy. MRI 6 weeks after the completion of proton therapy (first row), MRI 12 weeks after the completion of proton therapy (second row); MRI after 6 week of hyperbaric oxygen therapy (third row); MRI 2 years after proton therapy (fourth row)

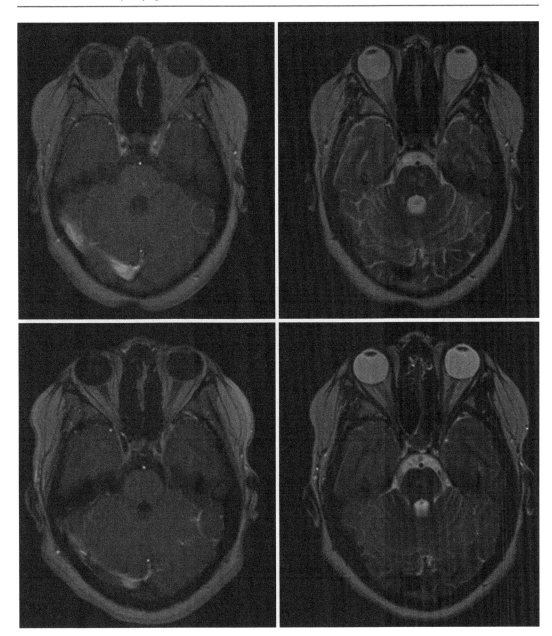

Fig. 12.7 (continued)

Fig. 12.8 Example of vasculopathy

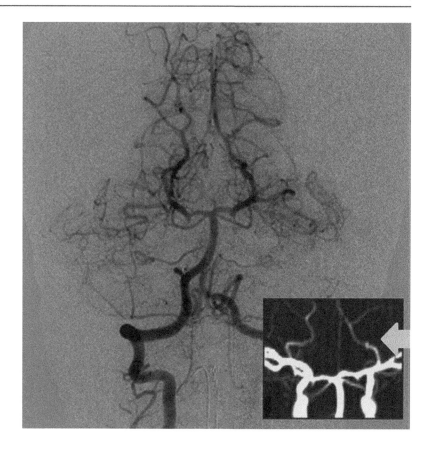

References

Alapetite C, Puget S, Ruffier A, Habrand JL, Bolle S, Noel G, Nauraye C, De Marzy L, Boddaert N, Brisse H, Sainte-Rose C, Zerah M, Boetto S, Laffond C, Chevignard M, Grill J, Doz F (2012) Proton therapy for craniopharyngioma in Children: Update of the Orsay Proton Center Experience. Neuro Oncol 14:i22–i5

Anastas JN, Moon RT (2013) WNT signalling pathways as therapeutic targets in cancer. Nat Rev Cancer 13:11–26

Ansari SF, Moore RJ, Boaz JC, Fulkerson DH (2016) Efficacy of phosphorus-32 brachytherapy without external-beam radiation for long-term tumor control in patients with craniopharyngioma. J Neurosurg Pediatr 17:439–445

Bartels U, Laperriere N, Bouffet E, Drake J (2012) Intracystic therapies for cystic craniopharyngioma in childhood. Front Endocrinol (Lausanne) 3:39

Bass JK, Hua CH, Huang J, Onar-Thomas A, Ness KK, Jones S, White S, Bhagat SP, Chang KW, Merchant TE (2016) Hearing loss in patients who received cranial radiation therapy for childhood cancer. J Clin Oncol 34:1248–1255

Baumert BG, Norton IA, Lomax AJ, Davis JB (2004) Dose conformation of intensity-modulated stereotactic photon beams, proton beams, and intensity-modulated proton beams for intracranial lesions. Int J Radiat Oncol Biol Phys 60:1314–1324

Beltran C, Naik M, Merchant TE (2010) Dosimetric effect of target expansion and setup uncertainty during radiation therapy in pediatric craniopharyngioma. Radiother Oncol 97:399–403

Bishop AJ, Greenfield B, Mahajan A, Paulino AC, Okcu MF, Allen PK, Chintagumpala M, Kahalley LS, McAleer MF, McGovern SL, Whitehead WE, Grosshans DR (2014) Proton beam therapy versus conformal photon radiation therapy for childhood craniopharyngioma: multi-institutional analysis of outcomes, cyst dynamics, and toxicity. Int J Radiat Oncol Biol Phys 90:354–361

Bitzer M, Topka H (1995) Progressive cerebral occlusive disease after radiation therapy. Stroke 26:131–136

Boehling NS, Grosshans DR, Bluett JB, Palmer MT, Song X, Amos RA, Sahoo N, Meyer JJ, Mahajan A, Woo SY (2012) Dosimetric comparison of three-dimensional conformal proton radiotherapy, intensity-modulated proton therapy, and intensity-modulated radiotherapy for treatment of pediatric craniopharyngiomas. Int J Radiat Oncol Biol Phys 82:643–652

Carpentieri SC, Meyer EA, Delaney BL, Victoria ML, Gannon BK, Doyle JM, Kieran MW (2003) Psychosocial and behavioral functioning among pediatric brain tumor survivors. J Neuro-Oncol 63:279–287

Cavazzuti V, Fischer EG, Welch K, Belli JA, Winston KR (1983) Neurological and psychophysiological sequelae following different treatments of craniopharyngioma in children. J Neurosurg 59:409–417

Crom DB, Smith D, Xiong Z, Onar A, Hudson MM, Merchant TE, Morris EB (2010) Health status in long-term survivors of pediatric craniopharyngiomas. J Neurosci Nurs 42:323–328. quiz 329–330

Devile CJ, Grant DB, Hayward RD, Stanhope R (1996) Growth and endocrine sequelae of craniopharyngioma. Arch Dis Child 75:108–114

Dhandapani S, Singh H, Negm HM, Cohen S, Souweidane MM, Greenfield JP, Anand VK, Schwartz TH (2017) Endonasal endoscopic reoperation for residual or recurrent craniopharyngiomas. J Neurosurg 126:418–430

Di Pinto M, Conklin HM, Li C, Merchant TE (2012) Learning and memory following conformal radiation therapy for pediatric craniopharyngioma and low-grade glioma. Int J Radiat Oncol Biol Phys 84:e363–e369

Dolson EP, Conklin HM, Li C, Xiong X, Merchant TE (2009) Predicting behavioral problems in craniopharyngioma survivors after conformal radiation therapy. Pediatr Blood Cancer 52:860–864

Drimtzias E, Falzon K, Picton S, Jeeva I, Guy D, Nelson O, Simmons I (2014) The ophthalmic natural history of paediatric craniopharyngioma: a long-term review. J Neuro-Oncol 120:651–656

Elliott RE, Wisoff JH (2009) Successful surgical treatment of craniopharyngioma in very young children. J Neurosurg Pediatr 3:397–406

Elliott RE, Moshel YA, Wisoff JH (2009) Minimal residual calcification and recurrence after gross-total resection of craniopharyngioma in children. J Neurosurg Pediatr 3:276–283

Elliott RE, Hsieh K, Hochm T, Belitskaya-Levy I, Wisoff J, Wisoff JH (2010) Efficacy and safety of radical resection of primary and recurrent craniopharyngiomas in 86 children. J Neurosurg Pediatr 5:30–48

Fange A, Iwarsson S, Persson A (2002) Accessibility to the public environment as perceived by teenagers with functional limitations in a south Swedish town centre. Disabil Rehabil 24:318–326

Fitzek MM, Linggood RM, Adams J, Munzenrider JE (2006) Combined proton and photon irradiation for craniopharyngioma: long-term results of the early cohort of patients treated at Harvard Cyclotron Laboratory and Massachusetts General Hospital. Int J Radiat Oncol Biol Phys 64:1348–1354

Goldman S (2013. ClinicalTrials.gov Identifier: NCT01964300. Phase II Study of Peginterferon Alfa-2b (PEGIntron) for pediatric patients with unresectable or recurrent craniopharyngioma. ClinicalTrials.gov Identifier: NCT01964300

Greenfield BJ, Okcu MF, Baxter PA, Chintagumpala M, Teh BS, Dauser RC, Su J, Desai SS, Paulino AC (2015) Long-term disease control and toxicity outcomes following surgery and intensity modulated radiation therapy (Imrt) in pediatric craniopharyngioma. Radiother Oncol 114:224–229

Habrand JL, Saran F, Alapetite C, Noel G, El Boustany R, Grill J (2006) Radiation therapy in the management of craniopharyngioma: current concepts and future developments. J Pediatr Endocrinol Metab 19(Suppl 1): 389–394

Harrabi SB, Adeberg S, Welzel T, Rieken S, Habermehl D, Debus J, Combs SE (2014) Long term results after fractionated stereotactic radiotherapy (FSRT) in patients with craniopharyngioma: maximal tumor control with minimal side effects. Radiat Oncol 9:203

Hoffman HJ (1985) Craniopharyngiomas. Can J Neurol Sci 12:348–352

Huang PP, Constantini S, Wisoff JH (1997) Etiology of an unusual visual field deficit associated with a craniopharyngioma: case report. Ophthalmologica 211:256–262

Ishikawa T, Houkin K, Yoshimoto T, Abe H (1997) Vasoreconstructive surgery for radiation-induced vasculopathy in childhood. Surg Neurol 48:620–626

Kiehna EN, Merchant TE (2010) Radiation therapy for pediatric craniopharyngioma. Neurosurg Focus 28:E10

Kiehna EN, Mulhern RK, Li C, Xiong X, Merchant TE (2006) Changes in attentional performance of children and young adults with localized primary brain tumors after conformal radiation therapy. J Clin Oncol 24:5283–5290

Lafay-Cousin L, Bartels U, Raybaud C, Kulkarni AV, Guger S, Huang A, Bouffet E (2007) Neuroradiological findings of bleomycin leakage in cystic craniopharyngioma. Report of three cases. J Neurosurg 107:318–323

Leroy R, Benahmed N, Hulstaert F, Van Damme N, De Ruysscher D (2016) Proton therapy in children: a systematic review of clinical effectiveness in 15 pediatric cancers. Int J Radiat Oncol Biol Phys 95:267–278

Lo AC, Howard AF, Nichol A, Sidhu K, Abdulsatar F, Hasan H, Goddard K (2014) Long-term outcomes and complications in patients with craniopharyngioma: the British Columbia Cancer Agency experience. Int J Radiat Oncol Biol Phys 88:1011–1018

Lui YW, Law M, Chacko-Mathew J, Babb JS, Tuvia K, Allen JC, Zagzag D, Johnson G (2007) Brainstem corticospinal tract diffusion tensor imaging in patients with primary posterior fossa neoplasms stratified by tumor type: a study of association with motor weakness and outcome. Neurosurgery 61:1199–1207

Lustig RH, Post SR, Srivannaboon K, Rose SR, Danish RK, Burghen GA, Xiong X, Wu S, Merchant TE (2003) Risk factors for the development of obesity in children surviving brain tumors. J Clin Endocrinol Metab 88:611–616

Luu QT, Loredo LN, Archambeau JO, Yonemoto LT, Slater JM, Slater JD (2006) Fractionated proton radiation treatment for pediatric craniopharyngioma: preliminary report. Cancer J 12:155–159

Macdonald RL, Hoffman HJ (1997) Subarachnoid hemorrhage and vasospasm following removal of craniopharyngioma. J Clin Neurosci 4:348–352

Martinez-Barbera JP (2015) Molecular and cellular pathogenesis of adamantinomatous craniopharyngioma. Neuropathol Appl Neurobiol 41:721–732

Merchant TE (2006) Craniopharyngioma radiotherapy: endocrine and cognitive effects. J Pediatr Endocrinol Metab 19(Suppl 1):439–446

Merchant TE, Goloubeva O, Pritchard DL, Gaber MW, Xiong X, Danish RK, Lustig RH (2002a) Radiation dose-volume effects on growth hormone secretion. Int J Radiat Oncol Biol Phys 52:1264–1270

Merchant TE, Kiehna EN, Sanford RA, Mulhern RK, Thompson SJ, Wilson MW, Lustig RH, Kun LE (2002b) Craniopharyngioma: the St. Jude Children's Research Hospital experience 1984–2001. Int J Radiat Oncol Biol Phys 53:533–542

Merchant TE, Williams T, Smith JM, Rose SR, Danish RK, Burghen GA, Kun LE, Lustig RH (2002c) Preirradiation endocrinopathies in pediatric brain tumor patients determined by dynamic tests of endocrine function. Int J Radiat Oncol Biol Phys 54:45–50

Merchant TE, Gould CJ, Xiong X, Robbins N, Zhu J, Pritchard DL, Khan R, Heideman RL, Krasin MJ, Kun LE (2004) Early neuro-otologic effects of three-dimensional irradiation in children with primary brain tumors. Int J Radiat Oncol Biol Phys 58:1194–1207

Merchant TE, Kiehna EN, Kun LE, Mulhern RK, Li C, Xiong X, Boop FA, Sanford RA (2006) Phase Ii trial of conformal radiation therapy for pediatric patients with craniopharyngioma and correlation of surgical factors and radiation dosimetry with change in cognitive function. J Neurosurg 104:94–102

Merchant TE, Hua CH, Shukla H, Ying X, Nill S, Oelfke U (2008) Proton versus photon radiotherapy for common pediatric brain tumors: comparison of models of dose characteristics and their relationship to cognitive function. Pediatr Blood Cancer 51:110–117

Merchant TE, Kun LE, Hua CH, Wu S, Xiong X, Sanford RA, Boop FA (2013) Disease control after reduced volume conformal and intensity modulated radiation therapy for childhood craniopharyngioma. Int J Radiat Oncol Biol Phys 85:e187–e192

Mori K, Takeuchi J, Ishikawa M, Handa H, Toyama M, Yamaki T (1978) Occlusive arteriopathy and brain tumor. J Neurosurg 49:22–35

Murakami N, Tsukahara T, Toda H, Kawakami O, Hatano T (2002) Radiation-induced cerebral aneurysm successfully treated with endovascular coil embolization. Acta Neurochir Suppl 82:55–58

Murphy ES, Chao ST, Angelov L, Vogelbaum MA, Barnett G, Jung E, Recinos VR, Mohammadi A, Suh JH (2016) Radiosurgery for pediatric brain tumors. Pediatr Blood Cancer 63:398–405

Netson KL, Conklin HM, Wu S, Xiong X, Merchant TE (2013) Longitudinal investigation of adaptive functioning following conformal irradiation for pediatric craniopharyngioma and low-grade glioma. Int J Radiat Oncol Biol Phys 85:1301–1306

Niwa J, Uede T, Ohtaki M, Ibayashi Y, Tanabe S, Hashi K (1996) Prognosis after total removal of craniopharyngiomas via the frontobasal interhemispheric approach. No Shinkei Geka 24:321–328

Ostrom QT, Gittleman H, Fulop J, Liu M, Blanda R, Kromer C, Wolinsky Y, Kruchko C, Barnholtz-Sloan JS (2015) CBTRUS statistical report: primary brain and central nervous system tumors diagnosed in the United States in 2008–2012. Neuro Oncol 17(Suppl 4):iv1–iv62

Palm L, Nordin V, Elmqvist D, Blennow G, Persson E, Westgren U (1992) Sleep and wakefulness after treatment for craniopharyngioma in childhood; influence on the quality and maturation of sleep. Neuropediatrics 23:39–45

Pereira P, Cerejo A, Cruz J, Vaz R (2002) Intracranial aneurysm and vasculopathy after surgery and radiation therapy for craniopharyngioma: case report. Neurosurgery 50:885–887

Poretti A, Grotzer MA, Ribi K, Schonle E, Boltshauser E (2004) Outcome of craniopharyngioma in children: long-term complications and quality of life. Dev Med Child Neurol 46:220–229

Puget S, Garnett M, Wray A, Grill J, Habrand JL, Bodaert N, Zerah M, Bezerra M, Renier D, Pierre-Kahn A, Sainte-Rose C (2007) Pediatric craniopharyngiomas: classification and treatment according to the degree of hypothalamic involvement. J Neurosurg 106:3–12

Rajan B, Ashley S, Gorman C, Jose CC, Horwich A, Bloom HJ, Marsh H, Brada M (1993) Craniopharyngioma—a long-term results following limited surgery and radiotherapy. Radiother Oncol 26:1–10

Riva D, Pantaleoni C, Devoti M, Saletti V, Nichelli F, Giorgi C (1998) Late neuropsychological and behavioural outcome of children surgically treated for craniopharyngioma. Childs Nerv Syst 14:179–184

Rosenfeld A, Arrington D, Miller J, Olson M, Gieseking A, Etzl M, Harel B, Schembri A, Kaplan A (2014) A review of childhood and adolescent craniopharyngiomas with particular attention to hypothalamic obesity. Pediatr Neurol 50:4–10

Rossi A, Cama A, Consales A, Gandolfo C, Garre ML, Milanaccio C, Pavanello M, Piatelli G, Ravegnani M, Tortori-Donati P (2006) Neuroimaging of pediatric craniopharyngiomas: a pictorial essay. J Pediatr Endocrinol Metab 19(Suppl 1):299–319

Sands SA, Milner JS, Goldberg J, Mukhi V, Moliterno JA, Maxfield C, Wisoff JH (2005) Quality of life and behavioral follow-up study of pediatric survivors of craniopharyngioma. J Neurosurg 103:302–311

Serman L, Nikuseva Martic T, Serman A, Vranic S (2014) Epigenetic alterations of the Wnt signaling pathway in cancer: a mini review. Bosn J Basic Med Sci 14:191–194

Shi Z, Esiashvili N, Janss AJ, Mazewski CM, Macdonald TJ, Wrubel DM, Brahma B, Schwaibold FP, Marcus RB, Crocker IR, Shu HK (2012) Transient enlargement of craniopharyngioma after radiation therapy: pattern of magnetic resonance imaging response following radiation. J Neuro-Oncol 109:349–355

Sutton LN (1994) Vascular complications of surgery for craniopharyngioma and hypothalamic glioma. Pediatr Neurosurg 21(Suppl 1):124–128

Uh J, Merchant TE, Li Y, Li X, Sabin ND, Indelicato DJ, Ogg RJ, Boop FA, Jane JA Jr, Hua C (2015) Effects of surgery and proton therapy on cerebral white matter of craniopharyngioma patients. Int J Radiat Oncol Biol Phys 93:64–71

Van Amerongen R, Nusse R (2009) Towards an integrated view of Wnt signaling in development. Development 136:3205–3214

Van Der Klaauw AA, Biermasz NR, Pereira AM, Van Kralingen KW, Dekkers OM, Rabe KF, Smit JW, Romijn JA (2008) Patients cured from craniopharyngioma or nonfunctioning pituitary macroadenoma (NFMA) suffer similarly from increased daytime somnolence despite normal sleep patterns compared to healthy controls. Clin Endocrinol 69:769–774

Weiner HL, Wisoff JH, Rosenberg ME, Kupersmith MJ, Cohen H, Zagzag D, Shiminski-Maher T, Flamm ES, Epstein FJ, Miller DC (1994) Craniopharyngiomas: a clinicopathological analysis of factors predictive of recurrence and functional outcome. Neurosurgery 35:1001–1010. discussion 1010–1011

Wen BC, Hussey DH, Staples J, Hitchon PW, Jani SK, Vigliotti AP, Doornbos JF (1989) A comparison of the roles of surgery and radiation therapy in the management of craniopharyngiomas. Int J Radiat Oncol Biol Phys 16:17–24

Winkfield KM, Linsenmeier C, Yock TI, Grant PE, Yeap BY, Butler WE, Tarbell NJ (2009) Surveillance of craniopharyngioma cyst growth in children treated with proton radiotherapy. Int J Radiat Oncol Biol Phys 73:716–721

Yang C, Liu F, Ahunbay E, Chang YW, Lawton C, Schultz C, Wang D, Firat S, Erickson B, Li XA (2014) Combined online and offline adaptive radiation therapy: a dosimetric feasibility study. Pract Radiat Oncol 4:e75–e83

Rare Embryonal Brain Tumours

13

Adriana Fonseca, Salma Al-Karmi,
Alexandre Vasiljevic, Andrew Dodghsun,
Patrick Sin Chan, Lucie Lafay Cousin,
Jordan Hansford, and Annie Huang

13.1 Introduction

Embryonal brain tumours comprise the largest category of malignant pediatric brain tumours in children 0–14 years of age (McKean-Cowdin et al. 2013; Smoll and Drummond 2012; Zhang et al. 2017), and span a wide spectrum with varying degrees of histologic differentiation. This group includes medulloblastoma (MB), the most

A. Fonseca · S. Al-Karmi · P. S. Chan · A. Huang (✉)
Pediatric Brain Tumour Program, Division of Hematology Oncology Hospital for Sick Children, Department of Pediatrics, University of Toronto, Toronto, ON, Canada
e-mail: annie.huang@sickkids.ca

A. Vasiljevic
Centre de Pathologie et Neuropathologie Est, Hospices Civils de Lyon, Bron, France

Université Claude Bernard Lyon 1, Lyon, France

A. Dodghsun
Christchurch Hospital, Christchurch, New Zealand

Department of Paediatrics, University of Otago, Christchurch, New Zealand

L. L. Cousin
Alberta Children's Hospital, Calgary, AB, Canada

J. Hansford
Children's Cancer Centre, Royal Children's Hospital Melbourne, Parkville, VIC, Australia

Murdoch Children's Research Institute, Parkville, VIC, Australia

Department of Paediatrics, University of Melbourne, Parkville, VIC, Australia

common pediatric embryonal tumour, as well as rarer tumours categorized under various labels based on tumour location or specific histopathologic features. These include tumours previously called central nervous system supratentorial primitive neuroectodermal tumours (CNS-PNET)/SPNETs—a particularly challenging diagnostic category, and CNS rhabdoid/atypical teratoid rhabdoid tumours (AT/RTs). In contrast to medulloblastoma, there has been relatively limited progress in the outcome of children with rare embryonal tumours, as both substantive biological and clinical studies have been difficult to conduct. Furthermore, recent studies indicate significant molecular heterogeneity among tumours diagnosed as "SPNET/CNS-PNETs" and AT/RTs, an apparent "monogenic" disease. This chapter will summarize current understanding of rare embryonal brain tumours in the context of recent molecular studies and postulate on the direction of future therapeutic approaches for these diseases.

13.2 CNS-PNETs

CNS-PNETs are rare, aggressive embryonal tumours predominantly arising in younger children and adolescents. Although epidemiological data are lacking, CNS-PNETs are estimated to comprise 3–5% of pediatric brain tumours (Louis et al. 2007; Rorke et al. 1997). These rare tumours have been associated with several cancer predisposition syndromes including the Li Fraumeni (Taylor et al. 2000) and DNA mismatch repair syndromes (Bakry et al. 2014), and have also been reported as secondary malignancies after cancer treatment (Leung et al. 2001).

Since their initial description (Hart and Earle 1973) as cerebral tumours with close histologic resemblance to medulloblastoma (MB), supratentorial PNETs /SPNETs have been contentious diagnoses, with frequently evolving classification. Diagnostic challenges have, in part, been due to lack of substantive clinical, histopathologic, and molecular studies of these rare tumours, inconsistent application of newer diagnostic tools that distinguish specific embryonal tumours, such as AT/RTs from SPNETs, and reports of "SPNET"/CNS-PNETs arising in non-cerebral locations. Clinical literature has also been difficult to interpret, since CNS-PNETs/SPNETs, pineoblastoma, medulloblastoma, and other embryonal tumours have been frequently lumped together based on proposed common cellular origins (Kleihues et al. 2002; Louis et al. 2007; Rorke 1983). Nonetheless, existing reported demographic data on non-pineal PNETs (91 cases) suggest most patients are young, with a median age at diagnosis of 3.7 years and with 44% less than 3 years of age. The majority of these lesions (83%) were reported in the cerebral hemispheres and a much smaller proportion (17%) arose in the brainstem or thalamus, with metastases reported in only 22% of patients at diagnosis (Table 13.1). Recent molecular studies have improved an evolving understanding of tumours encompassed under CNS-PNETs/SPNETs, and led to further diagnostic revisions in the current 2016 World Health Organization (WHO) CNS classification schema (Louis et al. 2016).

13.2.1 Molecular Features

Due to contentious histologic diagnoses, varying methods have been used to identify "CNS-PNETs/SPNETs" in different studies. Nonetheless, earlier molecular analyses of small

Table 13.1 Non-pineal PNET studies

	n = 91
Patient characteristics	
Age (years)	*n=88*
Median (years)	3.7
<3	39 (44%)
3–5	18 (20%)
5–10	15 (18%)
>10	16 (18%)
Gender	*n=29*
Female	11 (38%)
Male	18 (62%)
Location	*n=53*
Hemispheric	44 (83%)
Midline (brainstem and thalamic)	9 (17%)
Stage	*n=74*
M0	58 (78%)
M1-4	16 (22%)
Treatment characteristics	
Extent of surgical resection	*n=91*
Complete (GTR/<1.5 cm² residual tumour)	39 (42%)
Incomplete (STR, biopsy)	53 (58%)
Standard chemotherapy	*n=91*
Yes	78 (86%)
No	13 (14%)
High-dose chemotherapy	*n=91*
Yes	34 (37%)
No	57 (63%)
Radiotherapy	*n=91*
Yes	62 (68%)
CSI	53 (85%)
Focal only	5 (15%)
No	29 (32%)
Overall survival	*n=86*
24 months	53% (95% CI 41–63)
60 months	47% (95% CI 36–58)

GTR gross total resection, *STR* subtotal resection, *CSI* craniospinal irradiation, *CI* confidence interval

cerebral PNET cohorts established that they differed from MB based on lack of isochr17q alterations (Li et al. 2005) and unique gene expression signatures (Pomeroy et al. 2002). These findings were confirmed by larger PNET cohort studies (Li et al. 2009), which also revealed that a proportion of highly aggressive PNETs arising in younger children have recurrent amplification of

C19MC, a large miRNA cluster on chr19q13.41 (Li et al. 2009). These *C19MC* altered tumours, which encompass various rare histopathologic entities including ETANTRs, now represent a separate diagnostic category discussed later in this chapter.

To date, two large molecular studies of CNS-PNETs (Picard et al. 2012; Sturm et al. 2016) have been undertaken. In an initial study, Picard et al. (2012) reviewed 252 archived tumours with institutional diagnoses of CNS-PNETs, and excluded approximately 50% of archived CNS-PNETs after review of histopathology, tumour location, and SMARCB1/BAF47 testing, as they identified with other known diagnostic entities including high-grade gliomas (HGG), supratentorial ependymomas, pineoblastoma, AT/RTs, medulloblastoma or were tumours of uncertain histopathologic diagnoses. Based on transcriptional analyses, they proposed three molecular categories of cerebral PNETs. In addition to a group with primitive neural signatures and high LIN28 expression that corresponded to the *C19MC* associated CNS-PNETs (Li et al. 2009; Picard et al. 2012) and were named group 1 PNETs, they described a second group (group 2) enriched for oligoneural lineage with high OLIG2 expression and an OLIG2 negative subset (group 3) with mesenchymal transcriptional signatures; groups 2 and 3 were, respectively, correlated with a low and high incidence of metastases. Using methylation profiling of a large cohort of archived CNS-PNETs, Sturm et al. (Sturm et al. 2016) similarly showed that a substantial proportion of tumours with historical institutional diagnoses of CNS-PNETs identified with other histologically and molecularly defined brain tumours. They further reported the remaining tumours diagnosed as "CNS-PNETs" comprised four novel but distinct brain tumour entities characterized by *FOXR2*, *CIC*, and *MN-1* gene fusions and duplication of the *BCOR* loci; these were, respectively, designated CNS NB-*FOXR2*, CNS EFT-*CIC*, CNS HGNET-*MN1*, and CNS HGNET-*BCOR*, based on proposed histologic or molecular relatedness to neuroblastoma or Ewing sarcoma. CNS NB-*FOXR2* tumours have overlapping methylation profiles with the oligoneural group 2 PNETs described by Picard et al., while the *HGNET-MN1* tumours represent rarer entities and include tumours with classical histologic features of astroblastoma (Sturm et al. 2016). Their relationship to any of the prior reported PNET entities remains unclear. CIC fusions leading to ETS pathway upregulation (Huang et al. 2016; Peters et al. 2015; Yoshida et al. 2016), and *BCOR* exon 16 duplications (Kao et al. 2016) have been reported in various extracranial undifferentiated soft tissue sarcomas and suggest these CNS entities may actually represent intracranial, extra-parenchymal presentations of the same molecular disease.

In a move to incorporate molecular markers into brain tumour diagnoses, PNET has been removed as a diagnostic label in the 2016 WHO CNS classification (Louis et al. 2016). Group 1 and 2 PNETs described by Picard et al. are now, respectively, denoted as the *C19MC-* and *FOXR2*-associated tumours, and an additional category of CNS embryonal tumour NOS, without known genetic defining features, has been introduced. Interestingly, global methylation studies of pediatric embryonal and glial tumours suggest some of these tumours cluster with the previously designated *RTK* and *MYCN* groups of high-grade gliomas (Sturm et al. 2016). Furthermore, our studies suggest the RTK and MYCN high-grade gliomas are not genetically well-defined entities, but rather comprise tumours with substantial molecular heterogeneity without specific diagnostic genetic features (Norman et al., unpublished). These findings suggest that tumours diagnosed as "RTK/ MYCN" gliomas, mesenchymal "group 3 CNS-PNETs" (Picard et al. 2012), and "CNS embryonal tumours NOS" may arise from neural precursors on a spectrum of differentiation. More detailed studies of larger number of these tumours using deep functional genomics and genomic analyses will be important for understanding how these morphologic entities overlap at the molecular level, so that more precise diagnostic and treatment paradigms can be developed for these poorly defined "gliomas/PNETs."

13.2.2　Treatment Approaches and Prognostic Factors

Treatment and clinical prognostic data are difficult to interpret as no dedicated PNET therapeutic studies have been undertaken. CNS-PNET patients have historically been treated as high-risk embryonal brain tumours as per high-risk medulloblastoma protocols with augmented chemotherapy regimens and higher doses of brain and spine radiation. Although existing clinical data on CNS-PNETs predated the recent revised classification of these tumours, they nevertheless provide some useful insights into the prognostic role of specific therapeutic interventions for these rare diseases.

13.2.2.1　Surgical Resection

Published clinical data (Table 13.1) show gross total resection (GTR) is achieved in about 60% of patients and suggest extent of surgical resection is prognostic for CNS-PNETs. Albright et al. reported a 4-year postoperative survival of 40% and 13%, respectively, for patients with GTR and subtotal tumour resection (STR) in a small series of 27 children (Albright et al. 1995). Similar observations have also been reported in larger prospective European and North American collaborative group studies (Jakacki et al. 2015; Reddy et al. 2000), as well as smaller additional studies that employed various protocols (Chintagumpala et al. 2009; Friedrich et al. 2013, 2015; Johnston et al. 2008; Marec-Berard et al. 2002; Massimino et al. 2006; Sung et al. 2007; Thorarinsdottir et al. 2007) (Table 13.2) (Fonseca and Huang, unpublished), thus suggesting maximum safe surgical resection is important for patients with CNS-PNETs.

13.2.2.2　Radiation Therapy

Based on extrapolation from experience with MB therapy, whole brain and spine radiation has generally been prescribed for craniospinal prophylaxis and treatment in older children diagnosed with CNS-PNETs. Aggregate data from studies to date show 68% of patients with CNS-PNETs received some form of radiation therapy (RT); most (85%) received craniospinal irradiation (CSI), while a minority were treated with focal RT (Table 13.1). Although independent small cohort studies suggest incorporation of radiation early in treatment is important for survival (Jakacki et al. 1995; Marec-Berard et al. 2002; Reddy et al. 2000; Timmermann et al. 2002, 2006), the benefit of focal versus CSI has only been examined in limited cohorts of patients. Timmermann et al. (2002) reported a significantly poorer 3-year progression-free survival (PFS, 14.3%) for seven patients treated with only focal radiation in the HIT88/89 and 91 trials in contrast to superior 3 year PFS (43.7%) in 54 patients treated with CSI. However, 71% of disease recurrences were local, suggesting a multimodal approach is important in this disease (Table 13.2).

Various strategies have been used to postpone radiation in younger patients, or to deliver risk-adapted radiation for older children with CNS-PNETs. These include the use of hyperfractionated focal RT or reduced dose conventional CSI for nonmetastatic patients (Table 13.2). High-dose chemotherapy has been proposed as an important strategy to avoid or defer radiation in young children with CNS-PNETs (Chintagumpala et al. 2009; Cohen et al. 2015; Fangusaro et al. 2008a; Friedrich et al. 2013; Mason et al. 1998; Massimino et al. 2013). Of note, dismal outcomes have been reported in both smaller and consortia-based studies that employed conventional chemotherapy as a radiation avoidance strategy (Grundy et al. 2010; Marec-Berard et al. 2002; Strother et al. 2014). Important observations from the POG 8633 and HIT-SKK87 and 92 consortia-based studies indicate that, similar to young patients with MB, CNS-PNETs patients treated without radiation up-front may be successfully salvaged with craniospinal radiation (Wetmore et al. 2014).

In summary, cumulative literature suggests extent of surgery and radiation are important prognosticators for CNS-PNETs, and also indicate risk-adapted craniospinal radiation and high-dose chemotherapy may be an important strategy to defer, reduce, or avoid CSI, particularly in younger children.

Table 13.2 Summary of non-pineal PNET studies

Study	# patients	Age range (years)	Chemotherapy protocol		Radiation (RT)		DFS (years)	OS (years)	Prognostic findings
			Standard chemotherapy (SC)	HDC (# cycles)	CSI (Gy)	Focal only (Gy)			
High-dose chemotherapy (HDC)									
Mason et al. (1998)	14	0–6	VCR, CDDP, CPM, VP-16	CBDCA, TSPA, VP-16 (1)	No	No	43% (2)	64% (2)	RT can be deferred if using HDC
Fangusaro et al. (2008a, b)	30	0.1–6.9	HS I and HS II	CBDCA, TSPA, VP-16 (1)	No	No	48% (5)	60% (5)	RT can be deferred if using HDC
Chintagumpala et al. (2009)	9	3.8–12.9	SJMB06	CDDP, CPM (1)	SR:23.4 HR:36	No	SR: 75%; HR:60% (5)	SR: 88%; HR:58% (5)	HDC improve outcomes
Friedrich et al. (2013)	9	0–3.8	HIT2000	CDBCA, CPM (2)	24	No	50% (HDC); 9% (SC) (5)	67% (5)	HDC improve outcomes
Massimino et al. (2013)[a, b]	18	1.4–18	Milan protocol	TSPA (2)	31/39	No	53% (5)	52% (5)	Focal RT can be used in nonmetastatic disease when using HDC
Cohen et al. (2015)	9	0.5–3	CCG99703	CBDCA, TSPA (3)	No	No	29% (5)	41% (5)	HDC is tolerable and feasible
Adjuvant chemotherapy									
Cohen et al. (1995)	27	1.5–19.3	CCG921		36	No	45% (3)	57% (3)	8 in 1 more toxic with no survival benefit
Geyer et al. (2005)	36	0–3	CCG9921		36	54	17% (5)	31% (5)	No difference between induction regimens
Strother et al. (2014)[b, c]	38	0–3	POG9233/34		27/30/34	No	M0:40%; M+:10% (10)	M0:50%; M+:20% (10)	No benefit from intensified chemotherapy
Pre-irradiation chemotherapy									
Timmermann et al. (2002)	52	2.9–17.7	HIT 88/89 and 91		35	42	33.9% (3)	48% (3)	No benefit of pre-irradiation chemotherapy
Pizer et al. (2006)	54	2.9–16.6	PNET3		35	No	41% (5)	43% (5)	No benefit of pre-irradiation chemotherapy
Allen et al. (2009)[a]	28	3–20	CCG9931		40	No	46% (5)	48% (5)	No benefit of pre-irradiation chemotherapy

(continued)

Table 13.2 (continued)

Study	# patients	Age range (years)	Chemotherapy protocol		Radiation (RT)		DFS (years)	OS (years)	Prognostic findings
			Standard chemotherapy (SC)	HDC (# cycles)	CSI (Gy)	Focal only (Gy)			
Jakacki et al. (2015)	37	3–21	COG99701		36	No	45% (5)	50% (5)	CBDCA during RT is feasible
Radiation free									
Marec–Berard et al. (2002)	21	0–4	SFOP		No	No	2% (2)	14% (5)	RT confers survival benefit
Grundy et al. (2010)	11	0.1 3	UKCCSG/SIOP9204		No	No	0% (1)	9.1% (1)	RT confers survival benefit
Radiation deferral									
Duffner et al. (1993)	36	0–3	POG8633		35	No	19% (2)	21% (2)	Rads can be delayed until >36 months
Timmermann et al. (2006)	27	0–3	HIT-SKK87 and 92		35	No	15% (3)	17% (3)	RT confers survival benefit

OS overall survival, *DFS* disease-free survival, *VCR* vincristine, *CDDP* cisplatin, *CPM* cyclophosphamide, *CBDCA* carboplatin, *VP-16* etoposide, *TSPA* thiotepa
radiation therapy, *HR* high risk, *HDC* high-dose chemotherapy, *RT* free survival—reported as event-free survival and progression-free survival, *SR* standard risk, *HR* high risk
[a]Study used hyperfractionated radiation therapy
[b]Radiation dose was age dependent
[c]Study used focal radiation in nonmetastatic patients

13.2.2.3 Chemotherapy

Various adjuvant chemotherapy regimens have been used in CNS-PNET protocols across North American and European cooperative groups. Chemotherapy backbones have included various combination of vincristine, platinum compounds (cisplatinum and/or carboplatin), cyclophosphamide, and etoposide. To date, no specific regimen has been associated with better outcomes in the North American CCG921, CC992, and POG9233/34 trials. Of note, early disease progression has been reported in regimens that used pre-radiation chemotherapy (Allen et al. 2009; Pizer et al. 2006; Timmermann et al. 2006), indicating radiation delay is detrimental. As a result, with the exception of young children, radiation rather than chemotherapy has been the recommended first step in CNS-PNET therapy.

Similar to other embryonal brain tumours in young children, dose-intensified chemotherapy has been successfully employed to defer radiation in an attempt to mitigate the severe neurocognitive sequelae of irradiation at a young age (Chintagumpala et al. 2009; Friedrich et al. 2013, 2015; Johnston et al. 2008; Marec-Berard et al. 2002; Massimino et al. 2006; Sung et al. 2007; Thorarinsdottir et al. 2007).

In 2008, Fangusaro et al. reported relatively favorable 5-year event-free (EFS) and overall survival (OS) of 39% and 49%, respectively, in children treated with the dose intense Head Start I and II regimens (Fangusaro et al. 2008a). Similarly, results from the HIT 2000 trial demonstrated superior 5-year EFS (25%) and OS (40%) in patients treated with a short induction regimen combined with high-dose chemotherapy (HDC) versus a longer induction regimen (Friedrich et al. 2013). Notably, both studies reported long-term radiation-free survival in 18–50% of young children treated with HDC. This has led to the development of HDC-based protocols for infants with high-risk embryonal brain tumours in North America, including the CCG99703 and the more recent ACNS0334 protocols (Table 13.2).

13.2.3 Future Directions

Recent elucidation of several molecular entities under the previous umbrella term of "CNS-PNETs/SPNETs" represents an important step in studies of these rare tumours (Sturm et al. 2016). However, much work remains to fully elucidate the diagnostic and therapeutic significance of these recent findings in the context of previously described clinical and molecular entities. Preliminary data from retrospective and prospective studies suggest *FOXR2*-fused embryonal tumours have favorable biology with good outcomes when treated with high-risk MB type therapy. The relationship of *MN1* fused tumours and embryonal tumours NOS to other malignant neuroepithelial tumours, including the "*RTK/MYCN*" gliomas and previously reported CNS-PNET subcategories, remains less clear. Defining where these tumours fit on the spectrum of glial-neural tumours, and their specific clinical manifestations will have important practical therapeutic implications. In particular, re-examination of retrospective cohorts of malignant gliomas and CNS-PNET studies with molecular information will help guide and refine the application of glioma or embryonal brain tumour approaches to the spectrum of these poorly defined high-grade neuroepithelial tumours. Similarly, studying the intracranial tumours with *CIC* and *BCOR* fusions in the context of extra CNS soft tissue sarcomas with identical alterations will also be important to fully understand whether these warrant therapeutic approaches different from those already established for their extracranial counterparts.

13.3 C19MC Altered and Related Tumours

Historical classification of embryonal tumours/PNETs encompassed entities that had predominant primitive neural features but were distinguished by specific histologic features, including tumours called ependymoblastomas and medulloepitheliomas. In 2009, Gessi and colleagues (2009) added another histologic category to this spectrum of tumours that they named Embryonal Neoplasms with True Rosettes and Abundant Neuropil (ETANTR). However, the clinical and biological relationship between these various subcategories remained unclear until global molecular studies of CNS-PNETs reported that a subset of highly aggressive CNS-PNETs with variant histologic diagnoses, which arose in younger children, exhibited recurrent amplification of the oncogenic miRNA cluster on chr19q13.42 (Li et al. 2009). Many, but not all, of the tumours in the Li et al. study had features compatible with ETANTRs or ependymoblastoma. A series of studies have now confirmed that C19MC alterations identify a distinct clinical and molecular disease, which includes tumours with prior histologic diagnoses of ependymoblastoma, medulloepithelioma, and ETANTRs and thus a single, unifying histologic label, ETMRs, has been proposed. *C19MC* altered tumours and related molecular entities are now officially a distinct WHO diagnostic category (Louis et al. 2016).

C19MC associated tumours are distinctly aggressive brain tumours in younger children (Li et al. 2009; Spence et al. 2014a) with a median age of diagnosis at 24 months. While these tumours have been described in very young patients (<2–3 months of age), a majority (82%) of patients are 12–54 months old at diagnosis. Data from the rare tumour registry http://www.rarebraintumourconsortium.ca indicates tumours can arise in various CNS locations, with predominance in the cerebral hemispheres (59%). Although rapid disseminated progression has been reported in this disease, retrospective clinical data suggest most tumours (74%) are localized at the time of diagnosis. Epidemiological data for this relatively new category of disease remains to be established; however, studies from the Huang lab using fluorescence in situ hybridization (FISH) analyses in 500 malignant pediatric brain tumours diagnosed at a single institution indicate *C19MC* altered tumours may comprise up to 25% of cerebral CNS-PNETs (Li et al. 2009; Spence et al. 2014a). Notably, *C19MC* altered tumours can arise in pineal and cerebellar locations, and present as diffuse brain stem

lesions with a radiologic picture resembling diffuse intrinsic pontine glioma (DIPG). Rare *C19MC* altered tumours have also been reported in intraocular locations and need to be distinguished from other more benign lesions including medulloepitheliomas arising from the ciliary bodies (Jakobiec et al. 2015; Spence et al. 2014a). The young age of presentation for these tumours suggest a heritable association is likely; however, no specific germline alterations have been reported in this disease. Patient demographics from a series of studies are summarized in Table 13.3.

Table 13.3 C19MC altered and associated tumours

	$n = 75$
Patient characteristics	
Age (months)	*n=75*
Median (months)	24
<6	2 (3%)
6–12	12 (16%)
12–36	38 (51%)
>36	23 (31%)
Gender	*n=75*
Female	39 (52%)
Male	36 (48%)
Location	*n=74*
Cerebral hemispheres	44 (59%)
Midbrain, brainstem, thalamic	17 (23%)
Cerebellum	12 (16%)
Spinal	1 (1%)
Stage	*n=23*
M0	17 (74%)
M1-4	6 (26%)
Treatment characteristics	
Extent of surgical resection	*n=64*
Complete (GTR/<1.5 cm^2 residual tumour)	55 (86%)
Incomplete (STR, biopsy)	9 (14%)
Standard chemotherapy	*n=65*
Yes	54 (83%)
No	11 (17%)
Radiotherapy	*n=50*
Yes	20 (40%)
No	30 (60%)
Overall survival	*n=59*
24 months	25% (95% CI 12–40)
60 months	20% (95% CI 8–36)

GTR gross total resection, *STR* subtotal resection, *CSI* craniospinal irradiation, *CI* confidence interval

13.3.1 Molecular Features

Initial single-nucleotide polymorphism (SNP) arrays and FISH-based studies showed the *C19MC* locus is amplified or gained and overexpressed specifically in a subset of tumours with histopathologic features that include ependymoblastic rosettes, patterns of neuronal differentiation, including neurocytes, ganglion cells and neutrophil-like background classically described in ETANTRs or ependymoblastoma (Cervoni et al. 1995; Mork and Rubinstein 1985; Rubinstein 1970). With wider application of the *C19MC* FISH assays it is now clear that while ETANTRs characteristically exhibit C19MC copy number alterations, *C19MC* amplification or copy number changes can also be found in ~15–20% of tumours without classic histological features (Spence et al. 2014b). Gene expression studies showed that *C19MC* amplified tumours exhibit unique highly primitive transcriptional signatures, notably with elevated expression of *LIN28A and B*, both markers of pluripotency and upregulation of *SHH* and *WNT* developmental signaling (Li et al. 2009). Global methylation studies have now shown that ~20% of embryonal brain tumours that cluster with *C19MC* amplified tumours have no evidence of *C19MC* copy number alterations. They, however, exhibit high *LIN28* expression, similar gene expression profiles, and other copy number alterations including whole chr 2 gains (Spence et al. 2014b).

Biological understanding of *C19MC* altered and associated tumours have to date been derived from primary tumours and limited in vitro studies, as cell lines have been difficult to derive, and animal models have not yet been developed. To date, higher resolution genomic studies show only recurrent *C19MC* alterations in primary tumours, thus indicating *C19MC* as a major oncogenic driver in this disease. Although mechanisms by which *C19MC* promotes tumour formation remain to be elucidated, experimental studies show expression of a subset of *C19MC* miRs inhibits neural stem cell differentiation (Li et al. 2009). Significantly, RNA sequencing studies reveal tumours with *C19MC* amplification also exhibit gene fusions of *C19MC* with *TTHY1*, a primitive neural channel gene and increased expression of an embryonic-specific DNA methyl transferase 3B isoform. These studies suggest *C19MC* may also drive oncogenesis by regulating DNA methylation and promoting a transformation-prone epigenetic cell state (Kleinman et al. 2014). In addition to *C19MC*, experimental studies indicate *LIN28A/B*, which are highly expressed in all *C19MC* amplified and associated tumours, also drive tumour cell growth in part via regulation of the insulin and mTOR signaling pathways (Spence et al. 2014a).

13.3.2 Treatment Approaches and Prognostic Factors

Since *C19MC* altered and related tumours were only recently identified as a distinct disease, outcome data on a substantial group of uniformly treated patients are lacking. Similar to early reports on ETANTRs, Li et al. observed that among children with cerebral PNETs, presence of *C19MC* amplification correlated with a particularly dismal survival irrespective of treatment received (Li et al. 2009). The highly aggressive nature of this disease has now been borne out in approximately 80 cases reported in the literature (Gessi et al. 2009; Korshunov et al. 2010). Horowitz et al. (Horwitz et al. 2016) reported on the largest institutional series, and reported 1-year EFS of 36% and OS of 45% (Horwitz et al. 2016) in children treated with a variety of approaches. Overall it is estimated that long-term survival of children with these tumours is around 10%.

To date, no specific patient or tumour-related prognostic factors have been identified. It remains to be determined in larger studies where specific cellular morphology of tumours or presence or absence of C19MC amplification has prognostic significance. Although formal evaluation of different treatment modalities is not available, some reports suggest surgery, high-dose chemotherapy, and radiation offer survival benefits. However, data from the Rare Brain Tumour Registry suggests despite aggressive interventions, the majority of patients do not survive beyond 1 year. The apparent efficacy of radiotherapy and high-dose chemotherapy reported in retrospective series must thus be interpreted with caution. Cumulative reports suggest that early, rapid disease progression with tumour dissemination is frequently observed in children with *C19MC* altered and related tumours, indicating conventional embryonal brain tumour induction regimens are insufficient for tumour control even in the setting of complete tumour resection.

The identification of novel therapeutic agents for this disease has been difficult as only three cell lines have been reported to date (Kleinman et al. 2014; Schmidt et al. 2017; Spence et al. 2014a). Initial studies by the Huang group suggest epigenetic and metabolic pathways downstream of *C19MC* and *LIN28* hold promise as novel therapeutic targets (Sin-Chan and Huang 2014; Spence et al. 2014a). Notably, they demonstrated synergistic effects on a patient derived cell line with azacitidine and vorinostat. Interestingly, several case studies have reported maturation of residual tumour to a more differentiated cellular phenotype after conventional chemotherapy, and suggest drugs that induce cellular differentiation (Antonelli et al. 2015; Lafay-Cousin et al. 2014; Sin-Chan and Huang 2014; Spence et al. 2014a); such drugs as histone deactylaces and retinoids may be important therapeutic agents to include in the treatment of this disease. Two limited scope drugs screens have been reported using the three available *C19MC* altered cell lines (Schmidt et al. 2017; Spence et al. 2014a). In addition to drugs that target the metabolic pathway, these studies showed promising therapeutic effects of some conventional agents, including gemcitabine and topotecan, indicating these drugs may be important to incorporate into the future chemotherapeutic backbone for this disease. Given the young age of these patients and the propensity of these tumours to disseminate upon recurrence, it may also be important to incorporate intraventricular drug therapy into future trial design.

13.3.3 Future Directions

With the discovery of a specific genetic marker for *C19MC* altered tumours, the disease is now increasingly recognized and reported, suggesting the incidence of these tumours may be underestimated. Several different diagnostic methods have been used in the literature reports, including morphological descriptions compatible with ETANTR/ETMR/ependymoblastoma/medulloepithelioma, *C19MC* amplification, and/or *LIN28* IHC. While morphologic features of a classic ETANTR/ETMR are easily recognized, these may only be present in a subset of C19MC altered and related tumours; thus, histologic diagnoses should be augmented with molecular studies to distinguish tumours that may have overlapping histologic features, such as medulloepitheliomas arising in extracranial locations which are more benign. LIN28 immunopositivity is also not specific, but is reported in AT/RTs and high-grade gliomas (Spence et al. 2014a; Weingart et al. 2015). In order to robustly evaluate clinical and treatment-related prognostic factors, it will be important to adopt uniform methods for diagnosis. In our experience, a combination of tumour morphology, *LIN28* IHC, and FISH for *C19MC* alterations, which is highly specific for this group of tumours, is the best diagnostic combination. As a rare tumour, it is of utmost importance to create an international collaboration that allows the centralized collection of clinical information and biological material. The Rare Brain Tumour Consortium addresses this issue (http://www.rarebraintumourconsortium.ca). Ultimately, a clear clinical picture will only become apparent with prospective enrollment in clinical trials based on robust tumour diagnostics.

Drugs that inhibit DNA methylation/histone modifications and the IGF2/P13K metabolic pathway have been identified as biologically rational choices for therapy. Many of these have been in phase I/II trials in children and as such have safety profiles. Incorporating these into clinical trials, however, may prove challenging in this rare disease and will require international collaborations. Only by treating these tumours as a single diagnosis uniformly on clinical trials with biologically rational targets, will we start to change the outcome for these children.

13.4 Pineoblastoma

Pineoblastomas (PBs) are rare, aggressive embryonal tumours of the pineal region (Nakazato et al. 2007). They account for approximately 25% and are the most aggressive of pineal region neoplasms (Jouvet et al. 2000). They mainly occur during the two first decades of life and affect mainly children (Nakazato et al. 2007). Aggregate published studies indicate a median age at diagnosis of 4.3 years. There is a bimodal age distribution for PBs, with a peak around 3 years of age and a smaller peak at 9 years of age (Table 13.4), which is suggestive of biological heterogeneity in this disease. PBs are so rare that they were often included for convenience in the family of supratentorial PNETs for analysis. However, increasing molecular data suggest they represent distinct diseases. Robust epidemiological data are lacking; in addition to heritable association with retinoblastoma (de Jong et al. 2014), recent studies link defects in the microRNA biogenesis pathway with heritable PB (de Kock et al. 2014).

Histologically, PBs do not have specific immune-histochemical or morphological features (Jouvet et al. 2000; Schild et al. 1993). They share with other PNETs an appearance of highly cellular, proliferative small round blue cell tumours with diffuse, patternless sheets of poorly differentiated, neoplastic cells with a high nuclear-to-cytoplasmic ratio and a scant cytoplasm. Necrosis is common in these tumours, which typically exhibit high proliferative and mitotic counts (>20%) (Fevre-Montange et al. 2012). Homer-Wright pseudorosettes may be observed, but features of photoreceptor differentiation such as Flexner Wintersteiner rosettes or fleurettes are exceedingly rare. They show variable immunoexpression of neuronal markers, including synaptophysin and neurofilament protein. As a rule, they retain the expression of INI1, allowing differentiation from AT/RT (Miller et al. 2013), and lack *LIN28A* expression seen in *C19MC* associated tumours. Pineoblastomas should be distinguished from more differentiated pineal parenchymal tumours like pineocytoma and pineal parenchymal tumour of intermediate differentiation, which are less aggressive entities.

Table 13.4 Pineal PNET studies

	n = 28
Patient characteristics	
Age (years)	*n=28*
Median (years)	4.3
<3	12 (43%)
3–5	2 (11%)
5–10	7 (25%)
>10	6 (21%)
Gender	*n=12*
Female	7 (58%)
Male	5 (22%)
Stage	*n=25*
M0	18 (72%)
M1-4	7 (28%)
Treatment characteristics	
Extent of surgical resection	*n=27*
Complete (GTR/<1.5 cm^2 residual tumour)	8 (30%)
Incomplete (STR, biopsy)	19 (70%)
Standard chemotherapy	*n=26*
Yes	18 (69%)
No	8 (31%)
High-dose chemotherapy	*n=28*
Yes	13 (46%)
No	15 (54%)
Radiotherapy	*n=28*
Yes	17 (61%)
CSI	15 (88%)
Focal only	2 (12%)
No	11 (39%)
Overall survival	*n=28*
24 months	57% (95% CI 37–74)
60 months	48%(95% CI 28-66)

GTR gross total resection, *STR* subtotal resection, *CSI* craniospinal irradiation, *CI* confidence interval

13.4.1 Molecular Features

PBs may develop in the setting of germline RB-1 (retinoblastoma 1 gene located at position 13q14.2 on chromosome 13) defects, the co-occurrence of bilateral retinoblastoma and pineoblastoma being known as "trilateral retinoblastoma" (de Jong et al. 2014). Association with suparsellar/parasellar neuroectodermal tumours is more rarely described. Trilateral retinoblastoma has been especially described in patients harboring germline 13q deletion, in contrast with patients presenting *RB1* mutations (D'Elia et al. 2013). PB was recently recognized as one of the components of the *DICER1* syndrome (de Kock et al. 2014), which also predisposes to various tumours such as pleuropulmonary blastoma due to germline mutation of *DICER1* (located at position 14q32.13 on chromosome 14). Notably, *DICER1* RNA IIIb mutations, most commonly reported in other tumours (Heravi-Moussavi et al. 2012; Wang et al. 2015), are rare in PB. Nevertheless, loss of heterozygosity seems to be the main mechanism by which *DICER1* biallelic inactivation is achieved, indicating *DICER1* as an important tumour suppressor gene in the pineal gland.

Frequent other alterations in PB include various abnormalities of chromosome 1 and losses involving chromosomes 9, 16, 13, and 22 (Brown et al. 2006; Miller et al. 2011; Rickert et al. 2001; Russo et al. 1999). PBs, as well as other pineal parenchymal tumours and retinoblastomas, express CRX (Cone-Rod Homeobox), a transcription factor involved in the development of pineal and retinal lineages (Santagata et al. 2009). However, this expression is not specific as it is also found in some medulloblastomas, yet more focally. Some genes involved in various oncogenic processes such as invasion and growth (PRAME, CD24, POU4F2, and HOXD13) are overexpressed in PBs and high-grade pineal parenchymal tumour of intermediate differentiation (Fevre-Montange et al. 2006). The expression of O6-methylguanine-DNA-methyltransferase in all three PBs analyzed in one study may suggest resistance to temozolomide (Kanno et al. 2012).

13.4.2 Treatment Approaches and Prognostic Factors

Analysis of the optimal treatment for PBs is difficult. In clinical trials, PBs are often grouped together with other supratentorial PNETs, which makes it difficult to extract tumour-specific information. As in other embryonal tumours of the CNS, treatment of PB is multimodal and based upon combinations of surgery, chemother-

apy, and radiotherapy (Cohen et al. 1995). The first step in PB treatment usually consists of the acute management of obstructive hydrocephalus. The technique of choice is now endoscopic third ventriculostomy that allows CSF diversion and sampling as well as tumour biopsy in some cases (Tate et al. 2011). Precise histopathological diagnosis is also essential in the therapeutic management of patients with pineal parenchymal tumours (Fauchon et al. 2000). Surgical procedures in PB management include stereotactic biopsy, open surgical biopsy, and surgical removal. Complete surgical removal is usually difficult to achieve and requires experienced neurosurgeons. In our review, only 30% of the patients had complete surgical resection (Table 13.4). This may be explained by the deep-seated location of pineal region and by the network of major venous structures that are usually intimately associated with the neoplasm (Yamamoto 2001). Complete removal seems to be associated with a better prognosis in several studies (Jakacki et al. 2015; Kao et al. 2005; Lutterbach et al. 2002; Tate et al. 2012). Surgery is usually followed by RT in older children. RT has a positive impact on survival and includes CSI in order to prevent distant failure (Johnston et al. 2008; Timmermann et al. 2002). A majority of patients reported to date have received CSI RT (Table 13.4). In infants, RT cannot be safely applied without risk of severe neurocognitive impairment, but chemotherapy alone has proven to be ineffective (Duffner et al. 1995; Jakacki et al. 1995) (Table 13.5). The use of high-dose chemotherapy with autologous stem cell rescue may be a suitable procedure to improve survival in young children (Fangusaro et al. 2008b; Gururangan et al. 2003). The optimal regimen and drug association for chemotherapy in PBs is still unsettled. In older children, the adjunct of carboplatin during radiotherapy following by non-intensive chemotherapy was a feasible strategy and showed prolonged overall survival (81% at 5 years) (Jakacki et al. 2015).

Cumulative data suggest a generally poor outcome for PB with OS ranging between 10 and 81% (Fauchon et al. 2000; Jakacki et al. 2015).

Table 13.5 Summary of pineoblastoma studies

Study	# patients	Age range (years)	Chemotherapy protocol Standard chemotherapy (SC)	HDC (# cycles)	Radiation (RT) CSI (Gy)	Focal only (Gy)	DFS (years)	OS (years)
High-dose chemotherapy (HDC)								
Fangusaro et al. (2008)	13	0.1–6.9	HS I and HS II	CBDCA, TSPA, VP-16 (1)	No	No	15% (5)	23% (5)
Chintagumpala et al. (2009)	7	3.8–12.9	SJMB06	CDDP, CPM (1)	SR: 23.4; HR: 36	No	54% (5)	67% (5)
Massimino et al. (2013)[a,b]	9	1.4–18	Milan protocol	TSPA (2)	31/39	No	83% (5)	N/A[c]
Adjuvant chemotherapy								
Cohen et al. (1995)	17	1.5–19.3	CCG921		36	No	61% (3)	N/A[c]
Pre-irradiation chemotherapy								
Timmermann et al. (2002)	11	2.9–17.7	HIT 88/89 and 91		35	42	64% (3)	N/A[c]
Pizer et al. (2006)	14	2.9–16.6	PNET3		35	No	71% (5)	71% (5)
Allen et al. (2009)[a]	8	3–20	CCG9931		40	No	75% (5)	86% (5)
Jakacki et al. (2015)	23	3–21	COG99701		36	No	62% (5)	81% (5)
Radiation deferral								
Duffner et al. (1995)	11	0–3	POG8633		35	No	19% (2)	21% (2)

DFS disease-free survival—reported as event-free survival or progression-free survival, *SR* standard risk, *HR* high risk, *HDC* high-dose chemotherapy, *RT* radiation therapy, *VCR* vincristine, *CDDP* cisplatin, *CPM* cyclophosphamide, *CBDCA* carboplatin, *VP-16* etoposide, *TSPA* thiotepa
[a]Study used hyperfractionated radiation therapy
[b]Radiation dose was age dependent
[c]Overall survival (OS) provided for the entire group

Prognostic factors such as age, metastatic status at diagnosis, radiotherapy, and extent of surgery have been consistently identified across multiple studies. Young age (Cohen et al. 1995; Hinkes et al. 2007; Jakacki et al. 2015; Tate et al. 2012) and disseminated disease at diagnosis (Cohen et al. 1995; Farnia et al. 2014; Lutterbach et al. 2002; Tate et al. 2012) are negative prognostic indicators, whereas use of RT (Johnston et al. 2008; Parikh et al. 2017; Timmermann et al. 2002) and GTR have a positive impact. In children more than 18 months of age, prognosis of PBs may be better than that of other supratentorial PNETs (Cohen et al. 1995; Jakacki et al. 1995), whereas in infants a poorer prognosis in

PBs is found (Fangusaro et al. 2008a) (Table 13.5). Recently, Mynarek et al. (2017) published an analysis of 127 PB patients pooled from 10 European centers and the Head Start trial group in the US, and found similarly that younger children (<4 years old) had significantly poorer PFS and OS (11% and 12%, respectively) than patients over 4 years of age (72% and 73%, respectively), and had more rapid disease progression. Radiation therapy was the strongest risk factor for both PFS and OS in both age groups although the type of radiotherapy (conventional vs. hyperfractionated) did not impact survival. High-dose chemotherapy had limited impact on survival, but appeared to benefit older patients with metastatic disease. Notably, studies by Chintagumpala et al. (2009) suggest that HDC may allow risk-adapted reduced CSI in selected patients.

13.4.3 Future Directions

As with other embryonal tumours, it is clear that the diagnosis of PB in retrospective series may include a spectrum of other entities. Notably, in our studies archived pineoblastomas have included pineal region AT/RTs, *C19MC* altered tumours, high-grade gliomas, and germ cell tumours. Thus, the significance of various prognostic factors, particularly age, may be confounded by these misdiagnoses, and will require re-evaluation with incorporation of specific molecular diagnostic markers. Molecular characterization of large cohorts of pineoblastomas are currently being undertaken by several groups; thus, the full molecular spectrum of PB remains to be elucidated. Preliminary studies suggest that as is the case with other embryonal tumours, molecular subtypes of PB have emerged with global profiling studies (Li and Huang, unpublished).

Aggregate small studies suggest distinct association of PB subtypes with *DROSHA* or *DICER1* alterations, and potentially a third biological PB subtype. Future studies will help evaluate whether molecular subtypes of PB have distinct clinicopathologic correlates that will enable in risk and treatment stratification.

13.5 Atypical Teratoid Rhabdoid Tumours

Atypical teratoid rhabdoid tumour (AT/RT) is a malignant embryonal CNS tumour of early childhood with the most common characteristic being loss of function alterations of the *SMARCB1*, or more rarely the *SMARCA4*, tumour suppressor loci, which encode components of the ubiquitous SWI/SNF chromatin remodeling complex (Roberts 2016). Initially identified on the basis of histologic resemblance to malignant rhabdoid tumours of the kidneys, AT/RT was not appreciated as a distinct CNS entity until 1996 (Rorke

et al. 1996), and was included in the WHO classification of CNS tumours in 2000 (Gonzales 2001). Although historically considered a fatal disease, survival of AT/RT in children has improved in recent years. Significantly, recent global molecular analyses of large AT/RT cohorts indicate they comprise a biological spectrum with at least three different disease subtypes (Fig. 13.1) (Johann et al. 2016; Torchia et al. 2016). These studies suggest tumour biology may be combined with clinical factors to predict patient outcomes, thus raising exciting possibilities for risk and treatment stratification for AT/RTs in future trials.

The incidence of AT/RT has not been accurately defined, in part due to the large number of AT/RTs initially misdiagnosed as PNET or medulloblastoma (Burger et al. 1998; Rorke et al. 1996). With the discovery and development of highly portable immunohistochemical and genetic diagnostic tests, AT/RTs without classic histology are increasingly identified. As with medulloblastoma and ependymoma, there appears to be a slight male predominance of the disease (Biswas et al. 2009). AT/RT accounts for 1–2% of all pediatric CNS tumours with two-thirds diagnosed in children <3 years (Hilden et al. 2004; Picard et al. 2012; Tekautz et al. 2005). It represents the most common malignant CNS tumour in children less than 6 months of age (Fruhwald et al. 2016) with median age at diagnosis ranging from 1.2 to 2.3 years (Dufour et al. 2012; Pai Panandiker et al. 2012; von Hoff et al. 2011).

AT/RTs are observed in all CNS locations and arise most frequently in the cerebral hemispheres or posterior fossa (Table 13.6). Rare locations include the spine, which comprises 1–7% of reported cases (Athale et al. 2009; Picard et al. 2012; Tekautz et al. 2005), as well the pineal region and brain stem. Germline mutations of *SMARCB1* have been reported in up to 20–35% of patients with AT/RTs and are associated with the "rhabdoid tumour predisposition syndrome" (Biegel et al. 1999; Bourdeaut et al. 2011; Eaton et al. 2011; Sévenet et al. 1999), which predisposes to development of multiple intra- and extracranial tumours and tumour diagnosis at a younger age (Bourdeaut et al. 2011; Eaton et al. 2011; Kordes et al. 2010). *SMARCA4* (BRG1)

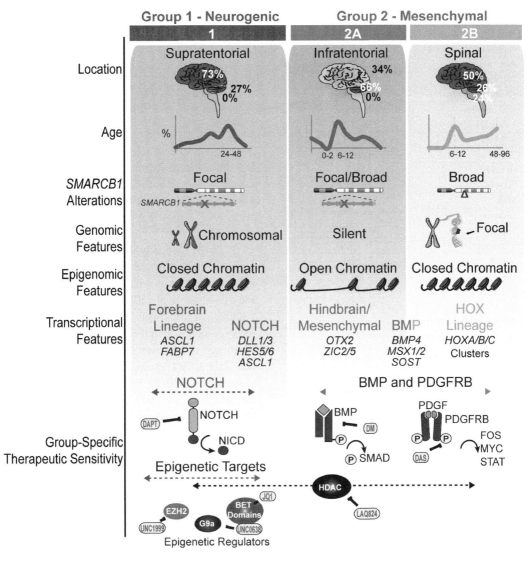

Fig. 13.1 Schematic of clinical and molecular features correlating with ATRT molecular subgroups. ATRTs segregate into two transcriptional subgroups: Group 1 with neurogenic signatures and Group 2 with mesenchymal signatures. Methylation profiling reveals three epigenetic subgroups: Group 1, Group 2a, and Group 2b. Classical tumour location, age distribution, genomic/epigenomic features, and epigenetic markers for the associated subgroups are shown (Torchia et al., 2015)

has also been linked to rare familial AT/RT (Hasselblatt et al. 2011).

AT/RTs exhibits diverse morphology with neuroepithelial, epithelial, and mesenchymal features. Although "rhabdoid" cells possessing eccentric nuclei and prominent nucleoli are considered classic features of AT/RTs, these are rare and most AT/RTs exhibit bland small blue cell morphology also seen in medulloblastoma and PNET (Bikowska et al. 2011). Loss of the *SMARCB1/INI1* or *SMARCA4* and negative

immunostaining for the respective gene products BAF47 and BRG1 are diagnostic for AT/RTs (Biegel 2006; Haberler et al. 2006).

13.5.1 Molecular Features of AT/RT

Early observation of chromosome 22 monosomy, and focal chr22q11.2 deletion/translocation (Rorke et al. 1996) led to identification of *SMARCB1* (Versteege et al. 1998) (also known as

Table 13.6 AT/RTs studies

	n = 619
Patient characteristics	
Age	*n=578*
Median (months)	19.2
≤6 months	82 (14%)
≤12 months	108 (19%)
1–3 years	235 (41%)
3–5 years	80 (14%)
ʾ5 years	73 (13%)
Gender	*n=567*
Female	231 (41%)
Male	336 (59%)
Location	*n=549*
Supratentorial	261 (48%)
Infratentorial	276 (50%)
Spinal	12 (2%)
Stage	*n=394*
M0	250 (63%)
M+	144 (37%)
Treatment characteristics	
Extent of surgical resection	*n=313*
Complete	137 (44%)
Incomplete	176 (56%)
High-dose chemotherapy	*n=315*
Yes	114 (36%)
No	201 (64%)
Radiotherapy	*n=298*
Yes	171 (57%)
No	127 (43%)
Overall survival	*n=278*
Median (months)	23.4
24 months	43% (95% CI 37–49)
60 months	37% (95% CI 29–45)

CI confidence interval

hSNF5/INI1/BAF47) as a critical etiologic tumour suppressor in all rhabdoid tumours, including AT/RTs. Recently, multiple high resolution genomic studies have shown the AT/RT genome is largely devoid of other recurrent coding mutations (Hasselblatt et al. 2013; Johann et al. 2016; Li et al. 2009; McKenna et al. 2008; Torchia et al. 2016), and have underscored the critical etiologic role of *SMARCB1/SNF5* in this disease. These observations have led to the proposal that AT/RT is a disease primarily driven by epigenetic mechanisms resulting from SNF 5 loss.

Cumulative global transcriptional and methylation studies now indicate AT/RT comprise a molecular heterogenous disease. Birks et al. first identified a subcluster of AT/RT with a high expression of the BMP pathway genes (i.e., *BMP4, SOST, BAMBI, MSX2*), which correlated with a worse prognosis (Birks et al. 2011). These studies were confirmed with larger cohort gene expression analyses, which showed AT/RT comprise at least two molecular subgroups with distinct anatomic and clinicopathologic correlations. Specifically, Torchia et al. reported a primarily supratentorial tumour group characterized by neurogenic differentiation, and high ASCL1 protein expression and a second primarily infratentorial tumour group with BMP signaling enrichments, which they respectively called group 1 and 2 AT/RTs (Torchia et al. 2015). Recently, two larger cohort studies indicate AT/RT may be further segregated into 3 epigenetic subtypes with distinct methylation profiles (Johann et al. 2016; Torchia et al. 2016). Although a consensus on AT/RT subtypes and direct comparison of the two study cohorts remain pending, a comparison of published data suggests the SHH AT/RT group reported by Johann et al. (Johann et al. 2016) corresponds to group 1 AT/RT, which are enriched for a pro-neural gene signature with prominent NOTCH as well as SHH signaling (group 1/AT/RT-SHH), while group 2a and b AT/RTs reported by Torchia et al. appear to (Torchia et al. 2016) have gene enrichment patterns corresponding to AT/RT-TYR and AT/RT-MYC groups, respectively. Significantly, Johann et al. correlated the presence of lineage-specific super-enhancers with group-specific signaling features (Johann et al. 2016), while Torchia et al. showed similar correlation of methylation status and gene expression levels at distinct lineage genes in an AT/RT subgroup specific manner (Torchia et al. 2016). Interestingly, in addition to location and patient age, both studies also reported an association of SMARCB1 genotypes with AT/RT molecular group. Specifically, they observed group 1/SHH-AT/RT had a higher frequency of focal *SMARCB1* alterations, including point mutations and deletions, whereas Group 2b/MYC AT/RT predominantly exhibited large deletions encompassing all of *SMARCB1* and neighboring genes. These collective data indicate SMARCB1 loss in AT/RTs may have different functional consequences, and suggest that a combination of tumour cell of origin and varying degrees of SWI/SNF dysfunction resulting from heterogenous genetic events targeting *SMARCB1* may underlie the molecular and clinical heterogeneity observed in AT/RTs. Significantly, consistent with these observations Torchia et al. showed AT/RT cell lines exhibit subgroup-specific sensitivity to various therapeutic compounds that target signaling and epigenetic pathways.

The substantial clinical and molecular heterogeneity observed in AT/RTs, a "monogenic" disease, is in keeping with earlier suggestions that deregulated epigenetic pathways resulting from loss of SNF5 and disruption of the ubiquitous and critical SWI/SNF chromatin remodeling complex is the major pathogenic driving mechanism in AT/RTs. Indeed, animal studies have shown that loss of *SMARCB1* potently induces rhabdoid tumour formation, and notably the molecular spectrum of human AT/RTs is recapitulated by conditional, temporal loss of *SMARCB1* in animal models (Han et al. 2016). Although mechanisms by which *SMARCB1* loss leads to tumour formation are incompletely elucidated, experimental studies point to upregulation of *EZH2* secondary to *SMARCB1* loss as a critical oncogenic event. Indeed, conditional double knockouts of *SMARCB1* and *EZH2* prevent tumour formation in murine models (Wilson et al. 2010).

13.5.2 Treatment Approaches and Prognostic Factors

To date, no standard treatment regimen has been established for AT/RT and the clinical prognoses of these patients are generally poor with median survival estimated at 1 year (Table 13.6) (Dufour et al. 2012; von Hoff et al. 2011). This may be ascribed to a combination of factors, including incorrect diagnoses prior to availability of a diagnostic marker. It has been shown that patients who were incorrectly diagnosed between 1996 and 2000 (prior to inclusion of AT/RT into the WHO classification) had significantly poorer survival ($p = 0.047$) (Woehrer et al. 2010). Today, multimodal therapies including surgery, chemotherapy, and radiotherapy have been associated with improved clinical outcomes (Chi et al. 2009), though the relative prognostic role of each modality has yet to be defined.

To date, there has only been one limited prospective AT/RT study reported, thus much of the clinical therapeutic literature is based on retrospective, often small, and heterogeneously treated cohorts (Table 13.7). Generally, studies have identified age, tumour location, and metastatic status at diagnosis as important prognostic factors. Age greater than 3 years at diagnosis has been reported in multiple studies to correlate with better prognosis (Bartelheim et al. 2016; Hilden et al. 2004; Ho et al. 2000; Tekautz et al. 2005). This may be due to a number of factors, including restricted use of radiation therapy (see below), higher incidence of metastatic disease (Chi et al. 2009; Dufour et al. 2012; Hilden 2004; Tekautz et al. 2005), and the potential negative prognostic impact of genetic predisposition syndromes in younger patients. However, a small study by Cohen et al. (Cohen et al. 2015) and Park et al. (2012) of younger patients showed 50% disease-free survival in contrast to only 16% of surviving young patients in a study by Zaky et al. (2014), while Dufour et al. (Dufour et al. 2012) identified age (<2 years) as a risk factor only in combination with M-stage and immunopositivity for claudin 6. Supratentorial tumour location has also been linked with favorable outcomes (Chi et al. 2009; Dufour et al. 2012; Pai Panandiker et al. 2012; von Hoff et al. 2011) whereas tumour metastases, estimated to be present in 14–21% of patients at diagnosis (Athale et al. 2009; Buscariollo et al. 2012; Hilden et al. 2004; Tekautz et al. 2005), has been reported to portend worse outcome.

Treatment factors implicated in AT/RT prognosis have included extent of surgery (Gardner et al. 2008; Hilden et al. 2004; Tekautz et al. 2005); Woehrer et al. (2010); (Zimmerman et al. 2005), with better outcomes reported for patients with GTR versus STR, near total (NR) or partial resections (PR) (Chi et al. 2009; Picard et al. 2012). Hilden et al. reported median EFS of 14 months and 9.25 months, respectively, for patients with GTR and PR. However, some studies have reported no prognostic impact of extent of surgery (Athale et al. 2009; Buscariollo et al.

Table 13.7 Summary of AT/RT studies

Study	# patients	Age range (years)	Chemotherapy protocol		Radiation (RT)		DFS (years)	OS (years)	Prognostic findings
			Standard chemotherapy (SC)	HDC (# cycles)	CSI (Gy)	Focal only (Gy)			
High-dose chemotherapy (HDC)									
Gardner et al. (2008)	13	0.3–4.3	HS I and HS II	CBDCA/TSPA or VP-16, MTX (1)	N/A	N/A	23% (3)[a]	23% (3)[a]	HD MTX prognostic
Zaky et al. (2014)	19	0–2.7	HS III	CBDCA/TSPA or VP-16, MTX (1)	18–36	59.4	21% (3)	26% (3)	Extent of surgery not prognostic
Tekautz et al. (2005)	31	N/A	Various (<3 year MOPP, CCG9921; >3 year SJ MB96, ICE)	CPM, Oxaliplatin/ TOPO	25–39.6	50.4–55.8	>3 years: 78% (2); <3 years: 11% (2)	>3 years: 89% (2); <3 years: 17% (2)	RT in younger patients improved survival outcome
Benesch et al. (2014)	19[b]	0–5.3	Rhabdoid 2007 or EU-RHAB	CBDCA/VP-16; CPM/TSPA (1–2)	24	54	29% (2)	50% (2)	RT prognostic
Intensive multimodal therapy									
Chi et al. (2009)	20	0.3–19.5	Modified IRSIII		36	54	53% (2)	70% (2)	Extent of surgery and tumour
Bartelheim et al. (2016)	31[b]	0–10	Rhabdoid 2007		24	54	45% (6)	46% (6)	Age (>3 years) and RT
Hilden et al. (2004)	42	0.1–9.8	Various (DFCI, CCG99703, CCG 9921, POG 9233, ICE, HS I, HS II)		23.4–36	45	Median: 10 months	Median: 17 months	Extent of surgery and RT prognostic; role of HDCT and IT unclear
von Hoff et al. (2011)	56	0.1–14	Various (HIT2000, HIT91, SKK87, SKK92)		23.4–36.8	44.5–59.4	13% (3)	22% (3)	Tumour location
Lafay-Cousin et al. (2012)	50	0–15.6	Various (ICE, Babybrain, DFCI, ACNS0333, CCG99703)		12–45	45–59	N/A	36% (2)[a]	Extent of surgery and HDCT
Radiation deferral									
Geyer et al. (2005)	28	<0.9–3	CCG9921 reg A/reg B		18–30.6	50.4–54	14% (5)	29% (5)	Extent of surgery not prognostic
Slavc et al. (2014)	22	0.17–22	Group A: MUV-ATRT (IRS III and HD MTX) Group B Various (HIT SKK, PEI)		N/A	40.6–54	53% (5)	56% (5)	HD MTX and IT beneficial
Proton therapy									
McGovern et al. (2014)	31	0.3–4.6	Various (DFCI, SJMB03,ACNS0333,EU-RHAB)		43.2–55.8	9–54	46% (2)	53% (2)	Metastatic status not prognostic

HDC high-dose chemotherapy, *RT* radiation therapy, *CPM* cyclophosphamide, *CBDCA* carboplatin, *VP-16* etoposide, *TSPA* thiotepa, *MTX* methotrexate, *TOPO* topotecan

[a]Predicted/projected

[b]Eight patients in common between Bartelheim et al. (2016) and Benesch et al. (2014)

2012; Hilden et al. 2004). Interestingly, Dufour et al. reported surgical treatment was significant in a univariate but not multivariate analyses (Dufour et al. 2012), again underscoring the interdependence of multiple clinical and treatment variables in disease prognostication.

13.5.2.1 Conventional-Dose Chemotherapy

Conventional-dose chemotherapy in first-generation studies has been generally unsuccessful in curing most AT/RT patients. Intensified chemotherapy regimens such as CCG 9921 and POG 9923 resulted in very poor outcomes with an EFS of <10%. The Intergroup Rhabdomyosarcoma Study protocol III (IRS-III), later modified by the Dana-Farber group to include doxorubicin and dactinomycin in a "modified IRS-III" regimen showed more promise and resulted in a 58% response rate prior to RT. The role of methotrexate- and anthracycline-based regimens is debatable, with some reports advocating their importance (Chi et al. 2009, Zimmerman 2005; Weinblatt 1992) and others noting no difference in survival (Finkelstein-Shechter et al. 2010). Platinum- and alkylator-based regimens have been favored (Lafay-Cousin and Strother 2009), although given the heterogenous and multi-agent therapies prescribed to AT/RT patients, the exact role of these drugs in therapeutic outcomes are unknown.

13.5.2.2 High-Dose Chemotherapy

High-dose chemotherapy followed by autologous stem cell rescue (ASCR) was initiated primarily as a method to circumvent irradiation in young children, but has been increasingly used and reported to be favorable for treatment of AT/RT patients (Finkelstein-Shechter et al. 2010; Gardner et al. 2008; Nicolaides et al. 2010; Shih et al. 2008). Regimens have varied in inclusion of high-dose methotrexate, as in the Head Start II study (Fangusaro et al. 2008a) in which methotrexate was used in the induction phase followed by consolidation therapy with one to three cycles of HDC with carboplatin, thiotepa, and etoposide. Notably, patients treated with an earlier HS I regimen fared worse than the HDC HS II regi-

men (6/6 patients died of disease [DOD] versus 3/7 patients alive with no evidence of disease [NED]). Particularly noteworthy is that none of the long-term survivors received RT. Two registry-based studies have also reported on the impact of HDC: Hilden et al. showed 46% of patients who received HDC were survivors with NED (Hilden 2004); 50% of survivors had complete surgery and only 33% were irradiated. In a Canadian registry study, HDC correlated with a survival benefit: 2-year OS of 47.9 ± 12.1% compared to 27.3 ± 9.5% for those who received conventional chemotherapy alone ($p = 0.036$) (Lafay-Cousin et al. 2012; Picard et al. 2012). However, the authors note that of the survivors who received HDC ($n = 9$), 55% (5/9) also had complete surgical resection and 67% (6/9) were not metastatic at diagnosis. Notably, preliminary reports of ACNS0333, the HDC-based prospective AT/RT trial protocol run by the Children's Oncology Group (COG), also suggest a significantly improved survival as compared to historical CCG9921 and POG9923 studies. Similar studies for older children conducted by the St Jude's group, which employed four tandem high-dose regimens and CSI for children over 3 years of age, has also reported superior survival compared to historical data (Tekautz et al. 2005).

For young patients with AT/RT, deferral or avoidance of RT and decreased dose or volume of RT has been frequently adopted to avoid neurocognitive toxicity, while risk-adapted RT has been applied in some protocols (Chi et al. 2009).

In a Canadian study, 54% (6/11) of patients were treated with HDC in the absence of RT and were long-term survivors (median follow up of 38.1 months) (Lafay-Cousin et al. 2012). In agreement with these reports, data from German studies have also shown no definitive evidence in support of RT favoring a survival benefit (von Hoff et al. 2011). Interestingly, von Hoff et al. described no survival benefit in patients who received focal ($n = 10$) versus those who received CSI ($n = 19$, $p = 0.578$), and up-front or salvage RT ($p = 0.314$). However, benefits of RT have been reported in a number of studies, including a meta-analysis by Athale et al., which showed a trend towards greater mean survival time in those who received RT (18.4 months versus 8.5 months) ($p = 0.097$) (Athale et al. 2009). Buscariollo et al. also demonstrated a survival benefit for AT/RT patients who received RT ($n = 144$, $p = 0.02$) (Buscariollo et al. 2012). In contrast, some retrospective studies found no significant difference in survival for AT/RT patients who received adjuvant radiotherapy compared to those who did not. It is important to note that surgical extent and accurate disease staging may have had a significant impact on the different observations in these retrospective studies.

13.5.2.3   Intrathecal Chemotherapy

A number of studies have explored intrathecal (IT) chemotherapy as an alternative option to irradiation for CNS axis treatment and prophylaxis in young AT/RT patients (Athale et al. 2009). Typically, IT methotrexate, cytarabine, and hydrocortisone alone or in combination have been incorporated into several treatment regimens, such as the German HIT SKK protocol (IT methotrexate) and the Dana-Farber Cancer Institute AT/RT protocol. While some studies, including a meta-analysis (Athale et al. 2009), have shown that IT correlated with survival benefits, contradictory findings have also been reported (Lafay-Cousin et al. 2012; Schrey et al. 2016; Tekautz et al. 2005). IT chemotherapy has been variably used either with mono- or multi-agents in various settings with conventional or HDC or with focal RT, thus making assessment of benefits difficult.

13.5.3   Future Directions

AT/RT is no longer a lethal disease, with substantial retrospective and emerging prospective data suggesting dose-intensification is beneficial and may even permit reduction or avoidance of RT in young children. However, overall outcomes for AT/RT patients remain poor, and current aggressive treatment regimens are reaching maximum tolerable toxicity. Substantial progress has been made in understanding impact of *SMARCB1* loss

on SWI/SNF function and downstream signaling effects, as well as the biological spectrum and heterogeneity that underlies the clinical phenotypes in AT/RTs.

The next challenge will be to integrate biologically informed strategies in selection of drugs and patients to improve efficacy while reducing toxicity of therapy.

Studies of the SWI/SNF complex have shown loss of *SNF5* leads to overexpression of *EZH2*, a histone methyl transferase of the repressive PRC2 complex, and aberrant activation of downstream signaling and cellular programs (Wilson et al. 2010). In addition to inhibitors of *EZH2*, several other components of the epigenetic machinery associated with SWI/SNF function, including inhibitors of G9a—a lysine methyl transferase—and BET/Bromodomain proteins, have emerged as promising drug targets (Tang et al. 2014; Torchia et al. 2016). Other promising pharmacologic targets implicated in signaling pathways downstream of SWI/SNF (Biegel et al. 2014; Kadoch et al. 2013) include cyclin D1 (Tsikitis et al. 2005), Aurora A kinase (Lee et al. 2011), insulin-like growth factor (Ogino et al. 2001) and PDGF (Torchia et al. 2016), for which repurposed or new drugs are available. Notably, Aurora kinase inhibitors have shown impressive monoagent effects on recurrent AT/RTs, while new cyclin D1 inhibitors have shown promising results as anti-proliferating agents (Knipstein et al. 2012; Maris et al. 2010).

With identification of AT/RT molecular subtypes, we may anticipate that new therapeutic agents with AT/RT subgroup sensitivity may be incorporated into the next generation AT/RT clinical trials. In addition to matching drugs to AT/RT subtypes, it will be important to evaluate and incorporate the prognostic impact of AT/RT subtypes with clinical risk factors to inform stratification in trials. Imminent questions that have arisen from studies to date are which group of patients can be treated without need for radiation or with less aggressive chemotherapy, and whether biological directed maintenance or IT therapy may be of benefit. To fully realize biology-tailored and risk-stratified therapy for AT/RT, development of robust subtyping tools and validation of the prognostic impact of tumour subtype biology in prospective cohorts will be critical.

13.6 Summary

The advent of high resolution genomic tools together with the establishment of international collaborative studies have significantly accelerated our understanding of the biological spectrum of rare embryonal brain tumours of childhood, and a refined classification of these previously challenging diagnostic entities (summarized in Figs. 13.2

and 13.3) has now emerged. The discovery of specific molecular markers for subcategories of tumours previously classified under the CNS-PNET umbrella will enable clinical studies of homogenous entities and permit more precise design of therapeutic approaches. Similarly, identification of molecular subtypes of AT/RTs will inform and refine selection of patients and therapies for future prospective trials. Development of robust, sensitive diagnostic tools not only for diagnosis but for evaluation and monitoring of therapeutic response and minimal molecular disease will be critical for future risk-stratified trials directed at harm reduction, without compromising efficacy, in these very young patients.

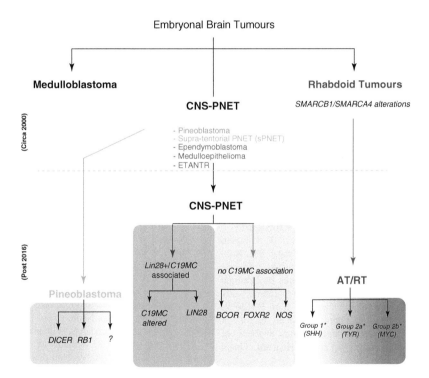

Fig. 13.2 Summary of embryonal brain tumour classification and corresponding molecular subtypes. Pineoblastoma, originally defined as a CNS-PNET tumour, is subdivided into DICER1 and RB1 mutated tumours with potentially other unidentified subgroups that have yet to be defined. Other tumours classified previously as CNS-PNET are further subdivided into two groups: Lin28+/C19MC associated tumours (ependy-

moblastoma, medulloepithelioma, ETANTRs) (Spence et al., 2014) and tumours with no C19MC association (sPNETs) subdivided into BCOR, FOXR2, and NOS (Norman et al., unpublished data). ATRT are divided into three epigenetic subgroups; group 1, 2a, and 2b (Torchia et al., 2016), respectively resembling ATRT-SHH, ATRT-TYR, and ATRT-MYC (Johann et al.) with distinct enhancer landscapes

	Pineoblastoma	ETMR		PNET			ATRT		
	DICER1/RB1	C19MC altered & related tumours		no C19MC association			SMARCB1/SMARCA4 alterations		
Subgroups/ Molecular entities	?	C19MC amp.	LIN 28 exp	BCOR	FOXR2	NOS	Group 1 (SHH)	Group 2a (TYR)	Group 2b (MYC)
Age distribution						?			
Reported location					?				
Oncogenic drivers	DICER/RB1	C19MC amp	LIN28	BCOR	FOXR2	?	NOTCH/SHH	BMP/PDGFRB/TYR	BMP/PDGFRB/MYC

0–2yrs 2–4yrs > 4yrs

Fig. 13.3 Schematic summary of rare embryonal brain tumours. Classical age distribution, tumor location, and known/proposed oncogenic drivers associated with each subgroup are shown. Primary tumor locations are indicated as circles where larger circles represent the predominant area of occurrence

References

Albright AL, Wisoff JH, Zeltzer P, Boyett J, Rorke LB, Stanley P, Geyer JR, Milstein JM (1995) Prognostic factors in children with supratentorial (nonpineal) primitive neuroectodermal tumors. A neurosurgical perspective from the Children's Cancer Group. Pediatr Neurosurg 22:1–7

Allen J, Donahue B, Mehta M, Miller DC, Rorke LB, Jakacki R, Robertson P, Sposto R, Holmes E, Vezina G et al (2009) A phase II study of preradiotherapy chemotherapy followed by hyperfractionated radiotherapy for newly diagnosed high-risk medulloblastoma/primitive neuroectodermal tumor: a report from the Children's Oncology Group (CCG 9931). Int J Radiat Oncol Biol Phys 74:1006–1011

Antonelli M, Korshunov A, Mastronuzzi A, Diomedi Camassei F, Carai A, Colafati GS, Pfister SM, Kool M, Giangaspero F (2015) Long-term survival in a case of ETANTR with histological features of neuronal maturation after therapy. Virchows Arch 466:603–607

Athale UH, Duckworth J, Odame I, Barr R (2009) Childhood atypical teratoid rhabdoid tumor of the central nervous system: a meta-analysis of observational studies. J Pediatr Hematol Oncol 31:651–663

Bakry D, Aronson M, Durno C, Rimawi H, Farah R, Alharbi QK, Alharbi M, Shamvil A, Ben-Shachar S, Mistry M et al (2014) Genetic and clinical determinants of constitutional mismatch repair deficiency syndrome: report from the constitutional mismatch repair deficiency consortium. Eur J Cancer 50:987–996

Bartelheim K, Nemes K, Seeringer A, Kerl K, Buechner J, Boos J, Graf N, Dürken M, Gerss J, Hasselblatt M et al (2016) Improved 6-year overall survival in AT/RT—results of the registry study Rhabdoid 2007. Cancer Med 5(8):1765–1775

Benesch M, Bartelheim K, Fleischhack G et al (2014) High-dose chemotherapy (HDCT) with auto-SCT in children with atypical teratoid/rhabdoid tumors (AT/RT): a report from the European Rhabdoid Registry (EU-RHAB). Bone Marrow Transplant 49(3):370–375

Biegel JA (2006) Molecular genetics of atypical teratoid/rhabdoid tumor. Neurosurg Focus 20:E11

Biegel JA, Busse TM, Weissman BE (2014) SWI/SNF chromatin remodeling complexes and cancer. Am J Med Genet C Semin Med Genet 166C:350–366

Biegel JA, Zhou JY, Rorke LB, Stenstrom C, Wainwright LM, Fogelgren B (1999) Germ-line and acquired mutations of INI1 in atypical teratoid and rhabdoid tumors. Cancer Res 59:74–79

Bikowska B, Grajkowska W, Jozwiak J (2011) Atypical teratoid/rhabdoid tumor: short clinical description and insight into possible mechanism of the disease. Eur J Neurol 18:813–818

Birks DK, Donson AM, Patel PR, Dunham C, Muscat A, Algar EM, Ashley DM, Kleinschmidt-Demasters BK, Vibhakar R, Handler MH, Foreman NK (2011) High expression of BMP pathway genes distinguishes a subset of atypical teratoid/rhabdoid tumors associated with shorter survival. Neuro Oncol 13:1296–1307

Biswas S, Burke A, Cherian S, Williams D, Nicholson J, Horan G, Jefferies S, Williams M, Earl HM, Burnet NG, Hatcher H (2009) Non-pineal supratentorial primitive neuro-ectodermal tumors (sPNET) in teenagers and young adults: time to reconsider cisplatin based chemotherapy after cranio-spinal irradiation? Pediatr Blood Cancer 52:796–803

Bourdeaut F, Lequin D, Brugieres L, Reynaud S, Dufour C, Doz F, André N, Stephan J-L, Pérel Y, Oberlin O et al (2011) Frequent hSNF5/INI1 germline mutations in patients with rhabdoid tumor. Clin Cancer Res 17:31–38

Brown AE, Leibundgut K, Niggli FK, Betts DR (2006) Cytogenetics of pineoblastoma: four new cases and a literature review. Cancer Genet Cytogenet 170:175–179

Burger PC, Yu IT, Tihan T, Friedman HS, Strother DR, Kepner JL, Duffner PK, Kun LE, Perlman EJ (1998) Atypical teratoid/rhabdoid tumor of the central nervous system: a highly malignant tumor of infancy and childhood frequently mistaken for medulloblastoma: a Pediatric Oncology Group study. Am J Surg Pathol 22:1083–1092

Buscariollo DL, Park HS, Roberts KB, Yu JB (2012) Survival outcomes in atypical teratoid rhabdoid tumor for patients undergoing radiotherapy in a Surveillance, Epidemiology, and End Results analysis. Cancer 118:4212–4219

Cervoni L, Celli P, Trillo G, Caruso R (1995) Ependymoblastoma: a clinical review. Neurosurg Rev 18:189–192

Chi SN, Zimmerman MA, Yao X, Cohen KJ, Burger P, Biegel JA, Rorke-Adams LB, Fisher MJ, Janss A, Mazewski C et al (2009) Intensive multimodality treatment for children with newly diagnosed CNS atypical teratoid rhabdoid tumor. J Clin Oncol 27:385–389

Chintagumpala M, Hassall T, Palmer S, Ashley D, Wallace D, Kasow K, Merchant TE, Krasin MJ, Dauser R, Boop F et al (2009) A pilot study of risk-adapted radiotherapy and chemotherapy in patients with supratentorial PNET. Neuro-Oncology 11:33–40

Cohen BH, Geyer JR, Miller DC, Curran JG, Zhou T, Holmes E, Ingles SA, Dunkel IJ, Hilden J, Packer RJ et al (2015) Pilot study of intensive chemotherapy with peripheral hematopoietic cell support for children less than 3 years of age with malignant brain tumors, the CCG-99703 phase I/II study. A report from the children's oncology group. Pediatr Neurol 53:31–46

Cohen BH, Zeltzer PM, Boyett JM, Geyer JR, Allen JC, Finlay JL, McGuire-Cullen P, Milstein JM, Rorke LB, Stanley P et al (1995) Prognostic factors and treatment results for supratentorial primitive neuroectodermal tumors in children using radiation and chemotherapy: a Childrens Cancer Group randomized trial. J Clin Oncol 13:1687–1696

D'Elia G, Grotta S, Del Bufalo F, De Ioris MA, Surace C, Sirleto P, Romanzo A, Cozza R, Locatelli F, Angioni A (2013) Two novel cases of trilateral retinoblastoma: genetics and review of the literature. Cancer Genet 206:398–401

de Jong MC, Kors WA, de Graaf P, Castelijns JA, Kivela T, Moll AC (2014) Trilateral retinoblastoma: a systematic review and meta-analysis. Lancet Oncol 15:1157–1167

de Kock L, Sabbaghian N, Druker H, Weber E, Hamel N, Miller S, Choong CS, Gottardo NG, Kees UR, Rednam SP et al (2014) Germ-line and somatic DICER1 mutations in pineoblastoma. Acta Neuropathol 128:583–595

Duffner PK, Horowitz ME, Krischer JP et al (1993) Postoperative chemotherapy and delayed radiation in children less than three years of age with malignant brain tumors. N Engl J Med 328(24):1725–1731

Duffner PK, Cohen ME, Sanford RA, Horowitz ME, Krischer JP, Burger PC, Friedman HS, Kun LE (1995) Lack of efficacy of postoperative chemotherapy and delayed radiation in very young children with pineoblastoma. Pediatric Oncology Group. Med Pediatr Oncol 25:38–44

Dufour C, Beaugrand A, Le Deley MC, Bourdeaut F, Andre N, Leblond P, Bertozzi AI, Frappaz D, Rialland X, Fouyssac F et al (2012) Clinicopathologic prognostic factors in childhood atypical teratoid and rhabdoid tumor of the central nervous system: a multicenter study. Cancer 118:3812–3821

Eaton KW, Tooke LS, Wainwright LM, Judkins AR, Biegel JA (2011) Spectrum of SMARCB1/INI1 mutations in familial and sporadic rhabdoid tumors. Pediatr Blood Cancer 56:7–15

Fangusaro J, Finlay J, Sposto R, Ji L, Saly M, Zacharoulis S, Asgharzadeh S, Abromowitch M, Olshefski R, Halpern S et al (2008a) Intensive chemotherapy followed by consolidative myeloablative chemotherapy with autologous hematopoietic cell rescue (AuHCR) in young children with newly diagnosed supratentorial primitive neuroectodermal tumors (sPNETs): report of the Head Start I and II experience. Pediatr Blood Cancer 50:312–318

Fangusaro JR, Jubran RF, Allen J, Gardner S, Dunkel IJ, Rosenblum M, Atlas MP, Gonzalez-Gomez I, Miller D, Finlay JL (2008b) Brainstem primitive neuroectodermal tumors (bstPNET): results of treatment with intensive induction chemotherapy followed by consolidative chemotherapy with autologous hematopoietic cell rescue. Pediatr Blood Cancer 50:715–717

Farnia B, Allen PK, Brown PD, Khatua S, Levine NB, Li J, Penas-Prado M, Mahajan A, Ghia AJ (2014) Clinical outcomes and patterns of failure in pineoblastoma: a 30-year, single-institution retrospective review. World Neurosurg 82:1232–1241

Fauchon F, Jouvet A, Paquis P, Saint-Pierre G, Mottolese C, Ben Hassel M, Chauveinc L, Sichez JP, Philippon J, Schlienger M, Bouffet E (2000) Parenchymal pineal tumors: a clinicopathological study of 76 cases. Int J Radiat Oncol Biol Phys 46:959–968

Fevre-Montange M, Champier J, Szathmari A, Wierinckx A, Mottolese C, Guyotat J, Figarella-Branger D, Jouvet A, Lachuer J (2006) Microarray analysis reveals differential gene expression patterns in tumors of the pineal region. J Neuropathol Exp Neurol 65:675–684

Fevre-Montange M, Vasiljevic A, Frappaz D, Champier J, Szathmari A, Aubriot Lorton MH, Chapon F, Coulon A, Quintin Roue I, Delisle MB et al (2012) Utility of Ki67 immunostaining in the grading of pineal parenchymal tumours: a multicentre study. Neuropathol Appl Neurobiol 38:87–94

Finkelstein-Shechter T, Gassas A, Mabbott D, Huang A, Bartels U, Tabori U, Janzen L, Hawkins C, Taylor M, Bouffet E (2010) Atypical teratoid or rhabdoid tumors: improved outcome with high-dose chemotherapy. J Pediatr Hematol Oncol 32:e182–e186

Friedrich C, von Bueren AO, von Hoff K, Gerber NU, Ottensmeier H, Deinlein F, Benesch M, Kwiecien R, Pietsch T, Warmuth-Metz M et al (2013) Treatment of young children with CNS-primitive neuroectodermal tumors/pineoblastomas in the prospective multicenter trial HIT 2000 using different chemotherapy regimens and radiotherapy. Neuro-Oncology 15:224–234

Friedrich C, Warmuth-Metz M, von Bueren AO, Nowak J, Bison B, von Hoff K, Pietsch T, Kortmann RD, Rutkowski S (2015) Primitive neuroectodermal tumors of the brainstem in children treated according to the HIT trials: clinical findings of a rare disease. J Neurosurg Pediatr 15:227–235

Fruhwald MC, Biegel JA, Bourdeaut F, Roberts CW, Chi SN (2016) Atypical teratoid/rhabdoid tumors-current concepts, advances in biology, and potential future therapies. Neuro-Oncology 18:764–778

Gardner SL, Asgharzadeh S, Green A, Horn B, McCowage G, Finlay J (2008) Intensive induction chemotherapy followed by high dose chemotherapy with autologous hematopoietic progenitor cell rescue in young children newly diagnosed with central nervous system atypical teratoid rhabdoid tumors. Pediatr Blood Cancer 51:235–240

Gessi M, Giangaspero F, Lauriola L, Gardiman M, Scheithauer BW, Halliday W, Hawkins C, Rosenblum MK, Burger PC, Eberhart CG (2009) Embryonal tumors with abundant neuropil and true rosettes. Am J Surg Pathol 33:211–217

Geyer JR, Sposto R, Jennings M et al (2005) Multiagent chemotherapy and deferred radiotherapy in infants with malignant brain tumors: a report from the Children's Cancer Group. J Clin Oncol 23(30):7621–7631

Gonzales M (2001) The 2000 World Health Organization classification of tumors of the nervous system. J Clin Neurosci 8:1–3

Grundy RG, Wilne SH, Robinson KJ, Ironside JW, Cox T, Chong WK, Michalski A, Campbell RH, Bailey CC, Thorp N et al (2010) Primary postoperative chemotherapy without radiotherapy for treatment of brain tumors other than ependymoma in children under 3 years: results of the first UKCCSG/SIOP CNS 9204 trial. Eur J Cancer 46:120–133

Gururangan S, McLaughlin C, Quinn J, Rich J, Reardon D, Halperin EC, Herndon J 2nd, Fuchs H, George T, Provenzale J et al (2003) High-dose chemotherapy with autologous stem-cell rescue in children and adults with newly diagnosed pineoblastomas. J Clin Oncol 21:2187–2191

Haberler C, Laggner U, Slavc I, Czech T, Ambros IM, Ambros PF, Budka H, Hainfellner JA (2006) Immunohistochemical analysis of INI1 protein in malignant pediatric CNS tumors: lack of INI1 in atypical teratoid/rhabdoid tumors and in a fraction of primitive neuroectodermal tumors without rhabdoid phenotype. Am J Surg Pathol 30:1462–1468

Han ZY, Richer W, Freneaux P, Chauvin C, Lucchesi C, Guillemot D, Grison C, Lequin D, Pierron G, Masliah-Planchon J et al (2016) The occurrence of intracranial rhabdoid tumors in mice depends on temporal control of Smarcb1 inactivation. Nat Commun 7:10421

Hart MN, Earle KM (1973) Primitive neuroectodermal tumors of the brain in children. Cancer 32:890–897

Hasselblatt M, Gesk S, Oyen F, Rossi S, Viscardi E, Giangaspero F, Giannini C, Judkins AR, Fruhwald MC, Obser T et al (2011) Nonsense mutation and inactivation of SMARCA4 (BRG1) in an atypical teratoid/rhabdoid tumor showing retained SMARCB1 (INI1) expression. Am J Surg Pathol 35:933–935

Hasselblatt M, Isken S, Linge A, Eikmeier K, Jeibmann A, Oyen F, Nagel I, Richter J, Bartelheim K, Kordes U et al (2013) High-resolution genomic analysis suggests the absence of recurrent genomic alterations other than SMARCB1 aberrations in atypical teratoid/rhabdoid tumors. Genes Chromosomes Cancer 52:185–190

Heravi-Moussavi A, Anglesio MS, Cheng SW, Senz J, Yang W, Prentice L, Fejes AP, Chow C, Tone A, Kalloger SE et al (2012) Recurrent somatic DICER1 mutations in nonepithelial ovarian cancers. N Engl J Med 366:234–242

Hilden JM (2004) Central nervous system atypical teratoid/rhabdoid tumor: results of therapy in children enrolled in a registry. J Clin Oncol 22:2877–2884

Hinkes BG, von Hoff K, Deinlein F, Warmuth-Metz M, Soerensen N, Timmermann B, Mittler U, Urban C, Bode U, Pietsch T et al (2007) Childhood pineoblastoma: experiences from the prospective multicenter trials HIT-SKK87, HIT-SKK92 and HIT91. J Neuro-Oncol 81:217–223

Ho DM, Hsu CY, Wong TT, Ting LT, Chiang H (2000) Atypical teratoid/rhabdoid tumor of the central nervous system: a comparative study with primitive neuroectodermal tumor/medulloblastoma. Acta Neuropathol 99:482–488

Horwitz M, Dufour C, Leblond P, Bourdeaut F, Faure-Conter C, Bertozzi AI, Delisle MB, Palenzuela G, Jouvet A, Scavarda D et al (2016) Embryonal tumors with multilayered rosettes in children: the SFCE experience. Childs Nerv Syst 32:299–305

Huang SC, Zhang L, Sung YS, Chen CL, Kao YC, Agaram NP, Singer S, Tap WD, D'Angelo S, Antonescu CR (2016) Recurrent CIC gene abnormalities in angiosarcomas: a molecular study of 120 cases with concurrent investigation of PLCG1, KDR, MYC, and FLT4 gene alterations. Am J Surg Pathol 40:645–655

Jakacki RI, Burger PC, Kocak M, Boyett JM, Goldwein J, Mehta M, Packer RJ, Tarbell NJ, Pollack IF (2015) Outcome and prognostic factors for children with supratentorial primitive neuroectodermal tumors treated with carboplatin during radiotherapy: a report from the Children's Oncology Group. Pediatr Blood Cancer 62:776–783

Jakacki RI, Zeltzer PM, Boyett JM, Albright AL, Allen JC, Geyer JR, Rorke LB, Stanley P, Stevens KR, Wisoff J et al (1995) Survival and prognostic factors following radiation and/or chemotherapy for primitive neuroectodermal tumors of the pineal region in infants and children: a report of the Childrens Cancer Group. J Clin Oncol 13:1377–1383

Jakobiec FA, Kool M, Stagner AM, Pfister SM, Eagle RC, Proia AD, Korshunov A (2015) Intraocular medulloepitheliomas and embryonal tumors with multilayered rosettes of the brain: comparative roles of LIN28A and C19MC. Am J Ophthalmol 159:1065–1074.e1

Johann PD, Erkek S, Zapatka M, Kerl K, Buchhalter I, Hovestadt V, Jones DTW, Sturm D, Hermann C, Segura Wang M et al (2016) Atypical teratoid/rhabdoid tumors are comprised of three epigenetic subgroups with distinct enhancer landscapes. Cancer Cell 29:379–393

Johnston DL, Keene DL, Lafay-Cousin L, Steinbok P, Sung L, Carret AS, Crooks B, Strother D, Wilson B, Odame I et al (2008) Supratentorial primitive neuroectodermal tumors: a Canadian pediatric brain tumor consortium report. J Neuro-Oncol 86:101–108

Jouvet A, Saint-Pierre G, Fauchon F, Privat K, Bouffet E, Ruchoux MM, Chauveinc L, Fevre-Montange M (2000) Pineal parenchymal tumors: a correlation of histological features with prognosis in 66 cases. Brain Pathol 10:49–60

Kadoch C, Hargreaves DC, Hodges C, Elias L, Ho L, Ranish J, Crabtree GR (2013) Proteomic and bioinformatic analysis of mammalian SWI/SNF complexes identifies extensive roles in human malignancy. Nat Genet 45:592–601

Kanno H, Nishihara H, Narita T, Yamaguchi S, Kobayashi H, Tanino M, Kimura T, Terasaka S, Tanaka S (2012) Prognostic implication of histological oligodendroglial tumor component: clinicopathological analysis of 111 cases of malignant gliomas. PLoS One 7:e41669

Kao C-L, Chiou S-H, Chen Y-J, Singh S, Lin H-T, Liu R-S, Lo C-W, Yang C-C, Chi C-W, Lee C-H, Wong T-T (2005) Increased expression of osteopontin gene in atypical teratoid/rhabdoid tumor of the central nervous system. Mod Pathol 18:769–778

Kao YC, Sung YS, Zhang L, Huang SC, Argani P, Chung CT, Graf NS, Wright DC, Kellie SJ, Agaram NP et al (2016) Recurrent BCOR internal tandem duplication and YWHAE-NUTM2B fusions in soft tissue undifferentiated round cell sarcoma of infancy: overlapping genetic features with clear cell sarcoma of kidney. Am J Surg Pathol 40:1009–1020

Kleihues P, Louis DN, Scheithauer BW, Rorke LB, Reifenberger G, Burger PC, Cavenee WK (2002) The WHO classification of tumors of the nervous system. J Neuropathol Exp Neurol 61:215–225. discussion 226–219

Kleinman CL, Gerges N, Papillon-Cavanagh S, Sin-Chan P, Pramatarova A, Quang DA, Adoue V, Busche S, Caron M, Djambazian H et al (2014) Fusion of TTYH1 with the C19MC microRNA cluster drives expression of a brain-specific DNMT3B isoform in the embryonal brain tumor ETMR. Nat Genet 46:39–44

Knipstein JA, Birks DK, Donson AM, Alimova I, Foreman NK, Vibhakar R (2012) Histone deacetylase inhibition decreases proliferation and potentiates the effect of

ionizing radiation in atypical teratoid/rhabdoid tumor cells. Neuro-Oncology 14:175–183

Kordes U, Gesk S, Fruhwald MC, Graf N, Leuschner I, Hasselblatt M, Jeibmann A, Oyen F, Peters O, Pietsch T et al (2010) Clinical and molecular features in patients with atypical teratoid rhabdoid tumor or malignant rhabdoid tumor. Genes Chromosomes Cancer 49:176–181

Korshunov A, Remke M, Gessi M, Ryzhova M, Hielscher T, Witt H, Tobias V, Buccoliero AM, Sardi I, Gardiman MP et al (2010) Focal genomic amplification at 19q13.42 comprises a powerful diagnostic marker for embryonal tumors with ependymoblastic rosettes. Acta Neuropathol 120:253–260

Lafay-Cousin L, Hader W, Wei XC, Nordal R, Strother D, Hawkins C, Chan JA (2014) Post-chemotherapy maturation in supratentorial primitive neuroectodermal tumors. Brain Pathol 24:166–172

Lafay-Cousin L, Hawkins C, Carret AS, Johnston D, Zelcer S, Wilson B, Jabado N, Scheinemann K, Eisenstat D, Fryer C et al (2012) Central nervous system atypical teratoid rhabdoid tumours: the Canadian paediatric brain tumour consortium experience. Eur J Cancer 48:353–359

Lafay-Cousin L, Strother D (2009) Current treatment approaches for infants with malignant central nervous system tumors. Oncologist 14:433–444

Lee S, Cimica V, Ramachandra N, Zagzag D, Kalpana GV (2011) Aurora A is a repressed effector target of the chromatin remodeling protein INI1/hSNF5 required for rhabdoid tumor cell survival. Cancer Res 71:3225–3235

Leung W, Ribeiro RC, Hudson M, Tong X, Srivastava DK, Rubnitz JE, Sandlund JT, Razzouk BI, Evans WE, Pui CH (2001) Second malignancy after treatment of childhood acute myeloid leukemia. Leukemia 15:41–45

Li M, Lee KF, Lu Y, Clarke I, Shih D, Eberhart C, Collins VP, Van Meter T, Picard D, Zhou L et al (2009) Frequent amplification of a chr19q13.41 microRNA polycistron in aggressive primitive neuroectodermal brain tumors. Cancer Cell 16:533–546

Li MH, Bouffet E, Hawkins CE, Squire JA, Huang A (2005) Molecular genetics of supratentorial primitive neuroectodermal tumors and pineoblastoma. Neurosurg Focus 19:E3

Louis DN, Ohgaki H, Wiestler OD, Cavenee WK, Burger PC, Jouvet A, Scheithauer BW, Kleihues P (2007) The 2007 WHO classification of tumors of the central nervous system. Acta Neuropathol 114:97–109

Louis DN, Perry A, Reifenberger G, von Deimling A, Figarella-Branger D, Cavenee WK, Ohgaki H, Wiestler OD, Kleihues P, Ellison DW (2016) The 2016 World Health Organization classification of tumors of the central nervous system: a summary. Acta Neuropathol 131:803–820

Lutterbach J, Fauchon F, Schild SE, Chang SM, Pagenstecher A, Volk B, Ostertag C, Momm F, Jouvet A (2002) Malignant pineal parenchymal tumors in adult patients: patterns of care and prognostic factors. Neurosurgery 51:44–55. discussion 55–56

Marec-Berard P, Jouvet A, Thiesse P, Kalifa C, Doz F, Frappaz D (2002) Supratentorial embryonal tumors in children under 5 years of age: an SFOP study of treatment with postoperative chemotherapy alone. Med Pediatr Oncol 38:83–90

Maris JM, Morton CL, Gorlick R, Kolb EA, Lock R, Carol H, Keir ST, Reynolds CP, Kang MH, Wu J et al (2010) Initial testing of the aurora kinase a inhibitor MLN8237 by the Pediatric Preclinical Testing Program (PPTP). Pediatr Blood Cancer 55:26–34

Mason WP, Grovas A, Halpern S, Dunkel IJ, Garvin J, Heller G, Rosenblum M, Gardner S, Lyden D, Sands S et al (1998) Intensive chemotherapy and bone marrow rescue for young children with newly diagnosed malignant brain tumors. J Clin Oncol 16:210–221

Massimino M, Gandola L, Biassoni V, Spreafico F, Schiavello E, Poggi G, Pecori E, Vajna De Pava M, Modena P, Antonelli M, Giangaspero F (2013) Evolving of therapeutic strategies for CNS-PNET. Pediatr Blood Cancer 60:2031–2035

Massimino M, Gandola L, Spreafico F, Luksch R, Collini P, Giangaspero F, Simonetti F, Casanova M, Cefalo G, Pignoli E et al (2006) Supratentorial primitive neuroectodermal tumors (S-PNET) in children: a prospective experience with adjuvant intensive chemotherapy and hyperfractionated accelerated radiotherapy. Int J Radiat Oncol Biol Phys 64:1031–1037

McGovern SL, Okcu MF, Munsell MF et al (2014) Outcomes and acute toxicities of proton therapy for pediatric atypical teratoid/rhabdoid tumor of the central nervous system. Int J Radiat Oncol Biol Phys 90(5):1143–1152

McKean-Cowdin R, Razavi P, Barrington-Trimis J, Baldwin RT, Asgharzadeh S, Cockburn M, Tihan T, Preston-Martin S (2013) Trends in childhood brain tumor incidence, 1973-2009. J Neuro-Oncol 115:153–160

McKenna ES, Sansam CG, Cho Y-J, Greulich H, Evans JA, Thom CS, Moreau LA, Biegel JA, Pomeroy SL, Roberts CWM (2008) Loss of the epigenetic tumor suppressor SNF5 leads to cancer without genomic instability. Mol Cell Biol 28:6223–6233

Miller S, Rogers HA, Lyon P, Rand V, Adamowicz-Brice M, Clifford SC, Hayden JT, Dyer S, Pfister S, Korshunov A et al (2011) Genome-wide molecular characterization of central nervous system primitive neuroectodermal tumor and pineoblastoma. Neuro-Oncology 13:866–879

Miller S, Ward JH, Rogers HA, Lowe J, Grundy RG (2013) Loss of INI1 protein expression defines a subgroup of aggressive central nervous system primitive neuroectodermal tumors. Brain Pathol 23:19–27

Mork SJ, Rubinstein LJ (1985) Ependymoblastoma. A reappraisal of a rare embryonal tumor. Cancer 55:1536–1542

Mynarek M, Pizer B, Dufour C, van Vuurden D, Garami M, Massimino M, Fangusaro J, Davidson T, Gilda-Costa MJ, Sterba J et al (2017) Evaluation of age-dependent treatment strategies for children and young adults with pineoblastoma: analysis of pooled European Society for Paediatric Oncology (SIOP-E) and US Head Start data. Neuro-Oncology 19:576–585

Nakazato Y, Jouvet A, Scheithauer B (2007) Pineal parenchymal tumour of intermediate differentiation. In: Louis DN, Ohgaki H, Wiestler OD, Cavenee WK (eds) WHO classification of tumors of the nervous system. IARC Press, Lyon, pp 122–127

Nicolaides T, Tihan T, Horn B, Biegel J, Prados M, Banerjee A (2010) High-dose chemotherapy and autologous stem cell rescue for atypical teratoid/rhabdoid tumor of the central nervous system. J Neuro-Oncol 98:117–123

Ogino S, Kubo S, Abdul-Karim FW, Cohen ML (2001) Comparative immunohistochemical study of insulin-like growth factor II and insulin-like growth factor receptor type 1 in pediatric brain tumors. Pediatr Dev Pathol 4:23–31

Pai Panandiker AS, Merchant TE, Beltran C, Wu S, Sharma S, Boop FA, Jenkins JJ, Helton KJ, Wright KD, Broniscer A et al (2012) Sequencing of local therapy affects the pattern of treatment failure and survival in children with atypical teratoid rhabdoid tumors of the central nervous system. Int J Radiat Oncol Biol Phys 82:1756–1763

Parikh KA, Venable GT, Orr BA, Choudhri AF, Boop FA, Gajjar AJ, Klimo P Jr (2017) Pineoblastoma—the experience at St. Jude Children's Research Hospital. Neurosurgery 81:120–128

Park ES, Sung KW, Baek HJ, Park KD, Park HJ, Won SC, Lim DH, Kim HS (2012) Tandem high-dose chemotherapy and autologous stem cell transplantation in young children with atypical teratoid/rhabdoid tumor of the central nervous system. J Korean Med Sci 27:135–140

Peters TL, Kumar V, Polikepahad S, Lin FY, Sarabia SF, Liang Y, Wang WL, Lazar AJ, Doddapaneni H, Chao H et al (2015) BCOR-CCNB3 fusions are frequent in undifferentiated sarcomas of male children. Mod Pathol 28:575–586

Picard D, Miller S, Hawkins CE, Bouffet E, Rogers HA, Chan TS, Kim SK, Ra YS, Fangusaro J, Korshunov A et al (2012) Markers of survival and metastatic potential in childhood CNS primitive neuro-ectodermal brain tumours: an integrative genomic analysis. Lancet Oncol 13:838–848

Pizer BL, Weston CL, Robinson KJ, Ellison DW, Ironside J, Saran F, Lashford LS, Tait D, Lucraft H, Walker DA et al (2006) Analysis of patients with supratentorial primitive neuro-ectodermal tumors entered into the SIOP/UKCCSG PNET 3 study. Eur J Cancer 42:1120–1128

Pomeroy SL, Tamayo P, Gaasenbeek M, Sturla LM, Angelo M, McLaughlin ME, Kim JYH, Goumnerova LC, Black PM, Lau C et al (2002) Prediction of central nervous system embryonal tumour outcome based on gene expression. Nature 415:436–442

Reddy AT, Janss AJ, Phillips PC, Weiss HL, Packer RJ (2000) Outcome for children with supratentorial primitive neuroectodermal tumors treated with surgery, radiation, and chemotherapy. Cancer 88:2189–2193

Rickert CH, Simon R, Bergmann M, Dockhorn-Dworniczak B, Paulus W (2001) Comparative genomic hybridization in pineal parenchymal tumors. Genes Chromosomes Cancer 30:99–104

Roberts CWM (2016) SWI/SNF (BAF) complex mutations in cancer. [abstract]. In: Proceedings of the AACR Special Conference on Advances in Pediatric Cancer Research: From Mechanisms and Models to Treatment and Survivorship; 2015 Nov 9-12; Fort Lauderdale, FL. Philadelphia (PA): AACR. Cancer Res 76(5 Suppl):Abstract nr IA12

Rorke LB (1983) The cerebellar medulloblastoma and its relationship to primitive neuroectodermal tumors. J Neuropathol Exp Neurol 42:1–15

Rorke LB, Packer RJ, Biegel JA (1996) Central nervous system atypical teratoid/rhabdoid tumors of infancy and childhood: definition of an entity. J Neurosurg 85:56–65

Rorke LB, Trojanowski JQ, Lee VM, Zimmerman RA, Sutton LN, Biegel JA, Goldwein JW, Packer RJ (1997) Primitive neuroectodermal tumors of the central nervous system. Brain Pathol 7:765–784

Rubinstein LJ (1970) The definition of the ependymoblastoma. Arch Pathol 90:35–45

Russo C, Pellarin M, Tingby O, Bollen AW, Lamborn KR, Mohapatra G, Collins VP, Feuerstein BG (1999) Comparative genomic hybridization in patients with supratentorial and infratentorial primitive neuroectodermal tumors. Cancer 86:331–339

Santagata S, Maire CL, Idbaih A, Geffers L, Correll M, Holton K, Quackenbush J, Ligon KL (2009) CRX is a diagnostic marker of retinal and pineal lineage tumors. PLoS One 4:e7932

Schild SE, Scheithauer BW, Schomberg PJ, Hook CC, Kelly PJ, Frick L, Robinow JS, Buskirk SJ (1993) Pineal parenchymal tumors. Clinical, pathologic, and therapeutic aspects. Cancer 72:870–880

Schmidt C, Schubert NA, Brabetz S, Mack N, Schwalm B, Chan JA, Selt F, Herold-Mende C, Witt O, Milde T et al (2017) Pre-clinical drug screen reveals topotecan, actinomycin D and volasertib as potential new therapeutic candidates for ETMR brain tumor patients. Neuro Oncol 19:1607–1617

Schrey D, Carceller Lechon F, Malietzis G, Moreno L, Dufour C, Chi S, Lafay-Cousin L, von Hoff K, Athanasiou T, Marshall LV, Zacharoulis S (2016) Multimodal therapy in children and adolescents with newly diagnosed atypical teratoid rhabdoid tumor: individual pooled data analysis and review of the literature. J Neuro-Oncol 126:81–90

Sévenet N, Sheridan E, Amram D, Schneider P, Handgretinger R, Delattre O (1999) Constitutional mutations of the hSNF5/INI1 gene predispose to a variety of cancers. Am J Hum Genet 65:1342–1348

Shih CS, Hale GA, Gronewold L, Tong X, Laningham FH, Gilger EA, Srivastava DK, Kun LE, Gajjar A, Fouladi M (2008) High-dose chemotherapy with autologous stem cell rescue for children with recurrent malignant brain tumors. Cancer 112:1345–1353

Sin-Chan P, Huang A (2014) DNMTs as potential therapeutic targets in high-risk pediatric embryonal brain tumors. Expert Opin Ther Targets 18:1103–1107

Slavc I, Chocholous M, Leiss U et al (2014) Atypical teratoid rhabdoid tumor: improved long-term survival with an intensive multimodal therapy and delayed radiotherapy. The Medical University of Vienna Experience 1992-2012. Cancer Med 3(1):91–100

Smoll NR, Drummond KJ (2012) The incidence of medulloblastomas and primitive neurectodermal tumors in adults and children. J Clin Neurosci 19:1541–1544

Spence T, Perotti C, Sin-Chan P, Picard D, Wu W, Singh A, Anderson C, Blough MD, Cairncross JG, Lafay-Cousin L et al (2014a) A novel C19MC amplified cell line links Lin28/let-7 to mTOR signaling in embryonal tumor with multilayered rosettes. Neuro-Oncology 16:62–71

Spence T, Sin-Chan P, Picard D, Barszczyk M, Hoss K, Lu M, Kim SK, Ra YS, Nakamura H, Fangusaro J et al (2014b) CNS-PNETs with C19MC amplification and/or LIN28 expression comprise a distinct histogenetic diagnostic and therapeutic entity. Acta Neuropathol 128:291–303

Strother DR, Lafay-Cousin L, Boyett JM, Burger P, Aronin P, Constine L, Duffner P, Kocak M, Kun LE, Horowitz ME, Gajjar A (2014) Benefit from prolonged dose-intensive chemotherapy for infants with malignant brain tumors is restricted to patients with ependymoma: a report of the Pediatric Oncology Group randomized controlled trial 9233/34. Neuro-Oncology 16:457–465

Sturm D, Orr BA, Toprak UH, Hovestadt V, Jones DT, Capper D, Sill M, Buchhalter I, Northcott PA, Leis I et al (2016) New brain tumor entities emerge from molecular classification of CNS-PNETs. Cell 164:1060–1072

Sung KW, Yoo KH, Cho EJ, Koo HH, Lim DH, Shin HJ, Ahn SD, Ra YS, Choi ES, Ghim TT (2007) High-dose chemotherapy and autologous stem cell rescue in children with newly diagnosed high-risk or relapsed medulloblastoma or supratentorial primitive neuroectodermal tumor. Pediatr Blood Cancer 48:408–415

Tang Y, Gholamin S, Schubert S, Willardson MI, Lee A, Bandopadhayay P, Bergthold G, Masoud S, Nguyen B, Vue N et al (2014) Epigenetic targeting of Hedgehog pathway transcriptional output through BET bromodomain inhibition. Nat Med 20:732–740

Tate M, Sughrue ME, Rutkowski MJ, Kane AJ, Aranda D, McClinton L, McClinton L, Barani IJ, Parsa AT (2012) The long-term postsurgical prognosis of patients with pineoblastoma. Cancer 118:173–179

Tate MC, Rutkowski MJ, Parsa AT (2011) Contemporary management of pineoblastoma. Neurosurg Clin N Am 22:409–412. ix

Taylor MD, Mainprize TG, Rutka JT (2000) Molecular insight into medulloblastoma and central nervous system primitive neuroectodermal tumor biology from hereditary syndromes: a review. Neurosurgery 47:888–901

Tekautz TM, Fuller CE, Blaney S, Fouladi M, Broniscer A, Merchant TE, Krasin M, Dalton J, Hale G, Kun LE et al (2005) Atypical teratoid/rhabdoid tumors (ATRT): improved survival in children 3 years of age and older with radiation therapy and high-dose alkylator-based chemotherapy. J Clin Oncol 23:1491–1499

Thorarinsdottir HK, Rood B, Kamani N, Lafond D, Perez-Albuerne E, Loechelt B, Packer RJ, MacDonald TJ (2007) Outcome for children <4 years of age with malignant central nervous system tumors treated with high-dose chemotherapy and autologous stem cell rescue. Pediatr Blood Cancer 48:278–284

Timmermann B, Kortmann RD, Kuhl J, Meisner C, Dieckmann K, Pietsch T, Bamberg M (2002) Role of radiotherapy in the treatment of supratentorial primitive neuroectodermal tumors in childhood: results of the prospective German brain tumor trials HIT 88/89 and 91. J Clin Oncol Off J Am Soc Clin Oncol 20:842–849

Timmermann B, Kortmann RD, Kuhl J, Rutkowski S, Meisner C, Pietsch T, Deinlein F, Urban C, Warmuth-Metz M, Bamberg M (2006) Role of radiotherapy in supratentorial primitive neuroectodermal tumor in young children: results of the German HIT-SKK87 and HIT-SKK92 trials. J Clin Oncol Off J Am Soc Clin Oncol 24:1554–1560

Torchia J, Golbourn B, Feng S, Ho KC, Sin-Chan P, Vasiljevic A, Norman JD, Guilhamon P, Garzia L, Agamez NR et al (2016) Integrated (epi)-genomic analyses identify subgroup-specific therapeutic targets in CNS rhabdoid tumors. Cancer Cell 30:891–908

Torchia J, Picard D, Lafay-Cousin L, Hawkins CE, Kim SK, Letourneau L, Ra YS, Ho KC, Chan TS, Sin-Chan P et al (2015) Molecular subgroups of atypical teratoid rhabdoid tumors in children: an integrated genomic and clinicopathological analysis. Lancet Oncol 16:569–582

Tsikitis M, Zhang Z, Edelman W, Zagzag D, Kalpana GV (2005) Genetic ablation of Cyclin D1 abrogates genesis of rhabdoid tumors resulting from Ini1 loss. Proc Natl Acad Sci U S A 102:12129–12134

Versteege I, Sévenet N, Lange J, Rousseau-Merck MF, Ambros P, Handgretinger R, Aurias A, Delattre O (1998) Truncating mutations of hSNF5/INI1 in aggressive paediatric cancer. Nature 394:203–206

von Hoff K, Hinkes B, Dannenmann-Stern E, von Bueren AO, Warmuth-Metz M, Soerensen N, Emser A, Zwiener I, Schlegel PG, Kuehl J et al (2011) Frequency, risk-factors and survival of children with atypical teratoid rhabdoid tumors (AT/RT) of the CNS diagnosed between 1988 and 2004, and registered to the German HIT database. Pediatr Blood Cancer 57:978–985

Wang Y, Chen J, Yang W, Mo F, Senz J, Yap D, Anglesio MS, Gilks B, Morin GB, Huntsman DG (2015) The oncogenic roles of DICER1 RNase IIIb domain mutations in ovarian Sertoli-Leydig cell tumors. Neoplasia 17:650–660

Weinblatt M, Kochen J (1992) Rhabdoid tumor of the central nervous system. Med Pediatr Oncol 20(3):258

Weingart MF, Roth JJ, Hutt-Cabezas M, Busse TM, Kaur H, Price A, Maynard R, Rubens J, Taylor I, Mao XG et al (2015) Disrupting LIN28 in atypical teratoid rhabdoid tumors reveals the importance of the mitogen activated protein kinase pathway as a therapeutic target. Oncotarget 6:3165–3177

Wetmore C, Herington D, Lin T, Onar-Thomas A, Gajjar A, Merchant TE (2014) Reirradiation of recurrent medulloblastoma: does clinical benefit outweigh risk for toxicity? Cancer 120:3731–3737

Wilson BG, Wang X, Shen X, McKenna ES, Lemieux ME, Cho Y-J, Koellhoffer EC, Pomeroy SL, Orkin SH, Roberts CWM (2010) Epigenetic antagonism between polycomb and SWI/SNF complexes during oncogenic transformation. Cancer Cell 18:316–328

Woehrer A, Slavc I, Waldhoer T, Heinzl H, Zielonke N, Czech T, Benesch M, Hainfellner JA, Haberler C, Austrian Brain Tumor R (2010) Incidence of atypical teratoid/rhabdoid tumors in children: a population-based study by the Austrian Brain Tumor Registry, 1996–2006. Cancer 116:5725–5732

Yamamoto I (2001) Pineal region tumor: surgical anatomy and approach. J Neuro-Oncol 54:263–275

Yoshida A, Goto K, Kodaira M, Kobayashi E, Kawamoto H, Mori T, Yoshimoto S, Endo O, Kodama N, Kushima R et al (2016) CIC-rearranged sarcomas: a study of 20 cases and comparisons with Ewing sarcomas. Am J Surg Pathol 40:313–323

Zaky W, Dhall G, Ji L, Haley K, Allen J, Atlas M, Bertolone S, Cornelius A, Gardner S, Patel R et al (2014) Intensive induction chemotherapy followed by myeloablative chemotherapy with autologous hematopoietic progenitor cell rescue for young children newly-diagnosed with central nervous system atypical teratoid/rhabdoid tumors: the Head Start III experience. Pediatr Blood Cancer 61:95–101

Zhang AS, Ostrom QT, Kruchko C, Rogers L, Peereboom DM, Barnholtz-Sloan JS (2017) Complete prevalence of malignant primary brain tumors registry data in the United States compared with other common cancers, 2010. Neuro-Oncology 19:726–735

Zimmerman MA, Goumnerova LC, Proctor M et al (2005) Continuous remission of newly diagnosed and relapsed central nervous system atypical teratoid/rhabdoid tumor. J Neurooncol 72(1):77–84

Cognitive Late Effects and Their Management

14

Heather M. Conklin, Jane E. Schreiber, and Ashley S. Fournier-Goodnight

14.1 Introduction

Brain tumors are the second most common malignancy among the pediatric population, impacting roughly three children per every 100,000 (Butler and Mulhern 2005; Mulhern and Butler 2004). Unlike other cancers involving the central nervous system (CNS; e.g., acute lymphoblastic leukemia [ALL]), brain tumors are heterogeneous in both neuroanatomical location and histology. With regard to location, tumors of the brain are often distinguished according to whether they occur above or below the tentorium, which refers to an extension of the dura that separates the cerebellum from the cerebrum. Tumors located above the tentorium are referred to as supratentorial and often result in seizures upon initial presentation, while those located below the tentorium are referred to as infratentorial and most commonly produce signs of increased intracranial pressure (i.e., headache, nausea, vomiting), imbalance, as well as cranial nerve dysfunction at initial presentation. Relatedly, infratentorial tumors are often denoted as tumors of the posterior fossa, which refers to the most inferior intracranial cavity containing the cerebellum and brainstem.

The varied location and histology of brain tumors are indicators for determining classification, grade, and treatment. Brain tumors are graded according to size, location, rate of growth, and other histopathological factors with more aggressive tumors receiving a higher grade. The most commonly occurring tumor type within the pediatric population is medulloblastoma (Butler and Mulhern 2005; Mulhern and Butler 2004). This is followed in incidence by astrocytoma and ependymoma, which are both broadly classified as gliomas, and then craniopharyngioma. Treatment can include different combinations of surgical resection, chemotherapy, and radiation therapy depending on child, disease, and familial factors. Various types of radiation therapy are used, which differ in radiation dose and margins and include craniospinal irradiation (CSI), whole-brain radiation therapy (WBRT), conformal radiation therapy or intensity modulated radiation therapy (CRT or IMRT) and proton beam therapy. The type of radiation therapy is selected again according to histology, location,

H. M. Conklin (✉)
Department of Psychology, St. Jude Children's Research Hospital, Memphis, TN, USA
e-mail: heather.conklin@stjude.org

J. E. Schreiber
Department of Child & Adolescent Psychiatry and Behavioral Sciences, The Children's Hospital of Philadelphia, Philadelphia, PA, USA

A. S. Fournier-Goodnight
Children's Healthcare of Atlanta, Division of Neurosciences, Department of Neuropsychology, Emory University School of Medicine, Atlanta, GA, USA

Department of Rehabilitation Medicine, Emory University School of Medicine, Atlanta, GA, USA

© Springer International Publishing AG, part of Springer Nature 2018
A. Gajjar et al. (eds.), *Brain Tumors in Children*, https://doi.org/10.1007/978-3-319-43205-2_14

age of the child, and other factors. Though children treated with adjuvant chemotherapy and/or radiation therapy are at greater risk for later cognitive deficits, children treated with surgical resection alone may also experience cognitive dysfunction (Ris and Noll 1994).

Overall prognosis is strongly associated with tumor type as this drives disease- and treatment-related risk factors (Butler and Mulhern 2005; Mulhern and Butler 2004). Children with medulloblastoma have a long-term survival rate of 70–80% while those with more aggressive tumors have a long-term survival rate ≤10% (Jemal et al. 2008; Mulhern et al. 2004a). However, advances in treatment have resulted in substantially improved prognosis over time and necessitate a focus upon enhancing overall quality of life including cognitive outcomes.

14.2 Cognitive Late Effects

Given that more children are surviving brain tumors and other cancers impacting the CNS, increasing numbers of children are experiencing long-term cognitive deficits associated with cancer and related treatments. This cognitive dysfunction has been termed cognitive late effects, which can be defined as deficits in core and secondary cognitive abilities that emerge about 2 years following diagnosis (Butler and Mulhern 2005; Mulhern and Butler 2004). These deficits are chronic and potentially progressive in course. Their prevalence is high among survivors of pediatric brain tumors in that they emerge in 40–100% of survivors depending upon the specific sample and the cognitive functions assessed (Castellino et al. 2014; Glauser and Packer 1991). Subsequently, quality of life is diminished such that survivors of pediatric brain tumors are less likely to meet milestones such as graduating from high school, maintaining employment, and getting married (Armstrong et al. 2009; Gurney et al. 2009).

Cognitive late effects are more prevalent among survivors of brain tumors as compared to those with ALL given the greater likelihood that the former population will receive large volume cranial radiation therapy such as CSI or WBRT (Butler and Mulhern 2005). These types of treat-

ments have been clearly associated with declines in global intellectual functioning as a result of a slower rate of acquisition of new cognitive abilities among brain tumor survivors in comparison to same-age, neurotypical peers (Palmer et al. 2001). Thus, survivors do not lose previous knowledge and skills, but demonstrate a more protracted development of new skills. In the case of standardized neuropsychological assessment, this manifests as an increase in raw scores (i.e., individual benchmarked scores) coupled with a decrease in scaled scores (i.e., peer benchmarked scores) on serial assessments.

Assessment of cognitive outcomes in patients treated for brain tumors and ALL has historically over-relied upon measures of global intelligence such as the overall intelligence quotient (IQ). However, more recent research related to neurocognitive outcomes focuses on assessing specific neurocognitive skills as a method of better understanding mechanisms of decline and identifying targets for intervention. The core cognitive deficits experienced by childhood brain tumor survivors most commonly include attention, processing speed, and executive functions (e.g., working memory or the mental manipulation of incoming information for the purpose of solving some problem) (Butler and Mulhern 2005; Mulhern and Butler 2004). These core cognitive abilities are important for overall intelligence in that they act in concert to facilitate or constrain global cognitive ability. Though attention can be considered the cornerstone of cognition, studies have demonstrated its importance specifically in the development of adequate working memory capacity (Cowan 2010; Oberauer and Bialkova 2009). Additionally, developmental improvements in processing speed have been shown to result in improvements in working memory, which accounts for much of the variance in global intelligence (Fry and Hale 1996, 2000a). In this way, attention, working memory, and processing speed function together to impact overall intelligence. However, the core deficits also result in secondary deficits, which include crystallized or knowledge-based abilities such as deficits in academic skills (Butler and Mulhern 2005; Mulhern and Butler 2004). Since crystallized abilities are also represented within global intelligence, secondary deficits impact overall cognitive ability as well.

A number of factors have been associated with risk for the development of cognitive late effects including those related to treatment, biology/genetics, and socioeconomic status (Table 14.1). Children treated with a higher dose and broader field of radiation therapy are at increased risk for experiencing later cognitive dysfunction (Ellenberg et al. 1987; Mulhern et al. 1998; Merchant et al. 2009). Reducing the dose of radiation therapy (i.e., from 36 Gy to 23.4 Gy) results in substantial sparing of global cognitive ability in randomized controlled trials (Mulhern et al. 1998). With regard to radiation field, those treated with CSI and WBRT are at greater risk in comparison to those treated with conformal or proton beam therapy (Castellino et al. 2014; Packer 2002; Merchant et al. 2008). While chemotherapy is generally considered less harmful than CSI and WBRT, agents administered intrathecally, such as methotrexate, are associated with some amount of later neurocognitive dysfunction (Copeland et al. 1996; Conklin et al. 2012). Time since treatment can be considered an additional treatment-related risk factor given that cognitive late effects gradually manifest starting about 2 years following diagnosis (Ellenberg et al. 1987;

Knight et al. 2014). Child variables that impact risk for development of neurocognitive late effects include age at treatment and biological sex (Ellenberg et al. 1987; Jannoun and Bloom 1990). Children who are younger when treated demonstrate weaker overall cognitive functioning in comparison to same-age, neurotypical peers. For example, children with a variety of brain tumors who were under 5 years of age during treatment with radiation therapy were found to have global cognitive ability that was borderline impaired (i.e., mean IQ of 72) while those between the ages of 6 and 11 as well as those over the age of 11 demonstrated average global cognitive functioning (Jannoun and Bloom 1990). In terms of biological sex, female patients more often experience cognitive late effects than male patients (Palmer et al. 2001). Genetic disorders that predispose children to cancer (e.g., neurofibromatosis type 1 [NF1], tuberous sclerosis) are also viewed as risk factors since the presence of cognitive deficits inherent to these disorders exacerbate cognitive late effects (Castellino et al. 2014; Ellenberg et al. 2009; Ullrich 2008). Additionally, later cognitive dysfunction has been associated with medical complications of disease and treatment such as seizure disorder, hydrocephalus, and cerebrovascular accidents

Table 14.1 Risk factors for cognitive late effects

Universal:	Higher treatment intensity (e.g., higher radiation therapy dose or broader therapy margins)	
	Medical complications (e.g., stroke, meningitis, seizure disorder)	
	Younger age at treatment (e.g., less than 5 years of age)	
	Longer time since treatment (i.e., emerge gradually over time)	
	Female sex	
Tumor specific:	Medulloblastoma	Higher dose craniospinal irradiation
		Posterior fossa syndrome
		Hearing loss
	Low-grade glioma	Adjuvant radiation therapy vs. surgery alone
		Supratentorial midline tumor location
		Neurofibromatosis type I
	Ependymoma	Broader margin radiation therapy vs. conformal radiation therapy
		Multiple resections
		Hydrocephalus and related interventions (e.g., shunt placement)
	Craniopharyngioma	Surgical approach/extent of resection
		Hydrocephalus and related interventions (e.g., shunt placement)
		Multiple endocrinopathies
	Germ cell tumor	Broader field radiation therapy vs. ventricular field irradiation
		Nongerminomatous germ cell vs. pure germinoma

(Ellenberg et al. 2009; Roncadin et al. 2008). There is evidence that variants of the methylene-tetrahydrofolate reductase (MTHFR) gene, which is important for the production of an enzyme that assists in the processing of amino acids, are associated with increased risk of cognitive dysfunction following treatment with CNS-directed therapies (Kamdar et al. 2011; Krull et al. 2008). This is also the case for children with specific variants of catechol-O-methyltransferase (COMT), an enzyme that metabolizes dopamine, such that those with the Met/Met or Val/Val genotype perform more poorly than those with the Met/Val genotype on tasks of working memory (Howarth et al. 2014). Finally, socioeconomic factors including maternal level of education have been associated with cognitive late effects in this population (Castellino et al. 2014; Waber et al. 2012).

The primary neurobiological substrate for cognitive late effects is believed to be treatment-related changes in white matter (Mulhern and Butler 2004). White matter tracts facilitate efficient communication between various regions of the brain and are susceptible to radiation necrosis resulting in demyelination following treatment (Burger and Boyko 1991; Soussain et al. 2009). Chemotherapeutic agents, such as methotrexate, have also been associated with white matter changes including leukoencephalopathy, which refers to necrotic lesions within white matter of the periventricular region (Hudson 1999). Oligodendrocytes work together with other cells to produce myelin in the brain; however, these cells are most sensitive to radiation therapy in comparison to other glial cells, resulting in cell death and subsequent demyelination (Soussain et al. 2009). Death of these cells indirectly initiates an inflammatory response that impairs neurogenesis. Demyelination and white matter necrosis ultimately result in a reduction in the overall volume of white matter (Mulhern et al. 2001; Reddick et al. 2003). Given the nature of these changes and the neurodevelopmental course of white matter, a context for specific risk factors such as time since treatment and younger age at treatment is provided. More specifically, the overall volume and distribution of white matter varies with age such that posterior regions of the brain (i.e., brain stem, cerebellum) myelinate first followed by anterior regions (i.e., cerebral hemispheres then frontal lobes). This process is protracted and continues into adulthood when some neurocognitive processes including executive functioning, are fully maturing. Thus, the core cognitive deficits that define cognitive late effects are delayed in their presentation as disruption to the development of white matter impacts the normal emergence and functioning of attention, processing speed, and working memory. Children who are younger at treatment evince greater disruption to white matter development, which more substantially impacts associated neurocognitive abilities resulting in lower overall intelligence (Reddick et al. 2003; Brinkman et al. 2012). The distribution of white matter also has implications for the specific neurocognitive functions impacted by CNS-directed therapies. White matter is particularly pronounced in the right frontal lobe, which is important for attention regulation; thus, disruptions in myelination in this region of the brain may explain attention deficits associated with cognitive late effects (Posner and Raichle 1994). White matter disruption in the corpus callosum and inferior frontooccipital fasciculus as evidenced by reduced fractional anisotropy on diffusion tensor imaging (DTI) is associated with decreased processing speed (Aukema et al. 2009). Decreased fractional anisotropy in the cerebellar region of the cerebello-thalamo-cerebral tracts in patients with tumors of the posterior fossa treated with surgical resection and radiation therapy is related to working memory deficits (Law et al. 2011). Though additional treatment-related changes, including surgical resection, microvascular occlusion, breakdown of the blood–brain barrier, and calcifications in cortical gray matter structures and basal ganglia, may account for aspects of cognitive late effects, white matter changes are considered the chief neurobiological underpinning for delayed neurocognitive dysfunction following CNS-directed treatments (Mulhern and Butler 2004).

14.3 Medulloblastoma

Medulloblastoma is the most common pediatric malignant brain tumor and accounts for 20% of all childhood brain tumors (Pui et al. 2011). Given the higher prevalence, much of the research examining neurocognitive late effects in brain tumor survivors has focused on patients with medulloblastoma. Moreover, medulloblastoma patients have required aggressive treatments that are particularly disruptive to neurodevelopment. The tumor is thought to arise from neural stem cell precursors in the granular cell layer of the cerebellum; however, the exact cellular origin is still debated (Crawford et al. 2007). Medulloblastoma is considered a heterogeneous disease due to multiple histological variants, which include classic, desmoplastic, anaplastic or large cell, and nodular variants (Louis et al. 2007). Most medulloblastomas are confined to the posterior fossa, but 11–43% of patients have disseminated disease along the craniospinal axis (Allen and Epstein 1982). Medulloblastoma can occur at any age but typically occurs before 10 years of age and has a peak incidence at 5 years of age. Approximately 25–35% of children with medulloblastoma are diagnosed at less than 3 years of age (Rutkowski et al. 2010). Medulloblastoma is diagnosed in boys almost twice as often as in girls (Gottardo and Gajjar 2006).

Prior to diagnosis, patients typically present with signs of increased intracranial pressure related to obstructive hydrocephalus due to location of the tumor in the posterior fossa and proximity to the third and fourth ventricles. These signs may include early morning headache with vomiting, irritability, and lethargy. Unsteady gate may also be a sign as many medulloblastomas arise in the cerebellar midline. Most contemporary treatment consists of surgical resection, CSI, and chemotherapy. Staging and risk stratification are important for determining treatment intensity. Staging requires analysis of cerebrospinal fluid (CSF) and magnetic resonance imaging (MRI) of the brain and spine to determine the presence of disseminated disease; up to 30% of pediatric patients have evidence of disseminated disease at presentation (Packer et al. 2003). Although treatment stratification will continue to change as we learn more about the biology of medulloblastoma, most contemporary treatment protocols have divided patients into risk-adapted treatment strata on the basis of age, the extent of residual tumor after surgical resection, and dissemination, as was done on a large ongoing prospective clinical trial (NCT00085202). On this trial, patients who were older than 3 years of age were assigned as average or standard risk if they had a gross total or near total resection (defined as ≤ 1.5 cm^2 of postoperative residual disease). Average risk patients account for 60–70% of cases (Gottardo and Gajjar 2006). Patients with disseminated disease at presentation or with residual disease >1.5 cm^2 were assigned as high risk. Patients younger than 3 years were treated using a different treatment scheme since they generally have worse outcomes due to increased risk of disseminated disease at presentation, increased rate of subtotal resection, and not receiving CSI (Crawford et al. 2007).

Surgical resection of the tumor is a fundamental part of treatment that has led to improved survival (Zeltzer et al. 1999; Grill et al. 2005). Depending on the exact location of the tumor, a ventricular shunt or third ventriculostomy might be needed to relieve increased intracranial pressure secondary to obstruction (Crawford et al. 2007). The extent of the surgical resection is thought to be a good prognostic marker of disease (Zeltzer et al. 1999), and thus neurosurgeons will often strive for a gross total resection whenever possible. Radiation therapy is another important part of treatment. In children less than 3 years of age, radiation therapy is usually delayed or not given at all because it can cause severe neurological impairments. In contemporary treatment protocols, patients at least 3 years of age receive CSI as well as a higher dose "boost" of radiation therapy directly to the posterior fossa or tumor bed. The intent of the CSI is to eliminate potential microscopic disease that was not previously detected. The damaging side effects of CSI, including neurocognitive decline, have led to a reduction in the dose given to patients with average risk medulloblastoma (Gajjar et al. 2006; Oyharcabal-Bourden et al. 2005; Deutsch et al. 1996; Thomas et al. 2000;

Packer et al. 2006). However, for patients with high-risk disseminated disease the dose or volume of CSI cannot be reduced without compromising chances of survival (Verlooy et al. 2006). Conformal radiation techniques have allowed for more specificity in directing the "boost" radiation therapy to within a 1–2 cm margin surrounding the tumor bed rather than irradiating the entire posterior fossa (Crawford et al. 2007). Finally, chemotherapy is deemed the standard of care for children in all risk groups and can be used to augment, delay, or avoid radiation treatment (Gottardo and Gajjar 2006). Dose intensive chemotherapy, using cisplatin, vincristine, and cyclophosphamide, has been found to be effective in modern risk-adapted treatment protocols with children at least 3 years of age (Gajjar et al. 2006). Infants and young children (less than 3 years of age) are typically treated with either reduced dose CSI and prolonged chemotherapy or combined systemic and intraventricular chemotherapy without any radiation therapy (Grill et al. 2005; Massimino et al. 2011; Rutkowski et al. 2005).

Multimodal risk-adapted treatment has been effective in improving cure rates. Five-year survival rates are up to 70% in patients with high-risk disease and up to 85% in patients with average risk disease (Gajjar et al. 2006). However, cure comes at a high price, and patients continue to experience long-term deficits in neurocognitive functioning as well as neuroendocrine problems, hearing loss, infertility, and poor cardiopulmonary fitness (Mulhern et al. 2004a; Laughton et al. 2008; Wolfe et al. 2012; Ness et al. 2006).

Neurocognitive difficulties are one of the most pervasive of all long-term effects and occur across all age groups (Palmer et al. 2007). Early studies examining neurocognitive late effects following treatment for medulloblastoma focused mainly on broad measures of overall intellectual functioning or IQ. Studies report that nearly 90% of medulloblastoma survivors have IQ scores that are below average (Dennis et al. 1996). Furthermore, intellectual ability appears to progressively deteriorate over time. In medulloblastoma survivors who were treated with 25–35 Gy of CSI therapy between the years of 1967 and 1987, 42% had IQ scores under 80 at 5 years after treatment and 85% had IQ scores under 80 ten years after treatment (Hoppe-Hirsch et al. 1990). Several subsequent studies have demonstrated a similar steady decline in intellectual ability over time (Mulhern et al. 1998, 2005; Schreiber et al. 2014). This decline in IQ is not the loss of previously acquired knowledge or skills, but rather the inability to acquire new information and skills at the same rate as healthy peers (Palmer et al. 2001). Several risk factors have been consistently associated with this decline in IQ, including younger age at diagnosis (Jannoun and Bloom 1990; Dennis et al. 1996; Hoppe-Hirsch et al. 1990), longer time since treatment (Dennis et al. 1996; Ellenberg et al. 1987), female sex (Ris et al. 2001), and intensity of radiation dose or volume (Grill et al. 1999). Hearing loss, a common side effect of treatment, has also been associated with significant decline in intellectual ability and academic skills (Schreiber et al. 2014).

Children treated with CSI for medulloblastoma also demonstrate worse academic performance and are more likely to utilize special education services (Hoppe-Hirsch et al. 1990; Seaver et al. 1994; Johnson et al. 1994). Approximately 75% of medulloblastoma survivors experience academic failure or report learning difficulties; this rate is three times the rate seen in survivors of cerebellar astrocytomas treated without radiation therapy (Dennis et al. 1996). Significant declines in the specific academic areas of spelling and reading skills were exhibited in both standard risk and high-risk medulloblastoma patients (Mulhern et al. 2005; Schreiber et al. 2014). Younger age at diagnosis was predictive of greater decline in these skills, lending support to the hypothesis that posterior fossa-directed irradiation at young ages may disrupt the normal patterns of brain development that underlie the acquisition of reading skills (Mulhern et al. 2005; Schreiber et al. 2014; Conklin et al. 2008).

More recent research on neurocognitive late effects in medulloblastoma survivors has suggested that impairment of a core set of foundational skills may be precursors to the declines in intellectual and academic skills (Dennis et al. 1998; Schatz et al. 2000; Nagel et al. 2006).

These core skills include attention (Reeves et al. 2006), working memory (Edelstein et al. 2011), and processing speed (Mabbott et al. 2008). Studies of healthy children revealed that age-related improvements in IQ can be attributed to developmental improvements in processing speed and working memory (Fry and Hale 2000b). A study of 163 medulloblastoma survivors who completed 514 prospective neurocognitive evaluations over 5 years following diagnosis and risk-adapted treatment revealed a significant decline in attention, working memory, and processing speed (Palmer et al. 2013). Patients were found to have the lowest scores on measures of processing speed, with scores dropping significantly below average, particularly for patients who were younger at diagnosis and had high-risk disease (i.e., received a higher dose of CSI). Thus, slowed processing speed may contribute to declines in intelligence and academic skills observed in medulloblastoma survivors.

CNS-directed cancer therapies are well-established causes of changes in cerebral white matter (Filley and Kleinschmidt-DeMasters 2001). Evidence suggests that reduced cerebral white matter accounts for a significant proportion of the observed decline in IQ among survivors of medulloblastoma. A comparison of 15 patients with medulloblastoma treated with tumor resection and CSI and 15 age-matched patients with low-grade astrocytoma of the posterior fossa treated with surgery alone found that all patients treated with CSI demonstrated significantly reduced white matter volume (Reddick et al. 1998). A related study indicated that the medulloblastoma survivors had significantly lower IQ scores that were associated with significantly reduced white matter volume (Mulhern et al. 1999). A longitudinal study found that medulloblastoma survivors experienced a significant loss of white matter volume during the 9 months following CSI (Reddick et al. 2000). Notably, the rate of white matter volume loss was 23% slower in patients who received a reduced dose of irradiation. Additional longitudinal studies examined change in the tissue volume of specific brain structures. A decline in corpus callosum volume over 4 years following diagnosis and risk-adapted treatment was identified in 35 medulloblastoma

survivors (Palmer et al. 2002), and an abnormal pattern of hippocampal development was identified in 25 pediatric medulloblastoma survivors during the 2–3 years following diagnosis and risk-adapted treatment (Nagel et al. 2004).

Reddick and colleagues suggested that reduced white matter volumes in brain tumor survivors resulted in decreased attention abilities, which eventually led to a decline in IQ and academic achievement (Reddick et al. 2003). In 40 long-term survivors, significant associations were found between white matter volume and both attention and intelligence. The final regression model that included white matter volume, attention, and IQ as predictors, explained at least 60% of the variance in academic skills. Mabbott and colleagues used DTI techniques to identify areas of tissue breakdown within *existing* white matter (Mabbott et al. 2006). Eight pediatric patients with medulloblastoma who were treated with CSI were compared with eight age-matched healthy control children on measures of DTI used to evaluate white matter integrity in multiple regions of interest in the cerebral hemispheres. Results showed associations between microscopic damage in existing white matter across multiple regions and poor intellectual outcomes in survivors of medulloblastoma relative to controls.

While most of the neurocognitive late effects literature has focused on the deleterious effects of CSI, it is also well established that tumor mass effect and surgical interventions are associated with neurocognitive risk (Di Rocco et al. 2010). One of the consequences of surgery in the posterior fossa region of the brain is posterior fossa syndrome (PFS), also sometimes referred to as cerebellar mutism. This syndrome occurs in up to 29% of patients with medulloblastoma following surgery (De Smet et al. 2007; Korah et al. 2010). Patients with PFS generally present with diminished speech or mutism that can be accompanied by ataxia, hypotonia, emotional lability, and other neurobehavioral abnormalities (Robertson et al. 2006; Gudrunardottir et al. 2011a). This syndrome is quite variable in presentation with a delayed onset of anywhere from 1 to 6 days following surgery and a limited duration of between 1 day and 4 months (Gudrunardottir et al. 2011a).

Recovery is often spontaneous but can be followed by a period of speech dysarthria (Robertson et al. 2006; Gudrunardottir et al. 2011a). Many patients continue to have long-term speech and language difficulties following the recovery from acute onset of symptoms (Robertson et al. 2006; Huber et al. 2006, 2007; Steinbok et al. 2003).

Although the cause of PFS is not well understood, evidence suggests that PFS is the result of bilateral damage to the proximal efferent cerebellar pathways along the dentarubrothalamocortical pathway (Patay et al. 2014; Miller et al. 2010). The cerebellum is thought to coordinate function, rhythm, articulation, and timbre but not language production (Robertson et al. 2006). Damage anywhere along the dentarubrothalamocortical pathway may lead to a speech disorder, and damage to the dentate nuclei in particular has repeatedly been cited as a cause of cerebellar mutism (Gudrunardottir et al. 2011b). Data from a prospective, longitudinal risk-adapted treatment study for pediatric medulloblastoma indicates that the experience of PFS is an additional risk factor for decline in intellectual ability and academic achievement (Schreiber et al. 2014), as well as working memory ability (Knight et al. 2014). In a cross-sectional analysis, neurocognitive function was examined at 12 months post-diagnosis in 17 pediatric medulloblastoma patients who experienced PFS compared with 17 medulloblastoma patients who did not experience PFS but were matched on age at diagnosis and risk status (Palmer et al. 2010). Results indicated that patients who experienced PFS had significantly lower performance on tests of processing speed, attention, working memory, executive processes, cognitive efficiency, reading, spelling, and math. A follow-up study examined the trajectory of general intellectual ability, processing speed, attention, and working memory ability in 29 patients who experienced PFS compared with 29 patients who did not experience PFS but were matched on age at diagnosis and risk status. Patients who experienced PFS had significantly lower estimated baseline scores and showed very little recovery in functioning over the 5 years following diagnosis (Schreiber et al. 2015).

Much has been learned regarding the late effects of treatment for medulloblastoma given the large focus on this particular patient population. Additionally, our understanding of medulloblastoma biology has substantially increased in the last decade. Currently, we know that medulloblastoma consists of four clinical and molecular subtypes: the WNT subtype, the sonic hedgehog, "group 3," and "group 4" (Gajjar and Robinson 2014; Ramaswamy et al. 2015; Northcott et al. 2012). Moreover, these four subtypes have different demographics, genetics, recurrence patterns, and outcomes (Ramaswamy et al. 2015). Most notably, prognosis differs dramatically across subtypes. Therefore, a new therapeutic strategy is being developed that aims to improve cure rates among patients with more aggressive subtypes and reduce treatment-related morbidities by tailoring treatment to match features of each subtype. For example, treatment intensity can be reduced for patients with subtypes that are predicted to have good outcomes, resulting in a low prevalence of treatment-related morbidities, and patients with a subtype that has more adverse prognostic features could receive more intensive treatment (Gajjar and Robinson 2014). This type of therapeutic strategy could potentially reduce the high rates of neurocognitive impairment that are typically seen in pediatric medulloblastoma survivors. A large phase II, multisite clinical trial that tailors therapy according to the molecular and clinical features of subgroups is currently underway (NCT01878617).

14.4 Other Tumors of Note

14.4.1 Low-Grade Glioma

Gliomas are tumors that arise from glial cells. Low-grade gliomas (LGG) refer to those with a grade of I or II, while those with a grade of III or IV are considered high grade. These tumors are also distinguished according to the type of glial cell from which they originate (i.e., astrocytes, oligodendrocytes, ependymocytes). The most common type arises from astrocytes and is referred to as pilocytic astrocytoma (Ris and Noll

1994; Aarsen et al. 2009; Ris and Beebe 2008). LGGs are well circumscribed and typically treated with complete surgical resection; however, adjuvant chemotherapy and/or radiation therapy is used in the setting of disease recurrence, progression, or inoperability based upon location. Though surgical resection alone is considered to result in fewer long-term sequelae, it is not completely void of cognitive risk.

LGGs of the infratentorium have received much attention in the literature such that neurocognitive sequelae associated with these tumors and various treatments have been well defined (Aarsen et al. 2009; Ris and Beebe 2008; Beebe et al. 2005; Levisohn et al. 2000). Cerebellar LGGs treated with complete surgical resection often result in executive dysfunction and deficits in visuospatial reasoning, expressive language, and verbal memory (Levisohn et al. 2000). Affective dysregulation consistent with cerebellar cognitive affective syndrome is also commonly noted. These deficits may be exacerbated in the setting of hydrocephalus. Infratentorial LGGs treated with radiation therapy result in poorer outcomes in comparison to those treated with surgical resection alone (Aarsen et al. 2009; Ris and Beebe 2008). For example, patients with low-grade cerebellar astrocytomas treated with radiation therapy demonstrated global cognitive functioning that was slightly more than one standard deviation below the mean, while those treated with surgical resection exhibited global intellectual ability that was solidly average (Chadderton et al. 1995). The use of CRT as opposed to WBRT and CSI results in improved outcomes with regard to cognitive and adaptive functioning (Merchant et al. 2009; Netson et al. 2013). In recognition of poorer outcomes associated with young age at the time of radiation therapy, chemotherapy is often used to delay this treatment. However, chemotherapy consisting of methotrexate in combination with other agents has been found to result in white matter disruption (Rutkowski et al. 2005). Additionally, treatment with chemotherapy prior to treatment with CRT resulted in greater deficits in learning and memory in comparison to patients with LGGs treated with CRT alone (Di Pinto et al. 2012).

LGGs of the supratentorium are often located within midline structures (i.e., optic chiasm, thalamus, hypothalamus), which limits treatment with total surgical resection (Ris and Beebe 2008). This is often the case in patients diagnosed with NF1 given that optic pathway gliomas are common in this population and frequently result in visual impairments. Patients with optic nerve involvement and involvement of other midline structures are therefore often treated with CRT. In addition to visual impairments associated with damage to the optic chiasm, nerve, and tract, midline LGGs often result in deficits in verbal learning and memory, which is consistent with disruption of diencephalic/temporal lobe structures that support these functions (Di Pinto et al. 2012; King et al. 2004). Endocrinopathies are also common secondary to disruption of the pituitary gland (Armstrong et al. 2011). These midline structures are damaged due to CRT as well as tumor mass effect, partial surgical resection, and hydrocephalus. Though LGGs arise in the cerebral hemispheres, less is known about neurocognitive functioning within this population (Ris and Beebe 2008; Turner et al. 2009). These tumors are typically treated with surgical resection alone and have better outcomes than midline LGGs, predominantly as a result of the stronger visuospatial reasoning and processing speed found among patients with hemispheric tumors (Ris and Beebe 2008). Additionally, LGGs arising in the left hemisphere have been associated with worse outcomes in comparison to those arising in the right hemisphere (Aarsen et al. 2009).

14.4.2 Ependymoma

Ependymomas are also gliomas that arise from ependymal cells lining the ventricles of the brain and the central canal of the spinal cord. These tumors can be low or high grade depending upon their rate of growth. Ependymomas are frequently treated with surgical intervention followed by radiation therapy since they have a tendency to metastasize (Landau et al. 2013). Given that ependymomas are comparatively localized, they are amenable to treatment with focal radiation therapy including CRT. Additionally, ependymomas are typically diagnosed at an earlier age in comparison to other focal tumors (i.e., astrocytoma) (Di Pinto et al. 2010). Overall, treatment with CRT has allowed for improvement in outcomes as well as cleaner investigation of the impact of biological, treatment, and medical factors upon those outcomes.

Ependymomas of the supratentorium are relatively rare; however, they result in cognitive dysfunction primarily in association with young age at the time of treatment with radiation therapy, female sex, and presence of a seizure disorder diagnosed at a young age (Landau et al. 2013). Infratentorial ependymomas are typically treated with CRT, which has done much to reveal the relationship between dose and volume of radiation and cognitive dysfunction (Merchant et al. 2014). In general, children treated with broader margin radiation therapy (i.e., WBRT, CSI) typically demonstrate declines in overall cognitive ability and learning (Di Pinto et al. 2010). While children treated with CRT do not demonstrate declines in global intellectual functioning, they may exhibit deficits in learning. Patients who are younger at the time of treatment often have an impaired rate of learning in comparison to same-age peers 5 years following treatment. Deficits in learning have been found prior to treatment with CRT (i.e., baseline) in children who have had multiple resections and shunts for the management of hydrocephalus; however, these deficits were largely transitory and improved secondary to alleviation of mass effect (Merchant et al. 2014). Use of chemotherapy prior to CRT has also resulted in poorer outcomes, particularly with regard to visual-auditory or paired-associates learning, which is a strong predictor of reading ability. Indeed, patients treated with CRT have experienced comparatively greater declines in reading versus mathematics and spelling (Conklin et al. 2008). Deficits in adaptive functioning have also been associated with younger age at treatment, use of chemotherapy prior to CRT, hydrocephalus and shunt placement, as well as surgical intervention (Netson et al. 2012). In summary, investigation of LGGs and

ependymomas has revealed that factors such as age at the time of treatment, tumor location, type of radiation therapy, number of surgical interventions, and medical complications (i.e., hydrocephalus, seizures) clearly have a synergistic effect upon cognitive outcomes. Neurocognitive processes including attention, processing speed, executive functioning, and learning are likely to be impacted with weaker functioning most probable in those treated at a younger age with broader field radiation therapy.

14.4.3 Craniopharyngioma

Craniopharyngioma is a slow-growing, extra-axial, calcified, and often cystic, tumor that occupies the sella/suprasellar brain region. It is relatively rare, accounting for 1–4% of all primary CNS tumors in children (Dolecek et al. 2012). Peak onset has a bimodal age distribution, with one peak during childhood at approximately 8–10 years of age and a second peak in middle age (Blaney et al. 2011). No biological sex predilection has been reported (Blaney et al. 2011). Prognosis is good with overall survival greater than 80% at 10 years post diagnosis (Rajan et al. 1993). Craniopharyngioma is benign in histology but behaves malignantly due to its location and tendency to progress after treatment. Among pediatric brain tumors, long-term morbidity including cognitive deficits is most closely associated with tumor location. Late effects result from tumor and treatment effect on surrounding brain structures and commonly include: (1) endocrinopathies, sleep disturbance and decreased fitness due to hypothalamic/pituitary damage; (2) visual disturbance due to mass effect on the optic chiasm; (3) hydrocephalus and resultant increased intracranial pressure due to compression of the third ventricle, and (4) memory difficulties due to disruption of Papez circuit including the mammillary bodies. General consensus is lacking regarding the best treatment approach for pediatric craniopharyngioma with some medical teams attempting gross total resection when damage to the anterior pituitary can be avoided and other medical teams preferring limited surgery, to increase CSF flow or restore vision, followed by radiation therapy. Radiation therapy is typically focal, including CRT or proton beam radiation therapy.

Not surprisingly, given tumor location, prior studies have reported frontal lobe dysfunction including impaired attention, perseveration, cognitive inflexibility, and decreased inhibitory control among childhood survivors of craniopharyngioma (Cavazzuti et al. 1983; Riva et al. 1998; Kiehna et al. 2006). There is some indication that impairment in frontal lobe functions may be greater following extensive tumor resection in comparison to irradiation with or without conservative surgical procedures (Cavazzuti et al. 1983). These findings are typically in the context of intact intellectual functioning. Multiple studies have reported memory impairment, particularly retrieval deficits, among survivors of craniopharyngioma (Cavazzuti et al. 1983; Carpentieri et al. 2001). Memory impairments have been found both among those patients undergoing extensive surgery as well as those with limited surgery and focal radiation therapy (Cavazzuti et al. 1983). Risk factors for declines in memory and learning may include hydrocephalus and shunt insertion for management of hydrocephalus (Di Pinto et al. 2012). There have also been reports of declines in adaptive functioning over time, with female sex and pre-irradiation chemotherapy (interferon) associated with a more rapid decline (Netson et al. 2013).While research suggests that emotional and behavioral outcomes are generally good, again there is indication that interventions to manage hydrocephalus, as well as endocrine dysfunction, may predict greater problems (Dolson et al. 2009). Taken together, attention, executive functions, and memory impairments may follow treatment for childhood craniopharyngioma, with likelihood of impairment related to surgical approach, need for hydrocephalus management, and the presence of endocrinopathies. Monitoring of adaptive functioning and emotional adjustment is also warranted given increased risk over time.

14.4.4 Germ Cell Tumors

Intracranial germ cell tumors develop when germ cells that normally form the reproductive organs fail to migrate appropriately. Germ cell tumors most frequently arise in the pineal and suprasellar brain regions. Infrequently, germ cell tumors are bifocal, occurring both in the pineal and suprasellar regions; it is unclear whether bifocal disease represents tumor metastases or simultaneous development in two sites. Intracranial germ cell tumors are rare, accounting for 3–6% of all brain tumors (Sands et al. 2001). Intracranial germinomas, a subtype of germ cell tumors, account for 0.5–2.5% of all intracranial tumors (O'Neil et al. 2011). Intracranial germ cell tumors arise most often in adolescence. Males are approximately two times more likely than females to develop germ cell tumors, with a higher male-to-female ratio for nongerminomatous germ cell tumors (i.e., germ cell tumors that are not pure germinomas) (Packer et al. 2000). Neuroimaging characteristics of germinomas and nongerminomatous germ cell tumors are not distinct enough to afford diagnostic certainty such that tissue confirmation via biopsy or measurement of specific tumor markers (e.g., β-human-chorionic-gonadotropin or α-fetoprotein) via blood and/or serum is often required. Clinical presentation is dependent on tumor location, tumor size, and patient age. Germ cell tumors of the pineal region most commonly present with symptoms of hydrocephalus, visual impairment including Parinaud's syndrome (i.e., vertical gaze palsy), reduced arousal, pyramidal tract signs, and ataxia (Packer et al. 2000). Those in the suprasellar region are often characterized by hypothalamic/pituitary involvement resulting in endocrinopathies (e.g., diabetes insipidus, hypopituitarism) at presentation. Radiation therapy has been the backbone of treatment for germ cell tumors; however, there is no consensus on dose or volume needed, especially if chemotherapy is used (Packer et al. 2000). Given the risk for cognitive late effects, there have been recent attempts to reduce radiation dose and/or volume, sometimes through the use of adjuvant chemotherapy.

Germinomas are associated with excellent prognosis, with most studies indicating 5-year progression-free survival rates over 90% (O'Neil et al. 2011; Packer et al. 2000). Nongerminomatous germ cell tumors have a poorer prognosis with reported survival rates between 40% and 70% (Packer et al. 2000).

Few studies have investigated neurocognitive outcomes following treatment for pediatric intracranial germ cell tumors. Merchant and colleagues reported no declines in intellectual functioning in eight children with assessments pre- and post-radiation therapy (CSI [median dose = 25.6 Gy] with a boost to the primary site [median dose = 50.4 Gy]) for intracranial germinoma, at a median age of 12 years (Merchant et al. 2000). Sands and colleagues reported findings from a feasibility trial of chemotherapy-based treatment for intracranial germ cell tumors; of note, the majority of these patients subsequently received radiation therapy at the time of recurrence (Sands et al. 2001). Twenty-two children completed cognitive assessments at an average age of 16 years and on average 6 years post diagnosis. Findings revealed full scale IQ, verbal IQ, reading, spelling, and math abilities all within the average range with low average range performance IQ (Sands et al. 2001). Age at diagnosis was positively correlated with all IQ scores and mathematics. Those children treated for pure germinomas significantly outperformed those with nongerminomatous germ cell tumors across measures of IQ and academic achievement; however, children with nongerminomatous germ cell tumors were significantly younger at diagnosis than those with pure germinomas. More recently, O'Neil and colleagues studied pediatric patients with newly diagnosed intracranial germinoma treated with four cycles of chemotherapy followed by reduced dose ventricular field irradiation (22.5–24 Gy) with simultaneous boost to the primary site (30 Gy) (O'Neil et al. 2011). Twenty patients, mean age of 14.4 years at diagnosis, participated in one to four cognitive assessments. Findings revealed average range performance on all measures with no decline over time (O'Neil et al. 2011). An improvement over time was found for nonverbal

reasoning, nonverbal memory, processing speed, working memory, response inhibition, and cognitive flexibility (O'Neil et al. 2011). There were no significant differences based on tumor location, age at diagnosis, or hydrocephalus at presentation. Taken together, these findings suggest children treated for intracranial germ cell tumors generally perform well cognitively, even years after treatment. In part, these positive findings may relate to an older age at diagnosis with some findings indicating greater risk for younger children and children treated for nongerminomatous germ cell tumors. New treatment approaches are under investigation (NCT01602666) that employ reduced radiation fields, which may offer better cognitive outcomes with similar survival rates.

14.4.5 Atypical Teratoid/Rhabdoid Tumors

Atypical teratoid/rhabdoid tumors (AT/RT) are rare, highly aggressive malignant rhabdoid tumors that occur within the CNS (Biggs et al. 1987). Morphologically, AT/RT resembles other embryonal tumors of the nervous system such as medulloblastoma, and is distinguished by a characteristic loss of the *SMARCB1* or *INI1* gene products (Squire et al. 2007; Strother 2005). Approximately 20% of CNS tumors in young children (less than 3 years of age) are AT/RT (Buscariollo et al. 2012), and AT/RT is one of the most common tumors arising in children younger than a year (Dolecek et al. 2012). Currently, AT/RT has no effective therapy and median event-free survival is less than 1 year (Tekautz et al. 2005). No large randomized clinical trials have been completed to establish a "standard of care" treatment for AT/RT. Current treatment strategies typically include surgical resection followed by intensive and/or high-dose chemotherapy and CSI for older patients (Strother 2005). Focal radiation therapy is sometimes used with younger patients.

Given such a poor survival rate, there is very limited information on neurocognitive outcomes. One study examined neurocognitive outcomes in four survivors of AT/RT (median age of

52 months) whose treatment included surgical resection followed by high-dose chemotherapy (Finkelstein-Shechter et al. 2010). All patients exhibited significant adaptive and neurocognitive delays even in the absence of radiation therapy. In a retrospective review, neurocognitive and/or academic achievement evaluations from eight survivors of AT/RT (median age of 7.6 years) were examined (Lafay-Cousin et al. 2015). Treatment included surgical resection and high-dose chemotherapy in all but one patient. Three patients also received radiation therapy. Five patients had IQ scores in the significantly impaired range and three were in the average to high average range. Despite the limited use of radiation therapy, the majority of patients exhibited significant neurocognitive impairment, suggesting that other tumor- or treatment-related factors must be contributing to poor neurocognitive outcomes. More clinical trials that focus solely on treatment for AT/RT are needed.

14.5 Interventions

As reviewed herein, neuro-oncologists and radiation oncologists have been working to reduce sources of known neurotoxicity as secondary prevention of cognitive late effects. For example, in young children, radiation therapy may be delayed through the use of surgery and/or chemotherapy to reduce risk of cognitive late effects (Lacaze et al. 2003; Rutkowski et al. 2009). There are also systematic efforts to reduce radiation dose and volume, while maintaining high survival rates through the use of CRT or IMRT, which have resulted in better preservation of intellectual functioning (Merchant et al. 2009), academic skills (Conklin et al. 2008), learning and memory (Di Pinto et al. 2010, 2012), and adaptive functioning (Netson et al. 2012, 2013). Proton beam radiation therapy offers even greater sparing of healthy surrounding brain tissue than conventional photon-based approaches, due to physical properties of protons, and is currently being investigated as a potential means to reduce cognitive late effects among children treated for brain tumors (Merchant et al. 2008; Greenberger et al. 2014; Macdonald

et al. 2013). Building on a growing research knowledge base, the hallmark of modern front-line treatment protocols for pediatric brain tumors is risk-adapted therapy whereby treatment exposure is reduced for those children with the best prognosis. While initial risk-adapted treatment schemas relied heavily on clinical factors such as extent of surgical resection or presence of metastatic disease, newer protocols are incorporating molecular and histological tumor features with demonstrated prognostic value in up-front treatment planning to offer even greater reduction in treatment burden.

It is important to realize even if cancer-directed therapy is fully optimized, the risk for cognitive late effects will remain. In the case of pediatric brain tumors, the impact of tumor mass effect cannot be eliminated. Further, for certain treatment approaches (surgical resection, radiation therapy) a plateau will be reached in the ability to limit treatment while still maintaining high survival rates. Despite the high prevalence of cognitive late effects among childhood cancer survivors and their known potential to negatively impact quality of life, there are few empirically validated interventions targeting these problems. The greatest research attention has been devoted to pharmacological approaches.

14.5.1 Pharmacotherapy

Early cognitive intervention studies with childhood cancer survivors were modeled after successful interventions for children diagnosed with attention-deficit/hyperactivity disorder (ADHD) given the overlap in attentional issues. The efficacy of stimulant medication is well established in addressing attention problems for otherwise healthy children diagnosed with ADHD. Methylphenidate (MPH), a mixed dopaminergic-noradrenergic agonist, is the most commonly prescribed stimulant medication for the treatment of ADHD with benefits demonstrated on performance measures of attention and concentration, as well as observable classroom and social behavior (Brown et al. 2005). However, the response rate and tolerability of stimulant medications may differ for brain tumor survivors secondary to compromised neurologic status. Findings from preliminary studies with childhood cancer survivors were mixed. Delong and colleagues studied 12 children with brain tumors or ALL treated with an "adequate trial" of MPH for a period lasting between 6 months and 6 years. Based on parent report, teacher report, and direct observation, response was indicated to be "good" for eight children, "fair" for two children, and "poor" for two children (DeLong et al. 1992). A second study of MPH response among six children who were experiencing attention, learning, and memory difficulties secondary to treatment with whole-brain irradiation for brain tumors revealed no improvements on attention or memory measures (Torres et al. 1996). Meyers and colleagues conducted an open-label trial of MPH with adults who had been treated for a brain tumor and found significant improvements in psychomotor speed, executive functions, and memory (Meyers et al. 1998). These studies tended to be limited by small sample sizes, poor sample characterization, lack of appropriate controls, and nonoptimal dosing, thus limiting conclusions.

The first randomized, double-blind, placebo-controlled trial of MPH with childhood cancer survivors was published by Thompson and colleagues in 2001 (Thompson et al. 2001). Thirty-two children with identified problems with attention and academic achievement were randomized to MPH (0.6 mg/kg) or placebo. Results revealed improved performance on a measure of sustained attention but not measures of verbal memory or visual-auditory learning. While encouraging, as a single dose trial this study lacked information regarding sustained response or performance in the naturalistic setting (school/home).

These findings led to a large multisite, multiphase MPH trial for brain tumor and ALL survivors who were between 6 and 18 years of age and at least 12 months from completion of cancer-directed treatment (Conklin et al. 2007, 2010a; Mulhern et al. 2004b). In the first (Screening) phase, patients who met eligibility criteria ($N = 469$) were assessed to identify those with adequate global cognitive functioning, attention problems, and academic difficulties. Patients who met screening criteria ($N = 210$) were offered participation in the second (In-Lab) phase, a 2-day, in-clinic, double-blind crossover trial during which they received MPH (0.6 mg/kg) and placebo in randomly assigned order. During the In-Lab phase, 134 patients were evaluated for acute neurocognitive response. Participants demonstrating adequate medication tolerance ($N = 132$) were offered participation in the third (Home Crossover) phase, a 3-week, randomized, double-blind, placebo-controlled, crossover trial consisting of placebo, low-dose MPH (0.3 mg/kg), and moderate-dose MPH (0.6 mg/kg). Of 122 patients participating in the Home Crossover phase, 91 demonstrated initial improvement on MPH relative to placebo based on parent and/or teacher report and were offered participation in the fourth and final (Maintenance) phase, a 12-month open-label MPH trial. Sixty-eight patients completed the Maintenance phase.

Findings from the Home Crossover phase revealed a significant improvement in attention regulation based on parent and teacher report for both MPH doses over placebo (Mulhern et al. 2004b). Teachers, but not parents, also reported a significant improvement in social and academic competence for both MPH doses (Mulhern et al. 2004b). The discrepancy in reporting across raters may be related to limited parental opportunity to observe children with their peers during a 1-week assessment period. Of note, across all outcome measures, there was no significant advantage for the higher (0.6 mg/kg) MPH dose over the lower (0.3 mg/kg) MPH dose, which is particularly relevant given different side effect risks as discussed below. Using a conservative, statistical approach to measuring medication response (reliable change index), the response rate during the Home Crossover phase, based on teacher report of attention skills, was 54% (Conklin et al. 2010b). While encouraging, this is significantly less than the 75–80% response rate typically reported in the ADHD literature (Barkley 1977; Efron et al. 1998). The only significant predictor of MPH response was higher levels of attention problems at study initiation; age, biological sex, diagnosis (brain tumor or

ALL), IQ, and time since treatment were not predictive of response (Conklin et al. 2010b). Findings from the yearlong Maintenance phase demonstrated sustained benefits in attention and behavioral improvements, often with normalization of performance by the end of the trial (Conklin et al. 2010a). Maintained benefits were seen on performance measures of sustained attention as well as parent-, teacher-, and self-report measures of behavior problems and social competencies. Notably, there were no improvements on academic measures that assessed reading and math abilities; however, parents reported that children received better school grades related to behaviors such as planning ahead for projects, studying in advance for tests, and remembering to turn in assignments (Conklin et al. 2010a).

The same study included assessment of MPH side effects, including growth effects. Overall, childhood cancer survivors tolerated MPH well (Conklin et al. 2009), with the frequency and severity of side effects similar to or less than those reported for children diagnosed with ADHD (Efron et al. 1998; Fine and Johnston 1993). A significantly higher frequency and severity of symptoms was confirmed for the higher (0.6 mg/kg) MPH dose. Female sex and lower IQ were the only child risk factors for increased side effects; childhood brain tumor survivors had similar frequency and severity of side effects as ALL survivors (Conklin et al. 2009). However, brain tumor survivors were more likely to discontinue MPH secondary to side effects. Stimulant medications have been associated with height and weight deceleration, which are of particular importance to childhood cancer survivors given risk for growth deficits secondary to disease- and treatment-related factors such as concomitant endocrinopathies. In comparison to childhood cancer survivors who were not taking MPH, survivors who took MPH over the yearlong Maintenance phase demonstrated a significant deceleration in body mass index and weight, but not height (Jasper et al. 2009). Factors predictive of growth deceleration included higher daily stimulant dose and loss of appetite. Of note, the cancer survivors in this study had body mass indices and weights significantly higher than age

based normative comparisons at study initiation with body mass index and weight closer to normative expectations at the end of the yearlong MPH trial.

Since this MPH study, investigators have been interested in the use of other psychostimulant medications for the management of cognitive late effects among childhood cancer survivors. Modafinil, a dopaminergic CNS stimulant developed for the treatment of narcolepsy, has been studied in adult cancer patients and cancer survivors. Multiple studies have reported improved fatigue/drowsiness (Blackhall et al. 2009; Lundorff et al. 2009; Gehring et al. 2012) and better mood (Blackhall et al. 2009; Lundorff et al. 2009; Gehring et al. 2012). Improved cognitive outcomes have also been reported, including findings from randomized, placebo-controlled trials that show improved attention and psychomotor speed (Lundorff et al. 2009) or improved attention and memory (Kohli et al. 2009); however, not all trials have found improved cognitive outcomes following treatment with modafinil with adult cancer survivors (Blackhall et al. 2009; Boele et al. 2013). A recent open-label, randomized, pilot trial comparing MPH and modafinil found differential outcomes based on medication with improved attention following treatment with MPH and improved processing speed following treatment with modafinil (Gehring et al. 2012). Currently, there is a randomized controlled trial investigating the safety and efficacy of modafinil use with survivors of pediatric brain tumors conducted through the Children's Oncology Group (NCT01381718).

Donepezil, an acetylcholinesterase inhibitor used to treat mild to moderate Alzheimer's dementia, has recently been used to manage cognitive late effects among survivors of cancer. Shaw and colleagues conducted a phase II, 24-week, open-label, dose escalation (5 mg/day for 6 weeks followed by 10 mg/day for 18 weeks) study with 34 adults who had received irradiation for primary brain tumors. Findings indicated improved attention, verbal memory, figural memory, mood, and health-related quality of life (Shaw et al. 2006). These results led to development of an ongoing phase III donepezil trial in survivors of adult brain tumors (NCT00369785). A feasibility trial is underway with childhood brain tumor survivors (NCT00452868) with encouraging initial findings. Castellino and colleagues reported preliminary findings from this trial, described as an open-label pilot study conducted with childhood brain tumor survivors who were at least 1 year from completion of cancer treatment. The medication was tolerated well and significant improvements were noted in executive function and memory following 24 weeks of donepezil (Castellino et al. 2012).

Taken together, findings from MPH trials reveal an intervention that is safe and beneficial for nearly half of childhood cancer survivors who are experiencing attention and learning problems. Clear benefits have been demonstrated on performance- and rater-measures of attention as well as rater-measures of social skills. While academic gains have not been demonstrated on standardized measures, parents indicated improved school grades related to better executive aspects of school performance. It should be noted that children were precluded from participating in these MPH trials for a number of possible medical contraindications (e.g., uncontrolled seizures and uncorrected hypothyroidism) and a significant proportion of children who qualified for the trial had parents refuse participation (36%) (Conklin et al. 2007). The most common reason cited for nonparticipation was concern about placing their child on a stimulant medication. These findings indicate there remains a significant proportion of children for whom MPH is not a viable treatment option because of medical exclusions, parental refusal, medication intolerance or poor response. Based on these findings, the investigation of different pharmacologic agents and the development of nonpharmacologic interventions for childhood cancer survivors is clearly a necessity.

14.5.2 Cognitive Remediation

Cognitive remediation refers to systematic attempts to improve cognitive skills following an acquired brain injury, often through massed practice and other psychology-based interventions (Butler and Namerow 1988). A primary tenet of cognitive remediation is that the brain is plastic and capable of functional reorganization following insult. The most comprehensive, therapist-delivered approach to cognitive remediation in survivors of childhood cancer was developed by Butler and Copeland (Butler and Copeland 2002). These researchers developed a tripartite model, Cognitive Remediation Program (CRP), which uses techniques from brain injury rehabilitation (e.g., repetitive exercises targeting sustained, selective and divided attention), special education (e.g., training in metacognitive strategies such as task preparedness and task monitoring), and clinical psychology (e.g., cognitive behavior therapy approaches such as reframing of cognitive struggles) (Butler et al. 2008). CRP includes 20 two-hour sessions, which are completed one-on-one with a child over 4 to 5 months. Butler and colleagues published findings from a multicenter, randomized, controlled trial of CRP with 167 survivors of childhood cancer who ranged in age from 6 to 17, were at least 1 year off treatment, and were experiencing attention problems. CRP participants experienced a significant improvement in academic skills, incorporated more metacognitive strategies in problem solving, and showed improvements on a parent-rated measure of attention (Butler et al. 2008). There were no significant differences between the group receiving CRP and controls on any measures of neurocognitive functioning, including attention, working memory, and episodic memory. Effect sizes were small to medium, ranging from 0.1 to 0.5, but comparable to other brain injury rehabilitation programs and psychological interventions (Cicerone et al. 2000; Anderson and Catroppa 2006). This study offered initial encouragement, particularly for improving academic skills in childhood cancer survivors.

Patel and colleagues conducted a single-arm, pilot study to evaluate the acceptance and impact of a brief (15 sessions/20 total child training hours over 3 to 4 months), clinic-based cognitive training program for childhood cancer survivors at least 6 months from completion of treatment (Patel et al. 2009). Remediation approaches were similar to Butler and Copeland's CRP and included five components: (1) general problem solving (learning to state the problem, generate and evaluate potential solutions), (2) study skills/metacognitive strategies (e.g., task preparedness and monitoring), (3) information processing techniques (e.g., grouping information into smaller chunks, mnemonic strategies, and visual imagery), (4) reviewing compensatory techniques (e.g., the SQ3R method that directs the child to survey, question, read, recite, and review assigned materials), and (5) collaborative contacts (e.g., teaching parents and teachers strategies to implement in the child's daily environment). Children were required to have a CNS-involved cancer or treatment, to be off treatment at least 6 months, and to have demonstrated attention and/or memory deficits. A total of 49 children met study eligibility criteria with 15 (31%) enrolling. Three children dropped out of the study within the first five training sessions resulting in 12 children in their final sample. As a group, children showed improvement across almost all performance-based cognitive measures, with two scores reaching significance reflecting improved written expression and social skills (Patel et al. 2009). Parents reported the strategies taught were useful. Although the majority of enrolled participants completed at least 70% of training sessions, the low participation rate among eligible families was notable, with families expressing concern regarding the inconvenience of traveling to the clinic after school hours. Further, study interpretations are limited by a small sample size and lack of a control group such that findings could be reflective of practice effects across assessments.

More recently, investigators have become interested in intervening earlier to be able to prevent rather than remediate cognitive late effects. Moore and colleagues conducted a randomized, controlled trial of mathematics intervention initiated during treatment for leukemia (Moore et al. 2012). Fifty-seven children with ALL were randomized to mathematics intervention or standard of care during the maintenance phase of chemotherapy. Participants completed cognitive assessments prior to the intervention, post-intervention, and 1 year later. The mathematics intervention

was based on Multiple Representation Theory and consisted of 40 to 50 hours of intervention delivered individually over the course of 1 year. The mathematics intervention sessions had the children explore, ask questions, solve problems, and explain their solutions using multi-modalities, such as pictures, abstract symbolism, contexts, mathematical language, and concrete manipulatives. Thirty-two of 57 children completed the study and were included in data analyses. The intervention group showed significant improvement in calculation skills and applied mathematics reasoning from pre- to post-intervention and also showed improvements in visual working memory (Moore et al. 2012). The findings suggested that intervention during cancer treatment is feasible and targeting a core skill like mathematics might have generalizable benefits to other skills.

Findings from therapist-delivered cognitive remediation studies with childhood cancer survivors have offered initial encouragement, particularly with respect to the ability to impact acquisition of academic skills. Parents and teachers appear to understand the cognitive strategies and their involvement, with ability to practice in the child's daily environment, might increase the potency of these interventions. Further, there are no medical concerns or contraindications as encountered with pharmacologic approaches. That said, these interventions require a considerable time investment from families and providers with the reviewed studies showing that family concerns about scheduling and travel can significantly diminish participation rates and adherence. Further, the benefits tend to be modest and most cancer survivors do not live near centers that offer cognitive remediation. Findings from these studies highlight the need for less time-intensive and portable cognitive interventions.

14.5.3 Computerized Cognitive Training

Computerized training refers to a group of computer software programs designed to exercise specified cognitive processes. Most rest on the principal of massed practice with repetition of similar exercises over multiple sessions. The difficulty of tasks is graded and increases with demonstrated success. Many programs require some level of "coaching" by a trained professional who provides feedback, trouble shoots problems, and assists in maintaining motivation. Research has shown the active ingredients for successful computerized cognitive training include intensity (number of sessions) and adaptivity (difficulty adjusted to participant's changing skill level). The benefits of adaptivity have been demonstrated in randomized, controlled trials comparing adaptive and non-adaptive administrations of the same computerized program (Chacko et al. 2013; Holmes et al. 2009; Klingberg et al. 2005) as well as by comparing adaptive computerized training to commercially available videogames (Thorell et al. 2009). Accordingly, not all computerized games/programs would be expected to be efficacious in addressing cognitive late effects.

The first computerized cognitive training study with childhood cancer survivors was a pilot study of *Captain's Log* with nine survivors of ALL and brain tumors with identified attention and working memory deficits (Hardy et al. 2011). This program (www.braintrain.com) consists of 33 multilevel, game-like exercises aimed at improving memory, attention, concentration, listening skills, self-control, patience, and processing speed. The investigators assessed the in-home use of the program for at least 50 min per week for 12 weeks. The intervention was associated with good feasibility and acceptability. Parents reported few technical problems. Participants completed between 9 and 53 training sessions (mean = 28.4) and from 3.7 to 20.8 training hours (mean = 11.4) (Hardy et al. 2011). While participants' working memory scores generally increased from baseline to immediate and 3 month post-intervention evaluations, only measures of attention (digit span and parent report) reached statistical significance. These findings offered initial encouragement for computerized cognitive training but the small sample size and single-arm design left open the possibility for parent rating bias or practice effects. Concerns have been noted with this program given the

graphical interface is simplistic relative to modern graphics with risk for boredom and difficulty standardizing administration across a large number of potential tasks.

A newer computerized program of interest is *Cogmed* (www.cogmed.com), a program created by neuroscience researchers and game developers to specifically train working memory. Cogmed is a manualized training program that consists of 25 sessions (15 to 45 minutes in duration depending on age/ability) completed at home over 5 to 9 weeks. Children are guided through rotating exercises that train visual-spatial and verbal working memory. As ability improves, exercises become more difficult. Compliance and performance is tracked over the internet with weekly telephone coaching. Hardy and colleagues conducted a randomized pilot study of Cogmed training with 20 survivors of pediatric brain tumors or ALL (Hardy et al. 2013). The majority of participants (85%) finished the required 20 of 25 sessions. Most parents (88%) rated themselves as "very" or "somewhat" satisfied with their child's training. This study also provided preliminary evidence for cognitive benefit. After controlling for baseline intellectual ability, survivors who completed the intervention demonstrated significant improvement in visual working memory and a reduction in parent report of learning problems relative to controls (Hardy et al. 2013). The working memory benefit showed a trend for maintenance of benefit following 3 month follow-up. While these findings are positive regarding feasibility and acceptability of Cogmed with childhood cancer survivors, the study was not powered (large enough) to measure efficacy, nor did the investigators use neuroimaging to assess brain-based changes associated with training.

Conklin and colleagues recently completed a randomized, controlled Cogmed intervention trial with childhood cancer survivors (Cox et al. 2015). Sixty-eight survivors of childhood ALL or brain tumor with identified working memory deficits were randomly assigned to Cogmed training or standard of care. Functional MRI (fMRI) was conducted pre- and post-intervention to assess neural correlates of cognitive change. Compliance was strong with 30 of 34 participants (88%) completing the intervention. Families had the necessary skills to use the computer program successfully (Cox et al. 2015). Caregivers reported that they were generally able to find training time (63%), viewed training as beneficial (70%), and would recommend this intervention to others (93%) (Cox et al. 2015). Survivors completing the intervention demonstrated greater improvements than control participants on measures of attention, working memory, and processing speed, and showed greater reductions in parent reported executive dysfunction (Conklin et al. 2015). FMRI revealed significant pre- to post-training reduction in activation of left lateral prefrontal and bilateral medial frontal areas (Conklin et al. 2015). These results replicated the earlier feasibility and acceptability study findings while providing evidence for efficacy, generalization of training benefits, and training-related neuroplasticity.

A single-arm pilot trial of *Lumosity* (www. lumosity.com), a home-based computerized cognitive rehabilitation curriculum designed to improve executive function skills, was conducted with childhood cancer survivors (Kesler et al. 2011). Twenty-three survivors of ALL or brain tumors who were exhibiting executive function deficits were assigned to complete Lumosity. Similar to other computerized training trials, compliance with training was good with 19 (83%) completing the entire curriculum (Kesler et al. 2011). While the program was designed to be 8 weeks, most children required longer time (mean = 14 weeks; SD = 7.5 weeks) citing forgetting, illness, vacation, and too much schoolwork as reasons for falling behind schedule. Intervention participants showed significant improvements in processing speed, cognitive flexibility, and memory following training (Kesler et al. 2011). There were no improvements in attention or working memory. FMRI revealed increased activation in inferior, middle, and superior frontal gyri and decreased reaction time from baseline to post training (Kesler et al. 2011). Findings suggest Lumosity may lead to improved executive and memory skills in childhood cancer survivors with evidence for associated neuroplasticity. While these findings are promising, the lack of a control group limits

interpretation with respect to potential for practice effects.

Palmer and colleagues completed a randomized controlled trial of computerized reading intervention (*Fast ForWord*; www.scilearn.com) with children undergoing radiation therapy for medulloblastoma (Palmer et al. 2014). Fast ForWord is a computerized program designed to improve phonological awareness, word reading, and reading comprehension. The investigators set a goal of 48 minutes of training per day, 5 days per week for 6 weeks. Children typically completed training in the hospital-based school. Of 85 eligible patients, 81 (95%) were randomized to reading intervention or standard of care, indicating a high acceptance rate (Palmer et al. 2014). Overall, the group completed a median of 27 sessions; however, there was large variability in training sessions completed with a range from 0 to 46 (SD = 10.71) and only 17 patients (40%) completed the target of 30 intervention sessions (Palmer et al. 2014). There was no significant difference in selected reading outcomes over time between the intervention and control groups. Of note, in contrast to the other computerized intervention studies, participants were not selected based on cognitive deficits in the targeted training area; participants in this study had average reading performance at baseline. Phone interviews conducted with a subset of these participants after study completion revealed some program-specific concerns (e.g., a reading intervention provided to fluid readers).

Taken together, computerized training with childhood cancer survivors is feasible and acceptable. When the program is targeted to a patient's areas of difficulty, there is evidence for efficacy as well as training-related neuroplasticity. Other benefits include the ability to standardize and titrate administration, which is particularly beneficial for research design. Programs can be administered remotely, extending intervention reach to individuals who often do not live in close proximity to providers. The time burden for training is reduced, for providers and families, relative to therapist-delivered cognitive remediation and there is greater flexibility to schedule around a patient's other obligations. Further, there are few medical contraindications, with possible concern related to photosensitive seizures. That being said, computerized programs that are commercially available are expensive and not yet covered by health insurance. Some individuals may lack requisite technology (i.e., computers or internet connection). Finally, additional research is required to demonstrate generalizability of benefits to untrained skills as well as maintenance of benefits over time.

14.5.4 Aerobic Exercise Training

The medical benefits of aerobic exercise are well established and include decreased risk for metabolic, cardiovascular, and metastatic disease (Powell and Blair 1994). Cognitive benefits are less established with emerging evidence to suggest improvements in learning and memory (Winter et al. 2007), delayed age-related memory decline or neurodegenerative disease (Laurin et al. 2001), promotion of recovery following acquired brain injury (Devine and Zafonte 2009), and mood enhancement (Lawlor and Hopker 2001). Correlational studies indicate children of higher cardiorespiratory fitness outperform lower fit children on laboratory cognitive tasks, academic measures, and complex real-world problem solving (Fedewa and Ahn 2011). An association between aerobic fitness and greater efficiency of neural networks underlying executive functions has been revealed by fMRI studies (Chaddock et al. 2012). One fMRI study of brain tumor survivors showed higher cardiorespiratory fitness was associated with better working memory performance, as well as more efficient functioning in frontal and parietal brain regions of interest (Wolfe et al. 2013).

Mabbott and colleagues recently examined the efficacy of a 12 week aerobic exercise intervention in long-term survivors of pediatric brain tumors treated with cranial radiation therapy (Mabbott et al. 2014). They conducted a controlled, crossover trial in which 18 brain tumor survivors were quasi-randomly assigned to either immediate exercise intervention or a waitlist control group. Intervention compliance was high as indicated by an 87% attendance rate and 100% retention. Exercise led to improved processing speed on a battery of computerized cognitive tasks (CANTAB), with waitlist participants showing an increase in mean latency time whereas exercise participants showed a decrease in mean latency across tasks of attention, reaction time, motor speed, and visual memory. There were no group differences in accuracy on computerized tasks. Examination of white matter changes with DTI revealed increased functional anisotropy, indicative of increased white matter integrity, in the corpus callosum and left central cerebral white matter following exercise training.

While randomized studies of exercise intervention in cancer survivors are rare, there is a large volume of literature demonstrating exercise benefits for cognitive functions in rodents, including improved spatial memory (Praag et al. 1999) and reduced age-related memory declines (Adlard et al. 2005). These studies provide clues regarding underlying mechanisms for exercise-related cognitive benefits including neurogenesis (Praag et al. 1999), synaptic plasticity (Farmer et al. 2004), angiogenesis (Pereira et al. 2007), and enhanced neurotransmitter functioning (Chaouloff 1989). Naylor and colleagues found voluntary running restored precursor cell and neurogenesis levels in the hippocampus of mice after a clinically relevant dose of irradiation (Naylor et al. 2008). Additionally, irradiation-induced behavior alterations were ameliorated by exercise. Wong-Goodrich and colleagues found daily running prevented a decline in spatial memory among mice receiving whole-brain irradiation; improved performance in behavioral paradigms was associated with restoration of newborn neurons in the hippocampal dentate gyrus (Wong-Goodrich et al. 2010).

Aerobic exercise is an exciting new intervention direction that may offer cognitive, in addition to cardiopulmonary, benefits to children treated for brain tumors. Exercise programs are relatively inexpensive and easy to implement. Further, candidate mechanisms underlying cognitive benefits have been identified by animal models. That said, there is not yet an established dose (i.e., type of exercise, duration, or intensity), and there may be physical limitations to aerobic

Table 14.2 Benefits and limitations of cognitive late effects interventions

Intervention type	Benefits	Limitations
Pharmacotherapy	• Improved attention and social skills	• Medical contraindications
	• Acceptable side effects profile	• High parental refusal
	• Widely available	• Lower response rate than with attention deficit hyperactivity disorder (ADHD)
Therapist-delivered cognitive remediation	• Improved metacognitive and academic skills	• High time investment/scheduling issues
	• Easily extends to home/school	• Modest effect sizes
	• No medical contraindications	• Limited availability of providers
Computerized cognitive training	• Improved attention and working memory	• Expensive/not covered by insurance
	• High acceptability and adherence	• Requisite technology (e.g., internet)
	• Remote administration/easy scheduling	• Need to demonstrate generalizability
Aerobic exercise training	• Cardiopulmonary and cognitive benefits	• Type/duration/intensity not established
	• Inexpensive and easy to implement	• Physical limitations among cancer survivors
	• Animal model support mechanisms	• Indirect cognitive benefits less robust

exercise among childhood brain tumor survivors, and reduced adherence to exercise routines. It is also likely that the cognitive benefits of aerobic exercise would be less robust than targeted cognitive interventions (Table 14.2).

14.5.5 Individualized Academic Supports

Although group-based intervention studies offer important direction for working with childhood cancer survivors experiencing cognitive late effects, one of the most common interventions is facilitated school reentry and development of individually customized academic support. It has been argued that children with cancer should return to normal activities, including school, as soon as medically possible. Regular school attendance facilitates learning and social involvement. Getting back to school has been associated with a better quality of life years after treatment (Hoffman 2011). Working with a hospital-based school liaison during treatment can facilitate continuation of educational services during treatment (e.g., home bound or hospital bound services), communication with the home school throughout treatment, and transition back to school following treatment. It may be possible to arrange for a school personnel workshop and/or a

presentation to peers to provide education about childhood cancer, treatment, and side effects. There are also written materials that may be of benefit for the school including *Helping Schools Cope with Childhood Cancer: Current Facts and Creative Solutions* (http://www.lhsc.on.ca/Patients_Families_Visitors/Childrens_Hospital/Programs_and_services/HelpingSchools.pdf) or *Educating the Child with Cancer (Hoffman 2011)*. Many children treated for a brain tumor will require academic accommodations and/or special education upon return to school. Special education services range from simple accommodations in the regular classroom to all-day placement in a resource room environment to instruction in the home or hospital. A school liaison can provide information regarding special education law and help advocate for appropriate services.

Three federal laws protect the rights of children between the ages of 3 and 21 with disabilities that impact their ability to profit from their education environment: Section 504 of the Rehabilitation Act of 1973, the Individuals with Disabilities Education Act (IDEA), and the Americans with Disabilities Act (Leigh et al. 2015). Any services required by a child returning to school, including classroom accommodations and special education, should be formalized with a written plan using Section 504 or IDEA. Section

504 of the Rehabilitation Act of 1973 is an anti-discrimination law that mandates that students with a mental or physical impairment be provided with a free and appropriate public education through use of classroom and instruction-based accommodations (http://www.parentcenterhub.org/reposoitory/section504). Section 504 is typically used for those children who are in need of accommodations in the regular classroom. This law applies to public schools as well as colleges, universities, and private schools that receive federal funds and is also a way for college students to receive accommodations. IDEA also mandates that students with a disability receive a free and appropriate public education; however, under IDEA students are provided with accommodations, modifications, and interventions based upon individual student need (http://www.parentcenterhub.org/repository/idea). To receive services under IDEA, a child must meet criteria for classification under one of 13 categories, with many brain tumor survivors qualifying under the category of Other Health Impaired. If deemed appropriate, an Individualized Education Program (IEP) will be developed for the child with goals and objectives reviewed annually and reassessment every 3 years. The Americans with Disabilities Act prohibits discrimination against persons with disabilities and applies to all state and local agencies (not just those receiving federal funds). It provides a second layer of protection, in addition to Section 504, to ensure schools provide reasonable accommodations.

The first step in developing individually customized academic support is a comprehensive assessment of cognitive abilities, preferably performed by a neuropsychologist with experience with the pediatric oncology population. Based on assessment findings, specific recommendations including accommodations and interventions for the school setting should be offered. Some examples of accommodations include preferential seating and frequent redirection/praise to address attention difficulties; increased time or shortened assignments to address slower processing speed; use of reference materials or multiple choice exams to address memory problems; and receiving a copy of teacher notes, tape

recording lectures, or using a word processor to reduce writing in children with fine motor difficulties. Interventions might include smaller group or one-to-one instruction with a special educator to address reading difficulties (e.g., greater instruction in phonological decoding), math difficulties (e.g., more frequent repetition of math concepts or greater use of manipulatives), executive dysfunction (e.g., explicit teaching of metacognitive skills such as task preparedness or task monitoring), or memory impairment (e.g., teaching of mnemonic strategies). Special education might also include related services such as speech-language therapy, occupational therapy, physical therapy, or school counseling as needed.

14.6 Future Directions

There has been notable progress in the treatment of childhood brain tumors with not only improved survival rates but also increased understanding and mitigation of neurotoxicity that contributes to cognitive late effects. Current knowledge affords the opportunity to risk-stratify patients prior to treatment to lessen treatment burden when positive prognostic factors exist. Risk-stratified treatment schemas have increased in sophistication, incorporating not only tumor type, extent of resection, and presence of post-surgical residual disease but also molecular subgrouping and histologic variants that can lead to significant reductions in standard treatment exposure. There has also been noteworthy growth in the development of novel drugs that target specific tumor signaling pathways, such as MEK inhibitors for the treatment of LGG (Sievert et al. 2013) or MET-targeted therapy for the treatment of sonic hedgehog driven medulloblastoma (Faria et al. 2015), which may offer greater ability to delay, dose reduce or, eventually, eliminate radiotherapy for certain tumor types. Improvements in neuroimaging and the delivery of radiation therapy have allowed for successively smaller radiation volumes and contoured margins that have significantly impacted cognitive outcomes with further refinement possible with proton beam therapy (Merchant et al. 2008). Cutting edge research, so far only with rodent models, has indicated a potential benefit of cranial transplantation of stems cells to reduce chemotherapy-induced cognitive dysfunction (Acharya et al. 2015). Currently, brain tumors in infancy remain one of the most challenging areas of care as these patients experience a significantly poorer response to treatment and increased treatment-related toxicities including cognitive late effects. Longitudinal trials evaluating risk-adapted therapy in young children that also include comprehensive, serial cognitive evaluation are greatly needed.

Cognitive intervention research in pediatric oncology has been building momentum over the past decade. There are now multiple pharmacologic and nonpharmacologic interventions with demonstrated feasibility and efficacy. That said, there is still much to be done to improve the quality of life of survivors. For those interventions that have demonstrated short-term efficacy, researchers need to evaluate maintenance of benefits over time as well as generalizability of benefits to skills that are functionally relevant (e.g., academic performance, independent living, career success). Moving outside of the clinic and into homes, schools, and community resource centers will also increase intervention reach to a growing number of survivors and hopefully improve enrollment and retention in intervention programs. Researchers need to intervene earlier to see if it is possible to prevent rather than remediate cognitive deficits. This applies to both pharmacologic and nonpharmacologic approaches. Prophylactic use of certain pharmacologic agents might offer neuroprotection prior to or during treatment. For example, Brown and colleagues completed a randomized placebo-controlled trial of memantine during radiotherapy for adults with brain metastases; findings indicated better cognitive outcomes over time in the group receiving memantine (Brown et al. 2013). Future studies should evaluate the ability of anti-inflammatory agents to attenuate loss of neuronal precursor cells and impact neurogenesis (Castellino et al. 2014). It is also time to start combining interventions such as medication and computerized training in order to capitalize on the synergism of different therapeutic modalities. It is unlikely that one intervention will be sufficient in isolation and most children will require a combined approach. Breakthroughs in genetics and neuroimaging should be exploited in order to identify early in treatment those children at greatest risk for cognitive late effects. These transdisciplinary efforts would increase our understanding of the mechanisms underlying cognitive late effects as well as eventually assist in selecting and/or tailoring interventions to the individual child. While recent findings provide reason for hope, clinicians and researchers cannot grow complacent with current successes, there are still many childhood brain tumor survivors for whom cognitive late effects negatively impact their ability to attain important milestones of adulthood. Working together, we can improve not only survival rates but also the quality of survivorship.

References

Aarsen FK et al (2009) Cognitive deficits and predictors 3 years after diagnosis of a pilocytic astrocytoma in childhood. J Clin Oncol 27(21):3526–3532

Acharya MM et al (2015) Stem cell transplantation reverses chemotherapy-induced cognitive dysfunction. Cancer Res 75(4):676–686

Adlard PA et al (2005) Voluntary exercise decreases amyloid load in a transgenic model of Alzheimer's disease. J Neurosci 25(17):4217–4221

Allen JC, Epstein F (1982) Medulloblastoma and other primary malignant neuroectodermal tumors of the CNS. The effect of patients' age and extent of disease on prognosis. J Neurosurg 57(4):446–451

Anderson VA, Catroppa C (2006) Advances in postacute rehabilitation after childhood-acquired brain injury: a focus on cognitive, behavioral, and social domains. Am J Phys Med Rehabil 85:767–778

Armstrong GA et al (2009) Long-term outcomes among adult survivors of childhood central nervous system malignancies in the Childhood Cancer Survivor Study. J Natl Cancer Inst 101(13):946–958

Armstrong GT et al (2011) Survival and long-term health and cognitive outcomes after low-grade glioma. Neuro Oncol 13(2):223–234

Aukema EJ et al (2009) White matter fractional anisotropy correlates with speed of processing and motor speed in young childhood cancer survivors. Int J Radiat Oncol Biol Phys 74(3):837–843

Barkley RA (1977) A review of stimulant drug research with hyperactive children. J Child Psychol Psychiatry 18(2):137–165

Beebe DW et al (2005) Cognitive and adaptive outcome in low-grade pediatric cerebellar astrocytomas: evidence of diminished cognitive and adaptive functioning in National Collaborative Research Studies (CCG 9891/POG 9130). J Clin Oncol 23(22):5198–5204

Biggs PJ et al (1987) Malignant rhabdoid tumor of the central nervous system. Hum Pathol 18(4):332–337

Blackhall L et al (2009) A pilot study evaluating the safety and efficacy of modafinal for cancer-related fatigue. J Palliat Med 12(5):433–439

Blaney SM et al (2011) Gliomas, ependymomas, and other nonembryonal tumors of the central nervous system. In: Pizzo P, Poplack D (eds) Principles and practice of pediatric oncology, 6th edn. Lippincott Williams & Wilkins, Philadelphia, PA, pp 717–771

Boele FW et al (2013) The effect of modafinil on fatigue, cognitive functioning, and mood in primary brain tumor patients: a multicenter randomized controlled trial. Neuro Oncol 15(10):1420–1428

Brinkman TM et al (2012) Cerebral white matter integrity and executive function in adult survivors of childhood medulloblastoma. Neuro Oncol 14(Suppl 4):iv25–iv36

Brown RT et al (2005) Treatment of attention-deficit/hyperactivity disorder: overview of the evidence. Pediatrics 115(6):e749–e757

Brown PD et al (2013) Memantine for the prevention of cognitive dysfunction in patients receiving whole-brain radiotherapy: a randomized, double-blind, placebo-controlled trial. Neuro Oncol 15(10):1429–1437

Burger PC, Boyko OB (1991) The pathology of central nervous system radiation injury. In: Leibel SA, Gutin PH, Sneline GE (eds) Radiation injury to the nervous system. Raven Press, New York, pp 3–15

Buscariollo DL et al (2012) Survival outcomes in atypical teratoid rhabdoid tumor for patients undergoing radiotherapy in a surveillance, epidemiology, and end results analysis. Cancer 118(17):4212–4219

Butler R, Copeland DR (2002) Attentional processes and their remediation in children treated for cancer: a literature review and the development of a therapeutic approach. J Int Neuropsychol Soc 8:115–124

Butler RW, Mulhern RK (2005) Neurocognitive interventions for children and adolscents surviving cancer. J Pediatr Psychol 30(1):65–78

Butler R, Namerow N (1988) Cognitive retraining in brain injury rehabilitation: a critical review. J Neurol Rehabil 2:97–101

Butler RW et al (2008) A multicenter, randomized clinical trial of a cognitive remediation program for childhood survivors of a pediatric malignancy. J Consult Clin Psychol 76(3):367–378

Carpentieri SC et al (2001) Memory deficits among children with craniopharyngiomas. Neurosurgery 49(5):1053–1057. discussion 1057–8

Castellino SM et al (2012) Toxicity and efficacy of the acetylcholinesterase (AChe) inhibitor donepezil in childhood brain tumor survivors: a pilot study. Pediatr Blood Cancer 59(3):540–547

Castellino SM et al (2014) Developing interventions for cancer-related cognitive dysfunction in childhood cancer survivors. J Natl Cancer Inst 106(8):1–16

Cavazzuti V et al (1983) Neurological and psychophysiological sequelae following different treatments of craniopharyngioma in children. J Neurosurg 59(3):409–417

Chacko A et al (2013) Cogmed Working Memory Training for youth with ADHD: a closer examination of efficacy utilizing evidence-based criteria. J Clin Child Adolesc Psychol 42(6):769–783

Chadderton RD et al (1995) Radiotherapy in the treatment of low-grade astrocytomas. II. The physical and cognitive sequelae. Childs Nerv Syst 11(8):443–448

Chaddock L et al (2012) A functional MRI investigation of the association between childhood aerobic fitness and neurocognitive control. Biol Psychol 89(1):260–268

Chaouloff F (1989) Physical exercise and brain monoamines: a review. Acta Physiol Scand 137(1):1–13

Cicerone K et al (2000) Evidence-based rehabilitation: recommendations for clinical practice. Arch Phys Med Rehabil 81:1596–1615

Conklin HM et al (2007) Acute neurocognitive response to methylphenidate among survivors of childhood cancer: a randomized, double-blind, cross-over trial. J Pediatr Psychol 32(9):1127–1139

Conklin HM et al (2008) Predicting change in academic abilities after conformal radiation therapy for localized ependymoma. J Clin Oncol 26(24):3965–3970

Conklin HM et al (2009) Side effects of methylphenidate in childhood cancer survivors: a randomized placebo-controlled trial. Pediatrics 124(1):226–233

Conklin HM et al (2010a) Long-term efficacy of methylphenidate in enhancing attention regulation, social skills, and academic abilities of childhood cancer survivors. J Clin Oncol 28(29):4465–4472

Conklin HM et al (2010b) Predicting methylphenidate response in long-term survivors of childhood cancer: a randomized, double-blind, placebo-controlled, cross-over trial. J Pediatr Psychol 35(2):144–155

Conklin HM et al (2012) Cognitive outcomes following contemporary treatment without cranial irradiation for childhood acute lymphoblastic leukemia. J Natl Cancer Inst 104(18):1386–1395

Conklin H et al (2015) Computerized cognitive training for amelioration of cognitive late effects among childhood cancer survivors: a randomized controlled trial. J Clin Oncol 33:3894–3902

Copeland DR et al (1996) Neuropsychologic effects of chemotherapy on children with cancer: a longitudinal study. J Clin Oncol 14:2826–2835

Cowan N (2010) Multiple concurrent thoughts: the meaning and developmental neuropsychology of working memory. Dev Neuropsychol 35(5):447–474

Cox LE et al (2015) Feasibility and acceptability of a remotely administered computerized intervention to address cognitive late effects among childhood cancer survivors. Neuro-Oncol Pract 2:78–87

Crawford JR, MacDonald TJ, Packer RJ (2007) Medulloblastoma in childhood: new biological advances. Lancet Neurol 6(12):1073–1085

De Smet HJ et al (2007) Postoperative motor speech production in children with the syndrome of 'cerebellar' mutism and subsequent dysarthria: a critical review of the literature. Eur J Paediatr Neurol 11(4):193–207

DeLong R et al (1992) Methylphenidate in neuropsychological sequelae of radiotherapy and chemotherapy of childhood brain tumors and leukemia. J Child Neurol 7(4):462–463

Dennis M et al (1996) Neuropsychological sequelae of the treatment of children with medulloblastoma. J Neurooncol 29(1):91–101

Dennis M, Hetherington CR, Spiegler BJ (1998) Memory and attention after childhood brain tumors. Med Pediatr Oncol 1(Suppl 1):25–33

Deutsch M et al (1996) Results of a prospective randomized trial comparing standard dose neuraxis irradiation (3,600 cGy/20) with reduced neuraxis irradiation (2,340 cGy/13) in patients with low-stage medulloblastoma. A Combined Children's Cancer Group-Pediatric Oncology Group Study. Pediatr Neurosurg 24(4):167–176. discussion 176–7

Devine JM, Zafonte RD (2009) Physical exercise and cognitive recovery in acquired brain injury: a review of the literature. PM R 1(6):560–575

Di Pinto M et al (2010) Investigating verbal and visual auditory learning after conformal radiation therapy for childhood ependymoma. Int J Radiat Oncol Biol Phys 77(4):1002–1008

Di Pinto M et al (2012) Learning and memory following conformal radiation therapy for pediatric craniopharyngioma and low-grade glioma. Int J Radiat Oncol Biol Phys 84(3):e363–e369

Di Rocco C et al (2010) Preoperative and postoperative neurological, neuropsychological and behavioral impairment in children with posterior cranial fossa astrocytomas and medulloblastomas: the role of the tumor and the impact of the surgical treatment. Childs Nerv Syst 26(9):1173–1188

Dolecek TA et al (2012) CBTRUS statistical report: primary brain and central nervous system tumors diagnosed in the United States in 2005–2009. Neuro Oncol 14(Suppl 5):v1–v49

Dolson EP et al (2009) Predicting behavioral problems in craniopharyngioma survivors after conformal radiation therapy. Pediatr Blood Cancer 52(7):860–864

Edelstein K et al (2011) Early aging in adult survivors of childhood medulloblastoma: long-term neurocognitive, functional, and physical outcomes. Neuro Oncol 13(5):536–545

Efron D, Jarman FC, Barker MJ (1998) Child and parent perceptions of stimulant medication treatment in attention deficit hyperactivity disorder. J Paediatr Child Health 34(3):288–292

Ellenberg L et al (1987) Factors affecting intellectual outcomes in pediatric brain tumor patients. Neurosurgery 21(5):638–644

Ellenberg L et al (2009) Neurocognitive status in long-term survivors of childhood CNS malignancies: a report from the Childhood Cancer Survivor Study. Neuropsychology 23(6):705–717

Faria CC et al (2015) Foretinib is effective therapy for metastatic sonic hedgehog medulloblastoma. Cancer Res 75(1):134–146

Farmer J et al (2004) Effects of voluntary exercise on synaptic plasticity and gene expression in the dentate gyrus of adult male Sprague-Dawley rats in vivo. Neuroscience 124(1):71–79

Fedewa AL, Ahn S (2011) The effects of physical activity and physical fitness on children's achievement and cognitive outcomes: a meta-analysis. Res Q Exerc Sport 82(3):521–535

Filley CM, Kleinschmidt-DeMasters BK (2001) Toxic leukoencephalopathy. N Engl J Med 345(6):425–432

Fine S, Johnston C (1993) Drug and placebo side effects in methylphenidate-placebo trial for attention deficit hyperactivity disorder. Child Psychiatry Hum Dev 24(1):25–30

Finkelstein-Shechter T et al (2010) Atypical teratoid or rhabdoid tumors: improved outcome with high-dose chemotherapy. J Pediatr Hematol Oncol 32(5):e182–e186

Fry AF, Hale S (1996) Processing speed, working memory, and fluid intelligence: evidence for a developmental cascade. Psychol Sci 7:237–241

Fry AF, Hale S (2000a) Relationships among processing speed, working memory, and fluid intelligence in children. Biol Psychol 7(4):734–740

Fry AF, Hale S (2000b) Relationships among processing speed, working memory, and fluid intelligence in children. Biol Psychol 54(1–3):1–34

Gajjar AJ, Robinson GW (2014) Medulloblastoma-translating discoveries from the bench to the bedside. Nat Rev Clin Oncol 11(12):714–722

Gajjar A et al (2006) Risk-adapted craniospinal radiotherapy followed by high-dose chemotherapy and stem-cell rescue in children with newly diagnosed medulloblastoma (St Jude Medulloblastoma-96): long-term results from a prospective, multicentre trial. Lancet Oncol 7(10):813–820

Gehring K et al (2012) A randomized trial on the efficacy of methylphenidate and modafinil for improving cognitive functioning and symptoms in patients with a primary brain tumor. J Neurooncol 107(1):165–174

Glauser TA, Packer RJ (1991) Cognitive deficits in long-term survivors of childhood brain tumors. Childs Nerv Syst 7(1):2–12

Gottardo NG, Gajjar A (2006) Current therapy for medulloblastoma. Curr Treat Options Neurol 8(4):319–334

Greenberger BA et al (2014) Clinical outcomes and late endocrine, neurocognitive, and visual profiles of proton radiation for pediatric low-grade gliomas. Int J Radiat Oncol Biol Phys 89(5):1060–1068

Grill J et al (1999) Long-term intellectual outcome in children with posterior fossa tumors according to radiation doses and volumes. Int J Radiat Oncol Biol Phys 45(1):137–145

Grill J et al (2005) Treatment of medulloblastoma with postoperative chemotherapy alone: an SFOP prospective trial in young children. Lancet Oncol 6(8):573–580

Gudrunardottir T et al (2011a) Cerebellar mutism: review of the literature. Childs Nerv Syst 27(3):355–363

Gudrunardottir T et al (2011b) Cerebellar mutism: definitions, classification and grading of symptoms. Childs Nerv Syst 27(9):1361–1363

Gurney JG et al (2009) Social outcomes in the Childhood Cancer Survivor Study cohort. J Clin Oncol 27(14): 2390–2395

Hardy KK, Willard VW, Bonner MJ (2011) Computerized cognitive training in survivors of childhood cancer: a pilot study. J Pediatr Oncol Nurs 28(1):27–33

Hardy KK et al (2013) Working memory training in survivors of pediatric cancer: a randomized pilot study. Psychooncology 22(8):1856–1865

Hoffman RI (ed) (2011) Educating the child with cancer: a guide for parents and teachers, 2nd edn. American Childhood Cancer Organization, Bethesda, MD

Holmes J, Gathercole SE, Dunning DL (2009) Adaptive training leads to sustained enhancement of poor working memory in children. Dev Sci 12(4):F9–F15

Hoppe-Hirsch E et al (1990) Medulloblastoma in childhood: progressive intellectual deterioration. Childs Nerv Syst 6(2):60–65

Howarth RA et al (2014) Investigating the relationship between COMT polymorphisms and working memory performance among childhood brain tumor survivors. Pediatr Blood Cancer 61(1):40–45

Huber JF et al (2006) Long-term effects of transient cerebellar mutism after cerebellar astrocytoma or medulloblastoma tumor resection in childhood. Childs Nerv Syst 22(2):132–138

Huber JF et al (2007) Long-term neuromotor speech deficits in survivors of childhood posterior fossa tumors: effects of tumor type, radiation, age at diagnosis, and survival years. J Child Neurol 22(7):848–854

Hudson M (1999) Late complications after leukemia therapy. In: Pui CH (ed) Childhood leukemias. Cambridge University Press, Cambridge, MA, pp 463–481

Jannoun L, Bloom HJ (1990) Long-term psychological effects in children treated for intracranial tumors. Int J Radiat Oncol Biol Phys 18(4):747–753

Jasper BW et al (2009) Growth effects of methylphenidate among childhood cancer survivors: a 12-month case-matched open-label study. Pediatr Blood Cancer 52(1):39–43

Jemal A et al (2008) Cancer statistics, 2008. CA Cancer J Clin 58(2):71–96

Johnson DL et al (1994) Quality of long-term survival in young children with medulloblastoma. J Neurosurg 80(6):1004–1010

Kamdar KY et al (2011) Folate pathway polymorphisms predict deficits in attention and processing speed after childhood leukemia therapy. Pediatr Blood Cancer 57(3):454–460

Kesler SR, Lacayo NJ, Jo B (2011) A pilot study of an online cognitive rehabilitation program for executive function skills in children with cancer-related brain injury. Brain Inj 25(1):101–112

Kiehna EN et al (2006) Changes in attentional performance of children and young adults with localized primary brain tumors after conformal radiation therapy. J Clin Oncol 24(33):5283–5290

King TZ et al (2004) Verbal memory abilities of children with brain tumors. Child Neuropsychol 10(2):76–88

Klingberg T et al (2005) Computerized training of working memory in children with ADHD--a randomized, controlled trial. J Am Acad Child Adolesc Psychiatry 44(2):177–186

Knight SJ, Conklin HM, Palmer SL, Schreiber JE, Armstrong CL, Wallace D, Bonner M, Swain MA, Evankovich KD, Mabbott DJ, Boyle R, Huang Q, Zhang H, Anderson VA, Gajjar A (2014) Working memory abilities among children treated for medulloblastoma: parent report and child performance. J Pediatr Psychol 39:501–511

Kohli S et al (2009) The effect of modafinil on cognitive function in breast cancer survivors. Cancer 115(12):2605–2616

Korah MP et al (2010) Incidence, risks, and sequelae of posterior fossa syndrome in pediatric medulloblastoma. Int J Radiat Oncol Biol Phys 77(1):106–112

Krull KR et al (2008) Folate pathway genetic polymorphisms are related to attention disorders in childhood leukemia survivors. J Pediatr 152(1):101–105

Lacaze E et al (2003) Neuropsychological outcome in children with optic pathway tumours when first-line treatment is chemotherapy. Br J Cancer 89(11):2038–2044

Lafay-Cousin L et al (2015) Neurocognitive evaluation of long term survivors of atypical teratoid rhabdoid tumors (ATRT): the Canadian registry experience. Pediatr Blood Cancer 62(7):1265–1269

Landau E et al (2013) Supratentorial ependymoma: disease control, complications, and functional outcomes after irradiation. Int J Radiat Oncol Biol Phys 85(4):e193–e199

Laughton SJ et al (2008) Endocrine outcomes for children with embryonal brain tumors after risk-adapted craniospinal and conformal primary-site irradiation and high-dose chemotherapy with stem-cell rescue on the SJMB-96 trial. J Clin Oncol 26(7):1112–1118

Laurin D et al (2001) Physical activity and risk of cognitive impairment and dementia in elderly persons. Arch Neurol 58(3):498–504

Law N et al (2011) Cerebello-thalamo-cerebral connections in pediatric brain tumor patients: impact on working memory. Neuroimage 56(4):2238–2248

Lawlor DA, Hopker SW (2001) The effectiveness of exercise as an intervention in the management of depression: systematic review and meta-regression analysis of randomised controlled trials. BMJ 322(7289):763–767

Leigh L, Conklin HM, Schreiber JE (2015) Educational issues for children with cancer. In: Pizzo P, Poplack D (eds) Principles and practice of pediatric oncology. Lippincott Williams & Wilkins, Philadelphia, PA

Levisohn L, Cronin-Golomb A, Schmahmann JD (2000) Neuropsychological consequences of cerebellar tumor resection in children: cerebellar cognitive affective syndrome in a pediatric population. Brain 123:1041–1050

Louis DN et al (2007) The 2007 WHO classification of tumours of the central nervous system. Acta Neuropathol 114(2):97–109

Lundorff LE, Jonsson BH, Sjogren P (2009) Modafinil for attentional and psychomotor dysfunction in advanced cancer: a double-blind, randomised, cross-over trial. Palliat Med 23(8):731–738

Mabbott DJ et al (2006) Diffusion tensor imaging of white matter after cranial radiation in children for medulloblastoma: correlation with IQ. Neuro Oncol 8(3):244–252

Mabbott DJ et al (2008) Core neurocognitive functions in children treated for posterior fossa tumors. Neuropsychology 22(2):159–168

Mabbott D et al (2014) NC-10 Training the brain to repair itself: an exercise trial in pediatric brain tumor survivors. Neuro Oncol 16(Suppl_5):v136

Macdonald SM et al (2013) Proton radiotherapy for pediatric central nervous system ependymoma: clinical outcomes for 70 patients. Neuro Oncol 15(11):1552–1559

Massimino M et al (2011) Childhood medulloblastoma. Crit Rev Oncol Hematol 79(1):65–83

Merchant TE et al (2000) CNS germinoma: disease control and long-term functional outcome for 12 children treated with craniospinal irradiation. Int J Radiat Oncol Biol Phys 46(5):1171–1176

Merchant TE et al (2008) Proton versus photon radiotherapy for common pediatric brain tumors: comparison of models of dose characteristics and their relationship to cognitive function. Pediatr Blood Cancer 51(1):110–117

Merchant TE et al (2009) Late effects of conformal radiation therapy for pediatric patients with low-grade glioma: prospective evaluation of cognitive, endocrine, and hearing deficits. J Clin Oncol 27(22):3691–3697

Merchant TE et al (2014) Effect of cerebellum radiation dosimetry on cognitive outcomes in children with infratentorial ependymoma. Int J Radiat Oncol Biol Phys 90(3):547–553

Meyers CA et al (1998) Methylphenidate therapy improves cognition, mood, and function of brain tumor patients. J Clin Oncol 16(7):2522–2527

Miller NG et al (2010) Cerebellocerebral diaschisis is the likely mechanism of postsurgical posterior fossa syndrome in pediatric patients with midline cerebellar tumors. Am J Neuroradiol 31(2):288–294

Moore IM et al (2012) Mathematics intervention for prevention of neurocognitive deficits in childhood leukemia. Pediatr Blood Cancer 59(2):278–284

Mulhern RK, Butler RW (2004) Neurocognitive sequelae of childhood cancers and their treatment. Pediatr Rehabil 7(1):1–14

Mulhern RK et al (1998) Neuropsychologic functioning of survivors of childhood medulloblastoma randomized to receive conventional or reduced-dose craniospinal irradiation: a Pediatric Oncology Group study. J Clin Oncol 16(5):1723–1728

Mulhern RK et al (1999) Neurocognitive deficits in medulloblastoma survivors and white matter loss. Ann Neurol 46(6):834–841

Mulhern RK et al (2001) Risks of young age for selected neurocognitive deficits in medulloblastoma are associated with white matter loss. J Clin Oncol 19(2):472–479

Mulhern RK et al (2004a) Late neurocognitive sequelae in survivors of brain tumours in childhood. Lancet Oncol 5(7):399–408

Mulhern RK et al (2004b) Short-term efficacy of methylphenidate: a randomized, double-blind, placebo-controlled trial among survivors of childhood cancer. J Clin Oncol 22(23):4795–4803

Mulhern RK et al (2005) Neurocognitive consequences of risk-adapted therapy for childhood medulloblastoma. J Clin Oncol 23(24):5511–5519

Nagel BJ et al (2004) Abnormal hippocampal development in children with medulloblastoma treated with risk-adapted irradiation. Am J Neuroradiol 25(9):1575–1582

Nagel BJ et al (2006) Early patterns of verbal memory impairment in children treated for medulloblastoma. Neuropsychology 20(1):105–112

Naylor AS et al (2008) Voluntary running rescues adult hippocampal neurogenesis after irradiation of the young mouse brain. Proc Natl Acad Sci U S A 105(38):14632–14637

Ness KK et al (2006) Physical performance limitations and participation restrictions among cancer survivors: a population-based study. Ann Epidemiol 16(3):197–205

Netson KL et al (2012) A 5-year investigation of children's adaptive functioning following conformal radiation therapy for localized ependymoma. Int J Radiat Oncol Biol Phys 84(1):217–223.e1

Netson KL et al (2013) Longitudinal investigation of adaptive functioning following conformal irradiation for pediatric craniopharyngioma and low-grade glioma. Int J Radiat Oncol Biol Phys 85(5):1301–1306

Northcott PA et al (2012) Medulloblastomics: the end of the beginning. Nat Rev Cancer 12(12):818–834

O'Neil S et al (2011) Neurocognitive outcomes in pediatric and adolescent patients with central nervous system germinoma treated with a strategy of chemotherapy followed by reduced-dose and volume irradiation. Pediatr Blood Cancer 57(4):669–673

Oberauer K, Bialkova S (2009) Accessing information in working memory: can the focus of attention grasp two elements at the same time? J Exp Psychol Gen 138:64–87

Oyharcabal-Bourden V et al (2005) Standard-risk medulloblastoma treated by adjuvant chemotherapy followed by reduced-dose craniospinal radiation therapy: a French Society of Pediatric Oncology Study. J Clin Oncol 23(21):4726–4734

Packer RJ (2002) Radiation-induced neurocognitive decline: the risks and benefits of reducing the amount of whole-brain irradiation. Curr Neurol Neurosci Rep 2(2):131–133

Packer RJ, Cohen BH, Cooney K (2000) Intracranial germ cell tumors. Oncologist 5(4):312–320

Packer RJ, Rood BR, MacDonald TJ (2003) Medulloblastoma: present concepts of stratification into risk groups. Pediatr Neurosurg 39(2):60–67

Packer RJ et al (2006) Phase III study of craniospinal radiation therapy followed by adjuvant chemotherapy for newly diagnosed average-risk medulloblastoma. J Clin Oncol 24(25):4202–4208

Palmer SL et al (2001) Patterns of intellectual development among survivors of pediatric medulloblastoma: a longitudinal analysis. J Clin Oncol 19(8):2302–2308

Palmer SL et al (2002) Decline in corpus callosum volume among pediatric patients with medulloblastoma: longitudinal MR imaging study. Am J Neuroradiol 23(7):1088–1094

Palmer SL, Reddick WE, Gajjar A (2007) Understanding the cognitive impact on children who are treated for medulloblastoma. J Pediatr Psychol 32(9):1040–1049

Palmer SL et al (2010) Neurocognitive outcome 12 months following cerebellar mutism syndrome in pediatric patients with medulloblastoma. Neuro Oncol 12(12):1311–1317

Palmer SL et al (2013) Processing speed, attention, and working memory after treatment for medulloblastoma: an international, prospective, and longitudinal study. J Clin Oncol 31(28):3494–3500

Palmer SL et al (2014) Feasibility and efficacy of a computer-based intervention aimed at preventing reading decoding deficits among children undergoing active treatment for medulloblastoma: results of a randomized trial. J Pediatr Psychol 39(4):450–458

Patay Z et al (2014) MR imaging evaluation of inferior olivary nuclei: comparison of postoperative subjects with and without posterior fossa syndrome. Am J Neuroradiol 35(4):797–802

Patel SK et al (2009) Cognitive and problem solving training in children with cancer: a pilot project. J Pediatr Hematol Oncol 31(9):670–677

Pereira AC et al (2007) An in vivo correlate of exercise-induced neurogenesis in the adult dentate gyrus. Proc Natl Acad Sci U S A 104(13):5638–5643

Posner MI, Raichle ME (1994) Images of mind. Scientific American Library, New York

Powell KE, Blair SN (1994) The public health burdens of sedentary living habits: theoretical but realistic estimates. Med Sci Sports Exerc 26(7):851–856

Praag Hv et al (1999) Running enhances neurogenesis, learning, and long-term potentiation in mice. Proc Natl Acad Sci U S A 96:13427–13431

Pui CH et al (2011) Challenging issues in pediatric oncology. Nat Rev Clin Oncol 8(9):540–549

Rajan B et al (1993) Craniopharyngioma—a long-term results following limited surgery and radiotherapy. Radiother Oncol 26(1):1–10

Ramaswamy V et al (2016) Medulloblastoma subgroup-specific outcomes in irradiated children: who are the true high-risk patients? Neuro Oncol 18(2):291–297

Reddick WE et al (1998) A hybrid neural network analysis of subtle brain volume differences in children surviving brain tumors. Magn Reson Imaging 16(4):413–421

Reddick WE et al (2000) Subtle white matter volume differences in children treated for medulloblastoma with conventional or reduced dose craniospinal irradiation. Magn Reson Imaging 18(7):787–793

Reddick WE et al (2003) Developmental model relating white matter volume to neurocognitive deficits in pediatric brain tumor survivors. Cancer 97(10):2512–2519

Reeves CB et al (2006) Attention and memory functioning among pediatric patients with medulloblastoma. J Pediatr Psychol 31(3):272–280

Ris MD, Beebe DW (2008) Neurodevelopmental outcomes of children with low-grade gliomas. Dev Disabil Res Rev 14(3):196–202

Ris MD, Noll RB (1994) Long-term neurobehavioral outcome in pediatric brain-tumor patients: review and methodological critique. J Clin Exp Neuropsychol 16(1):21–42

Ris MD et al (2001) Intellectual outcome after reduced-dose radiation therapy plus adjuvant chemotherapy for medulloblastoma: a Children's Cancer Group study. J Clin Oncol 19(15):3470–3476

Riva D et al (1998) Late neuropsychological and behavioural outcome of children surgically treated for craniopharyngioma. Childs Nerv Syst 14(4–5):179–184

Robertson PL et al (2006) Incidence and severity of postoperative cerebellar mutism syndrome in children with medulloblastoma: a prospective study by the Children's Oncology Group. J Neurosurg 105(6 Suppl):444–451

Roncadin C et al (2008) Adverse medical events associated with childhood cerebellar astrocytomas and medulloblastomas: natural history and relation to very long-term neurobehavioral outcome. Childs Nerv Syst 24(9):995–1002

Rutkowski S et al (2005) Treatment of early childhood medulloblastoma by postoperative chemotherapy alone. N Engl J Med 352(10):978–986

Rutkowski S et al (2009) Treatment of early childhood medulloblastoma by postoperative chemotherapy and deferred radiotherapy. Neuro Oncol 11(2):201–210

Rutkowski S et al (2010) Survival and prognostic factors of early childhood medulloblastoma: an international meta-analysis. J Clin Oncol 28(33):4961–4968

Sands SA et al (2001) Long-term quality of life and neuropsychologic functioning for patients with CNS germ-cell tumors: from the First International CNS Germ-Cell Tumor Study. Neuro Oncol 3(3):174–183

Schatz J et al (2000) Processing speed, working memory, and IQ: a developmental model of cognitive deficits following cranial radiation therapy. Neuropsychology 14(2):189–200

Schreiber JE et al (2014) Examination of risk factors for intellectual and academic outcomes following treatment for pediatric medulloblastoma. Neuro Oncol 16(8):1129–1136

Schreiber JE et al (2015) Posterior fossa syndrome and long-term neurocognitive problems among children treated for medulloblastoma on a multi-institutional, prospective study. J Int Neuropsychol Soc 20(S1):293

Seaver E et al (1994) Psychosocial adjustment in long-term survivors of childhood medulloblastoma and ependymoma treated with craniospinal irradiation. Pediatr Neurosurg 20(4):248–253

Shaw EG et al (2006) Phase II study of donepezil in irradiated brain tumor patients: effect on cognitive function, mood, and quality of life. J Clin Oncol 24(9):1415–1420

Sievert AJ et al (2013) Paradoxical activation and RAF inhibitor resistance of BRAF protein kinase fusions characterizing pediatric astrocytomas. Proc Natl Acad Sci U S A 110(15):5957–5962

Soussain C et al (2009) CNS complications of radiotherapy and chemotherapy. Lancet 374(9701):1639–1651

Squire SE, Chan MD, Marcus KJ (2007) Atypical teratoid/rhabdoid tumor: the controversy behind radiation therapy. J Neurooncol 81(1):97–111

Steinbok P et al (2003) Mutism after posterior fossa tumour resection in children: incomplete recovery on long-term follow-up. Pediatr Neurosurg 39(4):179–183

Strother D (2005) Atypical teratoid rhabdoid tumors of childhood: diagnosis, treatment and challenges. Expert Rev Anticancer Ther 5(5):907–915

Tekautz TM et al (2005) Atypical teratoid/rhabdoid tumors (ATRT): improved survival in children 3 years of age and older with radiation therapy and high-dose alkylator-based chemotherapy. J Clin Oncol 23(7):1491–1499

Thomas PR et al (2000) Low-stage medulloblastoma: final analysis of trial comparing standard-dose with reduced-dose neuraxis irradiation. J Clin Oncol 18(16):3004–3011

Thompson SJ et al (2001) Immediate neurocognitive effects of methylphenidate on learning-impaired survivors of childhood cancer. J Clin Oncol 19(6):1802–1808

Thorell L et al (2009) Training and transfer effects of executive functions in preschool children. Dev Sci 92(1–2):186–192

Torres CF et al (1996) Effect of methylphenidate in the postradiation attention and memory deficits of children. Ann Neurol 40:331

Turner CD et al (2009) Medical, psychological, cognitive and educational late-effects in pediatric low-grade glioma survivors treated with surgery only. Pediatr Blood Cancer 53(3):417–423

Ullrich NJ (2008) Inherited disorders as a risk factor and predictor of neurodevelopmental outcome in pediatric cancer. Dev Disabil Res Rev 14(3):229–237

Verlooy J et al (2006) Treatment of high risk medulloblastomas in children above the age of 3 years: a SFOP study. Eur J Cancer 42(17):3004–3014

Waber DP et al (2012) Neuropsychological outcomes of standard risk and high risk patients treated for acute lymphoblastic leukemia on Dana-Farber ALL constortium protocol 95-01 at 5 years post-diagnosis. Pediatr Blood Cancer 58(5):758–765

Winter B et al (2007) High impact running improves learning. Neurobiol Learn Mem 87(4):597–609

Wolfe KR et al (2012) Cardiorespiratory fitness in survivors of pediatric posterior fossa tumor. J Pediatr Hematol Oncol 34(6):e222–e227

Wolfe KR et al (2013) An fMRI investigation of working memory and its relationship with cardiorespiratory fitness in pediatric posterior fossa tumor survivors who received cranial radiation therapy. Pediatr Blood Cancer 60(4):669–675

Wong-Goodrich SJ et al (2010) Voluntary running prevents progressive memory decline and increases adult hippocampal neurogenesis and growth factor expression after whole-brain irradiation. Cancer Res 70(22):9329–9338

Zeltzer PM et al (1999) Metastasis stage, adjuvant treatment, and residual tumor are prognostic factors for medulloblastoma in children: conclusions from the Children's Cancer Group 921 randomized phase III study. J Clin Oncol 17(3):832–845

Long-Term Outcomes Among Survivors of Childhood Central Nervous System Malignancies: Late Mortality, Subsequent Neoplasms, Endocrine and Neurologic Morbidity

15

Gregory T. Armstrong, Raja B. Khan, and Wassim Chemaitilly

15.1 Introduction

According to the most recent estimates from the Surveillance, Epidemiology and End Results (SEER), 74% of children younger than 20 years of age diagnosed with a central nervous system (CNS) malignancy will become 5-year survivors (Howlader et al. 2012). Current therapy for children with CNS malignancies often includes both surgical resection and a combination of CNS-directed radiation therapy (RT) and chemotherapy. Among survivors of all primary pediatric cancers, survivors of CNS malignancies are at the highest risk for late mortality (Mertens et al. 2001; Taylor and Potish 1985; Dama et al. 2006). Furthermore, survivors of CNS malignancies are at risk for developing subsequent neoplasms and chronic endocrine and neurologic conditions (Neglia et al. 2001; Broniscer et al. 2004; Cardous-Ubbink et al. 2007; Duffner et al. 1998; Devarahally et al. 2003; Peterson et al. 2006; Jenkinson et al. 2004; Hammal et al. 2005; Oeffinger et al. 2006; Packer et al. 2003; Gurney et al. 2003a). Documenting the incidence of and risk factors for these conditions in the second, third, and fourth decades of survival in this aging population is essential as future efforts to reduce late morbidity and mortality through modification and risk stratification of primary therapy, screening and early detection of late effects, and interventions to reduce risk and impact of late effects are dependent on identifying populations at highest risk for poor outcomes. Thus, while 5-year survival has improved, the patterns of late morbidity and mortality after exposure to multimodal therapy are only now being established as this population ages. Future studies will need to identify whether exposure to modern therapies (including focal RT for embryonal CNS tumors in infants, whole ventricular volume RT for germ cell tumors, targeted therapies, and immunotherapy, among others) increases or decreases the risk of long-term morbidity and late mortality compared with patients treated in previous eras (Armstrong et al. 2009a).

G. T. Armstrong (✉)
Department of Epidemiology and Cancer Control,
St. Jude Children's Research Hospital,
Memphis, TN, USA
e-mail: greg.armstrong@stjude.org

R. B. Khan
Divisions of Neurology,
St. Jude Children's Research Hospital,
Memphis, TN, USA

W. Chemaitilly
Division of Endocrinology,
St. Jude Children's Research Hospital,
Memphis, TN, USA

© Springer International Publishing AG, part of Springer Nature 2018
A. Gajjar et al. (eds.), *Brain Tumors in Children*, https://doi.org/10.1007/978-3-319-43205-2_15

15.2   Late Mortality

Five-year overall survival has been the accepted benchmark for clinical trials, and yet it is now apparent that those who survive childhood cancer beyond the 5-year time point remain at significant risk for late mortality (Mertens et al. 2001, 2008; Armstrong et al. 2009b; Moller et al. 2001; Garwicz et al. 2012; Reulen et al. 2010; Cardous-Ubbink et al. 2004). Fewer studies have investigated late mortality specifically among central nervous system (CNS) tumor survivors, and many of those are limited by small population sizes from individual treatment institutions, short follow-up time, and lack of treatment exposure information (Morris et al. 2007; Jenkin 1996; Ning et al. 2015; Acharya et al. 2015; Perkins et al. 2013; Visser et al. 2010).

The most recent assessment of late-mortality among the 2821 5-year survivors of CNS tumors

diagnosed between 1970 and 1986 in the Childhood Cancer Survivor Study (CCSS) provides 30 years of follow-up (Armstrong et al. 2009a). Cumulative all-cause mortality rates among 5-year survivors were 13.5%, 17.1%, 21.5%, and 25.8% at 15, 20, 25, and 30 years, respectively (Fig. 15.1a); males had greater risk of death than females (28.1% vs. 23.1% at 30 years; $P < 0.001$). All-cause mortality at 30 years was higher in 5-year survivors of ependymoma (29.5%) and medulloblastoma (29.0%) than in 5-year survivors of astrocytoma and glial tumors (23.9%; $P < 0.001$ for both comparisons) (Fig. 15.1b) (Armstrong et al. 2009a).

Risk of death was 13-fold higher for survivors of central nervous system malignancies (SMR = 12.9, 95% CI = 11.8–14.0) compared to that of the age- and sex-specific general population. Survivors of medulloblastoma and primitive neuroectodermal tumors were at highest risk

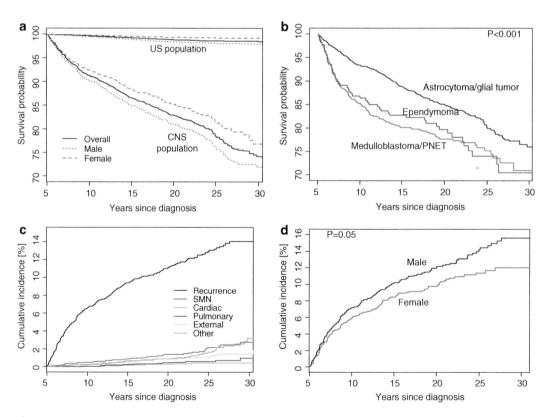

Fig. 15.1 (**a**) All-cause and sex-specific mortality: 5-year survivors of CNS tumors compared to age-adjusted U.S. population. (**b**) All-cause mortality by primary diagnosis.

(**c**) Cumulative cause-specific mortality. (**d**) Cumulative mortality attributable to recurrence by sex

(SMR = 17.4, 95% CI = 14.6–20.6). The most common cause of death was recurrence or progression of primary disease (61%), followed by medical causes of death (21%) that included death attributable to subsequent neoplasms (9%), cardiac disease (3%), and pulmonary disease (3%). Cumulative cause-specific mortality at 30 years (Fig. 15.1c) was highest for primary cancer progression or recurrence (14%), followed by subsequent malignant neoplasm (2.8%), pulmonary disease (1.0%), and cardiac disease (0.4%). Cumulative mortality due to recurrence was higher in males than females (15.6% vs. 12.1% at 30 years, $P = 0.05$) (Fig. 15.1d). Other studies have identified sepsis and metabolic death as significant causes as well (Morris et al. 2007). Notably, at 30 years from diagnosis the annual death rate from subsequent malignant neoplasms exceeds that of recurrence or progression of primary disease, suggesting that survivors face life-threatening consequences of their primary tumor for decades (Hawkins et al. 1990).

We can be optimistic, however, that survivors in more recent decades, where risk-stratification of therapeutic intensity has guided primary cancer treatment, may have better outcomes. In particular, among patients identified as having an excellent prognosis, such as those with low-grade astrocytoma, efforts have been directed toward use of chemotherapy to delay, and in some cases eliminate, use of radiotherapy. As a result, the CCSS recently reported that survivors of astrocytoma treated in the 1990s had a lower 15-year all-cause mortality than those from the 1970s (7.4% vs. 13.5%, $P < 0.001$). Most striking is that death due to late effects of cancer therapy was reduced (1.7% vs. 4.7%, $P = 0.02$). This was due to reduction in the 15-year cumulative mortality of death due to subsequent neoplasm (2.1–0.5%, $P = 0.02$) and pulmonary causes (0.5–0.2%, $P = 0.02$). During this time period, prevalence of RT exposure for treatment of astrocytoma was reduced from 55% of survivors in the 1970s to just 24% in the 1990s. Thus, it appears that efforts to reduce RT exposure in this population may now be extending the life span of survivors of astrocytoma (Armstrong GT et al. 2016). Given this finding, it becomes all the more essential to also improve the health span of these survivors so that those experiencing longer survival will be accompanied by good health status and high quality of life.

15.3 Subsequent Neoplasms

Development of subsequent neoplasms (SN) is an established late effect of childhood cancer therapy for which, unfortunately, the risk increases with time from diagnosis (Li et al. 1975; Neglia et al. 2001; Mike et al. 1982; Jenkinson et al. 2004; Cardous-Ubbink et al. 2007; Friedman et al. 2010). In addition, those who survive a first subsequent neoplasm remain at significant risk for multiple subsequent neoplasms (Armstrong et al. 2011b). Despite the large number of reports of subsequent malignancies from cohorts worldwide, fewer have explicitly focused on subsequent neoplasms specifically following a primary CNS tumor (Armstrong et al. 2009a; Broniscer et al. 2004; Duffner et al. 1998; Peterson et al. 2006; Devarahally et al. 2003; Stavrou et al. 2001; Hader et al. 2003; Tsui et al. 2015). Among 1877 survivors of CNS malignancies within the CCSS cohort, there were 76 subsequent malignant neoplasms (SMNs, self-reported, with histopathologic confirmation), occurring at a median of 16 years from diagnosis. This represents a fourfold increase over the general population (standardized incidence ratio [SIR] 4.1, 95% CI 3.2–4.2) (Armstrong et al. 2009a). Subsequent malignancies occurring in the CNS were most common (20 observed, SIR 25.3, 95% CI 15.5–39.1), followed by thyroid cancer (12 observed, SIR 11.2, 95% CI 5.8–19.6), soft tissue sarcomas (8 observed, SIR 8.4, 95% CI 3.6–16.5), and bone tumors (5 observed, SIR 15.1 95% CI 4.5–35.2). Notably, however, the most common subsequent cancers observed among survivors of CNS tumors were tumors for which SIRs cannot be easily estimated (due to lack of an available comparable rate in the general population): nonmelanoma skin cancers ($n = 112$, cumulative incidence 2.9% at 25 years) and benign meningiomas ($n = 59$, cumulative incidence 3.3% at 25 years). Notably, there has been no evidence for an increased risk for breast cancer among survivors who received craniospinal irradiaton (CSI) Moskowitz et al. (2015).

At 25 years from diagnosis of a primary CNS tumor, the cumulative incidence of all subsequent neoplasms is 10.7% (95% CI 8.8–12.6, Fig. 15.2a). Of concern, the incidence of meningiomas increases sharply with time such that even among patients who are meningioma-free at 25 years, the 30-year cumulative incidence is 3.5% (95% CI 0.9–6.1, Fig. 15.2b). This increased rate over time clarifies the need for long-term follow-up of these patients and raises suspicion that screening neuroimaging modalities should be employed well beyond the immediate post-diagnosis period (Bowers et al. 2013).

Radiation exposure has long been associated with an increased risk for subsequent neoplasms within the CNS. The association was first observed in children treated with low-dose cranial irradiation (mean 1.5 Gy) for tinea capitis (Ron et al. 1988). More recently, children with

computed tomography-based exposures were found to have increased risk for CNS tumors (Pearce et al. 2012). Likewise, the CCSS identified that survivors of CNS malignancies who received CNS-directed radiation >50 Gy had a cumulative incidence of a subsequent CNS neoplasm of 7.1% (95% CI 4.5–9.6) at 25 years compared to 1.0% (95% CI 0.0–2.3) among those who received no CNS radiation (Fig. 15.2c) (Armstrong et al. 2009a). Subsequent neoplasms that arise in the CNS in the first decade after RT exposure are most commonly high-grade gliomas, which have an extremely poor prognosis (5-year survival range 0–19.5%). Beyond that window, meningiomas (5-year survival range 69–100%) become more prevalent (Bowers et al. 2013). To further investigate the dose effect of RT on the development of subsequent CNS tumors, investigators used a nested case–control method

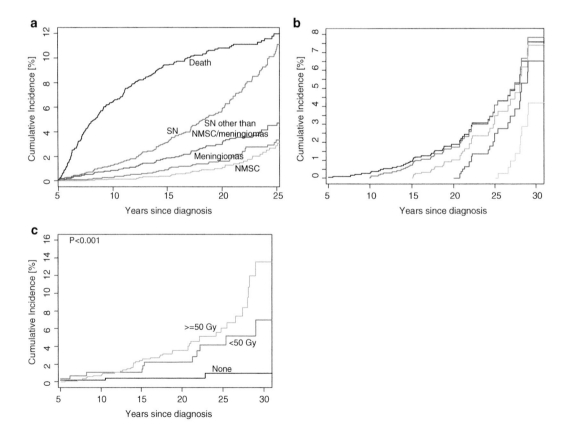

Fig. 15.2 (**a**) Cumulative incidence of subsequent neoplasms with death as competing risk. (**b**) Cumulative incidence of detected meningioma conditioned on menin-gioma-free survival at 5, 10, 15, 20 and 25 year survival. (**c**) Cumulative incidence of CNS second neoplasms by cranial RT dose

to match 116 individuals identified with a subsequent CNS neoplasm (from the entire CCSS cohort) with control subjects matched on age, sex, and time since original cancer diagnosis (Neglia et al. 2006). RT exposure was associated with an increased risk for any subsequent CNS malignant neoplasm, and specifically for subsequent gliomas (odds ratio [OR] = 6.78, 95% CI = 1.54–29.7) and meningiomas (OR = 9.94, 95% CI = 2.17–45.6). Importantly, linear dose–response relationships between RT dose and the development of both gliomas and meningiomas were identified and were statistically significant (Fig. 15.3). The excess relative risk per Gy, equal to the dose of the linear response function, was 0.33 (95% CI = 0.07–1.71) per Gy for gliomas, and 1.06 (95% CI = 0.21–8.15) per Gy for meningiomas. After adjustment of radiation dose, there were no statistically significant associations between chemotherapy exposure and the development of a CNS subsequent neoplasm (Neglia et al. 2006).

In the modern era of multimodal therapy, many survivors of CNS tumors have also received chemotherapy. With the well-established associations between alkylating agents, epipodophyllotoxins, and therapy-related acute myelogenous leukemia (t-AML), it is not surprising that increased rates of AML are present in CNS tumor survivors SIR 8.0, 95% CI 0.9–29.1 in CCSS (Armstrong et al. 2009a), and SIR 31.8, 95% CI 10.2–74.1 in a population of survivors from St. Jude Children's Research Hospital (Tsui et al. 2015). However, use of chemotherapy has often provided the opportunity for reduction of RT dose in standard risk populations, such as those with medulloblastoma; use of reduced RT plus chemotherapy has replaced use of cranospinal RT alone in these patients. A recent study by Tsui et al. (2015) observed no evidence for an increase in incidence of SNs in medulloblastoma/primitive neuroectodermal tumor (PNET) survivors treated with multimodal therapy compared to RT alone at 20 years from diagnosis (12% vs. 11.3%

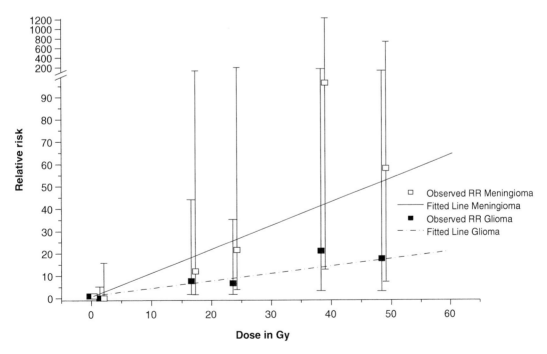

Fig. 15.3 Relative risk of subsequent glioma and meningioma within the Childhood Cancer Survivor Study cohort by radiation dose (open boxes, mean observed relative risk for meningioma; closed boxes, mean observed relative risk for glioma; solid line, fitted line for meningioma risk; hatched line, fitted line for glioma risk). $P < 0.001$ (likelihood ratio test, two-sided)

at 20 years), though the pattern of subsequent neoplasm appeared to differ. Furthermore, multivariable analysis of 2779 children with any type of CNS tumor identified no increase in risk for SNs among survivors who received multimodal therapy compared to those treated with RT but no chemotherapy (Tsui et al. 2015). This is important because previous studies have raised concern for an increased risk of SNs with multimodal therapy (Packer et al. 2013).

Because of the increased risk for subsequent cancers, the Children's Oncology Group has provided cancer surveillance recommendations for survivors of childhood cancer (Children's OG 2013). Specific recommendations for survivors exposed to CNS-directed radiotherapy are provided in Table 15.1. Given the paucity of evidence for the efficacy and cost-effectiveness of these recommendations, it remains unknown whether following such guidelines leads to improved outcomes; thus, future investigations to evaluate the efficacy of these guidelines should be a high priority.

15.4 Long-Term Endocrine Complications

Endocrine sequelae of cancer and cancer therapy are known to affect more than 50% of long-term survivors of childhood cancer (Chemaitilly and Sklar 2010; Mostoufi-Moab et al. 2016). Individuals with CNS tumors and those whose hypothalamus and/or pituitary regions (Fig. 15.4) were exposed to surgery or radiation are at particularly high risk for hypothalamic/pituitary dysfunction (Chemaitilly et al. 2015; Sklar and Constine 1995). Similarly, direct and indirect radiation exposures are known risk factors of primary thyroid and gonadal sequelae (Barnes and Chemaitilly 2014). High-dose chemotherapy regimens, such as those incorporating alkylating agents, are also known to cause gonadal damage (Barnes and Chemaitilly 2014). Finally, hormonal dysfunctions in childhood CNS tumor survivors can impact bone health and metabolism and hence potentially have lasting repercussions

on traditional cardiovascular risk factors and ultimately quality of life. The early recognition and expeditious treatment of endocrine disorders may reduce morbidity and improve overall state of health of this vulnerable group of individuals (Diller et al. 2009).

15.4.1 Hypothalamic/Pituitary Dysfunction

Hypothalamic/pituitary dysfunction may precede or appear acutely at the time of diagnosis of a CNS tumor or following surgical resection. In this context, hypothalamic/pituitary dysfunction is generally clinically evident and involves multiple hormonal systems from the outset. In contrast, radiation-induced hypothalamic/pituitary dysfunction often appears several years after the completion of therapy and rarely combines multiple hypothalamic/pituitary axes simultaneously from the outset, as the dose thresholds vary for the different anterior pituitary hormones. The pathophysiology of radiation-induced hypothalamic/pituitary deficits is not well understood. The nature (direct neuronal injury vs. neurovascular damage) and site (hypothalamic vs. pituitary) of the insult are not known with certainty (Chieng et al. 1991). The hypothalamus may have a higher degree of sensitivity to radiation compared to the pituitary (Schriock et al. 1984; Constine et al. 1993). Evidence supporting a hypothalamic origin for radiation-induced anterior pituitary hormone deficits includes the observation of hyperprolactinemia, attributed to the disruption of dopaminergic pathways within the hypothalamus, following radiation doses >50 Gy (Constine et al. 1993) and a preservation of growth hormone (GH) response to exogenous GH releasing hormone (GHRH) administration in certain individuals treated with radiotherapy (Schriock et al. 1984).

15.4.1.1 Growth Hormone Deficiency
Growth hormone deficiency (GHD) is the most common late effect after cranial RT and often only anterior pituitary deficiency is observed. In

Table 15.1 Children's Oncology Group surveillance recommendations for pediatric CNS tumor survivors at high risk of specific subsequent neoplasms

Subsequent neoplasm	High risk cancer treatment features	Surveillance recommendations	Comment
Brain tumor (benign or malignant)	High radiation dose (linear dose–response relationship), younger age at treatment, neurofibromatosis	History and physical exam yearly for new onset seizure, cognitive, motor or sensory neurologic symptoms, headache, vomiting	Brain MRI as clinically indicated for symptomatic patients
Colorectal cancer	Treatment with radiation ≥30 Gy potentially exposing colon/rectum with both dose and volume of bowel influencing risk	Colonoscopy every 5 years beginning 10 years after radiation or at age 35, whichever occurs last with frequency of surveillance informed by results (minimum every 5 years)	Due to lower prevalence of colorectal carcinoma and more limited information about it natural history in irradiated survivors, surveillance recommendation are linked to high-dose radiation exposure. Shared decision-making is advised regarding screening of individuals with radiation doses below 30 Gy until more definitive data is available
Oral cancer	Head/brain radiation, neck radiation, total body irradiation, acute/chronic graft vs. host disease	Yearly oral cavity exam	Head and neck and otolaryngology consultation as needed
Skin cancer	Any radiation treatment	Assessment of health risking and protective sun exposure behaviors. Skin examination yearly with particular attention to skin lesions and pigmented nevi in previous radiation treatment fields	Multiple occurrences of nonmelanoma skin cancers are commonly reported among childhood cancer survivors among survivors treated with radiation therapy. Clinicians should be aware that the occurrence of a nonmelanoma skin cancer as a first subsequent neoplasm appears to identify a population at subsequent risk for invasive subsequent neoplasms
Thyroid cancer	Thyroid gland in radiation field, risk increased up to 30 Gy with decreased risk above 30 Gy, >5 years after irradiation, total boy irradiation	Yearly thyroid exam	Ultrasound and fine needle aspiration for evaluation of palpable nodules. Surgical consultation for resection. Nuclear medicine consultation for ablation of residual disease. Endocrine consultation for postoperative medical management

a recent study of 748 adult survivors (mean age 34.2 years) of childhood cancer treated with cranial RT and followed for a mean 27.3 years, the prevalence of GHD was 46.5% (95% CI 42.9–50.2%) (Chemaitilly et al. 2015). This cohort included a majority of patients treated with cranial RT for acute lymphoblastic leukemia (ALL), most of whom were exposed to cranial RT at much lower doses (18 Gy) for CNS pro-phylaxis than those used for the treatment of CNS malignancies. The prevalence of GHD is even higher in cohorts of CNS tumor survivors. In a study of 88 survivors of childhood medullo-blastoma and embryonal tumors treated with CSI at 23.4–39.6 Gy, posterior fossa cranial RT dose of 55.8 Gy, and high-dose myeloablative chemo-therapy followed by autologous stem cell rescue, the cumulative incidence of GHD was 93 ± 4% at

4 years from diagnosis (Fig. 15.5) (Laughton et al. 2008). In a prospectively assessed cohort of 192 patients treated with conformal radiotherapy for localized primary brain tumors, GH secretion was shown to decrease in both a time- and dose-

dependent fashion, allowing the establishment of risk prediction models for GHD based on these two parameters (Fig. 15.6) (Merchant et al. 2011). In this study, a cumulative dose of 16.1 Gy to the hypothalamus was associated with a 50% risk of GHD after 5 years of follow-up. The risk of GHD is, indeed, known to increase at higher doses of radiation and with longer durations of follow-up (Merchant et al. 2011; Clayton and Shalet 1991a). Another risk factor for radiation-induced GHD is young age at exposure to radiotherapy, which has been suggested to have a significant role by some, but not all, investigators (Schmiegelow et al. 2000; Brauner et al. 1986).

The diagnosis of GHD in survivors of childhood CNS tumors is made using the same criteria as in the general population (Barnes and Chemaitilly 2014). However, in addition to GHD, multiple endocrine and non-endocrine factors could affect linear growth and need to be identified for diagnostic and prognostic considerations. Spinal radiotherapy affects growth by direct damage to the vertebral growth plates. As such, spinal growth is more severely affected than that of the limbs, causing survivors to have a relatively short truncus compared to the rest of their body (Shalet et al. 1987; Brauner et al. 1993;

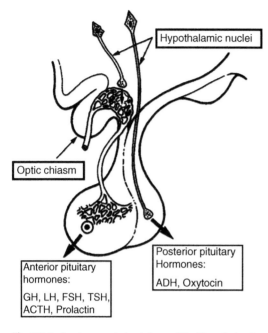

Fig. 15.4 Anatomy and physiology of the Hypothalamic-Pituitary system

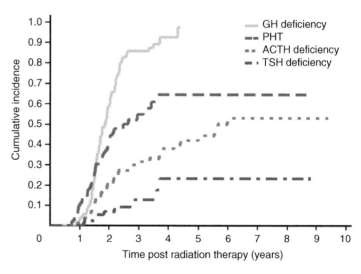

Fig. 15.5 Cumulative incidence of specific endocrine deficits following radiation therapy. *GH* growth hormone, *PHT* primary hypothyroidism, *ACTH* adrenocorticotropic hormone, *TSH* thyroid-stimulating hormone

No. at risk

GH deficiency	70	68	29	9	4				
PHT	87	78	40	16	8	4	3	2	2
ACTH deficiency	76	74	58	47	34	22	13	9	5	1
TSH deficiency	87	83	48	24	12	4	2	1	1

Fig. 15.6 Growth hormone secretion after irradiation of the hypothalamus/pituitary. Reproduced with permission from Merchant et al. (2011). ©2011 by American Society of Clinical Oncology

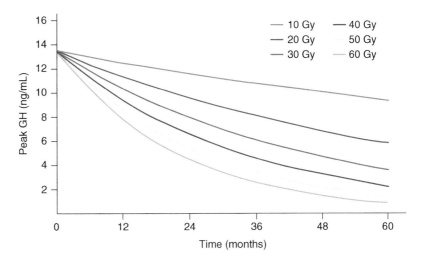

Thomas et al. 1993; Clayton and Shalet 1991b). This type of skeletal dysplasia can be unmasked by measuring the patient's sitting height and comparing it to the standing height using age- and sex-adjusted growth charts with values expressed in standard deviations (SD). A standing height (SD) out of proportion to the sitting height (SD) is generally suggestive of this type of skeletal dysplasia, although other factors such as scoliosis could also contribute to this discrepancy. Obesity (Iwayama et al. 2011) and disorders of puberty are additional factors that can affect both GH secretion and linear growth. Patients with GHD who are concomitantly experiencing central precocious puberty (CPP), a fairly common disorder in patients with hypothalamic or optic pathways tumors and those treated with cranial RT, may experience misleadingly "normal" prepubertal growth rates at the expense of a rapidly advancing bone maturation (Sklar and Constine 1995). Should this association of GHD and CPP go unnoticed, patients may incur an irreversible loss in growth potential (Sklar and Constine 1995). It is therefore of the utmost importance to closely monitor the pubertal status of brain tumor survivors during childhood and adolescence (Barnes and Chemaitilly 2014).

Given the pulsatile, and mostly nocturnal, nature of GH secretion, the diagnosis of GHD relies on the measurement of a plasma GH peak

level 2–3 h after the administration of a stimulating agent ("secretagogue"). While failing two different dynamic tests is necessary for the diagnosis of GHD in the general population, failing only one test was deemed sufficient in the consensus guidelines of the GH Research Society, given the higher likelihood of dysfunction following tumor- or treatment-related insults to the hypothalamus/pituitary (Consensus guidelines for the diagnosis and treatment of growth hormone (GH) deficiency in childhood and adolescence: summary statement of the GH Research Society. GH Research Society 2000). A variety of secretagogues are used in children and adults, the "gold standard" test being the insulin tolerance test (ITT). The combination of GHRH and arginine (GHRH-Arg), which is the most widely used test in adults assessed for GHD, cannot be used in brain tumor survivors exposed to cranial RT because of the likely hypothalamic origin of this disorder in this population (Ham et al. 2005; Darzy et al. 2003). Because of the risk of hypoglycemia associated with the ITT, glucagon has been suggested as an alternative (Conceicao et al. 2003). More stable markers of GH secretion, such as plasma IGF-1 and IGF binding protein-3 (IGFBP-3) levels may not be totally reliable when used as surrogate markers for GHD in individuals with a history of treatment with cranial RT. These markers were shown to remain normal in a subset of individuals who failed GH dynamic testing and their use may result in underdiagnosing GHD (Sklar et al. 1993; Weinzimer et al. 1999).

Treatment with human recombinant GH (hGH) can improve the growth potential of children with GHD (Beckers et al. 2010; Brownstein et al. 2004; Gleeson et al. 2003; Ciaccio et al. 2010). Children treated with CSI may not completely recover the loss in their growth potential, but it is possible that their height outcomes would be even worse without replacement with hGH (Brownstein et al. 2004; Ciaccio et al. 2010; Beckers et al. 2010). Given the in vitro proliferative and pro-mitogenic properties of GH and IGF-1, the safety of hGH in individuals with a history of cancers or brain tumors has come under scrutiny (Chemaitilly and Robison 2012). Use of hGH was not associated with cancer/tumor recurrence and/or death in large-scale studies conducted in long-term survivors of childhood cancers (Swerdlow et al. 2000; Packer et al. 2001; Sklar et al. 2002). However, there are data to suggest a small increase in the risk of any secondary solid tumor, specifically in survivors of ALL who received hGH therapy (Relative Risk [RR] 4.98 (95% CI 1.95–12.74) (Sklar et al. 2002; Ergun-Longmire et al. 2006). The association between second neoplasms and hGH was not found to be significant in a study comparing 110 survivors of childhood and adult cancers treated with hGH to 110 matched non-hGH-treated controls followed for a median of 14.5 years (Mackenzie et al. 2011). In a recent report from the CCSS, individuals treated with hGH during childhood did not have a higher risk of developing second CNS neoplasms when compared to others (Patterson et al. 2014). In summary, hGH can be offered by pediatric endocrinologists to children with GHD who have been in remission (for at least 1 year per expert opinion) after completing treatment for a brain tumor (Raman et al. 2015). Clearance should be sought from the treating oncologist, neurosurgeon, and other relevant providers following the individualized and multidisciplinary assessment of tumor recurrence and complication risks measured against potential benefits of hGH and provided that patients could

be closely monitored for potential risks during therapy (Raman et al. 2015). The recommendations of the medical team and the potential risk of subsequent neoplasms and anticipated benefits of treatment with hGH need to be reviewed in detail with the patients and their families prior to obtaining their consent for this therapy (Raman et al. 2015). Over the past 15–20 years, given the potential beneficial effects on body composition, plasma lipids, bone mass, and quality of life, therapy using hGH has been extended to adults with hypopituitarism (Link et al. 2004; Bakker et al. 2007; van den Heijkant et al. 2011; Elbornsson et al. 2012, 2013). There are, however, no studies specifically assessing the benefits and long-term risks associated with hGH use in adult survivors of childhood brain tumors; this continues to be an active area of research (Chemaitilly et al. 2015; van den Heijkant et al. 2011; Mukherjee et al. 2005; Murray et al. 2002; Follin et al. 2006).

15.4.1.2 Disorders of Luteinizing Hormone (LH) and Follicle Stimulating Hormone (FSH)

Central Precocious Puberty
Central precocious puberty (CPP) is the onset of puberty prior to the ages of 8 years in girls and 9 years in boys as a result of the early activation of the hypothalamic/pituitary-gonadal axis (Chemaitilly et al. 2001). CPP results in decreased adult height due to accelerated and premature closure of the skeletal growth plates. Poor psychosocial adjustment is associated with the early appearance of secondary sexual characteristics, especially menarche, and more so in survivors of childhood brain tumors with special needs (Chemaitilly et al. 2001). The exact prevalence of CPP among childhood brain tumor survivors is yet to be described. In a report from the CCSS, 14.5% of females exposed to cranial RT experienced menarche before the age of 10 years, which could be an indirect marker of CPP in this population (Armstrong et al. 2009c). Tumors in proximity to the hypothalamus and optic pathways, such as low-grade gliomas with or without neurofibromatosis type 1 (NF-1), and hypotha-

lamic cranial RT exposure are associated with an increased risk of CPP (Armstrong et al. 2009c; Oberfield et al. 1996). Additional risk factors include hydrocephalus, female sex, cranial RT before the age of 5 years, and increased BMI (Oberfield et al. 1996; Armstrong et al. 2009c).

The diagnosis of CPP relies on the identification of early and sustained pubertal development (Chemaitilly and Sklar 2010). In girls, the diagnosis is based on the presence of breast development. In boys treated with gonadotoxic treatments such as high-dose alkylating agents or direct testicular radiotherapy, clinicians should not rely on the measurement of testicular volume for the diagnosis of puberty because treatment-related germ cell injury can impair testicular growth without necessarily affecting the ability to produce testosterone. Other markers such as pubarche, scrotal thinning, and penile size can be useful. Laboratory markers of CPP include pubertal basal levels of LH and sex steroids (estradiol or testosterone). Basal, non-stimulated and random values may be inconclusive because of the pulsatile and circadian nature of gonadotropin secretion during the early stages of puberty. Gonadotropin Releasing Hormone agonists (GnRHa) are used in dynamic testing for the diagnosis of CPP (Carel et al. 2009). The impact of CPP on skeletal maturation and linear growth can be assessed using chronological age comparison standards for the X-ray of the left hand ("Bone Age") (Bayley and Pinneau 1952). Uterine length and ovarian volume measurements may also be helpful for establishing the diagnosis of CPP (de Vries et al. 2006).

Pubertal suppression using GnRHa can delay skeletal maturation and allow more time for skeletal growth (Carel et al. 2009). Patients with GHD in addition to CPP should also receive treatment with hGH (Gleeson et al. 2003). The duration of pubertal suppression depends on a variety of factors, including chronological age, bone age, mid-parental height, and psychosocial factors (Barnes and Chemaitilly 2014). Alternative approaches aimed at delaying skeletal maturation, such as the use of aromatase inhibitors, are of no proven benefit and remain experimental (Stephen et al. 2011).

LH/FSH Deficiency

Luteinizing hormone/follicle stimulating hormone deficiency (LH/FSHD), also known as hypogonadotropic hypogonadism, results in the decline or cessation of gonadal sex hormone production. The prevalence of LH/FSHD varies between 5 and 10% in long-term survivors who have been treated with cranial RT (Chemaitilly et al. 2015). It is the most common anterior pituitary deficiency after GHD in patients treated with cranial RT; it appears most commonly following radiation doses $\geq$30 Gy (Chemaitilly et al. 2015; Sklar and Constine 1995; Constine et al. 1993) and may possibly occur more frequently in males and Caucasians when compared to females and other races, respectively (Chemaitilly et al. 2015). The clinical manifestations of LH/FSHD vary depending on the age and pubertal stage at which the deficiency occurs. It can result in delayed (absence of pubertal signs after the ages of 12 and 13 years in girls and boys, respectively) or arrested pubertal development during childhood and in androgen insufficiency symptoms (decreased libido, fatigue, depression) in postpubertal males and secondary amenorrhea in postpubertal females (Barnes and Chemaitilly 2014). The treatment of the endocrine component of the gonadal failure secondary to LH/FSHD relies on sex hormone replacement therapy adjusted to pubertal stage. In postpubertal males and females, the stimulation of germ cells and follicular growth, respectively, when deemed appropriate, requires referral to reproductive medicine specialists (Kenney et al. 2012; Metzger et al. 2013).

15.4.1.3 Thyroid Stimulating Hormone (TSH) Deficiency (TSHD)

Deficiency in TSH, also known as central hypothyroidism, causes a decline of thyroid hormone production because of insufficient stimulation by the hypothalamus/pituitary. The prevalence of TSHD was estimated at 3.4–7.5% in large cohorts of childhood cancer and brain tumor survivors (Livesey and Brook 1989; Schmiegelow et al. 2003). The 4-year cumulative incidence of TSHD reached 28 ± 8% in childhood embryonal tumor survivors treated under a protocol combining

CSI, additional cranial RT to the posterior fossa and high-dose myeloablative chemotherapy followed by autologous stem cell rescue (Fig. 15.5) (Laughton et al. 2008). The main risk factor associated with TSHD is exposure to doses of cranial RT $\geq$ 30 Gy (Chemaitilly et al. 2015; Rose et al. 1999). Caucasians may also have a higher risk when compared to other races (Chemaitilly et al. 2015). The symptoms of TSHD are identical to those of primary hypothyroidism and include, in children, decreased stamina, decreased growth velocity, excessive weight gain, and delayed skeletal maturation. Other symptoms of hypothyroidism are constipation, cold intolerance, and depression. A plasma free T4 (FT4) below normal, coinciding with a low or "inappropriately" normal plasma TSH, is characteristic of TSHD (Barnes and Chemaitilly 2014). Replacement therapy with levothyroxine is the mainstay of the treatment of TSHD; doses should be adjusted to maintain FT4 values within mid to high normal ranges. In patients with TSHD, plasma TSH values are not helpful in monitoring the treatment of patients as they are expected to remain low, regardless of whether the doses of treatment are adequate or not (Barnes and Chemaitilly 2014).

15.4.1.4 Adrenocorticotropic Hormone (ACTH) Deficiency (ACTHD)

Deficiency in ACTH, also known as central adrenal insufficiency, causes insufficient glucocorticoid (cortisol) secretion by the adrenal glands due to inadequate stimulation by the hypothalamus/pituitary. Production of mineralocorticoid (aldosterone), which regulates electrolyte balance, is less commonly affected as it is largely controlled by the kidneys via the renin-angiotensin-aldosterone system. Estimates of the prevalence of ACTHD in survivors of childhood cancers and brain tumors have varied between 4 and 43% due to differences in the studied populations and testing modalities (Chemaitilly et al. 2015; Laughton et al. 2008; Rose et al. 2005). In the study of children with embryonal brain tumors treated with CSI, additional cranial RT to the posterior fossa and high-

dose myeloablative chemotherapy followed by stem cell rescue, the 4-year cumulative incidence of ACTHD was 38 ± 6% (Fig. 15.5) (Laughton et al. 2008). Symptoms of ACTHD include fatigue, weakness, decreased appetite, nausea, emesis, frequent illnesses, and vulnerability to infections. When exposed to a severe illness, patients with ACTHD may experience rapid clinical deterioration with hypoglycemia, seizures, and hypotensive shock if they are not treated with higher "stress" doses of intravenous or intramuscular glucocorticoids expeditiously. The diagnosis of ACTHD must be suspected in patients with 8 AM plasma cortisol levels <10 µg/dL. The confirmatory test most commonly used is the low-dose ACTH dynamic test. A peak cortisol value <16 µg/dL following the administration of 1 µg of ACTH is generally considered diagnostic of ACTHD (Chrousos et al. 2009). Patients with ACTHD should be treated with maintenance doses of hydrocortisone, generally close to 10 mg/m^2 per day given three times daily. The doses should be adjusted to respond to illness and patients should be treated with high doses of intravenous or intramuscular hydrocortisone in situations of severe illness or in preparation for significant medical procedures, such as those requiring sedation and/or general anesthesia (Chemaitilly and Sklar 2010). Patients and families should receive education on how to respond to moderate to severe illness by using higher doses of hydrocortisone ("stress dose teaching") orally or intramuscularly (in situations of emesis and severe diarrhea) until they can receive further medical advice. Patients should be instructed to carry some form of documentation that they have a diagnosis of adrenal insufficiency at all times (via cards, bracelets, etc.) in case they are found unconscious in the absence of their usual caregivers (Barnes and Chemaitilly 2014).

15.4.1.5 Hyperprolactinemia

Hyperprolactinemia can occur following disruptions of hypothalamic/pituitary connections because of the loss of hypothalamic inhibition on prolactin secretion (Constine et al. 1993). Tumor growth, surgical resections, and doses of radiotherapy >30–50 Gy can cause such disruptions and be associated with increased prolactin levels. Symptoms of hyperprolactinemia include galactorrhea and decreased sex hormone production (Barnes and Chemaitilly 2014). However, in childhood CNS tumor survivors, it tends to be asymptomatic and rarely warrants treatment given the high risks of concomitant LH/FSHD and gonadal dysfunction in this population.

15.4.1.6   Central Diabetes Insipidus

Central diabetes insipidus is defined by the inability to retain free water, with ensuing polyuria and polydipsia because of a deficit in the secretion and release of the antidiuretic hormone (ADH) by the hypothalamus and the posterior pituitary, respectively. Central diabetes insipidus is generally the consequence of an anatomical insult to the hypothalamus and/or pituitary and is not associated with cranial RT. It is usually present at the time of tumor diagnosis and/or surgical resection (Ramelli et al. 1998). However, central diabetes insipidus is frequently permanent, and is often among the more challenging endocrine dysfunctions in a large subset of brain tumor survivors (Barnes and Chemaitilly 2014). Certain tumors, such as germ cell tumors or hypophyseal non-Hodgkin lymphomas, can be revealed by diabetes insipidus (Ramelli et al. 1998; Silfen et al. 2001). This deficiency is, however, more commonly described in the context of panhypopituitarism accompanying sellar/supra-sellar tumors and/or the surgical resection required to remove them. Central diabetes insipidus is treated using desmopressin; replacement doses are adjusted by taking into account the patient's ability to sense thirst (which could be impaired due to hypothalamic injury), fluid intake, urine output and changes in body weight in order to maintain adequate hydration and avoid hyponatremia and seizures related to overtreatment (Di Iorgi et al. 2012; Mishra and Chandrashekhar 2011). The management of patients with altered thirst sensation usually requires the determination of a fixed daily fluid intake in addition to a fixed dose of desmopressin (Mishra and Chandrashekhar 2011).

15.4.2 Thyroid Disorders

Thyroid dysfunction is common following direct or indirect radiation exposures of the gland. In CNS tumor survivors, such exposures include scatter radiation from whole brain RT and CSI. Patients exposed to these treatments may develop primary hypothyroidism and thyroid cancer.

15.4.2.1   Hypothyroidism

The prevalence of primary hypothyroidism ranges between 41 and 51% among patients treated with CSI (Laughton et al. 2008; Livesey and Brook 1989; Schmiegelow et al. 2003). In a cohort of patients with medulloblastoma, the cumulative prevalence for this disorder reached 65 ± 7% by 4 years from diagnosis (Fig. 15.5) (Laughton et al. 2008). Significant associations with cranial RT alone were described by some, but not all, authors (Livesey and Brook 1989; Schmiegelow et al. 2003). A potentiating effect of chemotherapy along with CSI has been reported but not established (Schmiegelow et al. 2000; Livesey and Brook 1989; Ogilvy-Stuart et al. 1991). The majority of the cases reported in these studies had subclinical forms of primary hypothyroidism, in which thyroid hormone levels are normal but TSH levels are elevated (Barnes and Chemaitilly 2014). The reported prevalence of decompensated forms (i.e., patients with abnormally low FT4 and increased TSH levels) is much lower at 5.6–7.9% (Livesey and Brook 1989; Schmiegelow et al. 2003). Primary hypothyroidism may still occur decades after the exposure to radiation and patients at risk should have lifelong follow-up with yearly measurement of TSH and FT4 levels (Chemaitilly and Sklar 2010). The clinical symptoms are similar to those observed in patients with TSHD (see Sect. 17.4.1.3). The mainstay of replacement therapy is levothyroxine at doses maintaining plasma FT4 levels between the middle and the upper limit of the normal range while keeping plasma TSH levels within the normal range (in contrast to TSHD).

15.4.2.2 Thyroid Cancer

Thyroid cancer was the second most common subsequent neoplasm observed in a report on 455 survivors of childhood medulloblastoma followed for a mean 16 years; a mean latency period of 24.8 years was noted for thyroid cancer in this population (Ning et al. 2015). While this report does not specifically comment on the risk factors associated with thyroid cancer, it is likely related to exposure to CSI at a young age, given the established linear-exponential dose–response association relationship with RT exposure where risk increases linearly up to 30 Gy and doses >30 Gy actually provide decreased risk, consistent with a cell killing effect (Bhatti et al. 2010). The most common presentation for thyroid cancer is the presence of a palpable nodule or a cervical lymph node. The currently recommended screening modality in survivors deemed at risk of thyroid neoplasia by the Children's Oncology Group is yearly examination of the neck by an experienced provider, although significant controversy surrounds this subject with others suggesting the use of ultrasound (Li et al. 2014). The diagnosis is confirmed by a positive result on a fine needle aspiration biopsy of a suspected nodule; the treatment approach and prognosis are identical to thyroid cancer cases diagnosed in the general population (Acharya et al. 2003).

15.4.3 Disorders of the Gonads

Male survivors of childhood CNS tumors may experience primary testicular dysfunction because of the risk associated with alkylating agent chemotherapy regimens as well as scatter radiation exposure from CSI (Gleeson and Shalet 2004). The testes have two functional compartments with different susceptibilities to cancer treatments. The endocrine compartment, responsible for testosterone production, includes the Leydig cells. The reproductive compartment, responsible for sperm production, includes the germ cells and the Sertoli cells.

Testosterone production is impaired by the use of very high doses of alkylating agents, as demonstrated in other, non-CNS tumor survivor populations (Ridola et al. 2009; Bakker et al. 2004). Scatter radiation from CSI, however, has been shown not to significantly impact Leydig cell function (Schmiegelow et al. 2001; Ahmed et al. 1983). The clinical signs of low testosterone production are similar to those described in male patients with LH/FSHD. The laboratory diagnosis of Leydig cell failure relies on the measurement of a low AM plasma level of testosterone (normative ranges vary with age and depending on the assay) coinciding with an elevated plasma LH level (Barnes and Chemaitilly 2014). Treatment relies on replacement therapy using exogenous testosterone as described in patients with LH/FSHD (see Sect. 17.4.1.2).

In contrast to the testosterone-producing function, spermatogenesis may be affected by both chemotherapy and CSI regimens used to treat CNS tumors (Schmiegelow et al. 2001; Ahmed et al. 1983). The clinical examination of patients with primary germ cell failure may be remarkable for a small testicular volume, and laboratory testing may show increased plasma FSH and low inhibin B values (Schmiegelow et al. 2001). Nevertheless, the diagnosis of germ cell failure and/or abnormal spermatogenesis requires a semen analysis given the limited reliability of laboratory markers (Lopez Andreu et al. 2000). Patients who are capable of producing a semen sample should be offered the option of sperm banking prior to their exposure to potentially gonadotoxic treatments (Chemaitilly and Sklar 2010).

Endocrine and reproductive functions are closely interdependent in the ovarian follicle and the functional dichotomy (distinct endocrine and reproductive compartments) observed in the testes is not replicated in the ovaries. The ovaries have been shown to potentially incur damage from scatter radiation related to CSI (Livesey and Brook 1988) and from chemotherapy (Ahmed et al. 1983) in survivors of childhood brain tumors. In a report on 31 patients diagnosed with medulloblastoma during childhood, the prevalence of ovarian failure at a median age of 16.6 years was 25.8% (Balachandar et al. 2014). In this study, the main risk factor associated with ovarian failure was high-dose chemotherapy followed by autologous stem cell rescue; up to 60% of patients who received this treatment modality experienced ovarian failure, despite not being exposed to CSI. A higher percentage of patients treated with CSI at ≥35 Gy vs. ≤24 Gy experienced ovarian failure (22.2% vs. 5.9%) but this did not reach statistical significance, given the small number of patients in each group (Balachandar et al. 2014). These numbers likely underestimate the risk of ovarian failure in this population, as patients may still experience premature menopause during the course of their follow-up (Sklar et al. 2006). As with LH/FSHD (see Sect. 17.4.1.2) patients with primary ovarian failure may present with delayed or interrupted pubertal development or with primary or secondary amenorrhea in postpubertal females. Laboratory values combine low plasma estradiol and elevated FSH levels (Chemaitilly and Sklar 2010). Sex hormone replacement therapy is warranted in females with ovarian failure who would otherwise be at risk of poor bone mineral density, increased cardiovascular morbidity, and poor quality of life (Metzger et al. 2013). Mature oocyte cryopreservation may represent a viable option for young pubertal females prior to gonadotoxic therapies (Barnes and Chemaitilly 2014).

15.4.4 Abnormal Body Composition

15.4.4.1 Decreased Bone Mineral Density (BMD)

Survivors of childhood CNS tumors are susceptible to developing decreased BMD (Gurney et al. 2003a; Cohen et al. 2012). In a report compiling data on 1607 childhood brain tumor survivors and 3418 randomly selected sibling controls enrolled in the CCSS, the risk of low BMD was significantly higher in survivors vs. controls (RR = 24.7; 95% CI 9.9–61.4) (Gurney et al. 2003a). Several factors may contribute to this risk, including treatment toxicities, untreated hormonal deficiencies (GH, sex steroids), and rather sedentary lifestyles (Chemaitilly et al. 2015; Cohen et al. 2012). Optimizing bone health in this population requires adequate screening

and replacement of hormonal deficiencies, including vitamin D (Sala and Barr 2007). Patients should also engage in a healthy and active lifestyle, receive adequate amounts of calcium through diet, and refrain from smoking (Sala and Barr 2007).

15.4.4.2 Overweight and Obesity

The prevalence of obesity and overweight in the overall population of childhood CNS tumor survivors was reported as comparable to that observed in the general population in large cohort studies (Gurney et al. 2003b). However, patients with sellar/suprasellar tumors and those with hypothalamic injury do experience obesity at much higher rates and with higher degrees of severity (Lustig et al. 2003b; Muller 2014). The prevalence of severe obesity in patients with craniopharyngioma was reported at 55%, despite the adequate and complete substitution of all hormonal deficiencies (Muller 2014). These patients may experience "hypothalamic" or "central" obesity, which is characterized by hyperphagia and rapid weight gain (Lustig et al. 2003b). This phenomenon may be caused by increased parasympathetic tone and ensuing hyperinsulinemia (Lustig et al. 2003a). Treatment approaches for this particular type of obesity have included octreotide and dextroamphetamine (Lustig et al. 2003a; Mason et al. 2002). Octreotide allowed the stabilization of BMI over a period of 6 months in a randomized, double-blind placebo controlled study of 18 individuals with hypothalamic obesity (Lustig et al. 2003a). The use of dextroamphetamine allowed the stabilization of BMI over a period of 24 months in five children with hypothalamic obesity (Mason et al. 2002). The small number of patients in these studies and the cost and possible side effects of the treatments used, in addition to the limited data supporting long-term safety and efficacy, have limited the wider adoption of these treatment strategies.

Endocrine late effects are among the most commonly observed sequelae in survivors of childhood brain tumors. Endocrine complications may be present at the time of presentation in a child diagnosed with a brain tumor, and they may continue to appear years and decades following the initial diagnosis, throughout adulthood and middle age, potentially feeding into their increased risks of adverse long-term health outcomes. The importance of the long-term follow-up of this vulnerable group of patients cannot be overemphasized (Table 15.2).

15.5 Long-Term Neurologic Complications

Depending upon tumor location and histopathological diagnosis, varying combinations of treatment, including surgical resection, chemotherapy, and RT, are utilized to maximize 5-year survival in children with brain tumors. Neurologic deficits may develop at or prior to diagnosis due to tumor involving eloquent areas of the brain, or from effect of surgical resection. However, as survivors age, neurologic complications arising from acute and/or long-term effects of radiation and chemotherapy have become increasingly apparent.

15.5.1 Cerebrovascular Disease

Numerous reports provide evidence for an increased incidence of cerebrovascular disease among survivors of childhood CNS tumors (Bowers et al. 2006; Campen et al. 2012; Mueller et al. 2013; Noje et al. 2013). Many of these studies focused on symptomatic stroke (intracranial hemorrhage or ischemic infarct) and did not assess asymptomatic vascular stenosis, infarcts, or hemorrhages, nor did they confirm stroke based on CNS imaging. As a consequence, they likely underestimate the prevalence and incidence of cerebrovascular disease in CNS tumor survivors. The CCSS has provided the largest study to date, which includes 1871 survivors of childhood CNS tumors (Bowers et al. 2006). Data was collected via a self-reported questionnaire and included sibling controls. The incidence of late occurring stroke was 267.6/100,000 person-years and relative risk for first stroke of 29.0 (95% CI 13.8–60.6) compared to siblings. A relatively smaller single institution study of 431

childhood brain tumor survivors, which included a systematic chart and imaging review, reported an even higher incidence (548/100,000 person-years) of ischemic stroke or transient ischemic attack (Campen et al. 2012).

15.5.1.1 Types of Stroke

Both intracranial hemorrhage and ischemic stroke have been reported in approximately equal proportions in long-term survivors (Noje et al. 2013). Intracranial hemorrhage may be related to radiation-induced cavernous malformations, which have been described in adult and pediatric CNS tumor survivors (Duhem et al. 2005; Di Giannatale et al. 2014; Lew et al. 2006). Minor hemorrhage in a cavernous malformation is not uncommon and only rarely requires surgical intervention (Di Giannatale et al. 2014). Hemorrhage in a cavernous malformation is generally of low pressure, is self-limited, and rarely causes life-threatening complications, although it may be a nidus for seizures or new neurologic deficit. Survivors of CNS radiation therapy may also develop small (<0.5 cm) micro hemorrhages, which may be numerous and are best visible on susceptibility-weighted or gradient echo sequences on MRI (Fig. 15.7) (Kyrnetskiy et al. 2005). These likely represent micro bleeds in telangiectatic malformations. It is not clear if these increase the risk of symptomatic ischemic stroke or hemorrhage. However, in adults with no history of cancer, presence of micro hemorrhages is known to increase the risk for ischemic stroke (Boulanger et al. 2006).

15.5.1.2 Risk Factors

Radiation exposure has consistently been associated with an increased risk for stroke (Bowers et al. 2006; Campen et al. 2012; Duhem et al. 2005). One study suggested that exposure to alkylating agents increased stroke risk as well (Bowers et al. 2006). Time from radiation exposure may also increase the risk (Yuan et al. 2014). Animal studies suggest that radiation treatment promotes atherogenesis in irradiated arteries (Stewart et al. 2006; Hoving et al. 2008). Underlying pathophysiology has not been fully elucidated, but may include oxidative stress and

Table 15.2 Endocrine complications observed in survivors of childhood central nervous system tumors

Complication	Risk factors	Clinical symptoms	Evaluation/labs	Intervention
GH deficiency	– Damage to HPA by tumor growth and/or surgical resection – Radiotherapy to HPA >18 Gy	– Growth deceleration – Short stature	– Bone age X-ray, – IGF1, GH stimulation test	GH replacement
Central precocious puberty	– Tumor growth near HPA – Radiotherapy to HPA ≥18 Gy	– Puberty <8 years (girls) or 9 years (boys)	– Bone age X ray, – LH, FSH, sex hormones – GnRH agonist stimulation test	GnRH agonist
LH/FSH deficiency	– Damage to HPA by tumor growth and/or surgical resection – Radiotherapy to HPA ≥30 Gy	– Delayed puberty – Irregular menses – Low sex hormone signs	– Bone age X ray, – LH, FSH, sex hormones	Induction of puberty/ sex hormone replacement
TSH deficiency	– Damage to HPA by tumor growth and/ or surgical resection – Radiotherapy to HPA ≥30 Gy	Hypothyroidism	– Free T4 – TSH useful for diagnosis (low) but not follow up	Levothyroxine
ACTH deficiency	– Damage to HPA by tumor growth and/or surgical resection – Radiotherapy to HPA ≥30 Gy	Adrenal insufficiency	– 8 AM cortisol – Low dose ACTH stimulation test	Hydrocortisone and stress dose teaching
Central diabetes insipidus	– Damage to HPA by tumor growth and/or surgical resection	Polyuria, polydipsia	Monitor fluid intake/urine output; electrolytes, serum/ urine osmolality	Fluid management and DDAVP
Primary hypothyroidism	Indirect neck irradiation (CSI, CRT)	Hypothyroidism	TSH, Free T4	Levothyroxine
Thyroid neoplasms	Indirect neck irradiation (CSI, CRT)	Thyroid nodule or cervical lymph node	– Yearly palpation of neck – Thyroid ultrasound, FNAB	Per etiology
Leydig cell dysfunction	High dose alkylating agents	– Delayed puberty – Low sex hormone signs	8 AM testosterone, LH, FSH	Replacement therapy
Male germ cell dysfunction	– Indirect testicular irradiation – Alkylating agents	Male infertility	– Baseline FSH, inhibin B – Adults: Semen Analysis	Prevent infertility with sperm banking
Ovarian failure	– Indirect ovarian irradiation – Alkylating agents – Higher risk at older age	– Delayed puberty – Irregular menses – Female infertility	Baseline LH, FSH, estradiol	– Replacement therapy – Prevent infertility with oocyte cryopreservation
Osteoporosis	– Glucocorticoids, methotrexate – Untreated hormone deficiencies – Nutritional/lifestyle causes	Increased fracture risk	– BMD studies – Vitamin D 25 levels	Per etiology
Obesity, overweight, metabolic syndrome	– Hypothalamic damage due to tumor expansion and/ or surgery – CRT	Abnormal weight gain, obesity and overweight	– Waist to hip ratio – Fasting: glucose, lipids, insulin, HbA1c	– Lifestyle modifications- diet, physical activity – Per etiology

GH growth hormone, *HPA* hypothalamic pituitary axis, *IGF-1* insulin-like growth factor-1, *LH* luteinizing hormone, *FSH* follicle stimulating hormone, *TSH* thyroid stimulating hormone, *ACTH* corticotropin, *DDAVP* desmopressin, *CSI* cranio-spinal radiotherapy, *CRT* cranial radiotherapy, *FNAB* ultrasound guided fine needle aspiration biopsy, *BMD* bone mineral density

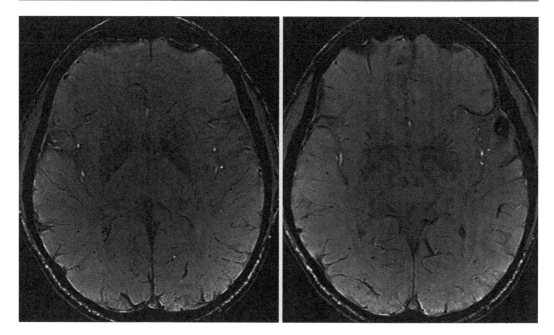

Fig. 15.7 Susceptibility-weighted images show multiple dark microhemorrhages in cortical and subcortical areas in both images. A left insular cavernoma is present in the right image

production of free radicals, endothelial cell stimulation, production of transcription factors, reduced responsiveness to nitrous oxide, and generation of inflammatory cytokines (Robbins and Zhao 2004; Halle et al. 2011; Sugihara et al. 1999; Napoli and Ignarro 2009; Hansson and Libby 2006; Krysiak et al. 2011). Radiation-induced risk for cerebrovascular disease is dose dependent with maximum risk for doses ≥50 Gy (Bowers et al. 2006; Campen et al. 2012; Mueller et al. 2013). Risk of symptomatic events may be increased if large arteries in the pre-pontine cistern or circle of Willis are irradiated (Bowers et al. 2006; Campen et al. 2012; Haddy et al. 2011). Risk of Moyamoya disease was 3.5% in a single institution cohort of 345 survivors (Ullrich et al. 2007). In addition to radiation dose, this study also found younger age at radiation treatment, a diagnosis of neurofibromatosis, and presence of optic pathway tumor as risk factors for development of vascular stenosis and Moyamoya disease.

Only a minority of survivors who are treated with cranial radiation develop clinical stroke. There are undoubtedly host factors that have not been adequately studied and identified. There may be a genetic disposition for development of intracranial vascular disease after exposure to radiation treatment. Indeed, a recent study suggested an increased tendency for development of carotid plaque when a certain haplotype was present in PON1, an anti-atherosclerotic gene (Yuan et al. 2015).

Migraine headaches, particularly those with an aura, are associated with an increased risk of ischemic stroke in non-cancer patients. Interestingly, a study of 265 pediatric patients with CNS tumors found a 19% prevalence of ischemic stroke in those with recurrent headaches compared to 3% in those without (hazard ratio 5.3, 95% CI 1.8–15.9) (Kranick et al. 2013). As survivors age, traditional cardiovascular risk factors may compound the risk for stroke. CCSS recently assessed diabetes, hypertension, smoking, and oral contraceptive use, and found a fourfold increased hazard of stroke in survivors with hypertension. This risk was even higher if hypertension coexisted with diabetes mellitus or black race (Mueller et al. 2013).

15.5.1.3 Management

There are no evidence-based guidelines for early detection or prevention of stroke. Generally, antiplatelet therapy is not recommended for asymptomatic smooth <50% narrowing of a major intracranial vessel, or asymptomatic periventricular hyperintense lesions on T2 MRI, or small periventricular lacunar infarcts. The latter represent small vessel hyalinosis likely not responsive to antiplatelet therapy. For a more severe or irregular stenosis, low dose daily or alternate day aspirin may be considered. In the presence of a severe asymptomatic stenosis antiplatelet therapy is reasonable when there is adequate collateralization seen on digital subtraction angiography. However, a surgical revascularization procedure in addition to antiplatelet therapy should be given strong consideration when there is severe or progressive vascular stenosis and inadequate cortical collateralization, or if a stenosis causes clinical stroke or TIA with inadequate cortical collateralization. Extradural arterial synangiosis is the procedure of choice and must be performed by an experienced neurosurgeon (Fig. 15.8). At least one study reported good long-term vascular outcome after this procedure (Scott et al. 2004). Finally, all conventional cerebrovascular risk factors must also be rigorously controlled. Management of cerebrovascular disease is largely empirical and further research is needed not only in acute management of stroke but also in primary and secondary prevention.

15.5.2 Seizure

Seizure as a presenting symptom of CNS tumor is less common in children compared to adults and this may reflect a dominance of posterior fossa tumors in children. Two separate studies reported 9% and 12% of childhood brain tumors presenting with seizures (Khan et al. 2005; Ibrahim and Appleton 2004). Seizure as a presenting symptom was similar (12.5%) in 280 children with low-grade brain tumors (Khan et al. 2006a). However, seizure frequency may approach 75–100% in glioneuronal tumors involving the temporal lobe (Wells et al. 2012). Overall seizure prevalence of 15–25% in children with CNS tumors is also lower compared to 30–50% in adults (Khan et al. 2005; Khan et al. 2006a; Packer et al. 2003). Most seizures develop at diagnosis or within the first few months after diagnosis of CNS tumor, but up to 6% of patients may develop late onset epilepsy after tumor diagnosis and treatment (Khan et al. 2005; Packer et al. 2003). Although a vast majority of patients with seizures have supratentorial tumors, particularly involving the cortex, seizures can develop in posterior fossa tumor as well (Khan et al. 2005). This is likely due to cortical dysfunction or injury from hydrocephalus, external ventricular drain, or a ventriculo-peritoneal shunt.

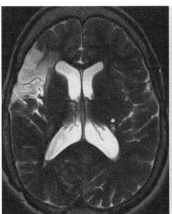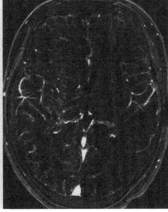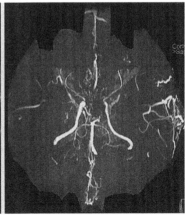

Fig. 15.8 T2-weighted image on the left shows a remote right frontal ischemic infarct and two left periventricular lacunes. T1 post contrast axial image after subtraction in the middle shows fine vascular blush in the basal ganglia area consistent with moyamoya disease. Prominent cortical circulation after extradural arterial synaniosis proce-dure can be seen bilaterally. MR angiogram in the right image shows intracranial termination of bilateral internal carotid arteries, absence of middle and posterior cerebral arteries, bilateral deep vascular blush of moyamoya, and cortical collateralization

15.5.2.1 Seizure Phenotype

The presentation of tumor-related seizures depends on the region of the brain involved. Seizure type may be simple-partial where there is no loss of awareness, or complex-partial when there is partial or complete loss of awareness, and either may progress to secondary generalization with loss of posture and tonic-clonic activity. A seizure may start as generalized tonic clonic, but a careful history will often reveal premonitory symptoms consistent with focal onset, such as head or eye deviation, speech arrest, paresthesia, or gustatory or olfactory hallucinations. Status epilepticus is uncommon but was reported in 3% in one study (Khan et al. 2005).

15.5.2.2 Pathophysiology

Underlying mechanisms of seizure generation in patients with CNS tumors is not completely understood. Pathological studies have demonstrated abnormal brain structure adjacent to tumor and in many cases frank cortical dysplasia is present (Prayson 2010). Molecular markers such as BRAF/V600, mammalian target of rapamycin (mTOR) activation, and IDH1/IDH2 mutations within the tumor have been evaluated and may be associated with higher risk of seizures (Ruda and Soffietti 2015). Improvement of intractable epilepsy with everolimus, an mTOR inhibitor, in patients with tuberous sclerosis lends support to this hypothesis (Krueger et al. 2013). Glutamate is an excitatory neurotransmitter and its release by glioma cells has been shown in preclinical models of glioma (Ruda and Soffietti 2015; Douw et al. 2013). However, the role of molecular factors contributing to seizure risk is not settled and further work is needed. Additionally, magnetic encephalogram studies have suggested altered peri-tumoral brain networks, and glioneuronal tumors may themselves have epileptogenic neurons within them (Douw et al. 2013; Douw et al. 2010).

15.5.2.3 Treatment

Prophylactic use of anti-seizure medications prior to development of seizures is not warranted in patients with CNS tumors, and anti-seizure drugs may be discontinued a week after the craniotomy if initiated in the absence of seizure. This was the position statement of the American Academy of Neurology steering committee on the subject after reviewing five randomized trials (Glantz et al. 2000). Because a second seizure may develop in up to 64–89% of children with CNS tumor after experiencing their first seizure (Khan et al. 2005; Khan et al. 2006a), most neuro-oncologists will start an anti-seizure medication after the first unequivocal seizure. Principles of seizure management are similar to those in non-cancer patients (i.e., use of single agent if possible, use of minimum dose needed, choice of second drug based on mechanism of action and drug interactions, and referral to an epilepsy center if seizures fail to control with two or more anti-seizure medications) (Engel et al. 2003). In patients with CNS tumors, complete surgical resection of the tumor improves seizure outcome (Ruda et al. 2012). It is still not established whether use of intraoperative electrocorticography improves seizure outcome over simple gross total lesionectomy (Ruda et al. 2012).

15.5.2.4 Choice of Anti-Seizure Medications

In 2000, a study showed adverse effect on overall survival if children with acute lymphoblastic leukemia were treated with enzyme inducing anti-seizure medications (Relling et al. 2000). There have been a number of other phase I studies confirming lower levels of many chemotherapeutic agents when treated concurrently with enzyme inducing anti-seizure medications (Yap et al. 2008; Prados et al. 2004). Cytochrome P450 enzymes of interest relevant to chemotherapy include CYP3A4, CYP2C9, and CYP2C19. Carbamazepine, phenytoin, oxcarbazepine, primidone, phenobarbital, prempanel, and high-dose topiramate induce these enzymes while valproic acid may suppress some of them. Other drugs like gabapentin, levetiracetam, lacosamide, zonisamide, and lamotrigine have none or few such effects. Two retrospective studies of children with CNS tumors and leukemia showed efficacy of gabapentin in controlling seizures (Khan et al. 2004, 2005). However, because of ease of use and availability of intravenous formulation, levetiracetam has become the first choice medication to treat seizures based on many observational studies (Bauer et al. 2014). Phenytoin or phenobarbital are reserved for status epilepticus that does not resolve after initial benzodiazepine and a loading dose of levetiracetam, and may be subsequently withdrawn when the patient stabilizes. Lacosamide has pharmacokinetic properties similar to levetiracetam and an intravenous formulation is available. It is an appropriate second line drug if levetiracetam fails or is not tolerated. Valproic acid, because of its ability to induce platelet dysfunction and thrombocytopenia, may be avoided. However, there are currently clinical trials looking at antitumor effect of valproic acid (Guthrie and Eljamel 2013; Kerkhof et al. 2013), and there is a suggestion of similar effect for levetiracetam as well (Bobustuc et al. 2010).

Approximately one-third of children with CNS tumors and seizures will continue to have breakthrough seizures or develop refractory intractable seizures (Khan et al. 2005). Referral to an epilepsy center for epilepsy surgery evaluation should be considered in these children after they have failed therapeutic trial with two or more anti-seizure medications. Epilepsy surgery in carefully selected patients can result in resolution or improvement of seizures in children with CNS tumors (Ojemann et al. 2012).

There has been only one study looking at withdrawal of anti-seizure medications in children with brain tumors (Khan and Onar 2006). In a relatively small study of 62 patients, the seizure recurrence rate of 27% was not different compared to a non-CNS tumor population with epilepsy. Most recurrent seizures developed in the first 6 months. Multiple tumor resections and whole brain radiation increased seizure risk while the presence of infrequent spikes on EEG did not. Seizure recurrence was also less likely in posterior fossa tumors. In carefully selected patients who have had long-standing seizure control, have required only single seizure medication, have not had frequent spikes on EEG,

and had few seizures before gaining control, it is reasonable to consider anti-seizure drug withdrawal.

Injury precautions, driving statutes, and potential for teratogenicity should be discussed with all survivors on seizure medications. There is a risk for osteoporosis with chronic use of anti-seizure medications and this risk may be enhanced in brain tumor survivors, especially if they have endocrine dysfunction. Vitamin D levels should be periodically checked in survivors taking anti-seizure medications and its deficiency should be appropriately treated. Physical activity should be encouraged in all survivors taking anti-seizure medications.

15.5.3 Headache

Although many children with CNS tumors will have headache as one of the presenting symptoms of their tumor (Wilne et al. 2007), prevalence, severity, types, outcome, and effect of headache on quality of life has been inadequately studied among long-term survivors. A Finnish study of 740 survivors found an elevated risk of headaches in survivors compared to healthy siblings (Gunn et al. 2015). Another retrospective study of 81 children found headache in 21% of medulloblastoma, 26% of pilocytic astrocytoma, and 56% of craniopharyngioma survivors (Johnson et al. 2009). A retrospective study of survivors of craniopharyngioma from St. Jude Children's Research Hospital reported that 68% had headaches prior to diagnosis, 78% during treatment, and only 25% still had headache at a median follow-up of more than 2 years (Khan et al. 2013). The majority fulfilled diagnostic criteria for migraine headaches, while 22% had episodic tension type headaches. Large tumor volume and distortion of circle of Willis were risk factors for frequent and severe headaches. The approach to treatment of headache in cancer survivors is similar to the general population. However, because of their potential to cause vasoconstriction, triptan drugs should be avoided when steno-occlusive vasculopathy is present.

15.5.4 Stroke-like Migraine After Radiation Treatment (SMART Syndrome)

Transient stroke-like symptoms and headaches in childhood cancer survivors were first reported in 1995 (Shuper et al. 1995). Stroke-like symptoms may develop with or without headaches and have been reported in children and adults (Armstrong et al. 2014). SMART syndrome develops usually a year or more after brain tumor radiation. A careful history may reveal that stroke-like symptoms develop more slowly over minutes to hours, may wax and wane, and may involve more than one vascular territory. There may or may not be an accompanying headache. MRI may reveal gyral swelling, cortical enhancement, patchy areas of diffusion restriction (Fig. 15.9), or may be normal (Armstrong et al. 2014). EEG may show focal slowing. Different treatments have been tried, including antiplatelet therapy, intravenous immunoglobulin, or high-dose steroids (Armstrong et al. 2014). Symptoms recover over a few days in most patients, but recovery is incomplete in some and laminar necrosis on MRI may develop (Black et al. 2013). Recurrent episodes may develop. SMART syndrome should be considered in the differential diagnosis of stroke in cancer survivors so that inappropriate thrombolytic therapy is avoided.

15.5.5 Sleep

Sleep control requires structures in hypothalamus, basal ganglia, and brain stem (Saper 2013). Orexin is a wakefulness-promoting hormone produced by cells in the lateral hypothalamus, and deficiency of this hormone is implicated in causation of narcolepsy (Krahn et al. 2002). One would expect increased or disturbed sleep if these structures are damaged with tumor or surgery, or if they receive high-dose radiation. Indeed many relatively smaller series have reported sleep disturbance or daytime sleepiness in childhood CNS tumor survivors (Mandrell et al. 2012; Rosen and

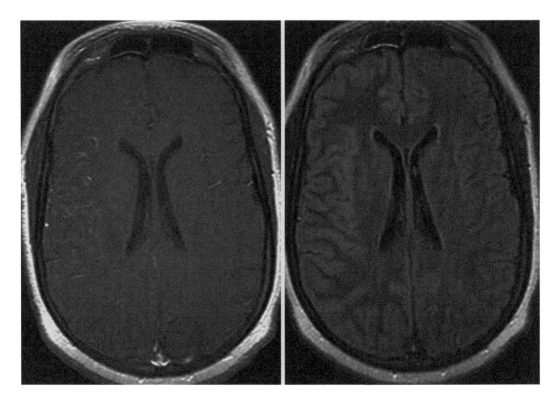

Fig. 15.9 T1-weighted post contrast image (right) of a patient with SMART syndrome shows cortical enhancement in the frontal, parietal, and occipital cortices. FLAIR image on the right shows gyral swelling in the corresponding areas

Brand 2011; Nolan et al. 2013). These studies of symptomatic patients revealed daytime sleepiness to be the most common symptom. Polysomnogram testing showed increased sleep latency, sleep-disordered breathing, obstructive sleep apnea, hypersomnia, and narcolepsy. Most of the CNS tumors in these studies were located in the sella–parasellar area, or in the brainstem. Paradoxically, a study of 299 brain tumor survivors and siblings did not find a meaningful difference in sleep disturbance or daytime sleepiness between the two groups based on Pittsburgh Sleep Quality Index and Epworth Sleepiness Scale (Mulrooney et al. 2008; Dewald-Kaufmann et al. 2014).

15.5.5.1 Management

Behavior therapy and management of underlying anxiety if present will help with delayed sleep latency (Dewald-Kaufmann et al. 2014). Although many clinicians prescribe melatonin, there is no evidence for its efficacy and no studies on its long-term toxicity. Obstructive sleep apnea should be managed with weight loss, evaluation by an ENT surgeon, posture control in sleep, and continuous positive airway pressure treatment when indicated. The latter will need supervision by a sleep specialist. Narcolepsy is treated with utilization of strategic naps and medications such as modafinil, armodafinil, and different stimulant medications. These are all schedule II drugs and require close monitoring by clinician for appetite suppression, hypertension, and other cardiovascular adverse effects.

15.5.6 Auditory and Visual Impairment

Medulloblastoma and ependymoma arise in the posterior fossa and are the two of the most common childhood CNS tumors. Both are treated with focal radiation and medulloblastoma with ototoxic cisplatin. A study of 78 children with posterior fossa tumors treated with radiation but no chemotherapy showed a low probability of hearing impairment if cochlear dose was <30 Gy, while the incidence of sensori-neural hearing loss progressively increased with radiation dose above 40 Gy (Hua et al. 2008). Overall 14% had hearing impairment which may develop within

few months after radiation or many years after completion of therapy. Another study of 72 children found that the need for ventriculo-peritoneal shunt and ototoxic chemotherapy both increased the risk of hearing loss (Merchant et al. 2004). Results from CCSS of more than 3000 adult survivors and a Finnish study of 740 survivors also showed an increased relative risk of hearing impairment, deafness, and need for hearing aid in adult survivors of childhood brain tumors compared to siblings (Packer et al. 2003; Whelan et al. 2011; Armstrong et al. 2011a). More than 50 Gy to the posterior fossa and temporal lobe tumor location were risk factors. There was also a suggestion that prevalence of hearing impairment increases with time, approaching 22% at 15 years from treatment (Armstrong et al. 2011a).

As for vision loss in the CCSS study, the relative risk of legal blindness in one or both eyes was 14.8 (Packer et al. 2003). This study also reported an elevated risk of cataracts and double vision. Another CCSS study of survivors of low-grade glioma reported an increasing risk of blindness with time approaching 18% at 15 years (Armstrong et al. 2011a). However, the majority of the tumors in this study involved the hypothalamus, optic chiasm, or thalamus. A study of 30 craniopharyngioma survivors treated with radiation reported visual acuity loss in one eye in at least 40% of survivors and visual field impairment in at least 67% (Merchant et al. 2002).

15.5.7 Neurologic Deficits and Motor Function

Survival of medulloblastoma and ependymoma depends on the extent of tumor resection. The need for aggressive surgical resection not infrequently results in injury to cranial nerves, sensory motor tracts, or cerebellum, and may result in impaired swallowing, need for airway protection with tracheostomy, hemiparesis, or ataxia (Morris et al. 2009). In one study of children with ependymoma, 79% of the 96 study participants had some neurologic functional deficit after surgery and radiation treatment (Morris et al. 2009). Neurologic deficits improved over time in most, even in those who had more severe deficits. Neurologic deficits were mild in those who survived to 60 months after surgery. Resection of supratentorial tumors when present close to eloquent structures may also cause motor weakness or sensory loss (Khan et al. 2006b). This study also reported improvement in deficits with time and that the presence of water diffusion restriction in a postoperative scan correlated with slower and incomplete recovery. The self-report based CCSS reported motor problems in 49% and coordination problems in 26% of 1607 survivors of CNS tumor (Packer et al. 2003). Radiation to frontal lobes was noted to be a risk factor for motor dysfunction.

A relatively small study of 52 survivors reported abnormal motor function in 50% and need for some assistance in activities of daily living in 13% (Pietila et al. 2012). A study of 78 adult survivors of childhood brain tumor and 78 normal controls from St. Jude Children's Research Hospital showed lower estimated grip strength, knee extension strength, and oxygen uptake in survivors compared to normal controls (Ness et al. 2010). Interestingly, this study also showed that lower physical performance correlated with not living independently. Impaired balance and coordination was also reported in a majority of survivors of posterior fossa tumors, especially in those with non-astrocytoma tumors. Frailty and pre-frailty, when defined based on presence of low muscle mass, exhaustion, low energy expenditure, slow walking speed, and weakness, was present in 40% of 148 survivors of childhood CNS tumors (Ness et al. 2013). Prevalence of frailty in survivors in this study was similar to that reported in 65 years and older population, suggesting CNS tumor survivors may be experiencing accelerated aging.

15.5.7.1   Management

There is little data on treatment or interventions to improve physical functioning in cancer survivors. Exercise, both aerobic and isometric, has been shown to improve frailty in older adults. There are studies looking at exercise as an intervention to improve motor function and endurance. In our opinion, it is appropriate to guide childhood brain tumor survivors toward a healthier eating and an appropriate graded exercise program.

References

Acharya S, Sarafoglou K, LaQuaglia M, Lindsley S, Gerald W, Wollner N, Tan C, Sklar C (2003) Thyroid neoplasms after therapeutic radiation for malignancies during childhood or adolescence. Cancer 97(10):2397–2403. https://doi.org/10.1002/cncr.11362

Acharya S, DeWees T, Shinohara ET, Perkins SM (2015) Long-term outcomes and late effects for childhood and young adulthood intracranial germinomas. Neuro-Oncology 17(5):741–746. https://doi.org/10.1093/neuonc/nou311

Ahmed SR, Shalet SM, Campbell RH, Deakin DP (1983) Primary gonadal damage following treatment of brain tumors in childhood. J Pediatr 103(4):562–565

Armstrong GT, Liu Q, Yasui Y, Huang S, Ness KK, Leisenring W, Hudson MM, Donaldson SS, King AA, Stovall M, Krull KR, Robison LL, Packer RJ (2009a) Long-term outcomes among adult survivors of childhood central nervous system malignancies in the Childhood Cancer Survivor Study. J Natl Cancer Inst 101(13):946–958. https://doi.org/10.1093/jnci/djp148

Armstrong GT, Liu Q, Yasui Y, Neglia JP, Leisenring W, Robison LL, Mertens AC (2009b) Late mortality among 5-year survivors of childhood cancer: a summary from the Childhood Cancer Survivor Study. J Clin Oncol 27(14):2328–2338. https://doi.org/10.1200/JCO.2008.21.1425

Armstrong GT, Whitton JA, Gajjar A, Kun LE, Chow EJ, Stovall M, Leisenring W, Robison LL, Sklar CA (2009c) Abnormal timing of menarche in survivors of central nervous system tumors: a report from the Childhood Cancer Survivor Study. Cancer 115(11):2562–2570. https://doi.org/10.1002/cncr.24294

Armstrong GT, Conklin HM, Huang S, Srivastava D, Sanford R, Ellison DW, Merchant TE, Hudson MM, Hoehn ME, Robison LL, Gajjar A, Morris EB (2011a) Survival and long-term health and cognitive outcomes after low-grade glioma. Neuro-Oncology 13(2):223–234. https://doi.org/10.1093/neuonc/noq178

Armstrong GT, Liu W, Leisenring W, Yasui Y, Hammond S, Bhatia S, Neglia JP, Stovall M, Srivastava D, Robison LL (2011b) Occurrence of multiple subsequent neoplasms in long-term survivors of childhood cancer: a report from the childhood cancer survivor study. J Clin Oncol 29(22):3056–3064. https://doi.org/10.1200/JCO.2011.34.6585

Armstrong AE, Gillan E, FJ DM Jr (2014) SMART syndrome (stroke-like migraine attacks after radiation therapy) in adult and pediatric patients. J Child Neurol 29(3):336–341. https://doi.org/10.1177/0883073812474843

Armstrong GT, Chen Y, Yasui Y, Leisenring W, Gibson TM, Mertens AC, Stovall M, Oeffinger KC, Bhatia S, Krull KR, Nathan PC, Neglia JP, Green DM, Hudson MM, Robison LL (2016) Reduction in late mortality among 5-year survivors of childhood cancer. N Engl J Med 374(9):833–842. https://doi.org/10.1056/NEJMoa1510795

Bakker B, Oostdijk W, Bresters D, Walenkamp MJ, Vossen JM, Wit JM (2004) Disturbances of growth and endocrine function after busulphan-based conditioning for haematopoietic stem cell transplantation during infancy and childhood. Bone Marrow Transplant 33(10):1049–1056. https://doi.org/10.1038/sj.bmt.1704481

Bakker B, Oostdijk W, Geskus RB, Stokvis-Brantsma WH, Vossen JM, Wit JM (2007) Growth hormone (GH) secretion and response to GH therapy after total body irradiation and haematopoietic stem cell transplantation during childhood. Clin Endocrinol 67(4):589–597. https://doi.org/10.1111/j.1365-2265.2007.02930.x

Balachandar S, Dunkel IJ, Khakoo Y, Wolden S, Allen J, Sklar CA (2014) Ovarian function in survivors of childhood medulloblastoma: impact of reduced dose craniospinal irradiation and high-dose chemotherapy with autologous stem cell rescue. Pediatr Blood Cancer 62:317–321. https://doi.org/10.1002/pbc.25291

Barnes N, Chemaitilly W (2014) Endocrinopathies in survivors of childhood neoplasia. Front Pediatr 2:101. https://doi.org/10.3389/fped.2014.00101

Bauer R, Ortler M, Seiz-Rosenhagen M, Maier R, Anton JV, Unterberger I (2014) Treatment of epileptic seizures in brain tumors: a critical review. Neurosurg Rev 37(3):381–388.; discussion 388. https://doi.org/10.1007/s10143-014-0538-6

Bayley N, Pinneau SR (1952) Tables for predicting adult height from skeletal age: revised for use with the Greulich-Pyle hand standards. J Pediatr 40(4):423–441

Beckers D, Thomas M, Jamart J, Francois I, Maes M, Lebrethon MC, De Waele K, Tenoutasse S, De Schepper J (2010) Adult final height after GH therapy for irradiation-induced GH deficiency in childhood survivors of brain tumors: the Belgian experience. Eur J Endocrinol 162(3):483–490. https://doi.org/10.1530/EJE-09-0690

Bhatti P, Veiga LH, Ronckers CM, Sigurdson AJ, Stovall M, Smith SA, Weathers R, Leisenring W, Mertens AC, Hammond S, Friedman DL, Neglia JP, Meadows AT, Donaldson SS, Sklar CA, Robison LL, Inskip PD (2010) Risk of second primary thyroid cancer after radiotherapy for a childhood cancer in a large cohort study: an update from the childhood cancer survivor study. Radiat Res 174(6):741–752. https://doi.org/10.1667/RR2240.1

Black DF, Morris JM, Lindell EP, Krecke KN, Worrell GA, Bartleson JD, Lachance DH (2013) Stroke-like migraine attacks after radiation therapy (SMART) syndrome is not always completely reversible: a case series. Am J Neuroradiol 34(12):2298–2303. https://doi.org/10.3174/ajnr.A3602

Bobustuc GC, Baker CH, Limaye A, Jenkins WD, Pearl G, Avgeropoulos NG, Konduri SD (2010) Levetiracetam enhances p53-mediated MGMT inhibition and sensitizes glioblastoma cells to temozolomide. Neuro-Oncology 12(9):917–927. https://doi.org/10.1093/neuonc/noq044

Boulanger JM, Coutts SB, Eliasziw M, Gagnon AJ, Simon JE, Subramaniam S, Sohn CH, Scott J, Demchuk AM (2006) Cerebral microhemorrhages predict new disabling or fatal strokes in patients with acute ischemic stroke or transient ischemic attack. Stroke 37(3):911–914. https://doi.org/10.1161/01.STR.0000204237.66466.5f

Bowers DC, Liu Y, Leisenring W, McNeil E, Stovall M, Gurney JG, Robison LL, Packer RJ, Oeffinger KC (2006) Late-occurring stroke among long-term survivors of childhood leukemia and brain tumors: a report from the Childhood Cancer Survivor Study. J Clin Oncol 24(33):5277–5282. https://doi.org/10.1200/JCO.2006.07.2884

Bowers DC, Nathan PC, Constine L, Woodman C, Bhatia S, Keller K, Bashore L (2013) Subsequent neoplasms of the CNS among survivors of childhood cancer: a systematic review. Lancet Oncol 14(8):e321–e328. https://doi.org/10.1016/S1470-2045(13)70107-4

Brauner R, Czernichow P, Rappaport R (1986) Greater susceptibility to hypothalamopituitary irradiation in younger children with acute lymphoblastic leukemia. J Pediatr 108(2):332

Brauner R, Fontoura M, Zucker JM, Devergie A, Souberbielle JC, Prevot-Saucet C, Michon J, Gluckman E, Griscelli C, Fischer A et al (1993) Growth and growth hormone secretion after bone marrow transplantation. Arch Dis Child 68(4):458–463

Broniscer A, Ke W, Fuller CE, Wu J, Gajjar A, Kun LE (2004) Second neoplasms in pediatric patients with primary central nervous system tumors: the St. Jude Children's Research Hospital experience. Cancer 100(10):2246–2252

Brownstein CM, Mertens AC, Mitby PA, Stovall M, Qin J, Heller G, Robison LL, Sklar CA (2004) Factors that affect final height and change in height standard deviation scores in survivors of childhood cancer treated with growth hormone: a report from the childhood cancer survivor study. J Clin Endocrinol Metab 89(9):4422–4427

Campen CJ, Kranick SM, Kasner SE, Kessler SK, Zimmerman RA, Lustig R, Phillips PC, Storm PB, Smith SE, Ichord R, Fisher MJ (2012) Cranial irradiation increases risk of stroke in pediatric brain tumor survivors. Stroke 43(11):3035–3040. https://doi.org/10.1161/STROKEAHA.112.661561

Cardous-Ubbink MC, Heinen RC, Langeveld NE, Bakker PJ, Voute PA, Caron HN, van Leeuwen FE (2004) Long-term cause-specific mortality among five-year survivors of childhood cancer. Pediatr Blood Cancer 42(7):563–573

Cardous-Ubbink MC, Heinen RC, Bakker PJ, van den Berg H, Oldenburger F, Caron HN, Voute PA, van Leeuwen FE (2007) Risk of second malignancies in long-term survivors of childhood cancer. Eur J Cancer 43(2):351–362

Carel JC, Eugster EA, Rogol A, Ghizzoni L, Palmert MR, Antoniazzi F, Berenbaum S, Bourguignon JP, Chrousos GP, Coste J, Deal S, de Vries L, Foster C, Heger S, Holland J, Jahnukainen K, Juul A, Kaplowitz P, Lahlou N, Lee MM, Lee P, Merke DP, Neely EK, Oostdijk W, Phillip M, Rosenfield RL, Shulman D, Styne D, Tauber M, Wit JM (2009) Consensus statement on the use of gonadotropin-releasing hormone analogs in children. Pediatrics 123(4):e752–e762. https://doi.org/10.1542/peds.2008-1783

Chemaitilly W, Robison LL (2012) Safety of growth hormone treatment in patients previously treated for cancer. Endocrinol Metab Clin N Am 41(4):785–792. https://doi.org/10.1016/j.ecl.2012.07.002

Chemaitilly W, Sklar CA (2010) Endocrine complications in long-term survivors of childhood cancers. Endocr Relat Cancer 17(3):R141–R159. https://doi.org/10.1677/ERC-10-0002

Chemaitilly W, Trivin C, Adan L, Gall V, Sainte-Rose C, Brauner R (2001) Central precocious puberty: clinical and laboratory features. Clin Endocrinol 54(3):289–294

Chemaitilly W, Li Z, Huang S, Ness KK, Clark KL, Green DM, Barnes N, Armstrong GT, Krasin MJ, Srivastava DK, Pui CH, Merchant TE, Kun LE, Gajjar A, Hudson MM, Robison LL, Sklar CA (2015) Anterior hypopituitarism in adult survivors of childhood cancers treated with cranial radiotherapy: a report from the St Jude Lifetime Cohort Study. J Clin Oncol 33:492–500. https://doi.org/10.1200/JCO.2014.56.7933

Chieng PU, Huang TS, Chang CC, Chong PN, Tien RD, Su CT (1991) Reduced hypothalamic blood flow after radiation treatment of nasopharyngeal cancer: SPECT studies in 34 patients. Am J Neuroradiol 12(4):661–665

Children's OG (2013) Children's Oncology Group long-term follow-up guidelines for survivors of childhood, adolescent, and young adult cancer. Children's Oncology Group. http://www.survivorshipguidelines.org/pdf/LTFUGuidelines_40.pdf

Chrousos GP, Kino T, Charmandari E (2009) Evaluation of the hypothalamic-pituitary-adrenal axis function in childhood and adolescence. Neuroimmunomodulation 16(5):272–283. https://doi.org/10.1159/000216185

Ciaccio M, Gil S, Guercio G, Vaiani E, Alderete D, Palladino M, Warman DM, Rivarola MA, Belgorosky A (2010) Effectiveness of rhGH treatment on adult height in GH-deficient childhood survivors of medulloblastoma. Horm Res Paediatr 73(4):281–286. https://doi.org/10.1159/000284393

Clayton PE, Shalet SM (1991a) Dose dependency of time of onset of radiation-induced growth hormone deficiency. J Pediatr 118(2):226–228

Clayton PE, Shalet SM (1991b) The evolution of spinal growth after irradiation. Clin Oncol (R Coll Radiol) 3(4):220–222

Cohen LE, Gordon JH, Popovsky EY, Sainath NN, Feldman HA, Kieran MW, Gordon CM (2012) Bone density in post-pubertal adolescent survivors of childhood brain tumors. Pediatr Blood Cancer 58(6):959–963. https://doi.org/10.1002/pbc.23300

Conceicao FL, da Costa e Silva A, Leal Costa AJ, Vaisman M (2003) Glucagon stimulation test for the diagnosis of GH deficiency in adults. J Endocrinol Invest 26(11):1065–1070

Constine LS, Woolf PD, Cann D, Mick G, McCormick K, Raubertas RF, Rubin P (1993) Hypothalamic-pituitary dysfunction after radiation for brain tumors. N Engl J Med 328(2):87–94

Dama E, Pastore G, Mosso ML, Ferrante D, Maule MM, Magnani C, Merletti F (2006) Late deaths among five-year survivors of childhood cancer. A population-based study in Piedmont Region, Italy. Haematologica 91(8):1084–1091

Darzy KH, Aimaretti G, Wieringa G, Gattamaneni HR, Ghigo E, Shalet SM (2003) The usefulness of the combined growth hormone (GH)-releasing hormone and arginine stimulation test in the diagnosis of radiation-induced GH deficiency is dependent on the post-irradiation time interval. J Clin Endocrinol Metab 88(1):95–102. https://doi.org/10.1210/jc.2002-021094

Devarahally SR, Severson RK, Chuba P, Thomas R, Bhambhani K, Hamre MR (2003) Second malignant neoplasms after primary central nervous system malignancies of childhood and adolescence. Pediatr Hematol Oncol 20(8):617–625

Dewald-Kaufmann JF, Oort FJ, Meijer AM (2014) The effects of sleep extension and sleep hygiene advice on sleep and depressive symptoms in adolescents: a randomized controlled trial. J Child Psychol Psychiatry 55(3):273–283. https://doi.org/10.1111/jcpp.12157

Di Giannatale A, Morana G, Rossi A, Cama A, Bertoluzzo L, Barra S, Nozza P, Milanaccio C, Consales A, Garre ML (2014) Natural history of cavernous malformations in children with brain tumors treated with radiotherapy and chemotherapy. J Neuro-Oncol 117(2):311–320. https://doi.org/10.1007/s11060-014-1390-9

Di Iorgi N, Napoli F, Allegri AE, Olivieri I, Bertelli E, Gallizia A, Rossi A, Maghnie M (2012) Diabetes insipidus—diagnosis and management. Horm Res Paediatr 77(2):69–84. https://doi.org/10.1159/000336333

Diller L, Chow EJ, Gurney JG, Hudson MM, Kadin-Lottick NS, Kawashima TI, Leisenring WM, Meacham LR, Mertens AC, Mulrooney DA, Oeffinger KC, Packer RJ, Robison LL, Sklar CA (2009) Chronic disease in the Childhood Cancer Survivor Study cohort: a review of published findings. J Clin Oncol 27(14):2339–2355

Douw L, van Dellen E, de Groot M, Heimans JJ, Klein M, Stam CJ, Reijneveld JC (2010) Epilepsy is related to theta band brain connectivity and network topology in brain tumor patients. BMC Neurosci 11:103. https://doi.org/10.1186/1471-2202-11-103

Douw L, de Groot M, van Dellen E, Aronica E, Heimans JJ, Klein M, Stam CJ, Reijneveld JC, Hillebrand A (2013) Local MEG networks: the missing link between protein expression and epilepsy in glioma patients? NeuroImage 75:195–203. https://doi.org/10.1016/j.neuroimage.2013.02.067

Duffner PK, Krischer JP, Horowitz ME, Cohen ME, Burger PC, Friedman HS, Kun LE (1998) Second malignancies in young children with primary brain tumors following treatment with prolonged postoperative chemotherapy and delayed irradiation: a Pediatric Oncology Group study. Ann Neurol 44(3):313–316

Duhem R, Vinchon M, Leblond P, Soto-Ares G, Dhellemmes P (2005) Cavernous malformations after cerebral irradiation during childhood: report of nine cases. Childs Nerv Syst 21(10):922–925. https://doi.org/10.1007/s00381-004-1120-2

Elbornsson M, Gotherstrom G, Bosaeus I, Bengtsson BA, Johannsson G, Svensson J (2012) Fifteen years of GH replacement increases bone mineral density in hypopituitary patients with adult-onset GH deficiency. Eur J Endocrinol 166(5):787–795. https://doi.org/10.1530/EJE-11-1072

Elbornsson M, Gotherstrom G, Bosaeus I, Bengtsson BA, Johannsson G, Svensson J (2013) Fifteen years of GH replacement improves body composition and cardiovascular risk factors. Eur J Endocrinol 168(5):745–753. https://doi.org/10.1530/EJE-12-1083

Engel J Jr, Wiebe S, French J, Sperling M, Williamson P, Spencer D, Gumnit R, Zahn C, Westbrook E, Enos B (2003) Practice parameter: temporal lobe and localized neocortical resections for epilepsy: report of the Quality Standards Subcommittee of the American Academy of Neurology, in association with the American Epilepsy Society and the American Association of Neurological Surgeons. Neurology 60(4):538–547

Ergun-Longmire B, Mertens AC, Mitby P, Qin J, Heller G, Shi W, Yasui Y, Robison LL, Sklar CA (2006) Growth hormone treatment and risk of second neoplasms in the childhood cancer survivor. J Clin Endocrinol Metab 91(9):3494–3498. https://doi.org/10.1210/jc.2006-0656

Follin C, Thilen U, Ahren B, Erfurth EM (2006) Improvement in cardiac systolic function and reduced prevalence of metabolic syndrome after two years of growth hormone (GH) treatment in GH-deficient adult survivors of childhood-onset acute lymphoblastic leukemia. J Clin Endocrinol Metab 91(5):1872–1875. https://doi.org/10.1210/jc.2005-2298

Friedman DL, Whitton J, Leisenring W, Mertens AC, Hammond S, Stovall M, Donaldson SS, Meadows AT, Robison LL, Neglia JP (2010) Subsequent neoplasms in 5-year survivors of childhood cancer: the Childhood Cancer Survivor Study. J Natl Cancer Inst 102(14):1083–1095. https://doi.org/10.1093/jnci/djq238

Garwicz S, Anderson H, Olsen JH, Winther JF, Sankila R, Langmark F, Tryggvadottir L, Moller TR (2012) Late and very late mortality in 5-year survivors of childhood cancer: changing pattern over four decades-experience from the Nordic countries. Int J Cancer 131(7):1659–1666. https://doi.org/10.1002/ijc.27393

Glantz MJ, Cole BF, Forsyth PA, Recht LD, Wen PY, Chamberlain MC, Grossman SA, Cairncross JG (2000) Practice parameter: anticonvulsant prophylaxis in patients with newly diagnosed brain tumors. Report of the Quality Standards Subcommittee of the American Academy of Neurology. Neurology 54(10):1886–1893

Gleeson HK, Shalet SM (2004) The impact of cancer therapy on the endocrine system in survivors of childhood brain tumours. Endocr Relat Cancer 11(4):589–602

Gleeson HK, Stoeter R, Ogilvy-Stuart AL, Gattamaneni HR, Brennan BM, Shalet SM (2003) Improvements in final height over 25 years in growth hormone (GH)-deficient childhood survivors of brain tumors receiving GH replacement. J Clin Endocrinol Metab 88(8):3682–3689

Growth Hormone Researhc Society (2000) Consensus guidelines for the diagnosis and treatment of growth hormone (GH) deficiency in childhood and adolescence: summary statement of the GH Research Society. GH Research Society. J Clin Endocrinol Metab 85 (11):3990–3993. doi:https://doi.org/10.1210/jcem.85.11.6984

Gunn ME, Lahdesmaki T, Malila N, Arola M, Gronroos M, Matomaki J, Lahteenmaki PM (2015) Late morbidity in long-term survivors of childhood brain tumors: a nationwide registry-based study in Finland. Neuro-Oncology 17(5):747–756. https://doi.org/10.1093/neuonc/nou321

Gurney JG, Kadan-Lottick NS, Packer RJ, Neglia JP, Sklar CA, Punyko JA, Stovall M, Yasui Y, Nicholson HS, Wolden S, McNeil DE, Mertens AC, Robison LL (2003a) Endocrine and cardiovascular late effects among adult survivors of childhood brain tumors: Childhood Cancer Survivor Study. Cancer 97(3):663–673

Gurney JG, Ness KK, Stovall M, Wolden S, Punyko JA, Neglia JP, Mertens AC, Packer RJ, Robison LL, Sklar CA (2003b) Final height and body mass index among adult survivors of childhood brain cancer: childhood cancer survivor study. J Clin Endocrinol Metab 88(10):4731–4739

Guthrie GD, Eljamel S (2013) Impact of particular antiepileptic drugs on the survival of patients with glioblastoma multiforme. J Neurosurg 118(4):859–865. https://doi.org/10.3171/2012.10.JNS12169

Haddy N, Mousannif A, Tukenova M, Guibout C, Grill J, Dhermain F, Pacquement H, Oberlin O, El-Fayech C, Rubino C, Thomas-Teinturier C, Le-Deley MC, Hawkins M, Winter D, Chavaudra J, Diallo I, de Vathaire F (2011) Relationship between the brain radiation dose for the treatment of childhood cancer and the risk of long-term cerebrovascular mortality. Brain 134(Pt 5):1362–1372. https://doi.org/10.1093/brain/awr071

Hader WJ, Drovini-Zis K, Maguire JA (2003) Primitive neuroectodermal tumors in the central nervous system following cranial irradiation: a report of four cases. Cancer 97(4):1072–1076

Halle M, Hall P, Tornvall P (2011) Cardiovascular disease associated with radiotherapy: activation of nuclear factor kappa-B. J Intern Med 269(5):469–477. https://doi.org/10.1111/j.1365-2796.2011.02353.x

Ham JN, Ginsberg JP, Hendell CD, Moshang T Jr (2005) Growth hormone releasing hormone plus arginine stimulation testing in young adults treated in childhood with cranio-spinal radiation therapy. Clin Endocrinol 62(5):628–632. https://doi.org/10.1111/j.1365-2265.2005.02272.x

Hammal DM, Bell CL, Craft AW, Parker L (2005) Second primary tumors in children and young adults in the North of England (1968–99). Pediatr Blood Cancer 45(2):155–161

Hansson GK, Libby P (2006) The immune response in atherosclerosis: a double-edged sword. Nat Rev Immunol 6(7):508–519. https://doi.org/10.1038/nri1882

Hawkins MM, Kingston JE, Kinnier Wilson LM (1990) Late deaths after treatment for childhood cancer. Arch Dis Child 65(12):1356–1363

van den Heijkant S, Hoorweg-Nijman G, Huisman J, Drent M, van der Pal H, Kaspers GJ, Delemarre-van de Waal H (2011) Effects of growth hormone therapy on bone mass, metabolic balance, and well-being in young adult survivors of childhood acute lymphoblastic leukemia. J Pediatr Hematol Oncol 33(6):e231–e238. https://doi.org/10.1097/MPH.0b013e31821bbe7a

Hoving S, Heeneman S, Gijbels MJ, te Poele JA, Russell NS, Daemen MJ, Stewart FA (2008) Single-dose and fractionated irradiation promote initiation and progression of atherosclerosis and induce an inflammatory plaque phenotype in ApoE(−/−) mice. Int J Radiat Oncol Biol Phys 71(3):848–857. https://doi.org/10.1016/j.ijrobp.2008.02.031

Howlader N, Noone AM, Krapcho M, Neyman N, Aminou R, Altekruse SF, Kosary CL, Ruhl J, Tatalovich Z, Cho H, Mariotto A, Eisner MP, Lewis DR, Chen HS, Feuer EJ, Cronin KA (eds) (2012) SEER cancer statistics review 1975–2009 (vintage 2009 populations). SEER Cancer Statistics Review (CSR). National Cancer Institute, Bethesda, MD

Hua C, Bass JK, Khan R, Kun LE, Merchant TE (2008) Hearing loss after radiotherapy for pediatric brain tumors: effect of cochlear dose. Int J Radiat Oncol Biol Phys 72(3):892–899. https://doi.org/10.1016/j.ijrobp.2008.01.050

Ibrahim K, Appleton R (2004) Seizures as the presenting symptom of brain tumours in children. Seizure 13(2):108–112

Iwayama H, Kamijo T, Ueda N (2011) Hyperinsulinemia may promote growth without GH in children after resection of suprasellar brain tumors. Endocrine 40(1):130–133. https://doi.org/10.1007/s12020-011-9493-y

Jenkin D (1996) Long-term survival of children with brain tumors. Oncology (Williston Park) 10(5):715–719. discussion 720, 722, 728

Jenkinson HC, Hawkins MM, Stiller CA, Winter DL, Marsden HB, Stevens MC (2004) Long-term population-based risks of second malignant neoplasms after childhood cancer in Britain. Br J Cancer 91(11):1905–1910. https://doi.org/10.1038/sj.bjc.6602226

Johnson AH, Jordan C, Mazewski CM (2009) Off-therapy headaches in pediatric brain tumor patients: a retrospective review. J Pediatr Oncol Nurs 26(6):354–361. https://doi.org/10.1177/1043454209340323

Kenney LB, Cohen LE, Shnorhavorian M, Metzger ML, Lockart B, Hijiya N, Duffey-Lind E, Constine L, Green D, Meacham L (2012) Male reproductive health after childhood, adolescent, and young adult cancers: a report from the Children's Oncology Group. J Clin Oncol 30(27):3408–3416. https://doi.org/10.1200/JCO.2011.38.6938

Kerkhof M, Dielemans JC, van Breemen MS, Zwinkels H, Walchenbach R, Taphoorn MJ, Vecht CJ (2013) Effect of valproic acid on seizure control and on survival in patients with glioblastoma multiforme. Neuro-Oncology 15(7):961–967. https://doi.org/10.1093/neuonc/not057

Khan RB, Onar A (2006) Seizure recurrence and risk factors after antiepilepsy drug withdrawal in children with brain tumors. Epilepsia 47(2):375–379. https://doi.org/10.1111/j.1528-1167.2006.00431.x

Khan RB, Hunt DL, Thompson SJ (2004) Gabapentin to control seizures in children undergoing cancer treatment. J Child Neurol 19(2):97–101

Khan RB, Hunt DL, Boop FA, Sanford RA, Merchant TE, Gajjar A, Kun LE (2005) Seizures in children with primary brain tumors: incidence and long-term outcome. Epilepsy Res 64(3):85–91. https://doi.org/10.1016/j.eplepsyres.2005.03.007

Khan RB, Boop FA, Onar A, Sanford RA (2006a) Seizures in children with low-grade tumors: outcome after tumor resection and risk factors for uncontrolled seizures. J Neurosurg 104(6 Suppl):377–382. https://doi.org/10.3171/ped.2006.104.6.377

Khan RB, Gutin PH, Rai SN, Zhang L, Krol G, DeAngelis LM (2006b) Use of diffusion weighted magnetic resonance imaging in predicting early postoperative outcome of new neurological deficits after brain tumor resection. Neurosurgery 59(1):60–66.; discussion 60-66. https://doi.org/10.1227/01.NEU.0000219218.43128.FC

Khan RB, Merchant TE, Boop FA, Sanford RA, Ledet D, Onar-Thomas A, Kun LE (2013) Headaches in children with craniopharyngioma. J Child Neurol 28(12):1622–1625. https://doi.org/10.1177/0883073812464817

Krahn LE, Pankratz VS, Oliver L, Boeve BF, Silber MH (2002) Hypocretin (orexin) levels in cerebrospinal fluid of patients with narcolepsy: relationship to cataplexy and HLA DQB1*0602 status. Sleep 25(7):733–736

Kranick SM, Campen CJ, Kasner SE, Kessler SK, Zimmerman RA, Lustig RA, Phillips PC, Beslow LA, Ichord R, Fisher MJ (2013) Headache as a risk factor for neurovascular events in pediatric brain tumor patients. Neurology 80(16):1452–1456. https://doi.org/10.1212/WNL.0b013e31828cf81e

Krueger DA, Wilfong AA, Holland-Bouley K, Anderson AE, Agricola K, Tudor C, Mays M, Lopez CM, Kim MO, Franz DN (2013) Everolimus treatment of refractory epilepsy in tuberous sclerosis complex. Ann Neurol 74(5):679–687. https://doi.org/10.1002/ana.23960

Krysiak R, Gdula-Dymek A, Okopien B (2011) Effect of simvastatin and fenofibrate on cytokine release and systemic inflammation in type 2 diabetes mellitus with mixed dyslipidemia. Am J Cardiol 107(7):1010–1018. e1011. https://doi.org/10.1016/j.amjcard.2010.11.023

Kyrnetskiy EE, Kun LE, Boop FA, Sanford RA, Khan RB (2005) Types, causes, and outcome of intracranial hemorrhage in children with cancer. J Neurosurg 102(1 Suppl):31–35. https://doi.org/10.3171/ped.2005.102.1.0031

Laughton SJ, Merchant TE, Sklar CA, Kun LE, Fouladi M, Broniscer A, Morris EB, Sanders RP, Krasin MJ, Shelso J, Xiong Z, Wallace D, Gajjar A (2008) Endocrine outcomes for children with embryonal brain tumors after risk-adapted craniospinal and conformal primary-site irradiation and high-dose chemotherapy with stem-cell rescue on the SJMB-96 trial. J Clin Oncol 26(7):1112–1118

Lew SM, Morgan JN, Psaty E, Lefton DR, Allen JC, Abbott R (2006) Cumulative incidence of radiation-induced cavernomas in long-term survivors of medulloblastoma. J Neurosurg 104(2 Suppl):103–107. https://doi.org/10.3171/ped.2006.104.2.103

Li FP, Cassady JR, Jaffe N (1975) Risk of second tumors in survivors of childhood cancer. Cancer 35(4):1230–1235

Li Z, Franklin J, Zelcer S, Sexton T, Husein M (2014) Ultrasound surveillance for thyroid malignancies in survivors of childhood cancer following radiotherapy: a single institutional experience. Thyroid 24(12):1796–1805. https://doi.org/10.1089/thy.2014.0132

Link K, Moell C, Garwicz S, Cavallin-Stahl E, Bjork J, Thilen U, Ahren B, Erfurth EM (2004) Growth hormone deficiency predicts cardiovascular risk in young adults treated for acute lymphoblastic leukemia in childhood. J Clin Endocrinol Metab 89(10):5003–5012

Livesey EA, Brook CG (1988) Gonadal dysfunction after treatment of intracranial tumours. Arch Dis Child 63(5):495–500

Livesey EA, Brook CG (1989) Thyroid dysfunction after radiotherapy and chemotherapy of brain tumours. Arch Dis Child 64(4):593–595

Lopez Andreu JA, Fernandez PJ, Ferris i Tortajada J, Navarro I, Rodriguez-Ineba A, Antonio P, Muro MD, Romeu A (2000) Persistent altered spermatogenesis in long-term childhood cancer survivors. Pediatr Hematol Oncol 17(1):21–30

Lustig RH, Hinds PS, Ringwald-Smith K, Christensen RK, Kaste SC, Schreiber RE, Rai SN, Lensing SY, Wu S, Xiong X (2003a) Octreotide therapy of pediatric hypothalamic obesity: a double-blind, placebo-controlled trial. J Clin Endocrinol Metab 88(6):2586–2592. https://doi.org/10.1210/jc.2002-030003

Lustig RH, Post SR, Srivannaboon K, Rose SR, Danish RK, Burghen GA, Xiong X, Wu S, Merchant TE (2003b) Risk factors for the development of obesity in children surviving brain tumors. J Clin Endocrinol Metab 88(2):611–616

Mackenzie S, Craven T, Gattamaneni HR, Swindell R, Shalet SM, Brabant G (2011) Long-term safety of growth hormone replacement after CNS irradiation. J Clin Endocrinol Metab 96(9):2756–2761. https://doi.org/10.1210/jc.2011-0112

Mandrell BN, Wise M, Schoumacher RA, Pritchard M, West N, Ness KK, Crabtree VM, Merchant TE, Morris B (2012) Excessive daytime sleepiness and sleep-disordered breathing disturbances in survivors of childhood central nervous system tumors. Pediatr Blood Cancer 58(5):746–751. https://doi.org/10.1002/pbc.23311

Mason PW, Krawiecki N, Meacham LR (2002) The use of dextroamphetamine to treat obesity and hyperphagia in children treated for craniopharyngioma. Arch Pediatr Adolesc Med 156(9):887–892

Merchant TE, Kiehna EN, Sanford RA, Mulhern RK, Thompson SJ, Wilson MW, Lustig RH, Kun LE (2002) Craniopharyngioma: the St. Jude Children's Research Hospital experience 1984-2001. Int J Radiat Oncol Biol Phys 53(3):533–542

Merchant TE, Gould CJ, Xiong X, Robbins N, Zhu J, Pritchard DL, Khan R, Heideman RL, Krasin MJ, Kun LE (2004) Early neuro-otologic effects of three-dimensional irradiation in children with primary brain tumors. Int J Radiat Oncol Biol Phys 58(4):1194–1207

Merchant TE, Rose SR, Bosley C, Wu S, Xiong X, Lustig RH (2011) Growth hormone secretion after conformal radiation therapy in pediatric patients with localized brain tumors. J Clin Oncol 29(36):4776–4780. https://doi.org/10.1200/JCO.2011.37.9453

Mertens AC, Yasui Y, Neglia JP, Potter JD, Nesbit ME Jr, Ruccione K, Smithson WA, Robison LL (2001) Late mortality experience in five-year survivors of childhood and adolescent cancer: the Childhood Cancer Survivor Study. J Clin Oncol 19(13):3163–3172

Mertens AC, Liu Q, Neglia JP, Wasilewski K, Leisenring W, Armstrong GT, Robison LL, Yasui Y (2008) Cause-specific late mortality among 5-year survivors of childhood cancer: the Childhood Cancer Survivor Study. J Natl Cancer Inst 100(19):1368–1379. https://doi.org/10.1093/jnci/djn310

Metzger ML, Meacham LR, Patterson B, Casillas JS, Constine LS, Hijiya N, Kenney LB, Leonard M, Lockart BA, Likes W, Green DM (2013) Female reproductive health after childhood, adolescent, and young adult cancers: guidelines for the assessment and management of female reproductive complications. J Clin Oncol 31(9):1239–1247. https://doi.org/10.1200/JCO.2012.43.5511

Mike V, Meadows AT, D'Angio GJ (1982) Incidence of second malignant neoplasms in children: results of an international study. Lancet 2(8311):1326–1331

Mishra G, Chandrashekhar SR (2011) Management of diabetes insipidus in children. Ind J Endocrinol Metab 15(Suppl 3):S180–S187. https://doi.org/10.4103/2230-8210.84858

Moller TR, Garwicz S, Barlow L, Falck Winther J, Glattre E, Olafsdottir G, Olsen JH, Perfekt R, Ritvanen A, Sankila R, Tulinius H (2001) Decreasing late mortality among five-year survivors of cancer in childhood and adolescence: a population-based study in the Nordic countries. J Clin Oncol 19(13):3173–3181

Morris EB, Gajjar A, Okuma JO, Yasui Y, Wallace D, Kun LE, Merchant TE, Fouladi M, Broniscer A, Robison LL, Hudson MM (2007) Survival and late mortality in long-term survivors of pediatric CNS tumors. J Clin Oncol 25(12):1532–1538. https://doi.org/10.1200/JCO.2006.09.8194

Morris EB, Li C, Khan RB, Sanford RA, Boop F, Pinlac R, Xiong X, Merchant TE (2009) Evolution of neurological impairment in pediatric infratentorial ependymoma patients. J Neuro-Oncol 94(3):391–398. https://doi.org/10.1007/s11060-009-9866-8

Moskowitz CS, Malhotra J, Chou JF, Wolden SL, Weathers RE, Stovall M, Armstrong GT, Leisenring WM, Neglia JP, Robison LL, Oeffinger KC (2015) Breast cancer following spinal irradiation for a childhood cancer: a report from the Childhood Cancer Survivor Study. Radiother Oncol 117(2):213–216. https://doi.org/10.1016/j.radonc.2015.09.016. Epub 2015 Sep 18

Mostoufi-Moab S, Seidel K, Leisenring WM, Armstrong GT, Oeffinger KC, Stovall M, Meacham LR, Green DM, Weathers R, Ginsberg JP, Robison LL, Sklar CA (2016) Endocrine abnormalities in aging survivors of childhood cancer: a report from the Childhood Cancer Survivor Study. J Clin Oncol 34:3240–3247

Mueller S, Fullerton HJ, Stratton K, Leisenring W, Weathers RE, Stovall M, Armstrong GT, Goldsby RE, Packer RJ, Sklar CA, Bowers DC, Robison LL, Krull KR (2013) Radiation, atherosclerotic risk factors, and stroke risk in survivors of pediatric cancer: a report from the Childhood Cancer Survivor Study. Int J Radiat Oncol Biol Phys 86(4):649–655. https://doi.org/10.1016/j.ijrobp.2013.03.034

Mukherjee A, Tolhurst-Cleaver S, Ryder WD, Smethurst L, Shalet SM (2005) The characteristics of quality of life impairment in adult growth hormone (GH)-deficient survivors of cancer and their response to GH replacement therapy. J Clin Endocrinol Metab 90(3):1542–1549. https://doi.org/10.1210/jc.2004-0832

Muller HL (2014) Craniopharyngioma. Endocr Rev 35(3):513–543. https://doi.org/10.1210/er.2013-1115

Mulrooney DA, Ness KK, Neglia JP, Whitton JA, Green DM, Zeltzer LK, Robison LL, Mertens AC (2008) Fatigue and sleep disturbance in adult survivors of childhood cancer: a report from the childhood cancer survivor study (CCSS). Sleep 31(2):271–281

Murray RD, Darzy KH, Gleeson HK, Shalet SM (2002) GH-deficient survivors of childhood cancer: GH replacement during adult life. J Clin Endocrinol Metab 87(1):129–135. https://doi.org/10.1210/jcem.87.1.8146

Napoli C, Ignarro LJ (2009) Nitric oxide and pathogenic mechanisms involved in the development of vascular diseases. Arch Pharm Res 32(8):1103–1108. https://doi.org/10.1007/s12272-009-1801-1

Neglia JP, Friedman DL, Yasui Y, Mertens AC, Hammond S, Stovall M, Donaldson SS, Meadows AT, Robison LL (2001) Second malignant neoplasms in five-year survivors of childhood cancer: childhood cancer survivor study. J Natl Cancer Inst 93(8):618–629

Neglia JP, Robison LL, Stovall M, Liu Y, Packer RJ, Hammond S, Yasui Y, Kasper CE, Mertens AC, Donaldson SS, Meadows AT, Inskip PD (2006) New primary neoplasms of the central nervous system in survivors of childhood cancer: a report from the Childhood Cancer Survivor Study. J Natl Cancer Inst 98(21):1528–1537

Ness KK, Morris EB, Nolan VG, Howell CR, Gilchrist LS, Stovall M, Cox CL, Klosky JL, Gajjar A, Neglia JP (2010) Physical performance limitations among adult survivors of childhood brain tumors. Cancer 116(12):3034–3044. https://doi.org/10.1002/cncr.25051

Ness KK, Krull KR, Jones KE, Mulrooney DA, Armstrong GT, Green DM, Chemaitilly W, Smith WA, Wilson CL, Sklar CA, Shelton K, Srivastava DK, Ali S, Robison LL, Hudson MM (2013) Physiologic frailty as a sign of accelerated aging among adult survivors of childhood cancer: a report from the st jude lifetime cohort study. J Clin Oncol 31(36):4496–4503. https://doi.org/10.1200/JCO.2013.52.2268

Ning MS, Perkins SM, Dewees T, Shinohara ET (2015) Evidence of high mortality in long term survivors of childhood medulloblastoma. J Neuro-Oncol 122(2):321–327. https://doi.org/10.1007/s11060-014-1712-y

Noje C, Cohen K, Jordan LC (2013) Hemorrhagic and ischemic stroke in children with cancer. Pediatr Neurol 49(4):237–242. https://doi.org/10.1016/j.pediatrneurol.2013.04.009

Nolan VG, Gapstur R, Gross CR, Desain LA, Neglia JP, Gajjar A, Klosky JL, Merchant TE, Stovall M, Ness KK (2013) Sleep disturbances in adult survivors of childhood brain tumors. Qual Life Res 22(4):781–789. https://doi.org/10.1007/s11136-012-0208-5

Oberfield SE, Soranno D, Nirenberg A, Heller G, Allen JC, David R, Levine LS, Sklar CA (1996) Age at onset of puberty following high-dose central nervous system radiation therapy. Arch Pediatr Adolesc Med 150(6):589–592

Oeffinger KC, Mertens AC, Sklar CA, Kawashima T, Hudson MM, Meadows AT, Friedman DL, Marina N, Hobbie W, Kadan-Lottick NS, Schwartz CL, Leisenring W, Robison LL (2006) Chronic health conditions in adult survivors of childhood cancer. N Engl J Med 355(15):1572–1582

Ogilvy-Stuart AL, Shalet SM, Gattamaneni HR (1991) Thyroid function after treatment of brain tumors in children. J Pediatr 119(5):733–737

Ojemann JG, Hersonskey TY, Abeshaus S, Geyer JR, Saneto RP, Novotny EJ, Kollros P, Leary S, Holmes MD (2012) Epilepsy surgery after treatment of pediatric malignant brain tumors. Seizure 21(8):624–630. https://doi.org/10.1016/j.seizure.2012.07.003

Packer RJ, Boyett JM, Janss AJ, Stavrou T, Kun L, Wisoff J, Russo C, Geyer R, Phillips P, Kieran M, Greenberg M, Goldman S, Hyder D, Heideman R, Jones-Wallace D, August GP, Smith SH, Moshang T (2001) Growth hormone replacement therapy in children with medulloblastoma: use and effect on tumor control. J Clin Oncol 19(2):480–487

Packer RJ, Gurney JG, Punyko JA, Donaldson SS, Inskip PD, Stovall M, Yasui Y, Mertens AC, Sklar CA, Nicholson HS, Zeltzer LK, Neglia JP, Robison LL (2003) Long-term neurologic and neurosensory sequelae in adult survivors of a childhood brain tumor: childhood cancer survivor study. J Clin Oncol 21(17):3255–3261

Packer RJ, Zhou T, Holmes E, Vezina G, Gajjar A (2013) Survival and secondary tumors in children with medulloblastoma receiving radiotherapy and adjuvant chemotherapy: results of Children's Oncology Group trial A9961. Neuro-Oncology 15(1):97–103. https://doi.org/10.1093/neuonc/nos267

Patterson BC, Chen Y, Sklar CA, Neglia J, Yasui Y, Mertens A, Armstrong GT, Meadows A, Stovall M, Robison LL, Meacham LR (2014) Growth hormone exposure as a risk factor for the development of subsequent neoplasms of the central nervous system: a report from the Childhood Cancer Survivor Study. J Clin Endocrinol Metab 99:2030–2037. https://doi.org/10.1210/jc.2013-4159

Pearce MS, Salotti JA, Little MP, McHugh K, Lee C, Kim KP, Howe NL, Ronckers CM, Rajaraman P, Sir Craft AW, Parker L, Berrington de Gonzalez A (2012) Radiation exposure from CT scans in childhood and subsequent risk of leukaemia and brain tumours: a retrospective cohort study. Lancet 380(9840):499–505. https://doi.org/10.1016/S0140-6736(12)60815-0

Perkins SM, Fei W, Mitra N, Shinohara ET (2013) Late causes of death in children treated for CNS malignancies. J Neuro-Oncol 115(1):79–85. https://doi.org/10.1007/s11060-013-1197-0

Peterson KM, Shao C, McCarter R, MacDonald TJ, Byrne J (2006) An analysis of SEER data of increasing risk of secondary malignant neoplasms among long-term survivors of childhood brain tumors. Pediatr Blood Cancer 47(1):83–88

Pietila S, Korpela R, Lenko HL, Haapasalo H, Alalantela R, Nieminen P, Koivisto AM, Makipernaa A (2012) Neurological outcome of childhood brain tumor survivors. J Neuro-Oncol 108(1):153–161. https://doi.org/10.1007/s11060-012-0816-5

Prados MD, Yung WK, Jaeckle KA, Robins HI, Mehta MP, Fine HA, Wen PY, Cloughesy TF, Chang SM, Nicholas MK, Schiff D, Greenberg HS, Junck L, Fink KL, Hess KR, Kuhn J (2004) Phase 1 trial of irinotecan (CPT-11) in patients with recurrent malignant glioma: a North American Brain Tumor Consortium study. Neuro-Oncology 6(1):44–54. https://doi.org/10.1215/S1152851703000292

Prayson RA (2010) Diagnostic challenges in the evaluation of chronic epilepsy-related surgical neuropathology. Am J Surg Pathol 34(5):e1–e13. https://doi.org/10.1097/PAS.0b013e3181d9ba38

Raman S, Grimberg A, Waguespack SG, Miller BS, Sklar CA, Meacham LR, Patterson BC (2015) Risk of neoplasia in pediatric patients receiving growth hormone therapy—a report from the Pediatric Endocrine Society Drug and Therapeutics Committee. J Clin Endocrinol Metab 100(6):2192–2203. https://doi.org/10.1210/jc.2015-1002

Ramelli GP, von der Weid N, Stanga Z, Mullis PE, Buergi U (1998) Suprasellar germinomas in childhood and adolescence: diagnostic pitfalls. J Pediatr Endocrinol Metab 11(6):693–697

Relling MV, Pui CH, Sandlund JT, Rivera GK, Hancock ML, Boyett JM, Schuetz EG, Evans WE (2000) Adverse effect of anticonvulsants on efficacy of chemotherapy for acute lymphoblastic leukaemia. Lancet 356(9226):285–290. https://doi.org/10.1016/S0140-6736(00)02503-4

Reulen RC, Winter DL, Frobisher C, Lancashire ER, Stiller CA, Jenney ME, Skinner R, Stevens MC, Hawkins MM (2010) Long-term cause-specific mortality among survivors of childhood cancer. JAMA 304(2):172–179. https://doi.org/10.1001/jama.2010.923

Ridola V, Fawaz O, Aubier F, Bergeron C, de Vathaire F, Pichon F, Orbach D, Gentet JC, Schmitt C, Dufour C, Oberlin O (2009) Testicular function of survivors of childhood cancer: a comparative study between ifosfamide- and cyclophosphamide-based regimens. Eur J Cancer 45(5):814–818. https://doi.org/10.1016/j.ejca.2009.01.002

Robbins ME, Zhao W (2004) Chronic oxidative stress and radiation-induced late normal tissue injury: a review. Int J Radiat Biol 80(4):251–259. https://doi.org/10.1080/09553000410001692726

Ron E, Modan B, Boice JD Jr, Alfandary E, Stovall M, Chetrit A, Katz L (1988) Tumors of the brain and nervous system after radiotherapy in childhood. N Engl J Med 319(16):1033–1039

Rose SR, Lustig RH, Pitukcheewanont P, Broome DC, Burghen GA, Li H, Hudson MM, Kun LE, Heideman RL (1999) Diagnosis of hidden central hypothyroidism in survivors of childhood cancer. J Clin Endocrinol Metab 84(12):4472–4479

Rose SR, Danish RK, Kearney NS, Schreiber RE, Lustig RH, Burghen GA, Hudson MM (2005) ACTH deficiency in childhood cancer survivors. Pediatr Blood Cancer 45(6):808–813. https://doi.org/10.1002/pbc.20327

Rosen G, Brand SR (2011) Sleep in children with cancer: case review of 70 children evaluated in a comprehensive pediatric sleep center. Support Care Cancer 19(7):985–994. https://doi.org/10.1007/s00520-010-0921-y

Ruda R, Soffietti R (2015) What is new in the management of epilepsy in gliomas? Curr Treat Options Neurol 17(6):351. https://doi.org/10.1007/s11940-015-0351-8

Ruda R, Bello L, Duffau H, Soffietti R (2012) Seizures in low-grade gliomas: natural history, pathogenesis, and outcome after treatments. Neuro-Oncology 14(Suppl 4):iv55–iv64. https://doi.org/10.1093/neuonc/nos199

Sala A, Barr RD (2007) Osteopenia and cancer in children and adolescents: the fragility of success. Cancer 109(7):1420–1431. https://doi.org/10.1002/cncr.22546

Saper CB (2013) The neurobiology of sleep. Continuum 19(1 Sleep Disorders):19–31. https://doi.org/10.1212/01.CON.0000427215.07715.73

Schmiegelow M, Lassen S, Poulsen HS, Feldt-Rasmussen U, Schmiegelow K, Hertz H, Muller J (2000) Cranial radiotherapy of childhood brain tumours: growth hormone deficiency and its relation to the biological effective dose of irradiation in a large population based study. Clin Endocrinol 53(2):191–197

Schmiegelow M, Lassen S, Poulsen HS, Schmiegelow K, Hertz H, Andersson AM, Skakkebaek NE, Muller J (2001) Gonadal status in male survivors following childhood brain tumors. J Clin Endocrinol Metab 86(6):2446–2452. https://doi.org/10.1210/jcem.86.6.7544

Schmiegelow M, Feldt-Rasmussen U, Rasmussen AK, Poulsen HS, Muller J (2003) A population-based study of thyroid function after radiotherapy and chemotherapy for a childhood brain tumor. J Clin Endocrinol Metab 88(1):136–140. https://doi.org/10.1210/jc.2002-020380

Schriock EA, Lustig RH, Rosenthal SM, Kaplan SL, Grumbach MM (1984) Effect of growth hormone (GH)-releasing hormone (GRH) on plasma GH in relation to magnitude and duration of GH deficiency in 26 children and adults with isolated GH deficiency or multiple pituitary hormone deficiencies: evidence for hypothalamic GRH deficiency. J Clin Endocrinol Metab 58(6):1043–1049. https://doi.org/10.1210/jcem-58-6-1043

Scott RM, Smith JL, Robertson RL, Madsen JR, Soriano SG, Rockoff MA (2004) Long-term outcome in children with moyamoya syndrome after cranial revascularization by pial synangiosis. J Neurosurg 100(2 Suppl Pediatrics):142–149. https://doi.org/10.3171/ped.2004.100.2.0142

Shalet SM, Gibson B, Swindell R, Pearson D (1987) Effect of spinal irradiation on growth. Arch Dis Child 62(5):461–464

Shuper A, Packer RJ, Vezina LG, Nicholson HS, Lafond D (1995) 'Complicated migraine-like episodes' in children following cranial irradiation and chemotherapy. Neurology 45(10):1837–1840

Silfen ME, Garvin JH Jr, Hays AP, Starkman HS, Aranoff GS, Levine LS, Feldstein NA, Wong B, Oberfield SE (2001) Primary central nervous system lymphoma in childhood presenting as progressive panhypopituitarism. J Pediatr Hematol Oncol 23(2):130–133

Sklar CA, Constine LS (1995) Chronic neuroendocrinological sequelae of radiation therapy. Int J Radiat Oncol Biol Phys 31(5):1113–1121

Sklar C, Sarafoglou K, Whittam E (1993) Efficacy of insulin-like growth factor binding protein 3 in predicting the growth hormone response to provocative testing in children treated with cranial irradiation. Acta Endocrinol 129(6):511–515

Sklar CA, Mertens AC, Mitby P, Occhiogrosso G, Qin J, Heller G, Yasui Y, Robison LL (2002) Risk of disease recurrence and second neoplasms in survivors of childhood cancer treated with growth hormone: a report from the Childhood Cancer Survivor Study. J Clin Endocrinol Metab 87(7):3136–3141

Sklar CA, Mertens AC, Mitby P, Whitton J, Stovall M, Kasper C, Mulder J, Green D, Nicholson HS, Yasui Y, Robison LL (2006) Premature menopause in survivors of childhood cancer: a report from the childhood cancer survivor study. J Natl Cancer Inst 98(13):890–896

Stavrou T, Bromley CM, Nicholson HS, Byrne J, Packer RJ, Goldstein AM, Reaman GH (2001) Prognostic factors and secondary malignancies in childhood medulloblastoma. J Pediatr Hematol Oncol 23(7):431–436

Stephen MD, Zage PE, Waguespack SG (2011) Gonadotropin-dependent precocious puberty: neoplastic causes and endocrine considerations. Int J Pediatr Endocrinol 2011:184502. https://doi.org/10.1155/2011/184502

Stewart FA, Heeneman S, Te Poele J, Kruse J, Russell NS, Gijbels M, Daemen M (2006) Ionizing radiation accelerates the development of atherosclerotic lesions in ApoE−/− mice and predisposes to an inflammatory plaque phenotype prone to hemorrhage. Am J Pathol 168(2):649–658. https://doi.org/10.2353/ajpath.2006.050409

Sugihara T, Hattori Y, Yamamoto Y, Qi F, Ichikawa R, Sato A, Liu MY, Abe K, Kanno M (1999) Preferential impairment of nitric oxide-mediated endothelium-dependent relaxation in human cervical arteries after irradiation. Circulation 100(6):635–641

Swerdlow AJ, Reddingius RE, Higgins CD, Spoudeas HA, Phipps K, Qiao Z, Ryder WD, Brada M, Hayward RD, Brook CG, Hindmarsh PC, Shalet SM (2000) Growth hormone treatment of children with brain tumors and risk of tumor recurrence. J Clin Endocrinol Metab 85(12):4444–4449. https://doi.org/10.1210/jcem.85.12.7044

Taylor DD, Potish RA (1985) Late deaths following radiotherapy for pediatric tumors. Am J Clin Oncol 8(6):472–476

Thomas BC, Stanhope R, Plowman PN, Leiper AD (1993) Growth following single fraction and fractionated total body irradiation for bone marrow transplantation. Eur J Pediatr 152(11):888–892

Tsui K, Gajjar A, Li C, Srivastava D, Broniscer A, Wetmore C, Kun LE, Merchant TE, Ellison DW, Orr BA, Boop FA, Klimo P, Ross J, Robison LL, Armstrong GT (2015) Subsequent neoplasms in survivors of childhood central nervous system tumors: risk after modern multimodal therapy. Neuro-Oncology 17(3):448–456. https://doi.org/10.1093/neuonc/nou279

Ullrich NJ, Robertson R, Kinnamon DD, Scott RM, Kieran MW, Turner CD, Chi SN, Goumnerova L, Proctor M, Tarbell NJ, Marcus KJ, Pomeroy SL (2007) Moyamoya following cranial irradiation for primary brain tumors in children. Neurology 68(12):932–938. https://doi.org/10.1212/01.wnl.0000257095.33125.48

Visser J, Hukin J, Sargent M, Steinbok P, Goddard K, Fryer C (2010) Late mortality in pediatric patients with craniopharyngioma. J Neuro-Oncol 100(1):105–111. https://doi.org/10.1007/s11060-010-0145-5

de Vries L, Horev G, Schwartz M, Phillip M (2006) Ultrasonographic and clinical parameters for early differentiation between precocious puberty and premature thelarche. Eur J Endocrinol 154(6):891–898. https://doi.org/10.1530/eje.1.02151

Weinzimer SA, Homan SA, Ferry RJ, Moshang T (1999) Serum IGF-I and IGFBP-3 concentrations do not accurately predict growth hormone deficiency in children with brain tumours. Clin Endocrinol 51(3):339–345

Wells EM, Gaillard WD, Packer RJ (2012) Pediatric brain tumors and epilepsy. Semin Pediatr Neurol 19(1):3–8. https://doi.org/10.1016/j.spen.2012.02.010

Whelan K, Stratton K, Kawashima T, Leisenring W, Hayashi S, Waterbor J, Blatt J, Sklar CA, Packer R, Mitby P, Robison LL, Mertens AC (2011) Auditory complications in childhood cancer survivors: a report from the childhood cancer survivor study. Pediatr Blood Cancer 57(1):126–134. https://doi.org/10.1002/pbc.23025

Wilne S, Collier J, Kennedy C, Koller K, Grundy R, Walker D (2007) Presentation of childhood CNS tumours: a systematic review and meta-analysis. Lancet Oncol 8(8):685–695. https://doi.org/10.1016/S1470-2045(07)70207-3

Yap KY, Chui WK, Chan A (2008) Drug interactions between chemotherapeutic regimens and antiepileptics. Clin Ther 30(8):1385–1407. https://doi.org/10.1016/j.clinthera.2008.08.011

Yuan C, Wu VW, Yip SP, Kwong DL, Ying M (2014) Predictors of the extent of carotid atherosclerosis in patients treated with radiotherapy for nasopharyngeal carcinoma. PLoS One 9(12):e116284. https://doi.org/10.1371/journal.pone.0116284

Yuan C, Yip SP, Wu VW, Kwong DL, Cheuk IW, Ying M (2015) Association between genetic polymorphisms and carotid atherosclerosis in patients treated with radiotherapy for nasopharyngeal carcinoma. Radiat Oncol 10:39. https://doi.org/10.1186/s13014-015-0341-8

Integrating Palliative Care into the Ongoing Care of Children with CNS Tumors

16

16.1 Introduction

Despite significant advances in the treatment of pediatric malignant tumors over the past several decades, cancer remains the leading cause of death by disease for children and adolescents in the United States (Arias et al. 2003). Brain tumors constitute a substantial proportion of childhood malignant neoplasms (Miltenburg et al. 1996), among which they have the highest disease-related mortality rate (Packer 1995). In addition to often facing a poor prognosis, children with brain cancer suffer from a distinct and significant constellation of symptoms secondary to both the primary disease and the acute and persistent sequelae of treatment (Hendricks-Ferguson 2008; Lannering et al. 1990), and these symptoms adversely affect the quality of life for both patients and their families (Wolfe et al. 2008). Additionally, the negative effects on the parents' long-term emotional and psychological well-being of inadequate communication and the insensitive delivery of bad news are well documented (Contro et al. 2004), and doctor–patient communication and continuity of care have been characterized as markers of high-quality physician care (Mack et al. 2005).

Palliative care for children is the active total care of the child's body, mind, and spirit while giving additional support to the family. This approach uses early identification and treatment of sources of physical, psychosocial, and spiritual distress to prevent and relieve suffering in patients with life-threatening illnesses and their families. The integration of palliative care principles and practices should begin when a serious disorder is diagnosed and should continue throughout the course of illness, regardless of whether or not a child receives treatment directed at the disease. The National Quality Forum (NQF), the Institute of Medicine (IOM), and the National Institutes of Health have identified palliative and end-of-life care as a national priority and have proposed that palliative care should be a key component of high-quality medical care for children with advanced illness. The NQF has outlined preferred practices to ensure that high-quality palliative care is provided (National Quality Forum 2006), and defined the role of the palliative care clinician and team to include addressing issues such as anticipatory counseling for end-of-life symptoms, symptom control, and emotional, social, spiritual, and bereavement care. This NQF-recommended interdisciplinary approach needs to be integrated early in the treatment process so that the interdisciplinary palliative care team can integrate with the primary oncology team as both work to support families and patients in defining goals of care near the end

J. N. Baker
Division of Quality of Life and Palliative Care,
Department of Oncology, St Jude Children's
Research Hospital, Memphis, TN, USA
e-mail: justin.baker@stjude.org

© Springer International Publishing AG, part of Springer Nature 2018
A. Gajjar et al. (eds.), *Brain Tumors in Children*, https://doi.org/10.1007/978-3-319-43205-2_16

379

of life and in determining the type of care that can best meet those goals.

Pediatric palliative care (PPC) has emerged as a multidisciplinary strategy to address and ease the suffering of children with life-threatening illness, as well as provide psychosocial support for their families (Waldman and Wolfe 2013), and there is a clear, growing recognition of the importance of integrating palliative care early as part of the overall management of children with cancer (Mack and Wolfe 2006). Experience and research demonstrate that children with cancer who receive optimal integrated palliative care have improved symptom control and experience less suffering (Pritchard et al. 2008; van der Geest et al. 2014; Zelcer et al. 2010). In light of accumulating data in support of PPC and strong recommendations from the IOM, the American Academy of Pediatrics (AAP), and the American Society of Clinical Oncology (ASCO), the early integration of PPC for children with especially life-threatening cancers and their families should be considered best practice within the field of pediatric neuro-oncology. Moreover, parents of children with cancer and other life-threatening conditions who are enrolled in PPC report significant improvements in their own quality of life, with decreased parental reporting of self-perceived burden and psychological stress (Groh et al. 2013a, 2013b). Even healthcare providers report significant improvements in all care domains after PPC is integrated into the care of complex patients before the end of life, particularly in the areas of cooperation, communication, and family support (Vollenbroich et al. 2012). Moreover, integrating PPC into the ongoing care of patients with high-risk disease across different care settings has been identified by PPC expert clinicians and researchers, parents of children with life-threatening illness, and bereaved parents as one of the top five research priorities that are integral to improving the quality of care for children with high-risk disease (Baker et al. 2015). Integrating high-quality PPC is particularly critical for individual practitioners or an institution caring for children with high-risk malignant CNS tumors. These children represent an especially vulnerable cohort, and early inte-

gration of palliative care is essential to manage their symptoms, coordinate the complex management required, and support their families in making difficult decisions throughout the illness trajectory and towards the end of life (Wolfe et al. 2008). Leaders in the field of PPC have advocated that an ideal model for compassionate care involves the early integration of palliative care principles by the primary neuro-oncology team in conjunction with parallel involvement of a subspecialty palliative care team, with both parties journeying cooperatively with the patient and family from the time of diagnosis to the end of life (Friebert and Osenga 2009).

In this chapter, the principles and practices that facilitate the integration of key palliative care concepts into the paradigm of caring for children with malignant CNS tumors will be described and discussed.

16.2 Models for Integrating Pediatric Palliative Care into Pediatric Neuro-Oncology

The individualized care planning and coordination (ICPC) model outlined in Fig. 16.1 was designed to facilitate the integration of PPC principles into the pediatric oncology paradigm (Baker et al. 2007, 2008; Kane and Himelstein 2007). The goal of individualized care planning is to value patient and family experiences and to use a patient- and family-centered approach to information delivery and needs assessment, thus enhancing communication about difficult issues by discerning the values and priorities of the patient and family before a crisis occurs or critical decision points are reached. Applying the ICPC model helps patients, families, and clinicians negotiate care options under uncertain conditions by assessing the patient's and family's understanding of the prognosis, elucidating their goals of care, and allowing them to choose from the available goal-directed treatment alternatives. At no time is use of the ICPC model more important than when caring for children with high-risk brain tumors, especially those who may die from their disease or its treatments.

Fig. 16.1 The individualized care planning and coordination (ICPC) model of care

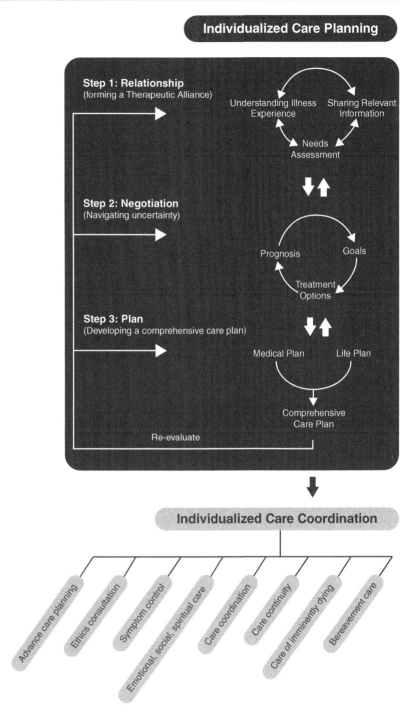

The provision of PPC for children with cancer has been described as "the total care of a child and family" (Waldman and Wolfe 2013). We believe that this total care philosophy should be guided by the primary oncology team, with collaboration from interdisciplinary clinicians and expert consultants as needed (Von Roenn 2011). Pediatric palliative care principles should be rooted in the culture of an institution (including formalized support of PPC education, policies, and resources), and should be integrated into patient care using specified mechanisms of support in predefined (trigger-based) or particularly challenging circumstances, as well as expert teams for consultation as needed (Fig. 16.2). In this system, the three tiers of PPC services function synergistically to maximize early provision of PPC to children with high-risk cancer and their families. We advocate that primary oncology teams should deliver the core elements of PPC from the time of diagnosis (Von Roenn 2011; von Gunten 2002) (e.g., symptom management and alignment of goals of care with treatment), reserving early subspecialty consultation for predefined high-risk scenarios (e.g., uniformly fatal diseases such as diffuse intrinsic pontine glioma or high-grade glioma) or more complex situations (e.g., managing refractory symptoms; mediating contentious or otherwise challenging family dynamics; or negotiating difficult conversations, such as those surrounding the discontinuation of life-sustaining therapies that are no longer beneficial, in which discordance emerges between the goals of patients/families and those of providers) (Quill and Abernethy 2013; Wentlandt et al. 2014). To capture a wider range of patients, PPC principles should emerge from the ground up, ideally being woven seamlessly into each aspect of the interdisciplinary care model. This may be achieved through institutionally supported didactics for nursing staff (ELNEC-Peds) (Ferrell et al. 2015), through cancer-specific PPC training models for clinicians, or by

embedding trained experts within outpatient and inpatient care settings to provide additional guidance and education as needed (Fig. 16.3) (Kaye et al. 2015).

Pediatric palliative care referral criteria for children were established through the Center to Advance Palliative Care (Friebert and Osenga 2009) and further modified for use in the pediatric oncology context (Kaye et al. 2015). The criteria offer optional guidelines for pediatric oncology teams to consider when triaging those patients and families who might benefit from early integration of PPC teams. Pediatric palliative care should be introduced early into the holistic cancer care plan for a child with a high-risk malignant CNS tumor, with the simple goal of familiarizing the child and family with basic PPC concepts and resources. The aims of this strategy, from the perspective of the patient and family, are threefold: (1) to establish the groundwork for PPC resources offered in parallel with cancer-directed therapy; (2) to demonstrate a collaborative partnership between the primary oncology team and PPC clinicians from the outset, with the mutual goal of supporting both the child and the family throughout the illness trajectory; and (3) to normalize PPC concepts for the child, family, and other members of the interdisciplinary team, thereby preempting stigmatizing language and other preconceived barriers to providing PPC. Additionally, with early PPC involvement, there are more opportunities for the child and family to benefit from

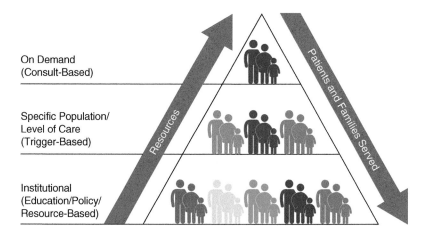

Fig. 16.2 Levels of integration of pediatric palliative care into oncology

On Demand
(Consult-Based)

Specific Population/
Level of Care
(Trigger-Based)

Institutional
(Education/Policy/
Resource-Based)

Resources

Patients and Families Served

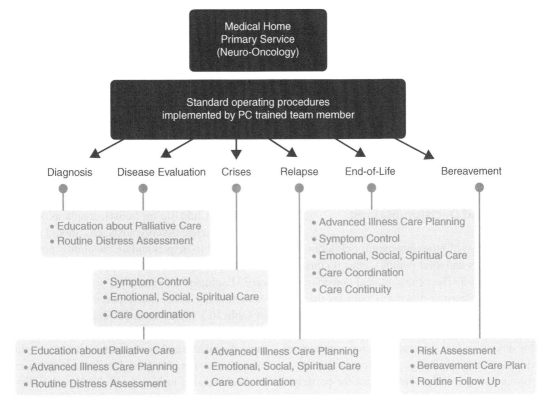

Fig. 16.3 The embedded expert model of pediatric palliative care

the continuity of care that PPC offers, including a range of flexible services and resources to link inpatient and outpatient care (Mack and Wolfe 2006; Kaye et al. 2015).

16.3 Barriers to Integrating Pediatric Palliative Care

Despite the increasing awareness of palliative care and support for its integration into the field of pediatric oncology, it is important to acknowledge that many patients, families, and healthcare providers retain the false perception of palliative care and disease-directed or cure-oriented therapy as being mutually exclusive (Davies et al. 2008; Knapp and Thompson 2012; Dalberg et al. 2013). As a result of this misconception, PPC is often offered at the end of an illness trajectory when no further curative or life-prolonging options exist. This phenomenon is particularly evident in the field of pediatric oncology, in

which the involvement of palliative care teams may be viewed as "giving up" (Dalberg et al. 2013). When PPC principles are introduced only late in the illness course, the patient and family are more likely to perceive PPC in a negative light, risking a fracturing of the therapeutic alliance. Two primary factors contribute to this adverse outcome: (1) after receiving extensive treatment and attention from the primary oncology team, the patient and family may perceive PPC consultation as representing abandonment by their primary caregivers; and/or (2) the patient and family might view the PPC team as a "second-best" resource employed as a last-resort strategy after all "real" diagnostic and treatment options have been exhausted. Patients and families with these perceptions may be more likely to have difficulty partnering with PPC clinicians to work collaboratively towards ameliorating symptoms or participating willingly in difficult decision-making processes. Pediatric palliative care should not be exclusive to the dying process;

rather, the goal is to honor the process of living in the face of childhood cancer. With this philosophy in mind, it stands to reason that the integration of palliative care into the ongoing care of children with malignant CNS tumors can and should begin at the time of diagnosis of high-risk disease and not be reserved exclusively for disease relapse, progression, or the end of life.

16.4 Ethical Considerations, Communication, and Decision-Making

In the context of providing care for children with brain tumors and their families, ethical considerations abound. The central ethical consideration of medical decision-making is built on the core palliative care concept of excellent communication. The majority of children with brain tumors by definition lack the capacity for autonomous decision-making, though children as young as 7 years of age can provide assent for participation, and assent is strongly recommended for enrolling adolescents in clinical research (Varma et al. 2008; Wiener et al. 2008). In clinical medicine, however, there is no standard for involving children in medical decision-making, even at critical junctures such as the end of life. Furthermore, there is no standard for advanced care planning with pediatric patients. Many advocate age-appropriate involvement of children in medical decision-making, especially at the end of life, by using developmentally appropriate means of communication (Bluebond-Langner et al.

2010). It is clear that children as young as 6 years of age can actively participate in complex end-of-life decision-making and play an influential role in those decisions when their preferences are considered (Hinds et al. 2005a; Nitschke et al. 2000; Nitschke 2000). Therefore, great attention should be paid to the child's preferences when working with children with malignant CNS tumors. A multidisciplinary approach to involving the child and promoting his/her participation in medical decision-making provides the greatest opportunity for successfully including the child's viewpoint. Child life specialists, chaplains, social workers, nurses, psychologists, etc. should all be encouraged to help elucidate the child's point of view and integrate it into the complex plan of care. Examples of empathic, exploratory, and validating questions and responses are presented in Table 16.1 (Baker et al. 2007).

Parents are the presumed decision-makers for these ill children and, in most cases, have the right to make decisions for them. Parental autonomy in medical decision-making for children with malignant CNS tumors is based on the premise that a child's parents are best able to judge what is in the child's best interest (Levine et al. 2012). With regard to decision-making for a child with incurable cancer, parents' choices are likely to be shaped by their own internal definition of being a "good parent to their ill child." This has been broadly defined as "one who makes informed, unselfish decisions in the child's best interest, meets the child's basic needs, remains at the child's side, shows the child love, protects the child's health, prevents suffering, teaches the child

Table 16.1 Examples of empathic, exploratory, and validating responses

Empathic statements	Exploratory questions	Validating responses
"I can see how upsetting this is to you."	"How do you mean?"	"I can understand how you felt that way."
"I can tell you weren't expecting to hear this."	"Tell me more about it."	"I guess anyone might have that same reaction."
"I know this is not good news for you."	"Could you explain what you mean?"	"You were perfectly correct to think that way."
"I'm sorry to have to tell you this."	"You said it frightened you?"	"Yes, your understanding of the reason for the tests is very good."
"This is very difficult for me also."	"Could you tell me what you're worried about?"	"It appears that you've thought things through very well."
"I was also hoping for a better result."	"Now, you said you were concerned about your children. Tell me more."	"Many other patients have had a similar experience."

moral values, and advocates for the child" (Hinds et al. 2009; Maurer et al. 2010). Considering that parents bear the burden of caring for their child and will be the most affected by the child's outcome, one question is whether weighing their own interests and those of the family can lead parents to make decisions that might not be solely in the child's best interest. Some maintain that it is well within the parents' rights to decide on behalf of their child while considering the interests of all affected members. Provided that parents are not clearly neglectful, are choosing within the range of medically acceptable options, and are not exposing the child to undue risk of harm, they are generally given broad latitude as the decision-makers for their children (Diekema 2004). Data demonstrate, however, that parents typically do not wish to bear the sole burden of medical decision-making and prefer to make medical decisions on behalf of their children in collaboration with their child's physicians (Mack et al. 2011; Pyke-Grimm et al. 1999).

The model of shared medical decision-making involves physicians presenting parents with a range of medically acceptable options and helping the family to prioritize them and choose a mutually agreeable plan (Levine et al. 2012). Building a relationship with the family and establishing trust is essential to arriving at medically sound and goal-directed care for each patient. Collaborative communication in this phase is critical for establishing clarity, understanding common goals, and developing mutual respect between the physician and the family (Feudtner 2007). Clear and concise language, as well as full prognostic disclosure, can increase clarity and comprehension while maintaining hope (Mack et al. 2007). Communication that is both informative and marked by active listening and sensitivity is associated with increased parental satisfaction with their role in the decision-making process. Developmentally appropriate communication with the pediatric patient, eliciting both the patient's preferences and their assent, is an important component of this process (Klick et al. 2014; Klick and Hauer 2010). For an adolescent or young adult patient, inclusion in medical decision-making, as well as open communication, is especially important in order to demonstrate respect for their desire for self-determination and enhance their overall care (Freyer 2004; Weaver et al. 2015).

Despite the earlier integration of palliative care and the emphasis on advance care planning, the process of caring for children at the end of life is not always without conflict. Occasionally, conflict may occur between family members, between staff, or between family members and staff about the goals of care or which treatments are in the best interest of the child. Conflicts may be highly emotional and result in moral distress. Often, these conflicts are the result of a breakdown in communication rather than a true ethical dilemma. Palliative care teams, with their expertise in family communication and shared decision-making, can often meet with individual family members or hold family care conferences and work through perceived conflicts about goals of care. Clinical ethics consultation may be helpful for difficult cases in which interdisciplinary team meetings or family care conferences have not resolved disagreements or in which a true ethical dilemma is felt to exist. When conflicts over goals of care occur within the care team and result in moral distress among clinical staff, ethics consultation can facilitate communication among the interdisciplinary team. This may be particularly helpful when the conflict involves ancillary staff who may feel excluded from primary decision-making. Clinical ethics consultations can help resolve conflicts, educate clinical staff on ethical issues, and provide a forum for discussing hospital policies (Johnson et al. 2015). Ethics consultations can often be used for "curbside" advice and can offer an opinion on the utility of a formal consultation. An ethics consultation may provide some reassurance for the family and staff when a medical decision involves a rarely used intervention (e.g., palliative sedation or withdrawal of artificial nutrition and hydration after a severe traumatic brain injury).

Life-sustaining medical treatments include all interventions that may prolong the life of a patient. They can range from technologically complex treatments (e.g., the use of a ventilator, dialysis, or vasoactive drugs) to less complex measures (e.g., antibiotics, insulin, or artificial nutrition and hydration) (Diekema and Botkin

2009). The decision to initiate, continue, or withdraw life-sustaining medical treatment most commonly involves a consideration of the benefits and burdens of the therapy in the context of the preferences and goals of the child and family. The *ability* to provide life-sustaining medical treatments (such as artificial nutrition and hydration) is not an *obligation* to do so, especially if the burdens of therapy are greater than the perceived benefits. It may be appropriate to limit or stop a life-sustaining medical treatment if it only preserves biological existence or if the goals of care have shifted from life prolongation to comfort-directed care (American Academy of Pediatrics Committee on Bioethics 1994). When the risk–benefit ratio of an intervention is unclear, a timed trial may be beneficial; the life-sustaining treatment can later be withdrawn if it fails to achieve the desired outcome. Withdrawing a life-sustaining medical treatment is ethically equivalent to withholding the treatment and is permissible if the treatment is not compatible with the goals of care, even if the withdrawal results in death. Discontinuing nonbeneficial life-sustaining medical treatments is within the scope of the parents' decision-making authority and should not be viewed as being inconsistent with a child's best interests. Clinicians who cannot participate in forgoing life-sustaining medical treatments must notify the family about their position and arrange for the transfer of care to another physician or care provider (American Academy of Pediatrics Committee on Bioethics 1994). Clinicians should override family wishes only when these wishes are in conflict with the best interests of the child. Clinical ethics consultation and input from other clinicians, such as palliative care specialists, is advisable in cases of conflict.

16.5　Symptom Management for Children with Malignant CNS Tumors

Caring for a child with cancer is difficult and emotionally charged, and few things are more heartrending than the suffering of a vulnerable young patient ravaged by cancer and its treatment. Integrating palliative care principles and practices into the mainstream of pediatric oncology programs requires appropriate attention to expected and unexpected symptoms from the point of diagnosis forward. The timely and skilled management of pain and symptoms is the cornerstone of palliation in the care of children facing life-threatening conditions (Himelstein et al. 2004). These symptoms may be disease-related, treatment-related, or both. The voice of the child has been noted as telling us that distressing symptoms are highly prevalent and of a high intensity level while the child is undergoing cancer treatment (Collins et al. 2000; Collins et al. 2002). The pediatric pain literature clearly demonstrates that "there is no such thing as a little stick" and that the effects of underdiagnosed and undertreated pain, as well as unrelieved procedural pain, are long lasting (Weisman et al. 1998; Berde and Sethna 2002). The same may be the case for many other symptoms that are yet to be studied in this manner. Furthermore, proper symptom management and attention to the suffering of children dying a cancer-related death must be comprehensively addressed, as pain and other symptoms continue to be prevalent and distressing in this setting (Goldman et al. 2006; Wolfe et al. 2000). The assessment and management of symptoms, including pain, are guided by age-adapted tools and principles, as well as by specific therapeutic parameters. In many cases, symptoms are not adequately addressed in pediatric patients with malignant CNS tumors (Hendricks-Ferguson 2008; Liben et al. 2008). The following briefly summarizes the symptoms that children with CNS tumors experience and provides clinical pearls for addressing them.

16.6　Pain

Pain is "an unpleasant sensory and emotional experience associated with actual or potential tissue damage, or described in terms of such damage" (Mack et al. 2011). Pain is subjective in nature. The experience of pain can be modulated by environmental, developmental, behavioral, psychological, familial, or cultural factors. Many children with malignant CNS tumors experience pain at some time during their course. Failure to relieve this pain can produce fear, mistrust, irritability, impaired coping, and other issues. Parents feel guilt and anger when pain is undertreated, and this may even lead them to consider euthanasia as a preferable alternative to watching their child's suffering (Dussel et al. 2010).

Clinical pearls

- Assessment is key
  Elements of the pain assessment should include the quality of the pain, its region and radiation, its severity, temporal factors, and provocative and palliative factors. Additional historical elements include the disease stage and context, fear of pain, the ability to take medication, prior analgesic use, the potential role of disease-specific treatment, the reactions of parents and family context, and other nonpain symptoms, including depression and/or anxiety, sleep disturbance, and, most importantly, interference with activities of daily life, including play.
- Identify the mechanism and pathophysiology of the pain
  Pain can be defined as either nociceptive or neuropathic; nociceptive pain can be further categorized as visceral or somatic pain. Mixed patterns of pain are common in the setting of metastatic solid malignant tumors, particularly when the tumors are invading nerves or nerve roots (Haanpää et al. 2011). Correctly assessing and characterizing pain may help in determining the appropriate first- and second-line treatments.
- Employ a stepwise approach using medications with different mechanisms of action
  In general, pain management should follow the World Health Organization's revised two-step approach, with low doses of a strong opioid for moderate pain. Medications for pain should be administered according to a regular schedule, with rescue doses being provided for intermittent or severe breakthrough pain. Pain medications should be given via the appropriate route for adequate treatment of pain, with frequent reassessment of the effectiveness of the medication, dose, and route of administration, and with tailoring of the treatment to meet the needs of the individual child. In general, the least invasive, most effective, and least painful

route of administration is to be preferred, making oral administration recommended if possible. When the oral route is unavailable, safe or effective alternative routes should be considered based on clinical judgment, preparation availability, and patient and family preference. Alternative routes include intravenous, subcutaneous, rectal, or transdermal administration. Intramuscular injections should be avoided in children, as they are associated with additional pain and may cause fear and anxiety, leading to children not requesting or receiving appropriate medications.

Pharmacologic management pearls

Opioids remain the mainstay of pain treatment in children with malignant CNS tumors. However, throughout the course of illness, nonpharmacologic options and nonopioid medications should be considered in addition to opioids. Nonopioid analgesics include acetaminophen, nonsteroidal anti-inflammatory drugs (NSAIDs), and selective cyclooxygenase 2 (COX-2) inhibitors. In children and adolescents who can take oral medications, acetaminophen and ibuprofen are the most frequently used nonopioid medications (Table 16.2).

- Adjuvant medications and neuropathic pain pharmacologic management pearls
  The term "adjuvant medications" refers to medications with a primary indication for pain and with analgesic properties in certain clinical circumstances; they have different mechanisms of action and are given in combination with analgesics to enhance and augment pain relief. The most commonly used adjuvant medications for pain in pediatrics are those used in treating neuropathic pain or specific disease-related pain, such as bone pain or pain associated with bladder, bowel, or muscle spasms. The medication algorithm and the order of medications used in treating neuropathic pain at our institution is as follows: (1) anticonvulsants (gabapentin, pregabalin); (2) tricyclic antidepressants (amitriptyline, nortriptyline); (3) methadone; and (4) other pharmacologic interventions (ketamine infusion, lidocaine infusion).

Table 16.2 Common medications and dosing in pediatric palliative care

Symptom	Medication	Pediatric dose (<60 kg)		Max. daily dose
Pain	Acetaminophen (mild pain)	10–15 mg/kg orally every 4–6 h		75 mg/kg/24 h
	Ibuprofen (mild pain)	5–10 mg/kg orally every 6–8 h		40 mg/kg/24 h
	Oxycodone	0.1 mg/kg/dose orally every 4 h		Patient dependent
	Morphine	0.3 mg/kg orally, SL, or PR every 3–4 h		Patient dependent
		0.1 mg/kg IV every 2–4 h		
	Sustained-release opioids (chronic severe pain)			
	Opioid/route	**Available dosages**		**Dosage frequency**
	Morphine (Kadian®)	10, 20, 30, 50 mg		Every 12 or 24 h
	Oxycodone/PO (Oxycontin®)	10, 20, 40, 80 mg		Every 12 h
	Fentanyl/transdermal (Duragesic® patches)	12.5, 25, 50, 75, 100 µg/h		Every 72 h
	Gabapentin (neuropathic pain)	Initially 5–10 mg/kg per day divided TID. Increase dose every 3 days		70 mg/kg/24 h or 3600 mg/24 h
	Amitriptyline (adjunct for neuropathic pain)	0.1 mg/kg orally at bedtime. Increase dose by doubling every 3–5 days		1 mg/kg/24 h
	PCA (severe pain)			
	Opioid	**Infusion**	**Boost dose**	**Interval between boosts**
	Morphine	0.02 mg/kg/h	0.02 mg/kg	15 min
	Hydromorphone	0.004 mg/kg/h	0.004 mg/kg	15 min
	Fentanyl	0.5 µg/kg/h	0.5 µg/kg	15 min
Symptom	**Medication**	**Pediatric dose (<60 kg)**		**Max. daily dose**
Constipation	Glycerin	<6 years: one infant suppository, one to two times or 2–5 mL as an enema		2 doses/day
		≥6 years: one adult suppository one to two times or 5–15 mL as an enema		
	Lactulose (can be diluted in water, juices, or milk)	<12 years: 7.5 mL orally; may be repeated after 2 h		60 mL/day
		>12 years: 15–30 mL orally; may be repeated after 2 h		
	Polyethylene glycol (mix in 4–8 oz. liquid)	½ to 1 packet (17 g) orally every day up to TID dosing		3 packets/day
	Docusate/senna (Senna-S)	2–6 years: ½ tab daily		1 tab BID
		6–12 years: 1 tab daily		2 tabs BID
		≥12 years: 2 tabs daily		4 tabs BID
Nausea/ vomiting	Ondansetron	0.15 mg/kg orally or IV every 6–8 h		8 mg/dose
	Promethazine	>2 years: 0.25 mg/kg/dose every 6–8 h orally or IV		1 mg/kg/24 h
	Scopolamine (transdermal)	8–15 kg: ½ patch every 3 days >15 kg: 1 patch every 3 days		1 patch every 3 days
Secretions	Hyoscyamine	2–12 years: 0.0625–0.125 mg orally or SL every 4 h		2–12 years: 0.75 mg/24 h
		>12 years: 0.125–0.25 mg orally or SL every 4 h		>12 years: 1.5 mg/24 h
	Glycopyrrolate	0.04–0.1 mg/kg orally every 4–8 h		1–2 mg/dose or 8 mg/day

Table 16.2 (continued)

Symptom	Medication	Pediatric dose (<60 kg)	Max. daily dose
Delirium Agitation	Haloperidol	0.01–0.02 mg/kg orally, SL, or PR every 8–12 h	0.15 mg/kg/day
Agitation Anxiety Seizures	Lorazepam	0.05 mg/kg orally, SL (preferred for seizure), or PR every 4–6 h	2 mg/dose
Pruritus	Diphenhydramine	0.5–1.0 mg/kg orally every 6–8 h	5 mg/kg/24 h or 400 mg/24 h
	Hydroxyzine	0.5–1.0 mg/kg orally every 6–8 h	4 mg/kg/24 h

Nonpharmacologic pain management

Psychosocial interventions represent an important approach to pain management throughout the course of treatment for children with malignant CNS tumors. These interventions are aimed at empowering the patient to gain a sense of control over their pain and decrease the experience and perception of pain. These techniques are adjuncts to appropriate analgesics for pain management. Psychosocial interventions can help alleviate pain by influencing how one interprets and experiences painful events and bodily sensations. Cognitive techniques focus primarily on altering how the patient thinks about, reacts to, and physically experiences pain, changing how the patient reacts to painful stimuli (by increasing pain tolerance while decreasing pain sensation). Behavioral approaches help the patient employ techniques and skills that alter the body's response to pain. When cognitive and behavioral techniques are combined, they form a highly effective treatment program. To be maximally effective, these techniques should be introduced early in the course of the pain management. Behavioral methods, such as deep breathing (blowing bubbles), progressive relaxation, and biofeedback, have a role in pain management for children. Physical methods, such as touch therapies (including massage), transcutaneous electrical nerve stimulation, physical therapy, heat/cold therapy, and acupuncture and/or acupressure, are helpful adjuncts. Cognitive modalities, including distraction, music, art, play, imagery, and hypnosis, are also effective in children. Studies have demonstrated the efficacy of many of these modalities alone or in combination with pharmacologic therapies (Mercadante and Giarratano 2014; Uman et al. 2013).

16.7 Dyspnea

Dyspnea is a term used to describe a feeling of breathlessness. It is a distressing symptom for children and their families and can be a major detriment to comfort and quality of life in advanced disease. In many cases, dyspnea is also associated with shorter survival. Measurement of dyspnea is difficult, as it is subjective and does not correlate well with respiratory rate, work of breathing, or oxygen level.

Clinical pearls

- Care of patients with dyspnea typically involves treating the underlying cause, if possible, and providing oxygen and/or oral and/or parenteral opiates and/or benzodiazepines (Ben-Aharon et al. 2008).
- Some patients may benefit from using a fan to blow cold air on their face, pulmonary rehabilitation, or chest physiotherapy to mobilize secretions (Bausewein et al. 2008).
- The use of supplemental oxygen has not been found to be more beneficial than air inhalation in adults with end-stage dyspnea, but there are no studies supporting the use of supplemental oxygen in children with malignant CNS tumors at the end of life. Clinical experience suggests that this treatment has additional psychological benefits for the parents and/or caregivers of the sick child.

16.8 Gastrointestinal Symptoms

Gastrointestinal symptoms are commonly seen in children with malignant CNS tumors. These include nausea and vomiting, constipation, and anorexia-cachexia syndrome. These symptoms cause considerable distress and diminish function and quality of life (Santucci and Mack 2007).

16.8.1 Nausea and Vomiting

Nausea may manifest as inactivity, weakness, irritability, and poor appetite. In older children, self-report is the preferred method of assessment. Nausea and vomiting in children with malignant CNS tumors may be secondary to medications (i.e., chemotherapy administration), gastrointestinal illness, such as gastroenteritis, constipation, gastric stasis, ileus, or obstruction, or increased intracranial pressure, as well as many other etiologies. Anticipatory nausea and vomiting may reflect the presence of anxiety and stress.

Clinical pearls

- Prokinetic agents, such as metoclopramide, are useful in treating ileus and intestinal hypomotility.
- Antihistamines (e.g., diphenhydramine, meclizine), phenothiazines (e.g., promethazine, chlorpromazine), and butyrophenones (e.g., haloperidol) are useful in treating centrally mediated nausea and vomiting.
- 5-HT3 antagonists (ondansetron and granisetron) are the treatment of choice for chemotherapy- and radiation therapy-induced and postoperative nausea and vomiting.
- Adding an oral neurokinin-1 antagonist, such as aprepitant, can provide superior protection against nausea and vomiting caused by highly emetogenic chemotherapy (Hesketh et al. 2003).
- Corticosteroids have intrinsic antiemetic properties and potentiate the effect of other antiemetics.
- Cannabinoids have antiemetic properties and may be beneficial to some pediatric patients.
- Benzodiazepines may reduce anxiety and the likelihood of anticipatory nausea.
- Nondrug measures for palliating nausea and vomiting that may enhance the effect of antiemetic drugs include acupuncture, psychological techniques, and transcutaneous electrical nerve stimulation (Burish and Tope 1992).

16.8.2 Constipation

Constipation may be defined as the passage of small, hard feces infrequently and with difficulty. Constipation can often be traced to an organic source, and the etiology should be investigated. On physical examination, clay-like masses may be palpated in a partially distended abdomen. Opioids, vincristine, and drugs with anticholinergic effects, such as phenothiazines and tricyclic antidepressants, may cause constipation. Other causes include malignant intestinal obstructions and metabolic conditions, such as dehydration and hypercalcemia. A spinal cord metastasis or other neuromuscular dysfunction may also be associated with constipation. Opioid-induced constipation is extremely common in children with malignant CNS tumors and results from the action of these medications on the peripheral mu receptors in the gastrointestinal tract. This action triggers delayed gastric emptying via constriction of the pyloric sphincter, decreased peristalsis and increased absorption of water and electrolytes from the gastrointestinal tract, and increased anal sphincter tone, all of which contribute to constipation development (Kyle 2011).

Clinical pearls

- Prophylactic measures are the first line of intervention. Prevention is the key concept when discussing constipation management.
- Mobility, adequate fluid intake, and increased fiber in the diet are helpful.
- Patients with hard stools can receive laxatives with a predominately softening action, such as lactulose or docusate sodium.
- A peristalsis-stimulating agent, such as senna or bisacodyl, can be combined with laxatives for improved effect.
- Osmotic laxatives, such as polyethylene glycol or magnesium citrate, can also be used in symptomatic children with severe constipation (Stevens et al. 1994).
- Prophylactic therapy is necessary for patients receiving opioids. Remember, prevention is the key.
- Methylnaltrexone has proven helpful in the treatment of opioid-induced constipation

(Laubisch and Baker 2013). This medication reacts only with gastrointestinal tract mu receptors, thus allowing analgesia centrally but lessening peripheral side effects. It is indicated for children who have opioid-induced constipation and cannot tolerate oral medications.

16.8.3 Anorexia and Cachexia

In patients with advanced disease, anorexia-cachexia syndrome often correlates with poor quality of life and poor outcome. Patients with anorexia-cachexia have diminished caloric intake, increased basal energy expenditure, progressive loss of lean body mass, and weight loss. Although decreased oral intake is often a natural development at the end of life, it can cause distress for children and their families because of the social associations of food preparation and eating (Santucci and Mack 2007). The underlying cause should be delineated in order to choose appropriate treatment, if indicated.

Clinical pearls

- Cyproheptadine can be used as an appetite stimulant and has proven helpful in preventing further weight loss in children with cancer-associated cachexia (Couluris et al. 2008).
- Corticosteroids and cannabinoids may also have a therapeutic role in some patients.
- Although a hypercaloric diet is not sufficient to reverse the syndrome, enteral nutritional supplementation may be appropriate in some cases.
- Parenteral nutrition support may be appropriate for patients in whom nutritional support is required for a short period of time or in patients for whom the enteral route is not feasible.

nature and the lack of confirmed physiologic or laboratory indicators. Symptoms of fatigue may include physical weakness, mental exhaustion, disruption of sleep, reduced energy, emotional withdrawal, decreased play, or reduced participation in usual activities. Some medications, including chemotherapeutic regimens used in treating cancer, can cause fatigue and generalized weakness (Bradshaw et al. 2005). Common causes of prolonged fatigue, such as anemia, hypothyroidism, sleep disturbances, anxiety, and depression, among others, should be excluded. A good history and physical examination may point to other potential causes that may respond to therapy.

Clinical pearls

- Treatment should be directed at the medical or psychiatric condition that is most likely associated with the fatigue.
- A gradual increase in exercise and rehabilitation may be helpful.
- Cognitive-behavioral approaches may also be an effective counseling technique to assist the child in switching to a more adaptive coping strategy.
- Reintegration with peer and school activities is recommended.
- The use of drugs has not been explored well in children. Steroids, transfusion of blood products, recombinant erythropoietin, and methylphenidate have been used in the treatment of fatigue with varying results (Mock et al. 2007).
- For children who are oversedated from opioid administration, adding adjuvant medications (see above) may permit dose reductions. Additionally, psychostimulants, such as methylphenidate or dexamphetamine, have been used empirically to improve quality of life.

16.9 Fatigue

Fatigue is one of the most prevalent symptoms in children dying with cancer (Dans et al. 2017). It is a nonspecific symptom that is difficult to measure and describe because of its subjective

16.10 Neurologic Symptoms

Some of the more common and distressing neurologic symptoms in children with malignant CNS tumors include seizures, headaches, sleep disturbances, and delirium.

16.10.1 Seizures

Seizures are often caused by primary or metastatic brain lesions or metabolic disturbances. They may also develop as a side effect of chemotherapy, radiotherapy, or medications. Maintenance medications are appropriate for children known to have seizures; for children who are at risk for seizures, it should be planned to have at least one anticonvulsant available in the home.

Clinical pearls

- For children who are unable to take medications orally, as is usually the case during a generalized seizure, it is possible to administer several agents by alternative routes: rectally for valproic acid, phenytoin, pentobarbital, lorazepam, and diazepam; sublingually for lorazepam; subcutaneously for midazolam and phenobarbital; and intramuscularly for fosphenytoin, phenobarbital, and lorazepam.
- Rectal diazepam gel provides premeasured medication in a convenient dose delivery device; its efficacy and safety in children have been demonstrated in randomized clinical trials (Dreifuss et al. 1998).

16.10.2 Headache

Headache is often multifactorial in nature. A careful history and examination of the child will often suggest the cause. In the preverbal child, increased intracranial pressure may result in symptoms associated with headache, such as nausea, vomiting, photophobia, lethargy, transient neurologic deficits, or severe irritability.

Clinical pearls

- Depending on the cause, increased intracranial pressure may be treated with surgery, chemotherapy, radiotherapy, steroids, or expectant management only.
- Immediate and aggressive use of analgesics, antiemetics, and, often, benzodiazepines is critical for managing rapidly escalating headache.

- Steroids may be the best medical management for headache related to tumor progression, but the positive clinical effects are relatively short-lived, and the side effect profile must be closely monitored.

16.10.3 Sleep Disturbance and Insomnia

Sleep disturbances and insomnia in children with malignant CNS tumors are often undetected unless specifically elicited in the history. The presence of other symptoms, such as pain or dyspnea, and emotional symptoms, such as anxiety, may be contributing factors and should be treated aggressively.

Clinical pearls

- Hypnotics are the mainstay of therapy for inadequate sleep.
- Low-dose tricyclic antidepressants, such as amitriptyline, may also be appropriate, particularly for children also presenting with neuropathic pain (Sheldon 2001).

16.10.4 Delirium

Delirium is a state of altered consciousness, confusion, and reversal of the sleep-wake cycle that develops acutely and may fluctuate throughout the day. It is fairly common in children with malignant CNS tumors because of the multiple inciting factors to which they are generally exposed. In our experience, delirium is frequently unrecognized by healthcare providers until it has been present for quite some time and is causing considerable distress. Delirium may be secondary to opioids or anticholinergics, infection, dehydration, renal or liver abnormalities, or psychosocial or spiritual distress.

Clinical pearls

- Elucidate and treat the underlying cause.
- Antipsychotic medications (e.g., haloperidol) are often helpful for managing agitation and mental confusion.

- Benzodiazepines (e.g., lorazepam) may exacerbate delirium. If agitation is not fully controlled with the antipsychotic medications, adding benzodiazepines may be warranted.

16.11 Anxiety

Children with malignant CNS tumors are under considerable personal and family strain and may experience symptoms of anxiety as a manifestation of psychological distress without meeting the criteria for diagnosis of an anxiety disorder. Working with the family system is the key way to decrease the anxiety symptoms experienced by the child. The aim of any intervention is to disrupt the dysfunctional patterns of interaction that promote family insecurity/instability.

Clinical pearls

- Attention to the child–parent relationship is vital to preventing and treating anxiety symptoms.
- Behavioral therapy, cognitive-behavioral therapy, and psychodynamic psychotherapy are useful for helping the child and family cope with the challenges of a life-limiting illness.
- Breakthrough medication with short-acting benzodiazepines may be useful in combination with nonpharmacologic techniques.
- Commonly selected medications for treating longer-standing anxiety symptoms include tricyclic antidepressants and selective serotonin reuptake inhibitors. These should be prescribed and monitored in collaboration with trained psychiatric personnel.

16.12 Depression

Fortunately, although children with malignant CNS tumors appear to be at slightly elevated risk for depression and have higher rates of maladjustment, most children with chronic disease are not depressed. The clinical picture of depression in children and adolescents varies considerably across different developmental stages.

Younger children may have more somatic complaints, auditory hallucinations, temper tantrums, and other behavioral problems, whereas older children may report low self-esteem, guilt, and hopelessness. The family relationships of youth with depressive symptomatology are frequently characterized by conflict, maltreatment, rejection, and problems with communication, with little expression of positive affect and support.

Clinical pearls

- The most important tool for diagnosing depression in children is a comprehensive psychiatric evaluation, which should be conducted by a trained clinician.
- The treatment of depressed children with malignant CNS tumors should not be based exclusively on pharmacotherapy.
- Treatment may include a combination of cognitive-behavioral therapy, interpersonal therapy, psychodynamic psychotherapy, and other psychotherapies.
- For patients requiring pharmacotherapy, drug-drug interactions and comorbidities must be considered before trialing any medications aimed at addressing the depression.
- Depressive symptoms may occur at the end of life as a normal reaction to grief. They could indicate the child's need to explore their fears and concerns and find support in the child's and the family's search for meaning and understanding of their disease, suffering, and imminent death.

16.13 Care of the Imminently Dying Child with a Malignant CNS Tumor

To best incorporate the principles and practices of palliative care into the care of children with cancer, processes to care for the imminently dying patient need to be included. Communication is key during the entire end-of-life process but has a heightened level of importance during the final days and hours of a child's life. As the symptoms progress and the child's condition deteriorates, the emotional and spiritual needs of both the patient and those caring for the patient increase. It is essential to continue to have frequent conversations about the prognosis and goals, as well as continuing the ongoing patient- and family-centered needs assessment. Open and honest communication can provide security in a situation that is filled with unknowns and fear for families.

Parents have a desire to be, and are appreciative of being, very involved in the decision-making during the final days of their child's care and treatment. They want to remain informed about the child's changes in condition and participate in the adjustments to the care plan. Parents report that receiving consistent information from a consistent team is very helpful during these distressing times (Contro et al. 2004). A coordinated effort, including a transdisciplinary approach and interdisciplinary participation in the child's care in order to provide consistent information, cannot be overemphasized, and an evidence-based standard operating procedure/checklist is probably the best way to accomplish this (Fig. 16.4) (Johnson et al. 2014).

1. This checklist has been adapted from the checklist used by the Quality-of-Life/Palliative Care Service at St. Jude Children's Research Hospital (2015).
2. The goal is to obtain items before the child enters the imminently dying phase of illness.
3. A column may be added to identify which staff members are assigned to follow up on an individual task

Parents report that end-of-life decisions are among the most difficult they face on behalf of their seriously ill child (Hinds et al. 2001). Some of the difficult decisions children, parents, and healthcare providers must face and their positive and negative aspects are outlined in Table 16.3. It is also complicated to decide the appropriate age at which to begin involving the child in end-of-life decision-making. Children as young as 9 years with progressive incurable cancer are able to complete a complex decision-making process and understand the ramifications of their decisions (Hays et al. 2006). In order to better support and understand decision-making in the care of the imminently dying child, an advanced

Checklist of Individualized Care Planning and Coordination Processes

Individualized care planning and coordination
- ☐ Comprehensive encounter completed and placed in medical record

Advanced Care Planning

- ☐ Participation of child and family in decision making
- ☐ Negotiation with family regarding plan of care
  - ☐ Prognosis and goal-directed treatment options ☐ Use of artificial hydration and nutrition
  - ☐ Use of artificial life-prolonging measures ☐ Use of transfusion therapies (platelets, RBCs, etc.)
  - ☐ Use of antibiotics ☐ Use of cancer-directed therapies (chemotherapy, radiation, surgery)
  - ☐ Admission to the critical care unit or transfer to the floor
- ☐ POST/POLST/DNaR signed and available in the medical record
- ☐ Advanced Care Plan/5 wishes/My wishes in chart, if applicable
- ☐ Unique patient/family requests identified and distributed to staff
- ☐ Appointment of health care agent in chart, if applicable
- ☐ Family conference offered to share the gravity of the patient's status with family members designated by primary care givers.
- ☐ Family notified that patient is imminently dying and medical decisions regarding care noted.
  - ☐ Medication review ☐ Need for vital signs
  - ☐ Discussed need for further diagnostic tests, invasive/painful procedures, and labs
- ☐ Nonessential equipment reviewed (e.g., monitors)
- ☐ Discussion complete on preferences of where death will occur
  ___Hospice care at home ___Inpatient hospice ___Hospital ___Home hospital ___ICU ___Other
- ☐ Ethical issues identified, Ethics Committee consulted (as needed)
- ☐ Autopsy discussion ☐ Organ donation
- ☐ Consent completed (autopsy or organ donation, when applicable)
  By whom? ______________________

Symptom Control

- ☐ Comfort optimized
  - ☐ Physical symptoms addressed ☐ Psychological symptoms addressed
  - ☐ Pain team notified of admission via pager, if applicable
  - ☐ Quality-of-Life Service notified of admission or via pager, if applicable

Fig. 16.4 Checklist of individualized care planning and coordination (ICPC) processes

☐ Function optimized
   ☐ Rehabilitation service notified of admission or via pager if applicable
☐ Signs and symptoms of imminently dying discussed with family (i.e., changes in vital signs, respiration, skin, neurologic response)
☐ Educational/resource materials provided

Emotional, Social, and Spiritual Care

☐ Assessments reviewed by family member
   ☐ Child's needs ☐ Siblings' needs ☐ Parents' needs
☐ Assessments reviewed by discipline
   ☐ Emotional needs ☐ Social needs ☐ Spiritual needs ☐ Cultural needs
☐ Sibling and patient relationship needs addressed (i.e., expressions of love, gratitude, forgiveness, and farewell)
☐ Family presence facilitated (e.g., Red Cross, military)
☐ Accommodations arranged for family gathering on unit (i.e., larger, quieter room)
☐ The need for calling cards addressed ☐ Family members contacted about status ___Yes ___ No ____N/A
   Contact made by: _____
☐ End-of-life cultural concerns addressed
☐ Financial burdens assessed ☐ Discussion of St. Jude's financial assistance complete
☐ Financial support optimized (i.e., Clayton Dabney)
☐ Servicesf/uneral arrangements ☐ Funeral home notified (name): _____
   Arrangements made by_____
   Funeral home contact person:_____
   Burial options - ☐ Cremation ☐ Burial
☐ Transportation home arranged ___Yes ___ No ___ N/A
Mode of transportation ____family car ____ambulance ____air ambulance
☐ Housing rule addressed _____N/A ☐ Extension given for housing _____
☐ Make-A-Wish or other wish agency contacted ___Yes ___No ____N/A

Care Coordination and Continuity

☐ Room flagged with symbol
☐ Social worker notified of admission via pager ☐ Child Life notified of admission via pager
☐ Chaplain notified of admission via pager ☐ Psychology notified of admission via pager ____N/A
☐ Primary Care Team emailed of admission for end-of-life care
☐ Plan for contacts at the time of death completed Plan: _____
☐ Identification of key health care member to contact in urgent situations
☐ Patient and family requesting notifications to ___ Family & friends ____Schools ____Church ____Other
☐ Notifications at time of death
   ☐ Other service providers
   ☐ Primary Care Physician_____
   ☐ Home hospital _____
   ☐ Referring physician _____
   ☐ Family members_____

☐ Postmortem packet stamped and placed in nursing binder
☐ Planned follow-up interdisciplinary care team meeting

Bereavement Care

☐ Anticipatory needs for bereavement process applied (i.e., assist family and staff with staying connected to the child, facilitated communication between child and family, addressed decisional regret, facilitated memorial objects/legacy items, educational/resource materials provided)
☐ Bereavement care of surviving family members
   ☐ Risk assessment for complicated bereavement
   ☐ Bereavement materials provided
☐ Sympathy Booklet in Nursing Binder for staff to sign
☐ Sympathy Booklet mailed
☐ Bereavement care of staff
   ☐ Debriefing scheduled

Signature/Initial:

FORMS: (Initial When completed)

_____ Record of Death
_____ Final Disposition
_____ Death Certificate
_____ Autopsy Consent

Fig. 16.4 (continued)

care planning process should be facilitated. This process will help ascertain the family's priorities, values, and goals. Advanced illness care planning has been demonstrated to improve aspects of quality of life and family satisfaction when implemented in the care of seriously ill children (Hinds et al. 2005a).

As the death becomes imminent, many parents feel that there is less interaction with the medical team. Certain members of the care team may become less visible as curative options are exchanged for comfort measures. This is difficult for families to comprehend, and parents report having feelings of abandonment when this occurs

Table 16.3 Specific decisions, along with their positive and negative aspects

Decision	Potential positive aspects	Potential negative aspects
Further cancer-directed therapy	Slow progression of the tumor Fulfills a need to continue to fight against the tumor	Introduces or increases suffering due to side effects Continued need for medical care, primarily provided through outpatient clinic or hospital setting, so less time to pursue other life goals
Enrollment in a Phase I study	Further understanding of how the medicine works Involvement in research → altruism; a chance to give back Closer monitoring of clinical status Fulfills a need to continue to fight against the tumor	No studies may be available Introduces or increases suffering due to side effects Continued need for medical care, primarily provided through outpatient clinic or hospital setting, so less time to pursue other life goals
Hospice enrollment	Home-based provision of care Expertise in pain and symptom management Interdisciplinary approach to care—availability of chaplain, physician, nurse, social worker, and volunteers 24/7 call coverage for symptom-related or other emergencies	May be viewed by others as "giving up"—seen as being for imminently dying people by public Another team working with you and your child; meeting new people may seem difficult May not allow for blood product transfusion or continuation of some cancer-directed therapies
Placement of a "Do Not Attempt Resuscitation" order	Allows recognition by all team members that the benefits of aggressive resuscitation efforts are outweighed by the suffering such efforts may inflict Focuses the final moments on comfort and mourning Can be rescinded/reversed at any point in time	May be viewed as "giving up" or not doing everything possible Because it is a piece of paper, it may not be followed unless presented to medical personnel at the point of death Can be a statement of acceptance that the end result will likely be death

(Hinds et al. 2005b). This may cause complicated grief issues following the death. Changing caregivers during the last and oftentimes most intense days of the illness can be stressful for both the patient and the parents; therefore, maintaining open communication is essential (Contro et al. 2004). A focus on care coordination and care continuity in the imminently dying pediatric cancer patient can help provide the much needed support and relationships sought by the families of these patients.

Imminently dying cancer patients experience many symptoms, such as pain, fatigue, behavior changes, breathing changes and dyspnea, reduced mobility, depression, anxiety, nausea and vomiting, anemia and bleeding, and loss of appetite (Wolfe et al. 2000; McCallum et al. 2000; Stevens et al. 1994; Wolfe et al. 2002; Jalmsell et al. 2006). As stated earlier, many of these symptoms are not treated, and even if treatment is instituted, it is frequently unsuccessful (Goldman et al. 2006; Wolfe et al. 2000). Addressing suffering and managing these symptoms is of paramount importance in that parents report fear of the child's physical symptoms as one of their main concerns at the end of life (Theunissen et al. 2007). Furthermore, parental report of unrelieved pain in their dying child has been linked to long-term distress in bereaved parents (Kreicbergs et al. 2005). There should be an ongoing comprehensive systematic symptom assessment of all children dying a cancer-related death. Those symptoms that are distressing to the child and/or parent should be addressed and treatment initiated.

Imminently dying children should not be allowed to experience suffering at the end of life. Clinicians have a clinical and ethical responsibility to their patients and should control symptoms with appropriate medical interventions. The rule of double effect and the principles that guide sedation of highly symptomatic adult patients with pain or dyspnea also apply in the care of children (Fleischman 1998). The goal of therapy is to relieve distressing symptoms and not to hasten death. Consultation with palliative care and pain teams can aid clinicians with symptom management at the end of life and is recommended.

Unfortunately, a small number of children with malignant CNS tumors will experience intractable physical suffering that is refractory to traditional medical interventions. Parents of seriously ill children may be willing to try a variety of approaches, some of which may be potentially harmful, hoping for benefit in a desperate situation, particularly when the condition imposes a heavy burden for which mainstream therapies are insufficient. Of note, although some alternative medicine practices in the care of seriously ill children may be justified, there are no published guidelines for using these practices in children. In these rare circumstances, palliative sedation therapy (PST) with medications achieving continuous deep sedation can be ethically permissible. Propofol is one such medication and has been demonstrated to reduce pain and suffering in pediatric patients. The indications for PST at the end of life include two core components: the presence of severe suffering that is refractory to standard palliative management and the primary aim of relief of distress. We recommend that traditional therapies be maximized under a time-limited trial and ethics consultation be obtained prior to initiating PST in pediatric patients (Anghelescu et al. 2012).

16.14 Psychosocial, Emotional, Cultural, and Spiritual Care

In addition to issues of pain and other physical symptoms, psychosocial and spiritual needs are consistently identified as being very important to patients and their families. These psychological and spiritual concerns are frequently left unattended but should be treated as aggressively as physical symptoms. Many clinicians are poorly trained with regard to the spiritual and religious concerns of patients and families. They may have an understanding of and a level of concern for the spiritual and religious needs of the patient, but this understanding does not translate into the interaction with the patient and their families (Grossoehme et al. 2007). A significant number of cancer patients report that spirituality/religion is important to them personally. Addressing these issues may lead to improved outcomes, in that there is an association between spirituality/religion and improved quality of life, as well as an increased ability to cope with the imminent death of a patient (Balboni et al. 2007).

In the ideal scenario, the end of a child's life will occur in the most comfortable manner possible, allowing the family and child to be together in their chosen place. More commonly, however, this ideal scenario is complicated by continuing advances in medical regimens that, although introduced with the hope of restoring function, may ultimately expose a child to overly aggressive treatments or interventions in the last days or weeks of life. This difficulty often occurs in the inpatient setting and may complicate the provision of end-of-life care that is inclusive of a family's personal, cultural, religious, or spiritual beliefs. Although commonly thought to be important, the role of these needs of families at the end of a child's life has been insufficiently studied in pediatric populations. Facilitating the expression of a family's religious or spiritual beliefs as a child approaches the end of life may provide comfort and a sense of meaning by supporting a sense of connection to a higher power. Parents often identify community religious figures as important members of their support system (Thiel and Robinson 1997). A community clergy person is typically more grounded in specific religious traditions and may already have an existing long-term relationship with the family. However, a hospital chaplain has more experience with counseling individuals through illness and death, so the ideal combination of resources may result from partnerships between the two. Therefore, the interdisciplinary team should include a trained and certified chaplain to address the religious and spiritual needs of dying children and their families. Chaplaincy services may be consulted to assist with assessing the religious and spiritual needs of a child and family

(Nelson-Becker 2013). Additionally, discussions with community-based religious leaders, interpreters, or other members of the cultural group can be informative. After the death of a child, parents are often asked to make difficult decisions about funeral, burial, or cremation plans. Families of children with malignant CNS tumors have probably already thought about the child's funeral and related plans before the death occurs as a part of anticipatory grief (Brown and Sourkes 2006). Various members of the interdisciplinary team, especially social workers and chaplains, may be helpful in supporting families and helping to make arrangements.

16.15 Bereavement Support

Bereavement is the objective situation of losing someone significant through death and the adjustment that follows (Bruce 2007). Grief refers to the distress resulting from bereavement and includes complex cognitive, emotional, and social difficulties. Together, these constitute the "grief process." The death of a child is one of the most intense and painful events that a parent can experience; parental grief is more intense and longer-lasting than other types of grief and is associated with increased risk of psychological and physical illness. Parents who survive their child's death experience higher intensities of grief than do adults who experience the death of a spouse or parent (Dans et al. 2017; Bradshaw et al. 2005; Sanders 1979). Bereaved parents have elevated risks of psychiatric hospitalizations, even 5 or more years after their child's death, and a higher risk of early death (Li et al. 2003, 2005). Pediatric cancer treatment places many burdens on families. Children receiving treatment for cancer are often hospitalized far from home for lengthy periods of time, and the geographic distance reduces the opportunity for social support from friends and extended family. Therefore, parents often come to depend upon the hospital staff for their psychosocial needs. When their child dies and these services are withdrawn, families may feel abandoned by the hospital staff (Truog et al. 2006). The majority of families desire some continued contact with the

members of their child's care team and report that such contact is meaningful to them (Hinds et al. 2005b; Contro et al. 2004; deCinque et al. 2004, 2006).

Bereaved parents may experience severe personal guilt in the years after their child's death, particularly if they did not expect their child to die during the week before their death (Surkan et al. 2006). When death is anticipated, it is important that the attending staff and other members of the interdisciplinary team clearly discuss the child's condition with the parents. Families who have access to and use psychological support during the last month of their child's life are more likely to work through grief, particularly if they have the opportunity to discuss their child's condition with the team (Kreicbergs et al. 2007). Healthcare professionals should display empathy and remain attentive to familial needs in a manner that is open and culturally sensitive. Families should be informed that there is no "right way" to feel or act at the time of death, and their privacy should be respected. Families should be allowed to spend as much time with their child as they need after death, and accommodations should be made to allow for personal, cultural, or spiritual needs within the hospital setting.

A practical approach to providing care for bereaved families begins when the child is first admitted for treatment. In these early stages of the child's treatment, important building blocks for future relationships are set in place. Using a "hope for the best, plan for the worst" approach enables care teams to help prepare a family for loss, which may lower the risk for psychological disturbances after the death. The goal to integrate bereavement care into the mainstream of the child's care also suggests the need to develop and implement effective evaluation tools that permit the team to identify families at risk for complicated bereavement. Initial assessments by the chaplaincy and social work departments can alert the team to families whose coping may be less than adaptive. Identifying disbelief, yearning, anger, or depression as negative grief indicators 6 months after the death of the child may identify those family members in need of further evaluation (Maciejewski et al. 2007). Individuals who lack a good social support network and those who have experienced a childhood history of neglect and abuse are at the highest risk for complicated bereavement. Individuals most at risk for complicated bereavement are often those who are the most reluctant to seek help, which can complicate attempts at intervention by clinicians (Zhang et al. 2006). There are seven symptoms that should serve as a warning signal to clinicians that a person may be experiencing complicated grief: trouble accepting the death, inability to trust others, excessive bitterness towards the death, uneasiness about moving on with life, detachment from other people to whom the person was previously close, the view that the future holds no prospect of fulfillment, and agitation since the death. These symptoms must be persistent and disruptive to the bereaved person and must have lasted for more than 6 months (Hawton 2007). Thus, in order to identify and help persons who may be suffering from complicated bereavement, a bereavement program must include regular contact between family members and trained staff over an extended period of time.

Conclusion

Despite advances in the field of neuro-oncology, children with brain tumors continue to experience high rates of morbidity and mortality and a substantial symptom burden, necessitating the integration of palliative care principles and practices throughout their illness trajectory. As a high-risk group, these patients experience a high number of hospital deaths, and there is often only a short interval between the initial palliative care consultation and death. The early introduction of palliative care for these patients is essential, and a broad-based approach that does not exclusively rely on consult-based palliative care services can help optimize the integration of palliative care into the continuum of care for pediatric neuro-oncology patients.

References

American Academy of Pediatrics Committee on Bioethics (1994) Guidelines on foregoing life-sustaining medical treatment. Pediatrics 93:532–536

Anghelescu DL, Hamilton H, Faughnan LG et al (2012) Pediatric palliative sedation therapy with propofol: recommendations based on experience in children with terminal cancer. J Palliat Med 15:1082–1090

Arias E, MacDorman MF, Strobino DM, Guyer B (2003) Annual summary of vital statistics—2002. Pediatrics 112:1215–1230

Baker JN, Barfield R, Hinds PS, Kane JR (2007) A process to facilitate decision making in pediatric stem cell transplantation: the individualized care planning and coordination model. Biol Blood Marrow Transplant 13:245–254

Baker JN, Hinds PS, Spunt SL et al (2008) Integration of palliative care practices into the ongoing care of children with cancer: individualized care planning and coordination. Pediatr Clin North Am 55:223–250. xii

Baker JN, Levine DR, Hinds PS et al (2015) Research priorities in pediatric palliative care. J Pediatr 167:467–470

Balboni TA, Vanderwerker LC, Block SD et al (2007) Religiousness and spiritual support among advanced cancer patients and associations with end-of-life treatment preferences and quality of life. J Clin Oncol 25:555–560

Bausewein C, Booth S, Gysels M, Higginson IJ (2008) Non-pharmacological interventions for breathlessness in advanced stages of malignant and non-malignant diseases. Cochrane Database Syst Rev (2):CD005623

Ben-Aharon I, Gafter-Gvili A, Paul M et al (2008) Interventions for alleviating cancer-related dyspnea: a systematic review. J Clin Oncol 26:2396–2404

Berde CB, Sethna NF (2002) Analgesics for the treatment of pain in children. N Engl J Med 347:1094–1103

Bluebond-Langner M, Belasco JB, DeMesquita WM (2010) "I want to live, until I don't want to live anymore": involving children with life-threatening and life-shortening illnesses in decision making about care and treatment. Nurs Clin North Am 45:329–343

Bradshaw G, Hinds PS, Lensing S et al (2005) Cancer-related deaths in children and adolescents. J Palliat Med 8:86–95

Brown MR, Sourkes B (2006) Psychotherapy in pediatric palliative care. Child Adolesc Psychiatr Clin N Am 15:585–596. viii

Bruce CA (2007) Helping patients, families, caregivers, and physicians, in the grieving process. J Am Osteopath Assoc 107:ES33–ES40

Burish TG, Tope DM (1992) Psychological techniques for controlling the adverse side effects of cancer chemotherapy: findings from a decade of research. J Pain Symptom Manag 7:287–301

deCinque N, Monterosso L, Dadd G et al (2004) Bereavement support for families following the death of a child from cancer: practice characteristics of Australian and New Zealand paediatric oncology units. J Paediatr Child Health 40:131–135

deCinque N, Monterosso L, Dadd G et al (2006) Bereavement support for families following the death of a child from cancer: experience of bereaved parents. J Psychosoc Oncol 24:65–83

Collins JJ, Byrnes ME, Dunkel IJ et al (2000) The measurement of symptoms in children with cancer. J Pain Symptom Manag 19:363–377

Collins JJ, Devine TD, Dick GS et al (2002) The measurement of symptoms in young children with cancer: the validation of the Memorial Symptom Assessment Scale in children aged 7–12. J Pain Symptom Manag 23:10–16

Contro NA, Larson J, Scofield S et al (2004) Hospital staff and family perspectives regarding quality of pediatric palliative care. Pediatrics 114:1248–1252

Couluris M, Mayer JL, Freyer DR et al (2008) The effect of cyproheptadine hydrochloride (periactin) and megestrol acetate (megace) on weight in children with cancer/treatment-related cachexia. J Pediatr Hematol Oncol 30:791–797

Dalberg T, Jacob-Files E, Carney PA et al (2013) Pediatric oncology providers' perceptions of barriers and facilitators to early integration of pediatric palliative care. Pediatr Blood Cancer 60:1875–1881

Dans M, Smith T, Back A, Baker JN et al (2017) NCCN guidelines insights: palliative care, version 2.2017. J Natl Compr Canc Netw 15(8):989–997. https://doi.org/10.6004/jnccn.2017.0132

Davies B, Sehring SA, Partridge JC et al (2008) Barriers to palliative care for children: perceptions of pediatric health care providers. Pediatrics 121:282–288

Diekema DS (2004) Parental refusals of medical treatment: the harm principle as threshold for state intervention. Theor Med Bioeth 25:243–264

Diekema DS, Botkin JR (2009) Committee on bioethics: clinical report—forgoing medically provided nutrition and hydration in children. Pediatrics 124:813–822

Dreifuss FE, Rosman NP, Cloyd JC et al (1998) A comparison of rectal diazepam gel and placebo for acute repetitive seizures. N Engl J Med 338:1869–1875

Dussel V, Joffe S, Hilden JM et al (2010) Considerations about hastening death among parents of children who die of cancer. Arch Pediatr Adolesc Med 164:231–237

Ferrell B, Malloy P, Virani R (2015) The end of life nursing education nursing consortium project. Ann Palliat Med 4:61–69

Feudtner C (2007) Collaborative communication in pediatric palliative care: a foundation for problem-solving and decision-making. Pediatr Clin North Am 54:583–607. ix

Fleischman A (1998) Commentary: ethical issues in pediatric pain management and terminal sedation. J Pain Symptom Manag 15:260–261

Freyer DR (2004) Care of the dying adolescent: special considerations. Pediatrics 113:381–388

Friebert S, Osenga K (2009) Pediatric palliative care referral criteria. Center to Advance Palliative Care, New York

van der Geest IM, Darlington AS, Streng IC et al (2014) Parents' experiences of pediatric palliative care and the impact on long-term parental grief. J Pain Symptom Manag 47:1043–1053

Goldman A, Hewitt M, Collins GS et al (2006) Symptoms in children/young people with progressive malignant disease: United Kingdom Children's Cancer Study Group/Paediatric Oncology Nurses Forum survey. Pediatrics 117:e1179–e1186

Groh G, Borasio GD, Nickolay C et al (2013a) Specialized pediatric palliative home care: a prospective evaluation. J Palliat Med 16:1588–1594

Groh G, Vyhnalek B, Feddersen B et al (2013b) Effectiveness of a specialized outpatient palliative care service as experienced by patients and caregivers. J Palliat Med 16:848–856

Grossoehme DH, Ragsdale JR, McHenry CL et al (2007) Pediatrician characteristics associated with attention to spirituality and religion in clinical practice. Pediatrics 119:e117–e123

von Gunten CF (2002) Secondary and tertiary palliative care in US hospitals. JAMA 287:875–881

Haanpää M, Attal N, Backonja M et al (2011) NeuPSIG guidelines on neuropathic pain assessment. Pain 152:14–27

Hawton K (2007) Complicated grief after bereavement. BMJ 334:962–963

Hays RM, Valentine J, Haynes G et al (2006) The Seattle Pediatric Palliative Care Project: effects on family satisfaction and health-related quality of life. J Palliat Med 9:716–728

Hendricks-Ferguson V (2008) Physical symptoms of children receiving pediatric hospice care at home during the last week of life. Oncol Nurs Forum 35:E108–E115

Hesketh PJ, Grunberg SM, Gralla RJ et al (2003) The oral neurokinin-1 antagonist aprepitant for the prevention of chemotherapy-induced nausea and vomiting: a multinational, randomized, double-blind, placebo-controlled trial in patients receiving high-dose cisplatin—the Aprepitant Protocol 052 Study Group. J Clin Oncol 21:4112–4119

Himelstein BP, Hilden JM, Boldt AM, Weissman D (2004) Pediatric palliative care. N Engl J Med 350:1752–1762

Hinds PS, Oakes L, Furman W et al (2001) End-of-life decision making by adolescents, parents, and healthcare providers in pediatric oncology: research to evidence-based practice guidelines. Cancer Nurs 24:122–134

Hinds PS, Drew D, Oakes LL et al (2005a) End-of-life care preferences of pediatric patients with cancer. J Clin Oncol 23:9146–9154

Hinds PS, Schum L, Baker JN, Wolfe J (2005b) Key factors affecting dying children and their families. J Palliat Med 8(Suppl 1):S70–S78

Hinds PS, Oakes LL, Hicks J et al (2009) "Trying to be a good parent" as defined by interviews with parents who made phase I, terminal care, and resuscitation decisions for their children. J Clin Oncol 27:5979–5985

Jalmsell L, Kreicbergs U, Onelöv E et al (2006) Symptoms affecting children with malignancies during the last month of life: a nationwide follow-up. Pediatrics 117:1314–1320

Johnson LM, Snaman JM, Cupit MC, Baker JN (2014) End-of-life care for hospitalized children. Pediatr Clin N Am 61:835–854

Johnson LM, Church CL, Metzger M, Baker JN (2015) Ethics consultation in pediatrics: long-term experience from a pediatric oncology center. Am J Bioeth 15:3–17

Kane JR, Himelstein BP (2007) Palliative care for children. In: Berger AM, Shuster JL, Von Roenn JH (eds) Principles and practice of palliative medicine and supportive oncology, 3rd edn. Lippincott Williams & Wilkins, Philadelphia, PA

Kaye EC, Rubenstein J, Levine D et al (2015) Pediatric palliative care in the community. CA Cancer J Clin 65:316–333

Klick JC, Hauer J (2010) Pediatric palliative care. Curr Probl Pediatr Adolesc Health Care 40:120–151

Klick JC, Friebert S, Hutton N et al (2014) Developing competencies for pediatric hospice and palliative medicine. Pediatrics 134:e1670–e1677

Knapp C, Thompson L (2012) Factors associated with perceived barriers to pediatric palliative care: a survey of pediatricians in Florida and California. Palliat Med 26:268–274

Kreicbergs U, Valdimarsdóttir U, Onelöv E et al (2005) Care-related distress: a nationwide study of parents who lost their child to cancer. J Clin Oncol 23:9162–9171

Kreicbergs UC, Lannen P, Onelov E, Wolfe J (2007) Parental grief after losing a child to cancer: impact of professional and social support on long-term outcomes. J Clin Oncol 25:3307–3312

Kyle G (2011) Constipation: symptoms, assessment and treatment. Br J Nurs 20:1432

Lannering B, Marky I, Lundberg A, Olsson E (1990) Long-term sequelae after pediatric brain tumors: their effect on disability and quality of life. Med Pediatr Oncol 18:304–310

Laubisch JE, Baker JN (2013) Methylnaltrexone use in a seventeen-month-old female with progressive cancer and rectal prolapse. J Palliat Med 16:1486–1488

Levine D, Cohen K, Wendler D (2012) Shared medical decision-making: considering what options to present based on an ethical analysis of the treatment of brain tumors in very young children. Pediatr Blood Cancer 59:216–220

Li J, Precht DH, Mortensen PB, Olsen J (2003) Mortality in parents after death of a child in Denmark: a nationwide follow-up study. Lancet 361:363–367

Li J, Laursen TM, Precht DH et al (2005) Hospitalization for mental illness among parents after the death of a child. N Engl J Med 352:1190–1196

Liben S, Papadatou D, Wolfe J (2008) Paediatric palliative care: challenges and emerging ideas. Lancet 371:852–864

Maciejewski PK, Zhang B, Block SD, Prigerson HG (2007) An empirical examination of the stage theory of grief. JAMA 297:716–723

Mack JW, Wolfe J (2006) Early integration of pediatric palliative care: for some children, palliative care starts at diagnosis. Curr Opin Pediatr 18:10–14

Mack JW, Hilden JM, Watterson J et al (2005) Parent and physician perspectives on quality of care at the end of life in children with cancer. J Clin Oncol 23:9155–9161

Mack JW, Wolfe J, Cook EF et al (2007) Hope and prognostic disclosure. J Clin Oncol 25:5636–5642

Mack JW, Wolfe J, Cook EF et al (2011) Parents' roles in decision making for children with cancer in the first year of cancer treatment. J Clin Oncol 29:2085–2090

Maurer SH, Hinds PS, Spunt SL et al (2010) Decision making by parents of children with incurable cancer who opt for enrollment on a phase I trial compared with choosing a do not resuscitate/terminal care option. J Clin Oncol 28:3292–3298

McCallum DE, Byrne P, Bruera E (2000) How children die in hospital. J Pain Symptom Manag 20:417–423

Mercadante S, Giarratano A (2014) Pharmacological management of cancer pain in children. Crit Rev Oncol Hematol 91:93–97

Miltenburg D, Louw DF, Sutherland GR (1996) Epidemiology of childhood brain tumors. Can J Neurol Sci 23:118–122

Mock V, Atkinson A, Barsevick AM et al (2007) Cancer-related fatigue. Clinical Practice Guidelines in Oncology. J Natl Compr Cancer Netw 5:1054–1078

National Quality Forum (2006) A National Framework and Preferred Practices for Palliative and Hospice Care Quality. http://www.qualityforum.org/Publications/2006/12/A_National_Framework_and_Preferred_Practices_for_Palliative_and_Hospice_Care_Quality.aspx

Nelson-Becker H (2013) Spirituality in end-of-life and palliative care: what matters? J Soc Work End Life Palliat Care 9:112–116

Nitschke R (2000) Regarding guidelines for assistance to terminally ill children with cancer: report of the SIOP working committee on psychosocial issues in pediatric oncology. Med Pediatr Oncol 34:271–273

Nitschke R, Meyer WH, Sexauer CL et al (2000) Care of terminally ill children with cancer. Med Pediatr Oncol 34:268–270

Packer RJ (1995) Brain tumors in children. Curr Opin Pediatr 7:64–72

Pritchard M, Burghen E, Srivastava DK et al (2008) Cancer-related symptoms most concerning to parents during the last week and last day of their child's life. Pediatrics 121:e1301–e1309

Pyke-Grimm KA, Degner L, Small A, Mueller B (1999) Preferences for participation in treatment decision making and information needs of parents of children with cancer: a pilot study. J Pediatr Oncol Nurs 16:13–24

Quill TE, Abernethy AP (2013) Generalist plus specialist palliative care—creating a more sustainable model. N Engl J Med 368:1173–1175

Sanders C (1979) A comparison of adult bereavement in the death of a spouse, child and parent. Omega 10:302–332

Santucci G, Mack JW (2007) Common gastrointestinal symptoms in pediatric palliative care: nausea, vomiting, constipation, anorexia, cachexia. Pediatr Clin North Am 54:673–689. x

Sheldon SH (2001) Insomnia in children. Curr Treat Options Neurol 3:37–50

Stevens MM, Dalla Pozza L, Cavalletto B et al (1994) Pain and symptom control in paediatric palliative care. Cancer Surv 21:211–231

Surkan PJ, Kreicbergs U, Valdimarsdóttir U et al (2006) Perceptions of inadequate health care and feelings of guilt in parents after the death of a child to a malignancy: a population-based long-term follow-up. J Palliat Med 9:317–331

Theunissen JM, Hoogerbrugge PM, van Achterberg T et al (2007) Symptoms in the palliative phase of children with cancer. Pediatr Blood Cancer 49:160–165

Thiel MM, Robinson MR (1997) Physicians' collaboration with chaplains: difficulties and benefits. J Clin Ethics 8:94–103

Truog RD, Meyer EC, Burns JP (2006) Toward interventions to improve end-of-life care in the pediatric intensive care unit. Crit Care Med 34:S373–S379

Uman LS, Birnie KA, Noel M, et al (2013) Psychological interventions for needle-related procedural pain and distress in children and adolescents. Cochrane Database Syst Rev (10):CD005179

Varma S, Jenkins T, Wendler D (2008) How do children and parents make decisions about pediatric clinical research? J Pediatr Hematol Oncol 30:823–828

Vollenbroich R, Duroux A, Grasser M et al (2012) Effectiveness of a pediatric palliative home care team as experienced by parents and health care professionals. J Palliat Med 15:294–300

Von Roenn JH (2011) Palliative care and the cancer patient: current state and state of the art. J Pediatr Hematol Oncol 33(Suppl 2):S87–S89

Waldman E, Wolfe J (2013) Palliative care for children with cancer. Nat Rev Clin Oncol 10:100–107

Weaver MS, Baker JN, Gattuso JS et al (2015) Adolescents' preferences for treatment decisional involvement during their cancer. In: Cancer, vol 121, pp 4416–4424

Weisman SJ, Bernstein B, Schechter NL (1998) Consequences of inadequate analgesia during painful procedures in children. Arch Pediatr Adolesc Med 152:147–149

Wentlandt K, Krzyzanowska MK, Swami N et al (2014) Referral practices of pediatric oncologists to specialized palliative care. Support Care Cancer 22:2315–2322

Wiener L, Ballard E, Brennan T et al (2008) How I wish to be remembered: the use of an advance care planning document in adolescent and young adult populations. J Palliat Med 11:1309–1313

Wolfe J, Grier HE, Klar N et al (2000) Symptoms and suffering at the end of life in children with cancer. N Engl J Med 342:326–333

Wolfe J, Friebert S, Hilden J (2002) Caring for children with advanced cancer integrating palliative care. Pediatr Clin North Am 49:1043–1062

Wolfe J, Hammel JF, Edwards KE et al (2008) Easing of suffering in children with cancer at the end of life: is care changing? J Clin Oncol 26:1717–1723

Zelcer S, Cataudella D, Cairney AE, Bannister SL (2010) Palliative care of children with brain tumors: a parental perspective. Arch Pediatr Adolesc Med 164:225–230

Zhang B, El-Jawahri A, Prigerson HG (2006) Update on bereavement research: evidence-based guidelines for the diagnosis and treatment of complicated bereavement. J Palliat Med 9:1188–1203

Global Challenges in Pediatric Neuro-Oncology

17

Simon Bailey, Jeannette Parkes, and Alan Davidson

17.1 Introduction

Eighty-five percent of the world's children live in areas of limited resources. The poorest continent, Africa, accounts for 23% of pediatric disease but only employs 1.3% of the world's health workers. Pediatric neuro-oncology requires highly specialized teams, and in countries where there are inadequate resources for even the most common diseases, such as infections, malnutrition, and HIV-related disease, it is understandable that children with central nervous system (CNS) tumors are not a priority.

According to the World Bank (TWB 2015a), there are 35 low income countries (LIC) with gross national income (GNI) per capita per year

"The rise of cancer in less affluent countries is an impending disaster" *Dr. Margaret Chan, WHO Director General 2008.*
"There is never nothing we can do" *Professor Elizabeth Molyneux OBE, Professor of Pediatrics,* Blantyre, Malawi *2010*

S. Bailey (✉)
Great North Children's Hospital and Newcastle University, Newcastle upon Tyne, United Kingdom
e-mail: simon.bailey@newcastle.ac.uk

J. Parkes
Groote Schuur Hospital and University of Cape Town, Cape Town, South Africa

A. Davidson
Red Cross War Memorial Children's Hospital and University of Cape Town, Cape Town, South Africa

(Atlas Method) of less than $1500, 56 lower middle income countries (LMIC) (GNI per capita of $1500–$3975), 54 upper middle income countries (UMIC, GNI per capita of $3976–$12,275), and 50 high income countries (HIC, GNI per capita of >$12,275), see Table 17.1 and Fig. 17.1. This is reflected in the health expenditure per capita (TWB 2015b) (Table 17.2), which varies as a percentage of gross domestic product (GDP) and ranges from $13 per person per year in the Central African Republics to $9715 per person per year in Norway. The inequity of financial resources is reflected in the availability of doctors and other health workers (Table 17.2) and certainly in the availability of pediatric neuro-oncology facilities. It is estimated that at least 80% of children with brain tumors in the world do not receive adequate treatment (Friedrich et al. 2015; Hadley et al. 2012; Barr et al. 2011) and major efforts would be required to reverse the current situation. Ensuring that all children of the twenty-first century are able to receive basic treatment in the neglected domain of CNS tumors should be a priority for all pediatric oncology health workers.

The number of children in the world under the age of 15 years presenting each year with any cancer is estimated to be 160,000 (Ferlay 2004; Howard et al. 2008), although the accuracy of this figure is questionable due to the uncertain incidence in many LMIC and LIC. Extrapolating from US data, about one-fifth of these cancers are CNS cancers (Howard et al. 2008). However, the

© Springer International Publishing AG, part of Springer Nature 2018
A. Gajjar et al. (eds.), *Brain Tumors in Children*, https://doi.org/10.1007/978-3-319-43205-2_17

Table 17.1 Tables showing countries in order as defined by Gross National Income (GNI) per capita

Rank	Country	GNI	Year
(a) High income countries			
1	Monaco	186,950	2008
2	Liechtenstein	116,030	2009
–	Bermuda (UK)	106,140	2013
3	Norway	103,050	2014
4	Switzerland	90,670	2013
5	Qatar	90,420	2014
–	Macau (China)	71,270	2013
–	Isle of Man (UK)	48,360	2007
6	Luxembourg	69,880	2013
7	Australia	64,680	2014
8	Sweden	61,600	2014
9	Denmark	61,310	2014
–	GuernseyJersey Channel Islands (UK)	65,440	2007
10	Kuwait	55,470	2013
11	United States	55,200	2014
12	Singapore	55,150	2014
–	Faroe Islands (Denmark)	NA	N/A
13	Canada	51,690	2014
14	San Marino	51,470	2008
15	Netherlands	51,210	2014
–	Cayman Islands (UK)	NA	N/A
16	Austria	50,390	2013
17	Finland	48,910	2013
18	Germany	47,640	2014
19	Iceland	47,640	2014
20	Belgium	47,030	2014
21	Ireland, Republic of	44,660	2014
22	United Arab Emirates	43,480	2014
23	France	43,080	2014
24	United Kingdom	42,690	2014
25	Japan	42,000	2014
26	Andorra	41,460	2013
–	Hong Kong (China)	40,320	2014
27	New Zealand	39,300	2013
28	Brunei Darussalam	36,710	2012
29	Israel	34,990	2014
30	Italy	34,280	2014
–	Curaçao (Netherlands)	NA	N/A
31	Spain	29,940	2013
–	Guam (USA)	NA	N/A
32	Korea, South	27,090	2014
33	Cyprus	26,370	2014
34	Saudi Arabia	26,340	2013
–	Greenland (Denmark)	26,020	2009
–	Aruba (Netherlands)	NA	N/A
–	Turks and Caicos Islands (UK)	NA	N/A
35	Slovenia	23,220	2013
36	Greece	22,090	2014

Table 17.1 (continued)

Rank	Country	GNI	Year
39	Portugal	21,320	2014
40	Bahrain	21,330	2013
41	Bahamas, The	21,010	2014
–	Sint Maarten (Netherlands)	NA	N/A
42	Malta	21,000	2013
43	Taiwan (TWB 2015b)	NA	N/A
–	Puerto Rico (USA)	19,310	2013
44	Czech Republic	18,970	2013
45	Estonia	18,530	2014
46	Oman	18,150	2013
47	Slovakia	17,810	2013
–	Saint Martin (France)	NA	N/A
48	Uruguay	16,360	2014
–	French Polynesia (France)	15,990	2000
49	Latvia	15,660	2014
50	Trinidad and Tobago	15,640	2013
51	Lithuania	15,380	2014
52	Barbados	14,880	2012
53	Chile	14,900	2014
54	Argentina	14,560	2014
55	Saint Kitts and Nevis	14,540	2014
–	New Caledonia (France)	14,020	2000
56	Seychelles	13,990	2014
57	Poland	13,730	2014
–	Virgin Islands, U.S. (USA)	13,660	1989
58	Hungary	13,470	2014
59	Antigua and Barbuda	13,360	2014
60	Equatorial Guinea	13,340	2014
61	Russia	13,210	2014
–	Northern Mariana Islands (USA)	NA	N/A
62	Croatia	13,020	2014
63	Venezuela	12,820	2014
(b) Upper middle income countries			
64	Brazil	11,760	2014
65	Kazakhstan	11,670	2014
66	Palau	11,110	2014
67	Panama	10,970	2014
–	World	10,858	2014
68	Turkey	10,850	2014
69	Malaysia	10,660	2014
70	Mexico	9980	2014
71	Lebanon	9880	2014
72	Costa Rica	9750	2014
73	Mauritius	9710	2014
74	Romania	9370	2014
75	Suriname	9370	2013
76	Gabon	9320	2014
–	American Samoa (USA)	NA	N/A
77	Turkmenistan	8020	2014

(continued)

Table 17.1 (continued)

Rank	Country	GNI	Year
78	Libya	7920	2014
79	Botswana	7880	2014
80	Grenada	7850	2014
81	Colombia	7780	2014
82	Azerbaijan	7590	2014
83	Bulgaria	7420	2014
84	China	7380	2014
85	Belarus	7340	2014
86	Maldives	7290	2014
87	Montenegro	7240	2014
88	Saint Lucia	7090	2014
89	Dominica	7070	2014
90	South Africa	6800	2014
91	Saint Vincent and the Grenadines	6560	2014
92	Iraq	6410	2014
93	Peru	6410	2014
94	Iran	6820	2013
95	Ecuador	6040	2014
96	Dominican Republic	5950	2014
97	Cuba	5910	2011
98	Tuvalu	5840	2013
99	Namibia	5820	2014
100	Serbia	5820	2014
101	Thailand	5410	2014
102	Algeria	5340	2014
103	Angola	5300	2014
104	Jamaica	5220	2013
105	Jordan	5160	2014
106	Macedonia, Republic of	5070	2014
107	Bosnia and Herzegovina	4770	2014
108	Fiji	4540	2014
109	Belize	4510	2013
110	Albania	4460	2013
111	Mongolia	4320	2014
112	Marshall Islands	4310	2013
113	Tonga	4280	2014
114	Tunisia	4210	2013
115	Paraguay	4150	2014
(c) Lower middle income countries			
116	Samoa	4050	2014
117	Kosovo	4000	2014
118	Guyana	3970	2014
119	Armenia	3810	2014
120	El Salvador	3780	2014
121	Georgia	3720	2014
122	Indonesia	3650	2014
123	Ukraine	3560	2014
124	Cabo Verde	3520	2014
125	Guatemala	3440	2014

Table 17.1   (continued)

Rank	Country	GNI	Year
126	Philippines	3440	2014
127	Sri Lanka	3400	2014
128	Egypt	3280	2014
129	Micronesia, Federated States of	3280	2013
130	Timor Leste	3120	2014
131	Vanuatu	3090	2013
132	Palestine	3060	2013
133	Morocco	3020	2013
134	Nigeria	2950	2014
135	Bolivia	2830	2014
136	Swaziland	2700	2014
137	Congo, Republic of the	2680	2014
138	Moldova	2550	2014
139	Bhutan	2390	2014
140	Kiribati	2280	2013
141	Honduras	2190	2014
142	Uzbekistan	2090	2014
143	Papua New Guinea	2020	2013
144	Vietnam	1890	2014
145	Syria	1850	2007
146	Nicaragua	1830	2014
147	Solomon Islands	1830	2014
148	Zambia	1760	2014
149	Sudan	1740	2014
150	Ghana	1620	2014
151	India	1610	2014
152	Laos	1600	2014
153	São Tomé and Príncipe	1570	2013
154	Côte d'Ivoire	1550	2014
155	Pakistan	1410	2014
156	Yemen	1370	2013
157	Cameroon	1350	2014
158	Lesotho	1350	2014
159	Kenya	1280	2014
160	Myanmar	1270	2014
161	Mauritania	1260	2014
162	Kyrgyzstan	1250	2013
163	Bangladesh	1080	2014
164	Tajikistan	1060	2014
165	Senegal	1050	2014
166	Djibouti	1030	2005
(d) Lower income countries			
67	Cambodia	1010	2014
168	Chad	1010	2014
169	South Sudan	960	2014
170	Tanzania	930	2014
171	Zimbabwe	860	2014
172	Comoros	840	2014
173	Haiti	830	2014

(continued)

Table 17.1 (continued)

Rank	Country	GNI	Year
174	Benin	810	2014
175	Nepal	730	2014
176	Mali	720	2014
177	Sierra Leone	720	2014
178	Burkina Faso	710	2014
179	Afghanistan	680	2014
180	Uganda	660	2014
181	Rwanda	650	2014
182	Mozambique	630	2014
183	Togo	580	2014
184	Guinea-Bissau	570	2014
185	Korea, North	500	2015
186	Ethiopia	550	2014
187	Eritrea	530	2014
188	Guinea	480	2014
189	Gambia	450	2014
190	Madagascar	440	2014
191	Niger	430	2014
192	Congo, Democratic Republic of the	410	2014
193	Liberia	400	2014
194	Central African Republic	330	2014
195	Burundi	270	2014
196	Malawi	250	2014
197	Somalia	150	1990

This is defined as the gross national income, converted to U.S. dollars using the World Bank Atlas method, divided by the midyear population. GNI is the sum of value added by all resident producers plus any product taxes (less subsidies) not included in the valuation of output plus net receipts of primary income (compensation of employees and property income) from abroad (TWB 2015a). (a) Shows high income countries, (b) upper middle income countries, (c) lower middle income countries, and (d) lower income countries. These are defined by the world bank as follows: low-income economies are those with a GNI per capita, calculated using the *World Bank Atlas* method, of $1045 or less in 2013; middle-income economies are those with a GNI per capita of more than $1045 but less than $12,746; high-income economies are those with a GNI per capita of $12,746 or more. Lower-middle-income and upper-middle-income economies are separated at a GNI per capita of $4125

actual incidence of brain tumors in LIC and LMIC is very difficult to ascertain. Many children and young people are not diagnosed for a variety of reasons, including late presentation and lack of neuroimaging facilities. In addition, there is frequently a lack of trained clinicians, including radiologists, pathologists, neurosurgeons, and oncologists (Barr 1994), which adversely affects the ability to adequately diagnose brain tumors. True numbers of subtypes of brain tumors may not be possible to determine since a tissue diagnosis is seldom achieved. The prevalence of the different CNS tumor types as well as the biological subgroups may differ in LIC and LMIC from HIC, but this information is

not readily available due to the factors mentioned above. In addition, a number of intracerebral lesions are labelled as brain tumors when in fact they are not (Mitra et al. 2012).

Globally, great advances have been made in the biological understanding of pediatric CNS tumors as well as treatment modalities and treatment stratification for children with CNS tumors, but these advances are not relevant to the majority of children with brain tumors in whom adequate access to the basic pillars of treatment are missing. Successful treatment of such children requires input from many different health professionals and is best coordinated by a formal and functioning multidisciplinary team. This can be

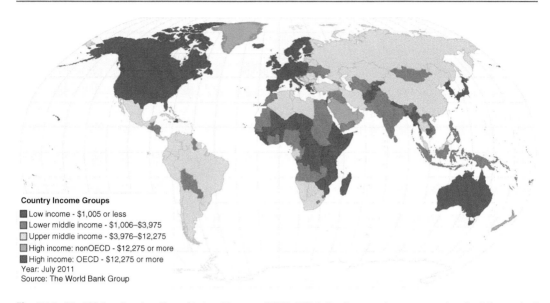

Country Income Groups
■ Low income - $1,005 or less
■ Lower middle income - $1,006–$3,975
☐ Upper middle income - $3,976–$12,275
■ High income: nonOECD - $12,275 or more
■ High income: OECD - $12,275 or more
Year: July 2011
Source: The World Bank Group

Fig. 17.1 World Map showing Gross National Income (GNI) (US dollars) per capita per year using the Atlas method (The World Bank 2015a)

difficult to achieve in LIC and LMIC where the number of health professionals varies widely (Table 17.2), with some countries having less than 0.2 doctors and 56 nurses per 100,000 population (TWB 2015b).

There are many factors important in setting up and maintaining a functioning program to adequately treat children with CNS tumors in LIC and LMIC. Some of these are outlined below.

17.2 Establishing a Neuro-Oncology Program in Low Income and Low Middle Income Countries

17.2.1 Political Will and Funding

Considerable investment is required to adequately care for children with brain tumors, but the commitment of different governments to their care varies. Not only are highly trained personnel required, but functioning tertiary facilities with adequate infrastructure and maintenance are needed as well. Nongovernmental organizations, including universities and charities from resource-rich countries, sometimes provide training, financial assistance, and equipment. However, the local government must be supportive in order to sustain effective programs.

Trained health professionals in some LIC and LMIC countries receive limited salaries for their public work, resulting in them seeking employment outside of their countries or in the private sector where they are better remunerated. This may result in less time for treating the majority of children who require their expertise. Some practitioners use income from their private practice to fund patients unable to afford treatment, and nongovernmental organizations and charities may supplement salaries of key personnel in order to ensure that more time is spent looking after those who are less advantaged. The requirement for patients to pay for part of their treatment or for certain drugs or treatment modalities varies from country to country and may also have an effect on the delivery of care.

17.2.2 The Importance of the Multidisciplinary Team

Early discussion of each child with a CNS tumor results in a higher standard of care and a better outcome (Parkes et al. 2015). There are many aspects of care requiring involvement from many

Table 17.2 Table showing health related parameters in countries as defined by the World Bank (TWB 2015b)

Country	Per capita	Health workers		Hospital beds
		Physicians	Nurses and midwives	
	$	per 1000 people	per 1000 people	per 1000 people
	2013	2007–13	2007–13	2007–12
Norway	9715	4.3	17.3	3.3
Switzerland	9276	4	17.4	5
United States	9146	2.5	9.8	2.9
Luxembourg	7980	2.9	12.6	5.4
Monaco	6993	7.2	17.2	13.8
Denmark	6270	3.5	16.8	3.5
Netherlands	6145	2.9	8.4	4.7
Australia	5827	3.3	10.6	3.9
Canada	5718	2.1	9.3	2.7
Sweden	5680	3.9	11.9	2.7
Austria	5427	4.8	7.9	7.6
Belgium	5093	4.9	16.8	6.5
Germany	5006	3.9	11.5	8.2
France	4864	3.2	9.3	6.4
Finland	4449	2.9	10.9	5.5
Ireland	4233	2.7	15.7	2.9
Iceland	4126	3.5	15.6	3.2
New Zealand	4063	2.7	10.9	2.3
Euro area	4018	3.9	7.5	5.6
Japan	3966	2.3	11.5	13.7
San Marino	3847	5.1	8.8	3.8
United Kingdom	3598	2.8	8.8	2.9
Italy	3155	3.8	0.3	3.4
Andorra	2948	4	4.8	2.5
Israel	2601	3.3	5	3.3
Spain	2581	4.9	5.7	3.1
Singapore	2507	2	5.8	2
Greece	2146	6.2	0.2	4.8
Slovenia	2085	2.5	8.5	4.6
Qatar	2043	7.7	11.9	1.2
Portugal	2037	4.1	6.1	3.4
Malta	1994	3.5	7.5	4.8
Korea, Rep.	1880	2.1	5	10.3
Cyprus	1866	2.3	4.5	3.5
Bahamas, The	1621	2.8	4.1	2.9
United Arab Emirates	1569	2.5	3.2	1.1
Kuwait	1507	2.7	4.6	2.2
Slovak Republic	1454	3.3	6.1	6
Uruguay	1431	3.7	5.5	2.5
Czech Republic	1367	3.6	8.4	6.8
Chile	1204	1	0.1	2.1
Brazil	1083	1.9	7.6	2.3
Argentina	1074	3.9		4.7
Estonia	1072	3.2	6.4	5.3
Bahrain	1067	0.9	2.4	2.1
Hungary	1056	3.1	6.5	7.2

Table 17.2   (continued)

Country	Per capita	Health workers		Hospital beds
		Physicians	Nurses and midwives	
	$	per 1000 people	per 1000 people	per 1000 people
	2013	2007–13	2007–13	2007–12
World	1048	1.5	3.3	
Palau	1008	1.4	5.7	4.8
Barbados	1007	1.8	4.9	6.2
Costa Rica	1005	1.1	0.8	1.2
Croatia	982	3	5.3	5.9
Brunei Darussalam	974	1.4	8	2.8
Lithuania	966	4.1	7.2	7
Trinidad and Tobago	965	1.2	3.6	2.7
Russian Federation	957	4.3	8.5	
Poland	895	2.2	6.2	6.5
Latvia	874	3.6	3.4	5.9
St. Kitts and Nevis	861			2.3
Saudi Arabia	808	2.5	4.9	2.1
Panama	796	1.7	1.4	2.2
Latin America and Caribbean	746	2	4.3	2
Maldives	720	1.4	5	4.3
Equatorial Guinea	714			2.1
Tuvalu	704	1.1	5.8	
Oman	678	2.4	5.4	1.7
Antigua and Barbuda	665			2.1
Mexico	664	2.1	2.5	1.5
Lebanon	631	3.2	2.7	3.5
Marshall Islands	630	0.4	1.7	2.7
St. Lucia	621	0.1		1.6
Turkey	608	1.7	2.4	2.5
Cuba	603	6.7	9.1	5.3
South Africa	593	0.8	5.1	
Kazakhstan	580	3.6	8.3	7.2
Bulgaria	555	3.9	4.8	6.4
Seychelles	551	1.1	4.8	3.6
Colombia	533	1.5	0.6	1.5
Romania	504	2.4	5.6	6.1
Grenada	499			3.5
Venezuela, RB	497			0.9
Upper middle income	479	1.8	2.7	3.4
Serbia	475	2.1	4.5	5.4
Belarus	463	3.9	10.6	11.3
Mauritius	463			3.4
Montenegro	461	2.1	5.4	4
Bosnia and Herzegovina	449	1.9	5.6	3.5
Suriname	445			3.1
Gabon	441			6.3
Azerbaijan	436	3.4	6.5	4.7
Europe and Central Asia	436	2.6	6	5.6
Libya	433	1.9	6.8	3.7
Iran, Islamic Rep.	432	0.9	1.4	0.1

(continued)

Table 17.2 (continued)

Country	Per capita	Health workers		Hospital beds
		Physicians	Nurses and midwives	
	$	per 1000 people	per 1000 people	per 1000 people
	2013	2007–13	2007–13	2007–12
Malaysia	423	1.2	3.3	1.9
Namibia	423	0.4	2.8	2.7
Dominica	417			3.8
Micronesia, Fed. Sts.	407	0.2	3.3	3.2
Botswana	397	0.3	2.8	1.8
Paraguay	395	1.2	1	1.3
China	367	1.9	1.9	3.8
Ecuador	361	1.7	2.2	1.6
Peru	354	1.1	1.5	1.5
Georgia	350	4.3	0.1	2.6
St. Vincent and the Grenadines	345			5.2
Jordan	336	2.6	4	1.8
Dominican Republic	315	1.5	1.3	1.7
Algeria	314	1.2	1.9	
Ukraine	313	3.5	7.7	9
Macedonia, FYR	312	2.6	0.6	4.5
Tunisia	309	1.2	3.3	2.1
Iraq	305	0.6	1.4	1.3
Jamaica	300	0.4	1.1	1.7
East Asia and Pacific	293	1.5	1.8	3.6
Samoa	271	0.5	1.9	
Angola	267	0.2	1.7	
El Salvador	266	1.6	0.4	1.1
Thailand	264	0.4	2.1	2.1
Moldova	263	3	6.4	6.2
Belize	262	0.8	2	1.1
Middle East and North Africa	260	1.4	2.1	0.8
Swaziland	256	0.2	1.6	2.1
Guyana	250	0.2	0.5	2
Mongolia	244	2.8	3.6	6.8
Albania	240	1.1	3.8	2.6
Guatemala	227	0.9	0.9	0.6
Tonga	204	0.6	3.9	2.6
Honduras	193			0.7
Fiji	189	0.4	2.2	2
Morocco	189	0.6	0.9	0.9
Bolivia	174	0.5	1	1.1
Kiribati	166	0.4	3.7	1.3
Cabo Verde	165	0.3	0.6	2.1
Armenia	159	2.7	4.8	3.9
Turkmenistan	158	2.4	4.4	4
Nicaragua	153			0.9
Egypt, Arab Rep.	151	2.8	3.5	0.5
Djibouti	137	0.2	0.8	1.4
Congo, Rep.	131	0.1	0.8	
Lesotho	123			

Table 17.2 (continued)

Country	Per capita	Health workers		Hospital beds
		Physicians	Nurses and midwives	
	$	per 1000 people	per 1000 people	per 1000 people
	2013	2007–13	2007–13	2007–12
Vanuatu	123	0.1	1.7	1.8
Philippines	122			1
Uzbekistan	120	2.5	11.9	4.4
Nigeria	115	0.4	1.6	
Sudan	115	0.3	0.8	0.8
Vietnam	111	1.2	1.2	2
Sao Tome and Principe	110			2.9
Indonesia	107	0.2	1.4	0.9
Sri Lanka	102	0.7	1.6	3.6
Sub-Saharan Africa	101	0.2	1.1	
Ghana	100	0.1	0.9	0.9
Solomon Islands	100	0.2	2.1	1.3
Sierra Leone	96	0	0.2	
Papua New Guinea	94	0.1	0.6	
Zambia	93	0.2	0.8	2
Bhutan	90	0.3	1	1.8
Lower middle income	88	0.8	1.8	
Cote d'Ivoire	87	0.1	0.5	
Kyrgyz Republic	87	2	6.2	4.8
Haiti	77			1.3
Cambodia	76	0.2	0.8	0.7
Yemen, Rep.	74	0.2	0.7	0.7
Rwanda	71	0.1	0.7	1.6
Tajikistan	70	1.9	5	5.5
Cameroon	67	0.1	0.4	1.3
India	61	0.7	1.7	0.7
Timor-Leste	59	0.1	1.1	5.9
Uganda	59	0.1	1.3	0.5
South Asia	56	0.7	1.4	0.7
Togo	54	0.1	0.3	0.7
Mali	53	0.1	0.4	0.1
Comoros	51			
Afghanistan	49	0.3	0.1	0.5
Tanzania	49	0	0.4	0.7
Burkina Faso	46	0	0.6	0.4
Senegal	46	0.1	0.4	0.3
Kenya	45	0.2	0.9	1.4
Liberia	44	0	0.3	0.8
Mauritania	44	0.1	0.7	
Syrian Arab Republic	43	1.5	1.9	1.5
Mozambique	40	0	0.4	0.7
Nepal	39			
Benin	37	0.1	0.8	0.5
Chad	37			
Pakistan	37	0.8	0.6	0.6
Bangladesh	32	0.4	0.2	0.6

(continued)

Table 17.2 (continued)

Country	Per capita	Health workers		Hospital beds
		Physicians	Nurses and midwives	
	$	per 1000 people	per 1000 people	per 1000 people
	2013	2007–13	2007–13	2007–12
Guinea-Bissau	32	0	0.6	1
Lao PDR	32	0.2	0.9	1.5
Gambia, The	29	0	0.6	1.1
Niger	27	0	0.1	
Malawi	26	0	0.3	1.3
Ethiopia	25	0	0.2	6.3
Guinea	25	0.1	0	0.3
Burundi	21			1.9
Madagascar	20	0.2		0.2
South Sudan	18			
Eritrea	17			0.7
Congo, Dem. Rep.	16			
Myanmar	14	0.6	1	
Central African Republic	13	0	0.3	1
Zimbabwe		0.1	1.3	1.7

Health expenditure per capita is the sum of public and private health expenditures as a ratio of total population. It covers the provision of health services (preventive and curative), family planning activities, nutrition activities, and emergency aid designated for health but does not include provision of water and sanitation. Values in US $. Nurses and midwives include professional nurses, professional midwives, auxiliary nurses, auxiliary midwives, enrolled nurses, enrolled midwives and other associated personnel, such as dental nurses and primary care nurses. Hospital beds include inpatient beds available in public, private, general, and specialized hospitals and rehabilitation centers. In most cases beds for both acute and chronic care are included

disciplines. Since they are interdependent, it is vital that coordinated care is discussed prior to definitive treatment. Interdisciplinary discussion is critical in order to maximize outcomes. An example of this is the decision to undertake curative surgery for a presumed medulloblastoma when there are no radiation facilities available. In some circumstances referral to the nearest tertiary unit with appropriate facilities should be encouraged. Lack of multidisciplinary team coordinated care is a major stumbling block to effective care in many LIC and LMIC centers.

17.2.3 The Value of Country-Wide Services and Common Protocols

Common treatment protocols used across a country or region allow a standard of care to be developed. Each LIC and LMIC should consider whether centralization of core neuro-oncology services, such as surgery and radiotherapy, would benefit the children of the region. A different solution may be necessary for each country or region. Twinning with regular online meetings with other centers or regions may also advance care. One such example is the weekly shared care telemedicine meeting run by the team at Red Cross Children's Hospital in Cape Town where sub-Saharan centers in Africa discuss difficult cases. Others include wider initiatives such as Asociacion de Hemato-Oncologia Pediatrica de Centro America (AHOPCA), which is a collaboration between many countries in Central America (Barr et al. 2014).

17.2.4 Outside Support, Including Twinning

The International Society of Paediatric Oncology (SIOP) has a subgroup named Paediatric Oncology in Developing Countries (PODC).

This latter group has been set up to aid health professionals working in the resource challenged world and to facilitate twinning between centers in resource challenged and resource rich countries. In addition, the development of treatment guidelines for specific tumor types appropriate to various settings is a priority. The first SIOP-PODC neuro-oncology guideline, namely that for standard risk medulloblastoma, was recently published (Parkes et al. 2015).

The American Society of Clinical Oncology (ASCO) has similar initiatives, as do a number of other organizations and institutions, particularly St. Jude Children's Research Hospital (Ribeiro et al. 2008; Ribeiro 2012) in Memphis and Sick Kids Hospital (Qaddoumi et al. 2008) in Toronto. The majority of these programs aim to enable the local hospitals to lead the process and to develop their own long-term clinical and funding strategies.

There are many other examples of twinning and many large institutions in HIC have twinning partners. Twinning is individualized according to the centers involved and most programs encompass the exchange of ideas, regular video conferencing or teleconferencing with multidisciplinary teams (Ribeiro et al. 2008; Ribeiro 2012; Qaddoumi et al. 2008) and remote pathological diagnosis (Mitra et al. 2012; Carey et al. 2014; Fischer et al. 2011; Gimbel et al. 2012; Sirintrapun et al. 2012).

17.2.5 Development of Essential Infrastructure

There are a number of core facilities and infrastructure requirements for treatment of children with CNS tumors. SIOP PODC has produced a guideline for determining settings according to the facilities and expertise available in order to facilitate decisions about what treatment should be offered (Parkes et al. 2015) (Table 17.3). The temptation to offer treatment conceived in HIC that requires a high level of supportive care may paradoxically worsen the outcome in LIC and LMIC, because excessive toxic mortality outweighs any survival advantage (Magrath et al.

2013). Some of the essential infrastructure required is outlined below.

17.2.5.1   Radiology

Accurate and detailed imaging is vital in diagnosis, decision-making, and follow-up of children with CNS tumors. The radiologist is a vital member of the multidisciplinary team. In most LIC and LMIC centers, reporting is done by a general radiologist. The experience of the radiologist may vary greatly depending on prior training opportunities. Hence, the guidance given to the surgeon, radiation oncologists, and oncologist varies. This must be taken into account when making decisions on when and how to treat children.

Diagnostic facilities vary greatly in LIC and LIMC. There may also be inequity in imaging facilities between the private and government sectors. In a survey of 104 SIOP PODC members, 93% of respondents had access to CT scans and 82% to MRI scans (77% in Africa, Table 17.4) (Parkes et al. 2015), but some of these centers did not have access to intravenous contrast agents. More refined techniques, such as magnetic resonance spectroscopy and diffusion weighted imaging were usually not available. Waiting times to access scans as well as the quality of the scans varies greatly. Twinning with a center in a HIC may be of some assistance since images may be shared and discussed remotely using telemedicine platforms (Mitra et al. 2012; Gimbel et al. 2012).

17.2.5.2   Neurosurgery

Neurosurgical expertise is vital for the safe treatment of children and adolescents with CNS tumors. Children with CNS tumors are usually referred directly to the neurosurgical service and the willingness and ability of surgeons to refer these patients on to other members of the multidisciplinary team, including oncologists, may determine the feasibility of further curative treatment. In the SIOP PODC survey, only 76% of respondents had neurosurgical and oncology facilities available within the same hospital network (Parkes et al. 2015). In addition, neurosurgeons in LMIC frequently did not have vital

Table 17.3 Infrastructural and personnel service line levels for selection of SIOP PODC adapted treatment regimens for standard risk medulloblastoma

Service	Level 0	Level 1	Level 2	Level 3	Level 4
Pediatric cancer unit description (multidisciplinary team operates at all levels)	Pilot project	Some basic oncology services	Established pediatric oncology program with most basic services and a few state-of-the-art services	Pediatric oncology program with all essential services and most state-of-the-art services	Pediatric oncology center of excellence with all state-of-the-art services and some highly specialized services (e.g., proton beam radiation therapy, MIBG therapy, access to phase I studies)
Typical settings	LIC in disadvantaged areas	LIC in larger healthcare centers, lower MIC in disadvantaged areas	Lower MIC in larger healthcare centers, upper MIC in disadvantaged areas	Upper MIC in larger healthcare centers, most centers in HIC	Selected tertiary and quaternary care centers in HIC
Medical facilities					
Ward	No pediatric oncology unit	Basic pediatric oncology service available to some patients	Pediatric oncology unit available to most patients; isolation rooms usually available for infected patients	Pediatric oncology unit with a full complement of fixed staff and available to all patients; isolation rooms always available for infected patients	Specialized pediatric oncology units for particular groups of patients (e.g., transplant, neuro-oncology, acute myeloid leukemia)
Diagnosis, staging, and therapeutic capabilities					
Pathology	None	Microscope, H&E staining, CSF cytology	Limited immunohistochemistry panel (disease-specific), Cytospin for CSF samples	Complete immunohistochemistry panel, molecular pathology for most diseases	Research diagnostics, whole genome sequencing, molecular pathology for all diseases
Diagnostic imaging	None	Radiographs, ultrasound	CT scan, bone scintigraphy, Gallium scintigraphy	Magnetic resonance imaging; PET-CT and MIBG may be available	Specialized imaging; advanced nuclear medicine applications, PET-CT and MIBG diagnostic
Antineoplastic availability	Access to a limited selection of oncology drugs	Access to a limited selection of oncology drugs	Access to almost all essential oncology drugs; occasional shortages	Access to almost all commercially available drugs; rare shortages	Access to all approved drugs, plus phase I and phase II studies
Radiation therapy facilities	None	Cobalt source; 2D planning	Cobalt source or linear accelerator; 2D or some 3D planning. Ability to plan craniospinal radiotherapy and deliver treatment on at least 4 days per week	Linear accelerator; full conformal therapy available. Intensity-modulated radiotherapy available	Intensity-modulated radiotherapy. Proton beam facility

Personnel					
Oncology team leader	Primary care physicians care for cancer and many other diseases	Primary care provider with interest in oncology	Primary care provider with pediatric oncology experience or some training, medical oncologist without pediatric expertise	Pediatric oncologist or medical oncologist with significant pediatric experience or training	Pediatric oncologist with highly disease-specific expertise
Oncology unit medical, nursing, and pharmacy staff	A few staff members with basic training	A few oncology personnel with some oncology training; trainees responsible for many aspects of patient care	Generally adequate numbers of oncology personnel; consistent supervision of any trainees involved in patient care	Full complement of oncology physicians; specialized oncology nurses; pharmacists with oncology training	Full complement of oncology personnel, including specialized physician extenders (e.g., nurse practitioners, hospitalists)
Surgery and surgical subspecialties relevant for each cancer	No surgeon	General surgeon or adult subspecialty surgeon (neurosurgeon, ophthalmologist, other)	Pediatric surgeon or subspecialty surgeon (neurosurgeon, ophthalmologist, other)	Pediatric cancer surgeon or pediatric subspecialty surgeon (neurosurgeon, ophthalmologist, other)	Pediatric cancer surgeon or subspecialty surgeon with highly specialized disease-specific expertise
Pathology	No pathologist	Pathologist available for some cases	Pathologist available for all cases	Hematopathologist and pediatric pathologist available	Pathologist with highly specialized disease-specific expertise
Radiation therapy	None	Radiation therapists with adult expertise	Radiation therapists with some pediatric experience	Radiation therapists with pediatric expertise	Pediatric radiation oncologist with highly specialized disease-specific expertise

This shows the suggested levels of infrastructure required for various levels of risk-adapted treatment and may be used as a model for deciding which CNS tumors are able to be treated in individual centers (Parkes et al. 2015)

LIC low income countries, *MIC* middle income countries, *H&E* *hematoxylin & eosin*, *CSF* cerebrospinal fluid, *PET* positron emission tomography, *MIBG* metaiodobenzylguanidine

Table 17.4 Online survey of resources available in low and low middle income countries with regards to services essential for a pediatric neuro-oncology service

Online survey via www.cure4kids.org in May and June 2013	
Total responses	104
Responses by continent	Africa 32%, Asia 30%, South and Central (S&C) America 33%
Respondents	Oncologists 58%, Neurosurgeons 15%, Radiation Oncologists 8%, Pediatricians 15%
Access to imaging	CT 93%, MRI 82% (Africa 77%)
Access to pathology	Morphologic diagnosis 96%, subtyping 53% Waiting time longer than 10 days 39%
On site neurosurgery	76%
VPS insertion	35% of 79 respondents reported that >50% of children had VPS
Access to ICU	80%
Referred to radiotherapy	Overall: 84% within 40 days: 74%
Access to CT planning	89%
Access to Linac	66% (Africa 48%) the rest have Cobalt
Access to craniospinal XRT	84%
Access to chemotherapy	79%
Vincristine with radiotherapy	63%
Chemotherapy pre-XRT	31% (1/3 routinely; 2/3 because of XRT delays)
Venous access devices (mostly portocaths)	45% (Africa 21%; Asia 41%; S&C America 64%)
Chemotherapy drug access	Lomustine 43% (Africa 44%; Asia 39%; S&C America 64%) Carboplatin 86% All other drugs >89%
Supportive care	Dedicated pediatric oncology ward 88% Nutritional support 72% and dietetics 67% Physiotherapy 78%; Occupational Therapy 47%; Play Therapy 33%
Access to a combined clinic	56%

VPS ventriculoperitoneal shunt, *ICU* intensive care unit, *Linac* linear accelerator, *XRT* external beam radiation therapy

equipment or adequate preoperative imaging, making definitive surgery more difficult. It may be appropriate in many LIC and LMIC centers to perform a temporary cerebrospinal fluid (CSF) diversion in order to enable transfer of the patient to another center with more expertise or facilities.

The experience and support of neurosurgeons varies greatly in terms of pediatric CNS tumor surgery in LIC and LMIC. Some surgeons may offer surgery without any knowledge of whether further treatment is available, and others may attempt surgery that is beyond the level of their expertise. The neuro-oncology units with the best

outcomes for children have a multidisciplinary team in which there is a close collaboration between the neurosurgeon and other members of the wider team.

17.2.5.3 Pathology

The pathological diagnosis of children's CNS tumors is complex. The majority of pathologists in LIC and LMIC are not subspecialized and see relatively few children's CNS tumors. In the SIOP PODC survey, 96% of centers had access to morphology and 53% to subtyping, but in 39% the waiting time for a result was longer than 10 days (Parkes et al. 2015). Many immunocytochemistry tests essential for accurate diagnosis are not routinely available in LIC and LMIC. With the increasing reliance on molecular testing and the likely inclusion of these tests in the new World Health Organization (WHO) tumor classification (Gottardo et al. 2014), this gap will only increase.

Some HIC services offer remote pathological advice through web-based systems such as with scanners or simple microscope cameras with dropboxes (Mitra et al. 2012; Carey et al. 2014; Fischer et al. 2011; Gimbel et al. 2012; Sirintrapun et al. 2012). The alternative is that specimens are sent by courier to other centers or countries, but this may lead to a delay in diagnosis.

17.2.5.4 Radiotherapy

Availability of radiotherapy requires considerable investment. Because of this, many LIC and LMIC have a single center or limited numbers of centers that cater to all patients requiring radiotherapy. Distances to access such centers are huge, and since most radiotherapy courses require daily treatments for up to 6 weeks, patients have to be accommodated in or close to the center. Small children requiring daily radiotherapy treatments require sedation or anesthetics. This is resource-intense and time consuming. For this reason,

some LIC and LMIC centers refer such cases to regional tertiary centers for treatment.

The radiotherapy technique used may determine the late side effect profile in the child. The ability to do at least 3-D conformal radiotherapy planning and treat patients on linear accelerators as opposed to 2-D planning and Cobalt treatment may significantly affect the future quality of life of survivors. Currently, less than 50% of centers within Africa are able to offer this (IAEA n.d.) (Fig. 17.2).

The ability to identify and manage late effects of radiotherapy may also be problematic in LIC and LMIC. Survivors of pediatric CNS tumors require long-term follow-up and management of various problems, including endocrinopathies, hearing and visual deficits, and neurocognitive problems. Poor diagnosis and management of these problems may impact significantly on quality of life for these patients.

17.2.5.5 Chemotherapy

Although surgery and radiotherapy are the mainstay of treatment for CNS tumors in children, chemotherapy plays an important role, especially in the very young and for chemosensitive tumors. Chemotherapeutic strategies need to be tailored in a risk-adapted way to take into account the

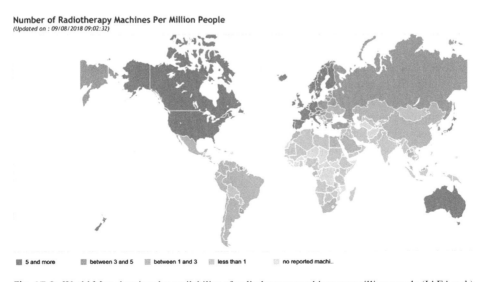

Number of Radiotherapy Machines Per Million People
(Updated on : 09/08/2018 09:02:32)

▇ 5 and more ▇ between 3 and 5 ▇ between 1 and 3 ▇ less than 1 ▢ no reported machi..

Fig. 17.2 World Map showing the availability of radiotherapy machines per million people (IAEA n.d.)

availability of drugs and the supportive care available. Skilled and knowledgeable staff are required to deliver chemotherapy that is often complex to administer and requires close monitoring. In 21% of centers surveyed, there was no access to chemotherapy necessary to treat pediatric CNS tumors (Parkes et al. 2015). Of the 79% of centers that used chemotherapy for brain tumors, carboplatin was available in 86% of centers but lomustine in only 43%. The regimens used varied widely; some centers used locally adapted regimens, some developed protocols in discussion with their twinning partners, and some attempted to use protocols developed in HIC. Treating children with chemotherapy is best undertaken when the potential consequences of toxicity can be adequately managed (e.g., hearing aids when cisplatin may lead to deafness).

17.2.5.6 Supportive Care

Advances in supportive care have enabled more intensive therapies to be delivered safely. This is not always the case in LIC and LMIC where levels of supportive care vary widely; therefore, it is vital that the intensity of treatment offered to patients does not exceed the level of supportive treatment available.

Supportive care has many facets, especially for children with CNS tumors, and includes both short- and long-term issues. In the immediate diagnostic and management period when the children may be extremely unwell, the ability to monitor electrolytes 24 h a day, perform blood counts and neurological observations, and have access to antibiotics and antifungals as well as blood products is essential to safe management. Children may have electrolyte instabilities, either as a presenting feature or as a consequence of their surgery. This, coupled with possible hormone disorders, such as antidiuretic hormone (ADH) deficiency (diabetes insipidus) or inappropriate ADH secretion, may require specialist endocrine input. Intracranial bleeding, CSF leaks, development of raised intracranial pressure, or deterioration in neurological state require rapid recognition and response,

especially in the acute setting. There needs to be rapid 24-h access to either CT or MRI scanning. Central venous catheters may need to be inserted to deliver some of this supportive care. The majority of children in the immediate postoperative phase are managed in an intensive care unit when the child is most susceptible to sudden deterioration. Supportive care drugs such as anti-emetics, opiates, and neuropathic analgesia play an important role in the comfort of the child.

After the immediate postoperative period, the ability to provide nutritional support (both enteral and parental) is an important adjunct to many treatment schedules and may limit the intensity of treatment that can be used. The access to visual and hearing aids for those children with compromised vision or hearing is necessary to ensure the quality of their life. The ability to measure and treat hormone deficiencies that were either present pre-surgery or developed post-surgery is essential.

In a survey by Parkes et al. (2015) (Table 17.4), only 45% of units surveyed were able to place central venous access devices (21% in Africa, 41% in Asia and 64% in Central and South America). Nutritional support was provided in 72% of centers and dietetic support in 67%. Physiotherapy was available in 78% of centers, occupational therapy in 47%, and play therapy in 33%. Dedicated pediatric oncology wards were present in 88%.

17.2.6 Developing Skills and Training Staff

Adequate training of all team members is one of the most vital aspects in both setting up a neuro-oncology service and in its continuing development. There are many training programs as well as twinning programs that are supported by governments from HIC or by nongovernmental organizations. It is important that the training should be appropriate to the setting in which the professionals are working and that specific issues relating to working in LIC and LMIC are addressed. Where training happens remotely, ongoing support from the host institutions must be provided in order to sustain this development.

In instances where expensive equipment needs to be procured for cancer services (e.g., radiotherapy equipment, neurosurgical equipment), it is prudent that the cost of training personnel, as well as the cost of maintaining such equipment, be included in the equipment tender. This requires commercial companies who supply such equipment to have a responsibility both in ensuring that the correct equipment is procured and that local staff are empowered to operate it optimally.

17.3 Factors Affecting the Program

17.3.1 Delayed Recognition

The successful treatment of CNS tumors is reliant on early diagnosis and timely intervention. Delays are more often the result of nonrecognition by medical personnel rather than nonpresentation by parents (Dang-Tan et al. 2007; Stefan et al. 2011; Abdelkhalek et al. 2014). It is important for the multidisciplinary team to work with the general pediatric and surgical services to continue to educate them about the warning signs of CNS tumors, and to be accessible to provide advice to referring centers as well as to expedite potential referrals.

17.3.2 Cultural Factors

In some poorly developed countries, prompt management is delayed due to families presenting to traditional healers first. However, traditional healers play an important role in many cultures and respect for these professionals must be maintained. Some countries, such as India, have chosen to promote such healers (Kumar 2000) and embed them in their health system. A

partnership with such healers may have multiple benefits, such as mutual respect and trust allowing for prompt referral in both directions. Gender bias in some societies may also be a barrier to effective and prompt treatment for some (Arora et al. 2010).

17.3.3 Financial Factors

The financial implications of having a child with a brain tumor cannot be overstated, especially in regions of extreme poverty. There is a wide variation within regions and countries as to the cost of healthcare to the patients themselves. Some countries have free healthcare but others require the parent to contribute, and often require them to pay for medications. This leads to further inequity of healthcare as the poorest families are not able to afford treatment.

Food and transport to and from the hospital is expensive. Since children with CNS tumors need to be treated at a central hospital, many parents in rural LMICs have to travel vast distances in order to be present for treatment. The child may require prolonged stays in the hospital with a caregiver present. This adds to the family's financial burden since the parent who is the primary caregiver is unable to work during this time. Additional caregivers may also need to be employed to care for siblings remaining at home.

17.3.4 Comorbidities

The treatment of children with CNS tumors in LMIC may be confounded by the presence of comorbidities making optimal treatment excessively toxic. Underlying nutritional status has major implications and although this has best been described for non-CNS tumors, the same principles apply (Israëls et al. 2008). There may be a decreased ability to tolerate some drugs, such as cardio- and nephrotoxic drugs. The children may also be unable to mount an adequate response to infection in the face of chemo- or radiotherapy-induced myelosuppression. Additionally, HIV infection is prevalent in many LIC and LMIC. It does not appear to play a major causative role in most primary pediatric CNS tumors, but it may significantly complicate the treatment of affected children.

17.4 Decision-Making and Service Development

17.4.1 Deciding Who to Treat and When

The key when developing a neuro-oncology service is to set realistic expectations and goals. One of the most challenging decisions is to decide what diagnoses are able to be treated safely and what level of treatment should be offered in a center. The balance of manageable toxicity versus potential curability needs to be carefully considered. It is tempting to try to offer advanced treatment to everyone in every setting, but the toxic death and morbidity rate may result in an overall poorer outcome. It is important that the whole team supports this concept. A suggestion would be that each unit uses setting tables such as those developed by SIOP PODC (Table 17.3) to realistically select the optimal treatment regimen for their patients. With limited resources, children who have tumors that are potentially curable should be prioritized. However, it is important that all children should be offered a good standard of clinical care, whether it be radical or palliative.

17.4.2 Preventing Treatment Abandonment

The failure to complete treatment for nonmedical reasons (also known as treatment abandonment) is a long-standing concern, especially in LIC and LMIC. In a recent survey it was estimated that 99% of cases in which children fail to complete treatment occur in LIC and LMIC (Friedrich et al. 2015). The number of children failing to complete

treatment is approximately equal to the number of children treated in HIC. There are many reasons, but the predominant ones are failure of caregivers to understand the reasons for treatment, financial concerns, need to care for other children, and lack of transport (Friedrich et al. 2015; Wang et al. 2015; Salaverria et al. 2015). There have been many efforts across many countries to tackle the issue of abandonment and great strides have been made. These are most successful when having government backing with national investment; an example is state-sponsored treatment for children with acute lymphoblastic leukemia in Mexico (Rivera-Luna et al. 2014). Since complex treatments and rehabilitation are required for many children with CNS tumors, active efforts must be made to address parents' concerns from the start of treatment.

17.4.3 Follow-Up and Management of Late Effects

One of the major challenges faced by units in LIC and LMIC is the ability to manage the late effects of treatment of children with CNS tumors. These children often have major difficulties in later life and it is crucial that support is available to help them. The tumors and treatment can cause a range of problems including motor difficulties, cognitive problems, hearing and visual deficits, endocrinopathies, and growth disturbances (Laughton et al. 2008; Palmer et al. 2013; Ullrich et al. 2007). These can significantly affect school performance, the ability to gain employment, interpersonal relationships, and reproductive ability. All of the above may result in depression and loss of self-worth requiring counselling and possibly intervention.

Treating the tumor is only the beginning of the child and family's journey. It is just as important that resources are used in this area as it is in the acute care of children with CNS tumors. However, many LIC and LMIC centers do not have the facilities, staffing levels, or training to provide follow-up.

17.4.4 Measuring Outcomes

Measuring outcomes is a fundamental cornerstone in developing and improving a neuro-oncology service. Outcomes should include not only survival but also morbidity and toxicity of treatment. Follow-up in LIC and LMIC can be challenging since patients may not return and considerable effort is required to make contact with the families in order to assess survival and impact of treatment. Many units employ a data manager or follow-up nurse/social scientist for this task. A robust and well backed-up database is essential and there are a number of web-based and stand-alone software solutions available (e.g., POND database from Cure 4 Kids based at St. Jude) (Quintana et al. 2013).

17.4.5 Registries and Tumor Banks

A national, regional, or even a center tumor registry is a worthwhile investment for the future. It allows the incidences of various CNS tumor types to be calculated, and records treatment details, toxicities, and outcomes. A registry takes a lot of effort, but is extremely beneficial in the long term. Similarly, although storing tumor samples for future research is a low priority for most LIC and LMIC, it is valuable for future translational research. It does need to go hand in hand with a tumor registry to ensure that appropriate clinical data is collected alongside the tumor sample. If possible, constitutional DNA in the form of blood should be collected at the same time.

17.4.6 Research

Research, mainly in the form of clinical trials or translational research, is an important aspect of the development of neuro-oncology services. Research conducted in resource-constrained countries fosters improved care and outcomes for children; most examples of this are found in leukemia (Carey et al. 2014; Magrath et al. 2005)

but it is just as important in children with CNS tumors. It has been well shown that participation in clinical trials improves the outcome of children with cancer (Magrath et al. 2013; Howard et al. 2005). While it is important to foster and encourage research in LIC and LMIC, this should not be the primary aim of a developing service. It is equally important that institutions from HIC do not use developing countries as testing grounds or a means of improving their institution's research portfolio and journal outputs. The local institution should have a local principal investigator who has equal rights, including senior authorship. The development of local principal investigators is important for long-term sustainability, growth, and ownership of neuro-oncology services.

Technological developments and equipment may help centers in LIC and LMIC, but these should be coupled with improvements in all aspects of care; for example, subgrouping of medulloblastoma is only of use if there is adequate surgery, radiotherapy, and supportive care. It is also important that any financial contribution from research to the care of the patients be spread among all the patients in the unit and not be used exclusively for those on the study, as this encourages differential levels of care.

17.4.7 The Wider Multidisciplinary Team

There are many other members of the wider multidisciplinary team who perform important roles in the functioning of a neuro-oncology service (Fig. 17.3). These may include physiotherapists and occupational therapists, dieticians, speech and language therapists, play therapists (very useful in helping children through various procedures and treatments such as radiotherapy), social workers, chaplains and equivalents in other religious faiths. A palliative care team that may double as a pain management team is vital in a context where a number of patients will not survive.

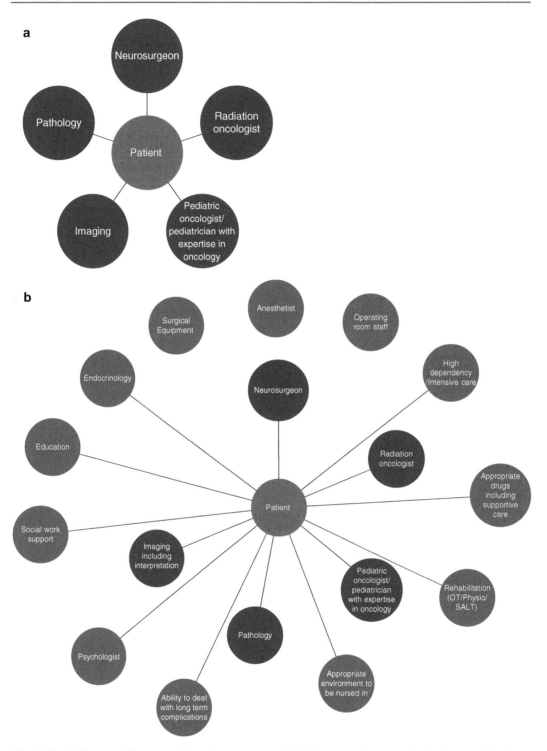

Fig. 17.3 (**a**) The essential core members of any neuro-oncology multidisciplinary team, ensuring that the patient is the focal point. (**b**) Suggested members of a wider mul-tidisciplinary team that can optimize therapy and outcome for children with CNS tumors

Conclusion

Treating children with CNS tumors in an LIC or LMIC setting is challenging, but with an effective multidisciplinary team and realistic decision-making the best possible outcomes can be achieved. Treating children with CNS tumors should only be undertaken if the side effects of treatment are manageable. Irrespective of experience, consulting with others outside one's own center is often beneficial.

References

Abdelkhalek E, Sherief L, Kamal N, Soliman R (2014) Factors associated with delayed cancer diagnosis in Egyptian children. Clin Med Insights Pediatr 8:39–44

Arora RS, Pizer B, Eden T (2010) Understanding refusal and abandonment in the treatment of childhood cancer. Indian Pediatr 47:1005–1010

Barr RD (1994) The challenge of childhood cancer in the developing world. East Afr Med J 71:223–225

Barr R, Antillon F, Agarwal B, Mehta P, Ribeiro R (2011) Pediatric oncology in countries with limited resources. In: Pizzo PA, Poplack DG (eds) Principles and practice of pediatric oncology. Lippincott Williams and Wilkins, Philadelphia, pp 1463–1473

Barr RD, Antillon Klussmann F, Baez F, Bonilla M, Moreno B, Navarrete M, Nieves R, Pena A, Conter V, De Alarcon P, Howard SC, Ribeiro RC, Rodriguez-Galindo C, Valsecchi MG, Biondi A, Velez G, Tognoni G, Cavalli F, Masera G (2014) Asociacion de Hemato-Oncologia Pediatrica de Centro America (AHOPCA): a model for sustainable development in pediatric oncology. Pediatr Blood Cancer 61:345–354

Carey P, Fudzulani R, Scholfield D, Chagaluka G, Tomoka T, Liombe G, Banda K, Wadehra V, Samarasinghe S, Molyneux EM, Bailey S (2014) Remote and rapid pathological diagnosis in a resource challenged unit. J Clin Pathol 67:540–543

Dang-Tan T, Franco EL, Dang-Tan T, Franco EL (2007) Diagnosis delays in childhood cancer: a review. Cancer 110:703–713

Ferlay J, Bray F, Pisani P, Parkin DM (2004) Cancer incidence. Mortality and prevalence worldwide. ARC Press, Lyon

Fischer MK, Kayembe MK, Scheer AJ, Introcaso CE, Binder SW, Kovarik CL (2011) Establishing telepathology in Africa: lessons from Botswana. [letter]. J Am Acad Dermatol 64(5):986–987

Friedrich P, Lam CG, Itriago E, Perez R, Ribeiro RC, Arora RS (2015) Magnitude of treatment abandonment in childhood cancer. PLoS One 10:e0135230

Gimbel DC, Sohani AR, Prasad Busarla SV, Kirimi JM, Sayed S, Okiro P, Nazarian RM (2012) A static-image telepathology system for dermatopathology consultation in East Africa: the Massachusetts General Hospital Experience. J Am Acad Dermatol 67:997–1007

Gottardo NG, Hansford JR, McGlade JP, Alvaro F, Ashley DM, Bailey S, Baker DL, Bourdeaut F, Cho YJ, Clay M, Clifford SC, Cohn RJ, Cole CH, Dallas PB, Downie P, Doz F, Ellison DW, Endersby R, Fisher PG, Hassall T, Heath JA, Hii HL, Jones DT, Junckerstorff R, Kellie S, Kool M, Kotecha RS, Lichter P, Laughton SJ, Lee S, McCowage G, Northcott PA, Olson JM, Packer RJ, Pfister SM, Pietsch T, Pizer B, Pomeroy SL, Remke M, Robinson GW, Rutkowski S, Schoep T, Shelat AA, Stewart CF, Sullivan M, Taylor MD, Wainwright B, Walwyn T, Weiss WA, Williamson D, Gajjar A (2014) Medulloblastoma down under 2013: a report from the third annual meeting of the International Medulloblastoma Working Group. Acta Neuropathol 127:189–201

Hadley LG, Rouma BS, Saad-Eldin Y (2012) Challenge of pediatric oncology in Africa. Semin Pediatr Surg 21:136–141

Howard SC, Ribeiro RC, Pui CH (2005) Strategies to improve outcomes of children with cancer in low-income countries. Eur J Cancer 41:1584–1587

Howard SC, Metzger ML, Wilimas JA, Quintana Y, Pui CH, Robison LL, Ribeiro RC (2008) Childhood cancer epidemiology in low-income countries. Cancer 112:461–472

IAEA (n.d.) Availability of radiation therapy. https://dirac.iaea.org/Query/Map2?mapld=0

Israëls T, Chirambo C, Caron HN, Molyneux EM (2008) Nutritional status at admission of children with cancer in Malawi. Pediatr Blood Cancer 51:626–628

Kumar S (2000) Indias government promotes traditional health practices. Lancet 355:1252

Laughton SJ, Merchant TE, Sklar CA, Kun LE, Fouladi M, Broniscer A, Morris EB, Sanders RP, Krasin MJ, Shelso J, Xiong Z, Wallace D, Gajjar A (2008) Endocrine outcomes for children with embryonal brain tumors after risk-adapted craniospinal and conformal primary-site irradiation and high-dose chemotherapy with stem-cell rescue on the SJMB-96 trial. J Clin Oncol 26:1112–1118

Magrath I, Shanta V, Advani S, Adde M, Arya LS, Banavali S, Bhargava M, Bhatia K, Gutiérrez M, Liewehr D, Pai S, Sagar TG, Venzon D, Raina V (2005) Treatment of acute lymphoblastic leukaemia in countries with limited resources; lessons from use of a single protocol in India over a twenty year period [corrected]. Eur J Cancer 41:1570–1583

Magrath I, Steliarova-Foucher E, Epelman S, Ribeiro RC, Harif M, Li CK, Kebudi R, Macfarlane SD, Howard SC (2013) Paediatric cancer in low-income and middle-income countries. Lancet Oncol 14:e104–e116

Mitra D, Kampondeni S, Mallewa M, Knight T, Skinner R, Banda K, Israels T, Molyneux E, Bailey S (2012) Central nervous system lesions in Malawian children: identifying the treatable. Trans R Soc Trop Med Hyg 106:567–569

Palmer SL, Armstrong C, Onar-Thomas A, Wu S, Wallace D, Bonner MJ, Schreiber J, Swain M, Chapieski L, Mabbott D, Knight S, Boyle R, Gajjar A (2013) Processing speed, attention, and working memory after treatment for medulloblastoma: an international, prospective, and longitudinal study. J Clin Oncol 31:3494–3500

Parkes J, Hendricks M, Ssenyonga P, Mugamba J, Molyneux E, Schouten-van Meeteren A, Qaddoumi I, Fieggen G, Luna-Fineman S, Howard S, Mitra D, Bouffet E, Davidson A, Bailey S (2015) SIOP PODC adapted treatment recommendations for standard-risk medulloblastoma in low and middle income settings. Pediatr Blood Cancer 62:553–564

Qaddoumi I, Musharbash A, Elayyan M, Mansour A, Al-Hussaini M, Drake J, Swaidan M, Bartels U, Bouffet E (2008) Closing the survival gap: implementation of medulloblastoma protocols in a low-income country through a twinning program. Int J Cancer 122:1203–1206

Quintana Y, Patel AN, Arreola M, Antillon FG, Ribeiro RC, Howard SC (2013) POND4Kids: a global web-based database for pediatric hematology and oncology outcome evaluation and collaboration. Stud Health Technol Inform 183:251–256

Ribeiro RC (2012) Improving survival of children with cancer worldwide: the St. Jude International Outreach Program approach. Stud Health Technol Inform 172:9–13

Ribeiro RC, Steliarova-Foucher E, Magrath I, Lemerle J, Eden T, Forget C, Mortara I, Tabah-Fisch I, Divino JJ, Miklavec T, Howard SC, Cavalli F (2008) Baseline status of paediatric oncology care in ten low-income or mid-income countries receiving My Child Matters support: a descriptive study. Lancet Oncol 9:721–729

Rivera-Luna R, Shalkow-Klincovstein J, Velasco-Hidalgo L, Cárdenas-Cardós R, Zapata-Tarrés M, Olaya-Vargas A, Aguilar-Ortiz MR, Altamirano-Alvarez E, Correa-Gonzalez C, Sánchez-Zubieta F, Pantoja-Guillen F (2014) Descriptive epidemiology in Mexican children with cancer under an open national public health insurance program. BMC Cancer 14:790

Salaverria C, Rossell N, Hernandez A, Fuentes Alabi S, Vasquez R, Bonilla M, Lam CG, Ribeiro RC (2015) Interventions targeting absences increase adherence and reduce abandonment of childhood cancer treatment in El Salvador. Pediatr Blood Cancer 62:1609–1615

Sirintrapun SJ, Cimic A (2012) Dynamic nonrobotic tele-microscopy via skype: A cost effective solution to tele-consultation. J Pathol Inform 3:28

Stefan DC, Siemonsma F (2011) Delay and causes of delay in the diagnosis of childhood cancer in Africa. Pediatr Blood Cancer 56:80–85

The World Bank (2015a) World Development Indicators. GNI per capita, Atlas method. https://data.worldbank.org/indicator/NY.GNP.PCAP.CD

The World Bank (2015b) World Development Indicators. Health expenditure per capita (US $). https://data.worldbank.org/indicator/SH.XPD.PCAP

Ullrich NJ, Robertson R, Kinnamon DD, Scott RM, Kieran MW, Turner CD, Chi SN, Goumnerova L, Proctor M, Tarbell NJ, Marcus KJ, Pomeroy SL (2007) Moyamoya following cranial irradiation for primary brain tumors in children. Neurology 68:932–938

Wang C, Yuan XJ, Jiang MW, Wang LF (2015) Clinical characteristics and abandonment and outcome of treatment in 67 Chinese children with medulloblastoma. J Neurosurg Pediatr:1–8

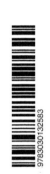

9783030132583